Chronic Pelvic Pain

Chronic Pelvic Pain

An Integrated Approach

John F. Steege, MD
Professor, Department of Obstetrics and Gynecology
Chief, Division of Gynecology
University of North Carolina at Chapel Hill School of Medicine
Chapel Hill, North Carolina

Deborah A. Metzger, PhD, MD
Clinical Associate Professor, Department of Obstetrics and Gynecology
Yale University School of Medicine
New Haven, Connecticut
Director, Reproductive Medicine Institute of Connecticut
Hartford, Connecticut

Barbara S. Levy, MD
Clinical Assistant Professor, Department of Obstetrics and Gynecology
University of Washington School of Medicine
Seattle, Washington
Chief of Staff, St. Francis Hospital
Federal Way, Washington

W.B. SAUNDERS COMPANY
A Division of Harcourt Brace & Company
Philadelphia London Toronto Montreal Sydney Tokyo

W.B. SAUNDERS COMPANY
A Division of Harcourt Brace & Company

The Curtis Center
Independence Square West
Philadelphia, Pennsylvania 19106

Library of Congress Cataloging-in-Publication Data

Chronic pelvic pain: an integrated approach / [edited by] John F. Steege, Deborah A. Metzger, Barbara S. Levy.—1st ed.

p. cm.

ISBN 0–7216–6529–2

1. Pelvic pain. I. Steege, John F. II. Metzger, Deborah A. III. Levy, Barbara S. [DNLM: 1. Pelvic Pain. 2. Chronic Disease. WP 155 C557 1998]

RG483.P44C47 1998 617.5′5—dc21

DNLM/DLC 97–7203

CHRONIC PELVIC PAIN: An Integrated Approach ISBN 0–7216–6529–2

Printed in the United States of America.

Last digit is the print number: 9 8 7 6 5 4 3 2 1

This book is dedicated to our patients and their families, who have endured much but have taught us even more.

Contributors

Gloria A. Bachmann, MD
Professor of Obstetrics and Gynecology
Professor of Medicine
University of Medicine and Dentistry of New Jersey–Robert Wood Johnson Medical School
Chief, Obstetrics and Gynecology Service
Robert Wood Johnson University Hospital
New Brunswick, New Jersey

Sexual Dysfunction

Patricia King Baker, MA, PT
Assistant Professor and Director of Distance Education
University of St. Augustine for Health Sciences
Institute of Physical Therapy
St. Augustine, Florida
Assistant Professor, Department of Physical Therapy
University of Tennessee, Memphis
Memphis, Tennessee
Clinical Faculty, Residency Program
Flagler Physical Therapy
St. Augustine, Florida

Musculoskeletal Problems

Robert A. Bashford, MD
Clinical Associate Professor
Departments of Psychiatry and Obstetrics and Gynecology
University of North Carolina at Chapel Hill School of Medicine
Chapel Hill, North Carolina

Psychiatric Illness

J. Thomas Benson, MD
Director, Urogynecology and Reconstructive Pelvic Surgery Fellowship
Clinical Professor of Obstetrics and Gynecology
Associate Director, OB/GYN Residency Program
Indiana University School of Medicine
Director, OB/GYN Education
Methodist Hospital of Indiana
Indianapolis, Indiana

Neuropathic Pain

William S. Blau, MD, PhD
Assistant Professor of Anesthesiology
University of North Carolina at Chapel Hill School of Medicine
Chapel Hill, North Carolina

Pain Medicine and the Role of Neurologic Blockade in Evaluation

Kristen Costello, PT, BCIAC
Women's Health Specialist
Federal Way, Washington

Myofascial Syndromes

Ibrahim Daoud, MD
Assistant Clinical Professor
University of Connecticut School of Medicine
Farmington, Connecticut
Attending Staff
St. Francis Hospital and Medical Center
Hartford, Connecticut

General Surgical Aspects

Maria C. DeNardis, PsyD
Private Practice
Columbus, Ohio

Sexual and Physical Abuse and Chronic Pelvic Pain

John M. Gibbons, Jr., MD
Professor of Obstetrics and Gynecology
University of Connecticut School of Medicine
Farmington, Connecticut
Senior Vice President for Medical Affairs
St. Francis Hospital and Medical Center
Hartford, Connecticut

Vulvar Vestibulitis

Gita P. Gidwani, MD
Staff, Departments of Gynecology and Obstetrics, and Pediatrics
The Cleveland Clinic Foundation
Cleveland, Ohio

Pelvic Pain in the Adolescent

Mary Casey Jacob, PhD
Associate Professor of Psychiatry and Obstetrics and Gynecology
University of Connecticut School of Medicine
Farmington, Connecticut

Sexual and Physical Abuse and Chronic Pelvic Pain; Pain Intensity, Psychiatric Diagnoses, and Psychosocial Factors: Assessment Rationale and Procedures

Barbara S. Levy, MD
Clinical Assistant Professor of Obstetrics and Gynecology
University of Washington School of Medicine
Seattle, Washington
Chief of Staff, St. Francis Hospital
Federal Way, Washington

History; Physical Examination; Diagnostic Studies; Miscellaneous Causes of Pelvic Pain; Taking Care of Patients: The Caregiver's Perspective

Marilynne McKay, MD
Professor of Dermatology and Gynecology/Obstetrics
Executive Director, CME and Biomedical Media
Emory University School of Medicine
Atlanta, Georgia

Vulvodynia

Deborah A. Metzger, PhD, MD
Clinical Associate Professor, Department of Obstetrics and Gynecology
Yale University School of Medicine
New Haven, Connecticut
Director, Reproductive Medicine Institute of Connecticut
Hartford, Connecticut

Laparoscopy in Diagnosis; An Integrated Approach to the Management of Endometriosis; Pelvic Congestion; Nerve Cutting Procedures for Pelvic Pain; Uterine Suspension; Research Directions

Jill M. Peters-Gee, MD
Assistant Professor
University of Connecticut Health Center
Farmington, Connecticut
Active Staff
Hartford Hospital
Hartford, Connecticut

Bladder and Urethral Syndromes

Nancy A. Phillips, MD
Assistant Professor, Department of Obstetrics and Gynecology
University of Medicine and Dentistry of New Jersey–Robert Wood Johnson Medical School
New Brunswick, New Jersey

Sexual Dysfunction

Robert M. Rogers, Jr., MD
Clinical Assistant Professor, Department of Obstetrics and Gynecology
University of Pennsylvania School of Medicine
Philadelphia, Pennsylvania
Attending Physician
Department of Obstetrics and Gynecology
The Reading Hospital and Medical Center
Reading, Pennsylvania

Basic Pelvic Neuroanatomy

Ellen S. Rome, MD, MPH
Clinical Instructor
Case Western Reserve University School of Medicine
Cleveland, Ohio
Clinical Assistant Professor
College of Medicine of the Pennsylvania State University
Hershey, Pennsylvania
Head, Section of Adolescent Medicine
The Cleveland Clinic Foundation
Cleveland, Ohio

Pelvic Pain in the Adolescent

Anne Shortliffe, BA, BSN
Nurse Education Clinician
University of North Carolina at Chapel Hill
Chapel Hill, North Carolina

One Patient's Experience

John F. Steege, MD
Professor, Department of Obstetrics and Gynecology
Chief, Division of Gynecology
University of North Carolina at Chapel Hill School of Medicine
Chapel Hill, North Carolina

Scope of the Problem; Basic Philosophy of the Integrated Approach: Overcoming the Mind-Body Split; Adhesions and Pelvic Pain; Pain After Hysterectomy; General Principles of Pain Management; Microlaparoscopy

William E. von Kaenel, MD
Assistant Professor of Anesthesiology
Dartmouth Medical School
Hanover, New Hampshire
Senior Medical Staff, Department of Anesthesiology
Lahey-Hitchcock Clinic
Arlington, Massachusetts

Pain Medicine and the Role of Neurologic Blockage in Evaluation

William E. Whitehead, PhD
Research Professor of Medicine, Division of Digestive Diseases and Nutrition
University of North Carolina at Chapel Hill School of Medicine
Chief, Gastrointestinal Motility Laboratory
University of North Carolina Hospital
Chapel Hill, North Carolina

Gastrointestinal Disorders

Foreword

Throughout the history of medicine, the evolution of knowledge and the acceptance of new ideas have required the courage of a few pioneers, systematic study by the curious, and passage of sufficient time so that new concepts might be accepted and practice patterns altered. In the gynecologic field of infertility, for example, this process took about 25 years to reach the current level of scientific exploration. However, this process is just beginning in the field of chronic pelvic pain.

It began in the second half of this century. Chronic pelvic pain underwent impressive early scientific scrutiny by such distinguished clinicians as Howard C. Taylor, Jr., in the United States and Marcel Renaer in Belgium, but despite the prestige of these pioneers, their discoveries about chronic pelvic pain had little impact on gynecology. Widespread use of the laparoscope ensued in the 1970s, and chronic pelvic pain soon was the indication for diagnostic and operative laparoscopy for about half of all procedures. Even with laparoscopy and other diagnostic tools, we have become aware of the critical need for new knowledge in this once obscure field.

This book comes at an appropriate time in the emergence of chronic pelvic pain as a clinical entity deserving scientific scrutiny. It thoroughly documents the current state of the art and knowledge in the diagnosis and management of this problem. Dr. John Steege, Dr. Deborah Metzger, and Dr. Barbara Levy, all well versed in both the psychosomatic and laparoscopic approaches to gynecologic conditions, consider all aspects of the problem in a balanced manner, including patients' concerns. An impressive mix of clinicians including a urologist, psychologist, psychiatrist, pediatrician, physical therapist, anesthesiologist, and general surgeon all appropriately contribute to this truly interdisciplinary integrated approach. The illustrations of anatomy and procedures are lucid. Historical credit is given to the old pioneers and their current disciples (e.g., Richet in 1857, Taylor in the 1950s, and Beard in the 1990s on pelvic congestion), a mark of scholarly thoroughness in this era of electronic review.

For today's clinicians, this book presents both the available hard scientific data and the softer clinical judgments necessary for treatment of today's patients. For tomorrow's investigators, it will serve as a database to explore the vast sea of unknowns surrounding the islands of knowledge presented here. The editors are aware that reliable data need to be gathered in many practical areas: prognostic factors of efficacy of therapy (such as location, extent and nature of adhesions causally related to pain), comparative costs of therapies (including quality of life lost), and effectiveness (in terms of long-term outcome) of the many therapeutic alternatives. It well fills these roles of serving today's and tomorrow's patients and should become a classic in the exciting evolution of the study of chronic pelvic pain into a modern clinical science.

Jaroslav F. Hulka, MD

Preface

From the beginnings of our clinical training, most of us were taught to adhere to the law of parsimony: Try to explain as many of a patient's symptoms and physical findings with the smallest number of identifiable disease processes and hence the fewest diagnostic labels. If our goal is to identify only concrete tissue changes, this remains an excellent guiding principle. If our goal is to understand a complex pain problem and assist in its resolution, the law of parsimony often fails us and, more importantly, our patients. This book suggests that careful review of all identifiable components of the problem, followed by practical therapeutic approaches launched simultaneously (or at least in rational sequence), is more likely to be helpful.

The purpose of this book is to attempt to convey to readers what we have learned from a collective 40 years of clinical experience in dealing with chronic pelvic pain; more importantly, it attempts to share what our patients have taught us about the complexities of pain and the nature of the suffering involved. Only a person who has had to endure chronic pain himself or herself can truly understand the experience, but we have been allowed by our patients to see the experience at close range for extended periods. Each of us has many tales to tell of personal courage shown by women (and their families) we have treated.

Each of us has learned that the more we know about pain, the less we know for certain. We have tried to be open to new ideas and new approaches, all the while keeping basic scientific principles in mind: the structure of how we know what we know. We have included many chapters dealing with topics not traditionally brought into the discussion of chronic pelvic pain, and we have included some information that may be seen as speculative (identified as such whenever possible). We invite readers to bring an open mind to the text.

The field of pain research in general is burgeoning. Application of new knowledge derived from animal research will beget new clinical treatments. At a clinical level, research in pelvic pain is just beginning. We have great hope for a future that will include ever more effective treatment approaches.

In the era of managed care, we would offer the thought that once a pain problem is recognized, it may be more cost-effective to change how we usually practice medicine. Rather than send patients through a series of organ-specific consultations and tests, perhaps it would be better to have patients seen in consultation by a pain specialist who might help develop an overall diagnostic and treatment plan. Perhaps this could be called the law of economic parsimony!

JOHN F. STEEGE, MD
DEBORAH A. METZGER, PhD, MD
BARBARA S. LEVY, MD

DRUG NOTICE

Gynecology is an ever-changing field. Standard safety precautions must be followed, but as new research and clinical experience broaden our knowledge, changes in treatment and drug therapy become necessary or appropriate. The editors of this work have carefully checked the generic and trade drug names and verified drug dosages to ensure that the dosage information in this work is accurate and in accord with the standards accepted at the time of publication. Readers are advised, however, to check the product information currently provided by the manufacturer of each drug to be administered to be certain that changes have not been made in the recommended dose or in the contraindications for administration. This is of particular importance in regard to new or infrequently used drugs. It is the responsibility of the treating physician, relying on experience and knowledge of the patient, to determine dosages and the best treatment for the patient. The editors cannot be responsible for misuse or misapplication of the material in this work.

THE PUBLISHER

Contents

1

Scope of the Problem

John F. Steege, MD

Gynecologists, internists, and family practitioners are very much aware that chronic pelvic pain (CPP) in women is a significant part of their practice. The majority of cases seem to occur during the reproductive years, although some particularly enigmatic pain syndromes may occur in young adolescents and others may occur after menopause and in the elderly.

Much of what has been said and written about CPP in women derives from the experience of tertiary care specialists or practitioners in various settings experienced in treating a particular facet of CPP, such as endometriosis, adhesions, pelvic congestion, or trigger points.[1] Two types of reporting bias emerge from this: (1) One etiology is emphasized above all others, and (2) optimistic treatment outcome statistics that may be reported may not apply to those with multifaceted problems.

The authors' initial hope in preparing this book is to equip readers with a broad understanding of the many aspects of CPP in the belief that early detection will lead to more effective treatment. Two further hopes are voiced in the term *integrated* in the title: First, that practitioners will consider many contributing factors in their conceptualization of the problem, and second, that practitioners will understand the roles that other professionals such as physical therapists, psychologists, and anesthesiologists may have in managing difficult CPP problems.

Definition

Most publications dealing with chronic pain of various types, including nongynecologic pain, use a duration of 6 months or more as a minimum definition of *chronic.* This cutoff point is arbitrary and lacks empirical validation in the area of CPP but nevertheless serves for purposes of discussion. Many of the behavioral, emotional, and biomechanical changes in victims of CPP after 6 months are similar to those in people coping with other types of pain. Certainly, some women with CPP develop a full-blown chronic pain syndrome (see Chapter 2) earlier in their illness, even when the pain is somewhat cyclic in nature, whereas others suffer pain much longer while continuing to function well in many aspects of life.

A perhaps more important part of defining CPP has to do with the traditional mind-body split of Western thinking that is often reflected in Western medicine. Many earlier studies of CPP expressed this anatomically: Only those with no evidence of physical pathology at laparotomy or laparoscopy were included. The converse presumption was often made in clinical practice—that if organic pathology *was* found, it was held responsible for the pain until proven otherwise.

A central premise of this book is that although all the common forms of gynecologic pathology (adhesions, endometriosis, fibroids, and so forth) are found more frequently in women with CPP, the development of pain is still very often likely to be multifactorial, especially in those who show signs of a chronic pain syndrome (see Chapter 2). Hence, when the hallmarks of a chronic pain syndrome begin to appear, clinical evaluation must be thorough from a medical, surgical, and psychologic standpoint. Published reports of treatment of pain associated with a particular form of pathology (e.g., endometriosis) are more informative if they include assessment of patients in terms of the many factors that may contribute to CPP, as reviewed in this book.

Prevalence and Impact

Although widely appreciated as common in clinical practice, true incidence and prevalence figures for CPP are lacking. The matter is of some importance from a public health point of view, as well as from a resource planning perspective, as the health care system evolves.

The prevalence no doubt varies depending on the setting examined. In a study of women attending two nongynecologic clinics in a university, 12% of women reported current CPP and 33% had experienced it at some point in their lives.[2] Jamieson and Steege[3] surveyed 581 women of reproductive age (patients and family members) attending primary care private practices. They found that 39.1% had pain (other than dysmenorrhea, dyspareunia, or bowel-related pain) at least some of the time and 11.7% had pain more than 5 days per month or lasting a full day or more each month. Pelvic pain was associated with high rates of health care resource use. A Gallup poll of 5325 women discovered that 16% of women reported problems with pelvic pain.[4] A total of 11% of this sample limited home activity because of CPP, and 11.9% limited sexual activity, 15.8% took medication, and 3.9% missed at least 1 day of work per month.

Data are not currently available for the frequency with which financial disability (Social Security and so on) is requested for CPP. In my own practice as a referral center physician, I am aware that requests for disability have increased from rare to only relatively uncommon. The problem has by no means reached the level in the practice of orthopedic surgery, but it seems likely to increase in the future.

If we generalize from the available literature dealing with other types of chronic pain, we would say that relief of CPP is less likely to occur when there are unresolved legal matters, such as workers' compensation, disability, and medicolegal actions. On the other hand, if disability is granted, in some cases this only serves to reinforce further a patient's role as a sick person and to undermine reasonable therapeutic efforts on the parts of both the patient and her physician. Used constructively, a period of disability can serve to address complex individual and family issues surrounding one family member's chronic pain problem. In the absence of data, the potential positive and negative effects of supporting a disability claim are left to the clinician's judgment.

Surgery

The indications for hysterectomy have been the subject of much critical discussion in recent years. Pelvic pain is the major indication for hysterectomy in approximately 12% of the approximately 600,000 hysterectomies performed annually in the United States.[5] In a study of hysterectomy for uterine pain, relief was obtained in 76% of patients regardless of whether or not uterine pathology was found.[6] In the Maine Women's Study, at 1 year of follow-up, 93% of women who underwent hysterectomy for various painful conditions reported good pain relief and satisfaction with having had the procedure.[7] A relatively small percentage of women developed new pain syndromes or other illnesses in the year after surgery. The study did not examine the question of whether this symptom substitution was more likely to develop in women who had no documented pathology. Medical treatment of pain was less successful than surgery; however, the study was observational (not randomized) and the selection factors that led to medical rather than surgical therapy were not described.

Laparoscopy is commonly performed to diagnose and treat CPP, with pain being the major indication for surgery in an estimated 15% to 40% of cases.[8] The success rates for surgical therapy vary with the procedure (see Chapter 13 regarding adhesions and Chapter 14 regarding endometriosis). The easier laparoscopy becomes and the more skilled we become at performing complex procedures, the more difficult the question becomes: How many conservative procedures should be carried out before extirpative surgery is performed? In the case of adhesions, if two laparoscopies are better than one, how many should be performed? Ironically, it almost seems that our best surgical tool (laparoscopy) can become a patient's worst enemy if it is used excessively and leads both patients and physicians to exclude thorough evaluation and treatment of musculoskeletal, functional, and emotional components. A normal-appearing pelvis at laparoscopy does not mean that the pain problem is all psychologic in nature: In a study of 122 women with a nondiagnostic laparoscopy, 47% were believed to have some somatic cause of pain.[1] When used as an initial diagnostic step in the evaluation of pelvic pain, laparoscopy is less revealing than one might think. In one randomized trial of traditional treatment versus an interdisciplinary pain evaluation and treatment program, laparoscopy by itself was less successful in relieving pain.[10] The procedure seems to be most worthwhile when used selectively and incorporated into a well-planned treatment program.[11] Perhaps the value of laparoscopy can be augmented with the new approach of conscious pain mapping described in Chapter 34.

The challenge to physicians is to subject common beliefs about the effectiveness of treatment to careful examination and to balance patient and physician preferences against the need to demonstrate the cost-effectiveness of the treatments we offer.

Types of Chronic Pelvic Pain

This book discusses the spectrum of pelvic pain problems that affect any of the components of the female reproductive tract, as well as those that may involve surrounding viscera, the musculoskeletal system, and other systems. Almost all syndromes include at least some demonstrable organic or physiologic change, yet none of the organic changes discussed inevitably cause symptoms in every individual who has them. Clinicians must carefully judge the probable role that any identified pathology may have in the development of a pain problem. This can only be done with the help of thorough structural and functional evaluation of all potentially involved organ systems.

To make matters more complex, it is not uncommon for more than one type of CPP problem to present in the same person (see Chapter 4). A woman with vulvar vestibulitis (see Chapter 20) may develop vaginismus (see Chapter 9) that may persist even after successful medical or surgical treatment of the original problem. Patients with proven endometriosis (see Chapter 14) may develop irritable bowel syndrome (see Chapter 23) or pelvic floor muscle dysfunction (see Chapter 24), to cite just a few examples.

In the presence of chronic pain, patients often experience depression. In the population with pelvic pain, this may first appear as a mild sleep disturbance without evidence of anorexia or weight loss. In my experience, the depression seems to coevolve with the pain as both worsen simultaneously. A person with a genetic predisposition to affective disorder may be more prone to developing a chronic pain problem when faced with a physical illness, there seems to be little direct evidence to show that pain grows entirely from a primary problem of depression (see Chapters 2, 8, and 27). True conversion disorders exist, and those with true somatization disorder may develop pelvic pain as one of many problems, but these together make up a small minority of patients with CPP.

An additional major problem in women with CPP is sexual dysfunction. Indeed, in my experience, a major motivation for compliance with referral to a pain clinic is the hope that comfortable coitus will be restored and a relationship saved. Sexual dysfunction may lead to CPP (e.g., vaginismus to levator spasm, absent response to deep dyspareunia), but far more often, some organic change (e.g., endometriosis, pelvic adhesions) produces discomfort that blocks sexual response, and functional disorders follow (e.g., levator spasm, vaginismus). Over time, everything hurts, and the patient loses the ability to discriminate one source from another.

Evaluation

Classic teaching in medicine holds that the history (see Chapter 6) and physical examination (see Chapter 7) reveal the nature of the patient's problem in 90% of cases. In no case is this axiom more true than in the case of CPP.

When the type of patient described earlier first visits the physician's office, the clinician must first obtain a detailed picture of the systems involved in the problem in the present. The greater challenge in understanding the history in such a case, however, is to examine the *chronology* of the pain: Which components were added at what times and in association with what physical and psychosocial or psychosexual events. Attention to this level of detail validates the patient's concerns, conveys understanding of the problem, and often helps the clinician develop a comprehensive list of helpful suggestions (see Chapter 2).

The physical examination for a pain problem should be more thorough and more detailed than an ordinary office pelvic examination (see Chapter 7). Depending on the nature of evidence emerging from the history, surrounding organ systems are evaluated in appropriate detail. Interpretation of examination findings requires understanding of common visceral-somatic referral patterns (see Chapters 5, 7, 24, 25).

Treatment

In the case of CPP, the reductionist approach (i.e., an attempt to render a single diagnosis and hence a single treatment) often simply does not apply. Medical management works best when all identified components are treated simultaneously (see Chapter 2, 4, 28), as opposed to offering one treatment after another in a series.

The selection and timing of surgical intervention are often equally problematic. When should repeat laparoscopy be performed when monitoring someone with endometriosis whose pain does not respond to initial treatment? If multiple components are present, should the nongynecologic ones be treated before or after the gynecologic surgery is completed? This book attempts to provide the informational background needed to make these difficult clinical judgments.

Patient and Physician Success

It is difficult for a clinician to deal with seemingly intractable problems in patients with diverse life stresses that stretch their coping abilities and support systems to their limits. Success for patients and professional gratification for physicians depend on establishing realistic therapeutic goals, making a thorough and thoughtful evaluation, and developing effective collaborative relationships with other helping professionals. Our purpose in preparing this book is to offer information and guidance that will facilitate this ongoing process.

References

1. Steege JF, Stout AL, Somkuti S: Chronic pelvic pain: Toward an integrative model. Obstet Gynecol Surv 1993;48:95.
2. Walker EA, Katon WJ, Jemelka R, et al: The prevalence of chronic pelvic pain and irritable bowel syndrome in two university clinics. J Psychosom Obstet Gynecol 1991;12(Suppl):77.
3. Jamieson DJ, Steege JF: The prevalence of dysmenorrhea, dyspareunia, pelvic pain, and irritable bowel syndrome in primary care practices. Obstet Gynecol 1996;87:55.
4. Mathias SD, Kupperman M, Liberman RF, et al: Chronic pelvic pain: Prevalence, health-related quality of life, and economic correlates. Obstet Gynecol 1996;87:321.
5. National Center for Health Statistics, Graves EJ: National Hospital Discharge Survey: Annual Summary, 1990. Vital and Health Statistics. DHHS publication (PHS) 92-1773. Series 13, No. 112. Washington, DC, US Government Printing Office, 1992.
6. Stovall TG, Ling FL, Crawford DA: Hysterectomy for chronic pelvic pain of presumed uterine etiology. Obstet Gynecol 1990;75:676.
7. Carlson KJ, Miller BA, Fowler FJ: The Maine Women's Health Study: II. Outcomes of nonsurgical management of leiomyomas, abnormal bleeding, and chronic pelvic pain. Obstet Gynecol 1994;83:566.
8. Hulka JF, Peterson HB, Phillips JM, Surrey MW: Operative laparoscopy: American Association of Gynecologic Laparoscopists 1991 membership survey. J Reprod Med 1993;38:569.
9. Reiter RC: Occult somatic pathology in women with chronic pelvic pain. Clin Obstet Gynecol 1991;33:154.
10. Peters AAW, van Dorst E, Jellis B, et al: A randomized clinical trial to compare two different approaches in women with chronic pelvic pain. Obstet Gynecol 1991;77:740
11. Howard FM: The role of laparoscopy in chronic pelvic pain: Promise and pitfalls. Obstet Gynecol Surv 1993;48:357.

2

Basic Philosophy of the Integrated Approach: Overcoming the Mind-Body Split

John F. Steege, MD

Most clinicians dealing with the problem recognize chronic pelvic pain (CPP) as a complex set of difficulties without easy solutions. Although aware of the many physical and emotional/psychologic components of chronic pain, many clinicians trained in Western medicine embark on the evaluation with an agenda: To decide how much of the problem is physically based and how much might have its roots in psychologic conflict or distress (i.e., the mind-body split). Similarly, many patients struggling with a CPP problem develop their own assumptions about the cause of the pain and choose their health care providers accordingly: Those thinking in more psychologic terms seek mental health help, whereas those who interpret pain as physically caused seek gynecologic evaluation. When the evaluation begins, this often tacit agreement about the likely cause continues, as both patient and health care provider tend to focus on information that supports their preconceptions.

Referral to a pain specialist can result in a fresh look at the complexities involved. In the field of gynecology, some pain specialists, however, tend to emphasize one potential cause over others: Those with a special interest in pelvic congestion tend to see many pelvic congestion patients, and those with an interest in endometriosis interpret most symptoms in someone with the disease as secondary to endometriosis. Similarly, a neurologist or anesthesiology pain specialist may focus on neuropathic or musculoskeletal factors while having less intuitive feel for the impact of gynecologic disease.

The intent of this book is twofold: (1) to present a balanced discussion of the major entities discussed as causes of CPP and (2) to encourage an approach that recognizes mind and body as one functioning unit rather than separate components of a person. We would like to call this the *integrated approach*.[1]

Integrated Approach

We intend the term *integrated* in this context to mean an approach to clinical evaluation that has as its goal an understanding of (1) the subtle interactions among disease states, physical sensations, and psychologic/emotional processes that exist in the present and (2) how the pain problem started and how it gradually reached its present condition in each of these dimensions. Understanding the evolution and chronology of the pain and its impact often both provides clues to diagnosis and suggests avenues for intervention more readily than does focusing largely on the present condition.

Integrated in this sense does not necessarily mean *interdisciplinary* or *multispecialty*. The integrated approach may be carried out entirely by one provider or may require multiple clinicians, depending on the severity and complexity of the problem. Consultation with various specialists can be approached in one of two ways. First, if the goal is simply to rule out organic disease in an organ system, then endoscopy by a urologist or gastroenterologist may provide that information, and that may be all you wish to accomplish through the consultation. If you as the primary physician plan to be the primary pain manager and to take responsibility for understanding the details, you may not wish to complicate the picture by having two or three other clinicians also trying to establish the same type of relationship with the patient. On the other hand, a consultant who takes the time to understand the chronology and evolution of the problems relevant to his or her organ system specialty will be in a better position to offer ongoing management suggestions that will make sense to the patient. Before the consultation, it is useful to clarify which of these two roles you wish the consultant to have. After all consultations are completed, it is useful for the physicians involved to communicate directly to decide which one is to be the main provider, with the others receding into a more advisory role. This is especially important when prescribing controlled drugs (see Chapter 28).

Integrated in our approach also means that body and mind are regarded as a functioning unit. It does not make sense to ask that a person be "cleared" medically before psychologic approaches should begin, any more than it is possible to clear a person psychologically in order to urge further medical work-up. In the vast majority of cases of CPP, physical and emotional/psychologic processes make ongoing contributions to the problem.

Chronic Versus Acute Pain

Central to this discussion is the notion that chronic pain is qualitatively different from acute pain: It is not simply acute pain that has not yet been cured. The task of this chapter is to define the difference in biologic, behavioral, and psychologic terms. This discussion naturally begins with a review of the theories used to explain pain.

The theoretic constructs needed to explain acute pain phenomena are relatively straightforward: Centrally perceived pain originates from painful stimuli from damaged or irritated tissue; pain intensity is roughly proportional to tissue damage. In the case of pelvic pain, physical examination, laboratory tests, imaging techniques, or laparoscopy can usually detect enough pathology to explain the pain. In this setting, taking a patient's personality and medical or psychiatric status into consideration may be part of delivering care in a sensitive manner but does not influence the choice of treatments. (Vaginitis still is treated with the appropriate drug, pelvic inflammatory disease is treated with antibiotics, and so on.)

In the case of chronic pain, it is most often difficult to find enough pathology to explain the pain. In fact, I am not aware of a single chronic clinical problem associated with pain in which pain is seen as proportional to tissue damage. To explain this apparent anomaly, most clinicians would agree that a pain victim's psychologic status has a great deal to do with chronic pain. Perhaps most commonly, patients with pain are described as having a significant psychologic (emotional, psychiatric) overlay. This seems to mean that a pain stimulus-perception system fundamentally similar to that in acute pain is still going on but is obscured by complicating emotional factors. The clinician's task is framed in terms of the need to figure out how much of the patient's distress is due to true organic pathology ("real" pain) and how much arises from the overlay ("unreal" pain?).

I would suggest that this way of looking at chronic pain does not make any sense to patients because it does not reflect physiologic or psychologic reality or their personal subjective experience. When the problem is viewed this way, clinicians and patients are starting out with fundamental disagreements that hamper their relationship and compromise the evaluation and treatment of the problem.

More recent (and more involved) theories of pain perception attempt to integrate physical and psychologic elements into a single functional whole.[2] To provide the background for their discussion, a more detailed review of pain theories is useful.

Pain Theories

Cartesian Theory

Also called *specificity theory*, this way of explaining pain was formulated largely by the 17th century French philosopher and physician René Descartes.[3] He reasoned that dedicated tubular structures throughout the body were responsible for the conduction of pain signals to the brain. His theory stimulated extensive neuroanatomic work aimed at discovering the fibers he described. Although skin structures that were discovered were thought to be specific for certain sensations (e.g., pacinian corpuscles for vibration or deep pressure), none clearly specific for pain were ever found.

Cartesian theory holds that pain signals travel to the brain essentially unimpeded. The intensity of the pain felt is proportional to the tissue damage at the periphery (the law of proportionality). Any pain modulation or the ability to block it out completely is attributed to central psychologic processes. Information travels in one direction only.

In fairness, although Descartes is most remembered for his hypothesized tubules, he was keenly aware of the complexity of pain perception and was very much the descendant of the ancient Greek physicians who viewed pain as one of the emotions. The general public view of pain was not so different, with the exception that for many centuries control of this ethereal emotion was believed to be held by spiritual forces beyond the comprehension of the individual. Before it became possible to alter pain with medication, it was perhaps much more accepted as a natural and expected part of human existence. From a historical perspective, the notion that life should be largely pain free is a rather recent idea.

Gate Control Theory

The inability to identify specific pain fibers led to a somewhat more complex theory, perhaps best elaborated by Melzack and Wall in the mid-1960s (Fig. 2–1). Signals from the periphery are conducted to the spinal cord by poorly myelinated A fibers and unmyelinated C fibers, the latter responding to heat, mechanical pressure, or the chemical mediators of inflammation. At this level, signals are described as *nociceptive* and are not yet labeled *pain*, because this term is reserved for the sensation after it reaches consciousness.

After entering the spinal cord, nociceptive signals may be modulated by feedback loops entirely within the spinal cord, with signals mediated within these loops by various neurotransmitters. The nociceptive signals may stop completely at this point, or they may ascend via the lateral spinothalamic tracts.

Based on extensive animal research, Melzack[2] suggested that modulation of nociceptive transmission through the spinal cord was also mediated by descending signals from higher centers in the brain, again using various neurotransmitters. The spinal cord thus acts as though it contained a gate to allow variable amounts of nociceptive signals to pass through.

The ability of higher brain centers to modulate spinal cord gating activity adds a new and very important element to pain theory. It suggests that information is transmitted in both directions, not just in the single direction from damaged tissue up to the brain.

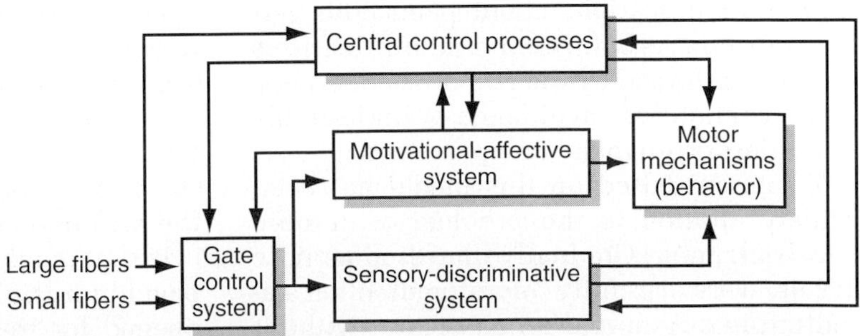

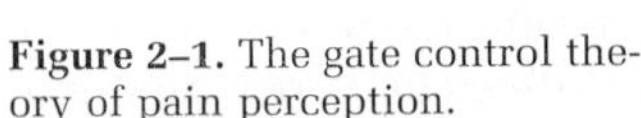
Figure 2–1. The gate control theory of pain perception.

The significance of this addition is hard to overemphasize. It provides a sound basis for the notion that neurotransmitter states in the brain (the emotions?) may have direct, chemically mediated effects on the ability of the spinal cord gating mechanism to block the cephalad transmission of nociceptive signals. To the degree that this is true, direct and tangible links are formed between body and mind. For example, much clinical and research evidence suggests that the presence of depression may be associated with lower thresholds for pain perception and lower levels of pain tolerance.[4] Gate control theory allows for the possibility that neurochemical changes associated with depression may truly alter the victim's modulation of pain at a spinal cord level, thus placing an additional burden on central systems in ignoring, blocking, or coping with the pain. Research suggests that pain originally prompted by peripheral nociceptive signals can, over time, become centralized—that is, intrinsic to other brain and spinal cord structures with little or no ongoing input from peripheral tissue damage (see Chapter 25). The clinical implications of this are discussed later.

The gate control theory has been challenged and modified in its particulars and almost certainly oversimplifies the complex phenomenon of pain perception. It remains a useful framework for discussing body-mind synthesis and serves a useful educational function in talking with patients.

Operant Conditioning Model

The inability to objectively measure or observe pain led Fordyce[5] and others to emphasize the importance of pain behaviors and communications about pain, both verbal and nonverbal. Such communications can be reinforced by the responses of others, such as attention; avoidance of undesirable activities; or financial compensation.

Treatment based on this model has been widely applied to the problem of chronic low back pain.[6] Gradually increased activity levels were carefully monitored, often resulting in substantial rehabilitation without increased pain. Many of these programs required inpatient hospitalization.

A number of ideas emerging from this approach have application to the problem of CPP. For example, if pain medication is prescribed on a set schedule (as opposed to as needed), the patient is less likely to demonstrate increased pain behaviors (grimacing, resting, voicing complaint) to justify the use of the medication. At the same time, the surrounding family members are less likely to feel the need to respond to the pain behaviors/complaints in some fashion. Medication taken on an as-needed basis ironically can become a powerful reinforcer of the pain itself: It conditions patients to experience continued pain. A set schedule for medication diminishes this reinforcing effect.

A second idea central to the operant conditioning model that is applicable to many types of clinical pain is the notion that improvement is in large part due to the patient's own efforts, not to a specific medicine or surgery. Finally, successful patients in these programs accepted the idea that the pain may not disappear completely but that it can be better managed. These last two ideas are perhaps the most difficult for a woman and her family to accept. Again ironically, when this acceptance occurs, the best progress is made toward minimizing the impact of pain on a person's life.

Cognitive-Behavioral Theory

An outgrowth of the gate control theory is the cognitive-behavioral theory.[7] This holds that how one thinks about pain and the impact of these cognitions on behavior (activity level, investment in relationships, and so on) influence the intensity of the pain itself. Clearly, this theory fits neatly with the downward transmission pathways from the brain to the spinal cord that are part of the gate control theory. It emphasizes the importance of a patient's internal conceptualizations of the pain's cause, the prognosis, and the likelihood that treatment will be helpful.

If such cognitions are important in some psychophysiologic way, new avenues are opened for treatment of pain through conscious, intentional altering of the cognitions held by an individual. On the downside, it may also explain the frustrating failure of well-designed and conscientiously applied treatment programs among those who cannot escape seeing themselves as ill and disabled.

This theory raises some troublesome and tantalizing questions about the impact of cognitions on illness in a general sense. Are the cognitions that a person has about her body an active ingredient in the intensity of pain? If a woman with endometriosis or adhesions fears their continued growth, will this make her pain worse, not simply in the sense of psychologic distress but by truly changing her pain perception mechanisms in a neurotransmitter-driven biologic sense? Does the experience of sexual or physical abuse condition the pain perception mechanism to develop hyperalgesic syndromes when stressed? If so, is this mediated by a sense of oneself as damaged and vulnerable?

If one is willing to go beyond the Cartesian model at all, then one recognizes that the pain felt by an individual is always real pain; she (in the case of pelvic pain) indeed experiences the pain. The attempt to decide if the pain is physically or psychologically based has less and less meaning and utility. Certainly, reporting to a patient that the pain is in her head makes no sense to her at all.[8]

Recognizing the Chronic Pain Syndrome

Every clinician has seen patients who are afflicted with chronic pain and who steadfastly maintain their ability to perform everyday functions without showing signs of clinical depression and without worsening of the pain. They have learned to live with it in the best sense of the phrase. In many others, function gradually declines, depression worsens, and pain spreads. Some risk factors for these developments are obvious, but the transition into this chronic pain syndrome is often subtle. The following suggested operational definitions for some of the risk factors appear to be useful in recognizing the syndrome (Table 2–1).[9]

Table 2–1. **CHARACTERISTICS OF THE CHRONIC PAIN SYNDROME**

Duration of 6 months or more
Incomplete relief by previous treatments
Pain out of proportion to tissue damage
Loss of physical function
Vegetative signs of depression
Altered family dynamics

Duration of Symptoms

In many types of clinical pain, chronic changes begin to appear after 4 to 6 months, although in a more vulnerable individual, they may certainly appear earlier. When a person has some respite from the pain, for example in the case of cyclic pain of early endometriosis, signs of a chronic pain syndrome may take longer to develop or may not develop at all. As the pain becomes more constant, the victim begins to wonder if it will ever go away, and coping strategies such as diversion, relaxation, exercise, and so on lose their power.

Even in the healthiest of individuals, physically and psychologically speaking, a chronic pain syndrome may appear if the pain has enough impact on function. The syndrome's development may be hastened in the more vulnerable, but it can happen to the most emotionally robust.

Incomplete Effectiveness of Previous Treatments

Many forms of pain treatment may seem to provide relief initially, only to lose their effectiveness gradually over time. This may happen for one or more of the following reasons: (1) A true placebo effect has occurred, (2) tachyphylaxis has occurred (in the case of medication treatment), or (3) the treatment has addressed only one of several components of the pain. For example, a person who has irritable bowel syndrome and who also has some element of sacroiliitis may notice that previously effective bowel management becomes less effective when the back pain is worse. If pain persists because all components have not been addressed, the treatments that have been given may be inappropriately discredited by the patient.

In assessing the effectiveness of treatments for someone with chronic pain, a clinician must question the patient carefully about the degree of relief obtained. For example, a pain victim often reports that the new analgesic prescribed did "no good at all" because the pain came back after 4 to 6 hours, when this would be expected based on the pharmacodynamics of the drug. In this way, helpful and rational treatments can come to be discounted when they actually could contribute to an effective overall management program.

Another common facet of this problem is the gradual escalation of use of analgesic medication despite the absence of clear organic deterioration. Again, pain associated with endometriosis and pain due to adhesions are common examples.

Pain Out of Proportion to Tissue Damage

Most clinicians intuitively or by training look for enough pathology to explain the pain. With chronic pain, this proportionality simply does not exist. This is true of all chronic pain problems, not just chronic gynecologic pain. For example, the most common forms of pathology found in women with CPP are endometriosis and pelvic adhesions. In both of these disorders, studies have demonstrated that in most instances, the location of the pain is close to the location of the physical pathology but the intensity of the pain is not consistently related (either directly or inversely) to the apparent degree of tissue damage.[10, 11]

Loss of Physical Function

Recreation is often the first activity to be given up: Swimming, cycling, playing ball with the kids, and conditioning exercise are forsaken. Physical function at work may be sacrificed next: The patient may request a note restricting lifting on the job, or some other adjustment may seem necessary.

In a referral center pain clinic setting, a common loss of function that prompts patients to ask for or accept referral is loss of sexual function. In the presence of chronic pain, orgasmic response may first decline, followed by progressive loss of response and interest. This happens more rapidly, of course, if dyspareunia is part of the pain problem from the start (see Chapter 9).

Vegetative Signs of Depression

The three classic vegetative signs of depression are anorexia, sleep disturbance, and psychomotor retardation. Of these, disturbed sleep is by far the most common sign to appear in a person with CPP. The others are far less common in my experience. It may be that when all three are present, the depression is obvious to all involved, and referring physicians may turn to mental health professionals rather than a gynecologic pain clinic.

The most common type of sleep disturbance is early morning awakening. In this case, patients often awaken 1 to 3 hours earlier than would be necessary for their usual routine and find it difficult or impossible to get back to sleep. Close questioning or prospective diary keeping may be needed to decide if pain is awakening a patient or if she awakens first and then happens to notice the pain. This distinction is usually possible. When this symptom is present, the need for intervention is urgent and there is good reason to begin antidepressant medication (see Chapter 28).

Altered Family Dynamics

When a woman and her family come to feel that the pain has become like another family member (not necessarily wanted) who has moved in, then a chronic pain syndrome has likely developed. Put another way, if a patient and her family label the pain problem as the most important problem that the family has, then family dynamics have most likely been substantially altered.

In the early stages of a pain problem, family members commonly offer supportive help: taking over responsibilities, trying to reduce stress in the family, and so on. When the pain does not go away, the family's mode of helping often does not change. With time, a pain victim finds her roles taken over, her authority undermined, and her sense of usefulness and self-worth eroded. Unresolved family conflicts are not discussed out of consideration for the sick person, so they remain shelved, and emotional distance can increase.

In a dysfunctional family, these changes may serve a need. A daughter with a medical (pain) problem may serve as a buffer between feuding parents or may (unconsciously) find that her pain problem provides a reason to remain dependent on her parents. Having someone in the family with a chronic illness may provide opportunities for members of an extended family to nurture and care for someone when they have not been able to be close in other ways. There are probably as many maladaptive roles for pain as there are families, but suffice it to say that when pain has been a part of the family structure for years, the resulting alterations in the family are very difficult to change. As one patient said (see Chapter 4), "My family has seen me sick for so long, I'm not sure they're really going to let me get well."

Evolution from Acute to Chronic

The types of changes described earlier most often occur slowly and gradually. The patient herself and her family may to some extent recognize that they cannot keep dealing with the pain in the same way and function well as a family, but they see no way out of it. They are more likely to continue to see the pain as having a single cause and to hope and search for a single solution.

The types of complaints offered during office visits and the style in which those problems are communicated may evolve very gradually. New symptoms may appear but often serve to distract the patient and clinician into thinking a new (acute?) problem has occurred rather than promote the recognition of a growing chronic pain syndrome. The patient described in Chapter 4 provides a good example of how many organ systems can come to be involved in a person's pain over time. The six criteria listed earlier can serve to promote the recognition of a true chronic pain syndrome.

Implications for Diagnosis and Treatment

Once a chronic pain syndrome is recognized, the first step in treatment is a meeting with the patient and, ideally, at least one family member, for the purpose of education. A longer visit such as this is time well spent, serving to make a patient and her family aware that the nature of her pain has fundamentally changed. Further, you can emphasize that because of this change, subsequent diagnostic and therapeutic efforts need to be different.

The first educational point is that the pain is no longer caused by a single problem. Regardless of what triggered the pain initially, other components have joined the original cause. Treatment of the original cause may untangle the syndrome and relieve the pain, but the added components often develop a life of their own and persist (see Chapter 4).

If several causes are present, many treatments may be necessary. Included in the list of treatments may be medications or a surgical procedure aimed at the physical changes (e.g., endometriosis), other measures designed to treat functional disorders (e.g., physical therapy for piriformis or levator spasm), and still others to modulate the central processing of nociceptive signals (e.g., antidepressants). These treatments often work best when used simultaneously. When one thing is tried at a time, a patient may experience only partial relief, leading her to discredit the treatment and spiral further down into the chronic pain syndrome.

Particularly when the discussion of causes is led by one who performs surgery (a gynecologist), a surgical procedure must be described as just one of a number of possible or necessary treatments. This cannot be emphasized too strongly, because those who seek help from a physician who performs surgery often do so because of their own personal belief that of all treat-

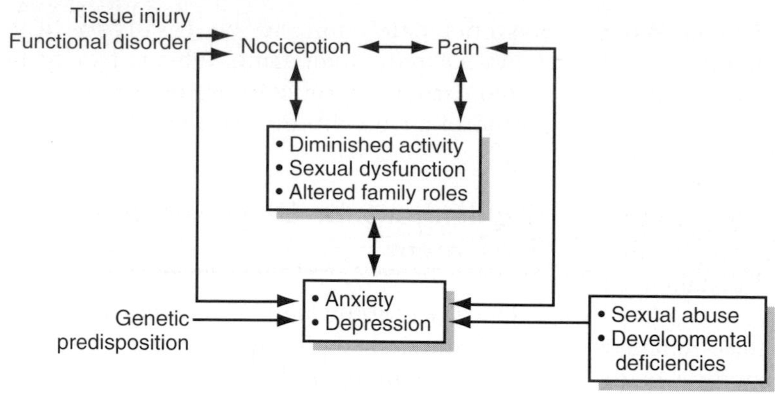

Figure 2–2. An integrative model of chronic pelvic pain, including elements of gate control theory, cognitive-behavioral theory, and the operant conditioning model.

ments, surgery works best. The surgeon, naturally, concurs.

Chapter 28 further discusses general techniques of chronic pain management.

Summary

This chapter ends as it began, with the following idea. According to prevailing theories of pain perception, it no longer makes theoretic or practical sense to try to categorize pain as either physical or psychologic in origin. The traditional Western mind-body split simply does not serve to explain chronic pain. Rather, chronic pain often has multiple organic roots and simultaneously has emotional, central biochemical, and behavioral components, all of which need attention. Figure 2–2 summarizes the integration of these components. The integrated approach regards the components of chronic pain as integrated into one pain process; hence, they demand well-considered simultaneous attention to as many components as practically possible. The ongoing care required presents an opportunity to promote patients' realization that chronic pain is the integrated product of body and mind.

References

1. Steege JF, Stout AL, Somkuti SG: Chronic pelvic pain: Toward an integrative model. Obstet Gynecol Surv 1993;48:95.
2. Melzack R: Neurophysiologic foundations of pain. In Sternbach RA (ed): The Psychology of Pain. New York, Raven Press, 1986, p 1.
3. Descartes R: "L'Homme" (Paris, 1644) (Foster M, translator). In Lectures on the History of Physiology During the 16th, 17th, and 18th Centuries. Cambridge, UK, Cambridge University Press, 1901.
4. Romano JM, Turner JA: Chronic pain and depression: Does the evidence support a relationship? Psychol Bull 1985;97:18.
5. Fordyce WE: Behavioral methods of control of chronic pain and illness. St. Louis, CV Mosby, 1976.
6. Sternbach RA: The Psychology of Pain. New York, Raven Press, 1986.
7. Rudy TE, Kerns RD, Turk DC: Chronic pain and depression: Toward a cognitive-behavioral mediation model. Pain 1988;35:129.
8. Engel G: "Psychogenic" pain and the pain-prone patient. Am J Med 1959;26:899.
9. Steege JF, Stout AL: Resolution of pain following laparoscopic adhesiolysis. Am J Obstet Gynecol 1991;165:278.
10. Fedele L, Parazzini F, Bianchi S, et al: Stage and localization of pelvic endometriosis and pain. Fertil Steril 1990;53:155.
11. Stout AL, Steege JF, Dodson WC, et al: Relationship of laparoscopic findings to self-report of pelvic pain. Am J Obstet Gynecol 1991;164:73.

3

Sexual and Physical Abuse and Chronic Pelvic Pain

Mary Casey Jacob, PhD, and Maria C. DeNardis, PsyD

It has been noted for some time that women with a history of sexual abuse may be overrepresented in the population of women with chronic pelvic pain (CPP) who seek help; this may also be true of women with a history of physical abuse.[1–4] (The relationship of emotional abuse to pelvic pain conditions has not been addressed.) Making sense of this correlation is a task that continues to challenge practitioners, and methods of using this information in a way that is helpful to patients have not been satisfactorily addressed.

Incidence of Abuse Histories in Women with Chronic Pelvic Pain

In a study of 36 women with CPP, Toomey and colleagues found that 53% reported a history of sexual or physical abuse during childhood (11%), adulthood (17%), or both (25%).[5] Walker and coworkers compared 25 women with CPP with 30 women needing laparoscopy for other reasons. They found that 64% of the women with CPP experienced sexual abuse by age 14 years and 48% experienced sexual abuse after age 14.[6] Reiter and Gambone studied 106 women with CPP with no identifiable organic cause and found that 48% reported a history of "major psychosexual trauma."[3] Walling and associates found that 56% and 50% of their sample of 64 women with CPP reported a lifetime history of sexual abuse or physical abuse, respectively.[7] Forty-two percent report a history of both. Thus, in these few studies, abuse prevalence rates range from 48% to 56%. Keep in mind that standard definitions of abuse were not used, and in some cases, *abuse* referred to sexual *or* physical abuse.

Also of interest is a study of 66 women currently or very recently (within the past year) living in physically abusive relationships, compared with matched controls. The abused women were identified after they sought either emergency medical care or help from a women's refuge center. Forty-eight percent of the abused women reported suffering pelvic pain, compared with 21% of the controls.[8]

General Prevalence of Abuse

To interpret the foregoing information, we must turn to data on the general prevalence of abuse. For example, epidemiologic surveys identify the incidence of child abuse. In a review of 19 retrospective surveys of adults, Finkelhor found that at least 20% of American women reported being sexually abused as children.[9] Finkelhor's review also notes that 90% of sexual abuse is perpetrated by men, 70% to 90% of the perpetrators are known to the child, and 33% to 50% of girl victims are assaulted by family members.[9] Russell surveyed 932 women and found that 20% reported being victims of incest and 38% described being victims of other sexual abuse.[10] A 1989 survey of the nation's child protective agencies found that

This chapter is based in large part on "The Relationship Between Chronic Pelvic Pain and Childhood Abuse," a clinical research project completed by Maria C. DeNardis in partial fulfillment of the requirements for the PsyD degree from the Illinois School of Professional Psychology, Chicago, 1994.

of 2.5 million reports of child abuse, the distribution of types of abuse was 25% physical abuse, 55% neglect, and 20% sexual abuse.[11] Emotional abuse was not reported as a separate category. It is generally believed that surveys such as these underreport the actual incidence of abuse,[12] and it has even been argued that as much as 98% of sexual abuse is unreported.[10] Retrospective surveys of adults suggest that 16% to 27% of girls and 15% of boys are abused, usually by a family member, by their 18th birthdays.[13]

When we compare these numbers with those given for prevalence of abuse histories among women with CPP, it does indeed appear that women who have been victimized in these ways are overrepresented in the CPP population. How does that information influence the care these women receive?

Theoretic Explanations

Psychodynamic Perspective

At about the time that Engel was writing of psychogenic pain and the pain-prone personality,[14] Gidro-Frank and colleagues studied 40 women with CPP and postulated that all were unable to fulfill their female roles without conflict.[15] It was thought that these women were so anxious about the typical female functions ("homemaking, relating affectionately to a husband, performing sexually, menstrually, gestationally") that only repression and denial allowed them to enter into marriage. When those defenses failed, pelvic pain was thought to develop. Twenty years later, Gross and coworkers proposed that the coexistence of CPP and an abuse history denoted a psychogenic origin of the pain.[1] They argued that the physical pain was an unconscious expression of psychic pain resulting from the abuse. Similarly, Walker and colleagues emphasized the unconscious but symbolic nature of the pain and argued that their data support Gidro-Frank and associates' hypothesis that CPP removes a woman from the responsibilities of traditional female tasks and responsibilities.[6]

Psychodynamic researchers have also proposed that the coexistence of psychiatric disorders, often personality disorders, argues for making a psychogenic diagnosis for the pain.[1] However, this broad assumption lacks empirical support and offers no guidance to physicians and others seeking to rehabilitate these patients.

Family Systems Perspective

Many researchers have noted the coexistence of variables such as depression and substance abuse with sexual abuse, and some have hypothesized that the presence of these multiple problems points to a dysfunctional family-of-origin structure, an unpredictable family life, inadequate protection, and lack of care. Walker and colleagues[6] have proposed that these variables cause not only the pelvic pain but the concomitant sexual difficulties. Although nonsupportive family relationships may have a role in the development or expression of pelvic pain, several problems exist with this cause-effect assumption. First, the correlational nature of the studies precludes making this assumption. It is interesting to note that Walker and associates[6] observe that "a serious flaw in many previous studies was the assumption that there was a cause-effect relationship between pathology and pain," and yet they make this same mistake in discussing their psychosocial findings. Second, this simplistic understanding of the implications of psychosocial history overlooks the facts that not all children in these dysfunctional families are sexually abused or develop chronic pain and that family variables are just as likely to buffer a child from the effects of abuse or other family dysfunction. It also presumes a level of expertise about child development that not even experts in child development and sexual abuse believe they have attained. It is clearly worth continuing to put effort into understanding the links between family history and CPP, but caution and appropriate methods must be used.

Cognitive-Behavioral Perspective

Rapkin and colleagues[2] have applied a cognitive-behavioral approach to understanding the link between an abuse history and CPP. They suggest that natural responses to pain include fear, loss of control, anger, and helplessness. These feelings are similar to what an abused child might experience, and in this way pain might reactivate old feelings and old coping responses. Responses such as passivity and withdrawal might have been life saving to an abused child, but they are less functional for an adult in pain.

Diathesis-Stress Model

Kerns and Jacob have proposed a model for understanding the development of chronic pain called the diathesis-stress model.[16–18] This model suggests that some people have preexisting congenital or learned *vulnerabilities* that heighten their risk for developing chronic pain. These vulnerabilities may be in *cognitive* (e.g., low self-esteem), *affective* (e.g., trait anger), *biologic* (e.g., endogenous depression), or *behavioral* (e.g., poor communication in relationships, resulting in little social support) *domains* or may be present in the individual's *family and social milieu* (for example, when a girl learns from her mother to stay home from school when she has cramps). This diathesis-stress model emphasizes the temporal and social contexts in which pain becomes chronic. It specifically hypothesizes that the experience of pain may persist and that disability and distress may develop when there is a match between a preexisting vulnerability and a specific *challenge* associated with acute pain. Three examples of challenges are physical impairment, activation of central monoamine and endorphin systems, and fear. Additionally, the model emphasizes the likely moderating role of social support. As an example of the vulnerability/challenge relationship, consider how a woman with a history of abuse may have low self-esteem and may be depressed. These conditions may reduce her tolerance for distress and prevent her from developing a self-management approach to chronic pain.

History of Abuse and Chronic Nonpelvic Pain

In addition to looking at the frequency of the coexistence of CPP and a history of abuse in the context of abuse epidemiology, it is illuminating to investigate other branches of medicine to determine whether other specialists have noted similar relationships. Outside the pelvic pain arena, Haber and Roos were perhaps the first to publish a report examining the relationship between chronic pain and a history of abuse.[19] Fifty-three percent of 151 consecutively evaluated women presenting to a chronic pain clinic reported histories of physical or sexual abuse in childhood or adulthood, with 41% having suffered both types of abuse. Several years later, Domino and Haber[20] studied 30 women who had chronic headache and who were referred to an interdisciplinary pain management center by their primary care physicians for help after conventional therapies failed. Sixty-six percent of the women reported more than one incident of physical or sexual abuse. The abused women reported greater pain intensity, more medical problems, and more lifetime operations than did the nonabused controls.

Drossman and colleagues studied 206 consecutive patients at a gastroenterology clinic. They found that 44% reported some type of sexual or physical abuse during childhood or adulthood.[21] Patients with functional disorders (e.g., irritable bowel syndrome, nonulcer dyspepsia) were more likely to report histories of abuse than patients with organic disorders (e.g., Crohn's disease, ulcerative colitis). Patients with a history of abuse were more likely to report pelvic pain and many somatic symptoms and to have had more operations. In a separate study of 239 gastrointestinal patients at the same site, 66.5% of the patients reported a history of sexual or physical abuse, and those abused as children did not differ from those abused as adults in terms of health.[22] Walker and associates also studied patients in a gastroenterology clinic and found that 48% of their female sample reported severe victimization.[23] Drossman reports that the literature on abuse supports the notion that the most common somatic complaints of girls and adult women who have been abused are gastrointestinal and genitourinary symptoms.[24]

In a creative study, Karol and coworkers[25] investigated the prevalence of physical, sexual, and emotional abuse histories in patients with back pain (n = 174) and in female health care providers/staff working in the area of chronic pain management, with no history of back pain treatment (n = 33). (Male providers were recruited but responded in such small numbers that their data were not included in the analyses.) Importantly, in addition to asking if one had been abused, the study also asked about perpetration of abuse. Female and male patients and providers/staff reported abuse histories in these percentages, respectively: physical abuse, 27%, 16%, 36%; sexual abuse, 28%, 6%, 33%; and emotional abuse, 36%, 23%, 55%. Note that the providers reported a higher incidence in each category. Additionally, female and male patients and providers/staff reported being perpetrators of physical, sexual, or emotional abuse in these percentages, respectively: physical abuse, 4%, 10%, 15%; sexual abuse, 1%, 3%, 3%; and emotional abuse, 12%, 9%, 12%. Thirty-seven percent of abuse victims were also perpetrators, and 94% of perpetrators were also victims. In this study, the only between-groups comparison that was statistically different was the rate of sexual abuse for male and female patients. As Karol and colleagues point out, however, the fact that other group differences were not statistically significant is beside the point when the prevalence rates are so high.

Rapkin and associates studied both women with pelvic pain (n = 31) and those with other types of chronic pain (n = 141), all of whom presented to a pain management center for help. They found that of the patients with CPP and other chronic pain, 39% and 28%, respectively, reported histories of physical abuse, and 26% and 19% reported histories of sexual abuse.[2] They argue that the greater prevalence of a history of physical abuse in women with CPP negates the traditional psychodynamic hypotheses that sexual trauma uniquely leads to psychosomatic gynecologic problems. This argument is supported by the work of Walling and coworkers, who found that a history of childhood sexual abuse did not predict depression, anxiety, or somatization but that a history of physical abuse did.[4] They hypothesize that the observed relation of sexual abuse to these outcome variables is a result of its likely association with physical abuse. Finally, in a fairly comprehensive review of the literature, Fry found that the data do not support the notion that a history of sexual abuse leads to specific somatic concerns such as pelvic pain but rather that abuse and neglect generally put people at risk for many sorts of health problems.[26] More data are needed to clarify these issues, but certainly, the high rates of physical abuse experiences in these populations do undermine psychodynamic arguments about sexual abuse causing pelvic pain.

Sequelae of Abuse

How can we use knowledge of an abuse history to understand our patients better and help them more effectively? We can usefully start by understanding what is known about the sequelae of abuse generally. Importantly, perhaps as many as one third of victims of childhood abuse do not suffer obvious difficulties in the 12 to 18 months after the abuse.[27] For the remainder, however, although studies have shown links between a history of abuse and varied psychiatric and psychosocial difficulties,[27–30] *for boys as well as girls*,[27] no one set of symptoms has been identified as uniquely characteristic.[27] Although persons with a history of abuse share these common vulnerabilities, evidence suggests that certain forms and conditions of abuse put people at greater or lesser risk for these vulnerabilities individually.[31] When studied as adults, fewer than 20% of victims of child sexual abuse demonstrate *serious* psychopathology. Keep in mind that because of the difficulty and expense of longitudinal studies, most of the information that we have merely shows the coexistence of a history of abuse and life difficulties; we do not yet have proof that the former causes the latter. Similarly, we do not yet have evidence that the one third of childhood sexual abuse victims who appear relatively unscathed at the time of their abuse remain so.

Psychiatric Diagnoses

Evidence suggests a greater than chance association between a history of abuse and the following diagnoses: depression, generalized anxiety disorder, phobias, obsessive-compulsive disorder, panic disorder, dissociative personality disorder (formerly multiple personality disorder), borderline personality disorder, posttraumatic stress disorder, somatoform disorders, eating disorders, and substance abuse.[28, 30–33]

Mood disorders are perhaps the most commonly identified problems in victims of abuse.[29, 34–36] Browne and Finkelhor have written about this link as a consequence of being stigmatized[29] and relate it to low self-esteem, and Gold[35] and Barlow[37] relate it to feelings of loss of control.

Both general community surveys and studies of persons seeking care have identified an association between substance abuse in adulthood and a history of abuse.[33, 38–42] Ongoing substance use for many survivors is a form of self-medication, allowing them to withdraw psychologically from the environment, to dull painful internal states, and to blur distressing memories.[30]

Avoidance of memories of abuse and of other concomitant symptoms is a common coping strategy. Related to the psychiatric conditions under discussion, suicidal thoughts, feelings, and actions are the ultimate attempt at avoidance. Victims of abuse are significantly more likely to have attempted suicide than are nonabused controls.[42, 43]

In addition to data on related formal psychiatric conditions, evidence suggests that victims of abuse are at greater risk for a broad range of general vulnerabilities, including general psychologic distress, cognitive distortions and low self-esteem, difficulties with sexual adjustment, impaired interpersonal relationships, revictimization, and somatic concerns.[28–30, 36, 40, 44–46]

Cognitive Distortions and Low Self-Esteem

For all of us, childhood experience plays a significant role in how we now see the world and our own place in it. The experiences of abuse victims can easily lead them to see the world as a dangerous and negative place and to see themselves as worthless. Feelings of hopelessness and helplessness make perfect sense in this context. Without significant corrective experiences, these cognitive distortions are likely to follow child victims into adulthood.[35]

Impaired Interpersonal Relationships

Community surveys support the notion that victims of sexual abuse feel isolated and stigmatized as adults.[29] Women sexually abused in childhood report difficulties relating to both men and women, ongoing problems in relationships with their own parents, and difficulties in being parents themselves.[29] Why is this? As much as 85% of sexual abuse is perpetrated by someone known to the victim,[27] and the same scenario is most likely with physical and emotional abuse. The violation and betrayal of boundaries that occur during abuse is hypothesized to create ambivalence about and fear of interpersonal vulnerability.[30] Loss of trust may be especially prominent when an abused child discloses to an adult and is not believed or is made to feel guilty.[44] Interpersonal difficulties are especially prominent in survivors when the victimization began early in life, was ongoing, and occurred within the nuclear family.[47]

Feelings of powerlessness, often accompanied by low self-esteem, may express themselves in several ways. A woman may perceive herself as overly dependent and vulnerable and yet appear to others as overcontrolling.[48] Caring for others from positions of power (see Karol and colleagues[25]) and compulsive caregiving, even when it puts one's own health at risk, are examples of this.[48] Abusing others is another expression of feeling powerless, and we know that about one third of abused children become perpetrators.[49] Thinking from a perspective of chronic pain management, we might assume that women who feel powerless will find it more difficult to participate in a self-management approach to rehabilitation.

Physical abuse has been linked to aggression toward others and to criminality.[50, 51] Adult sexual abuse survivors score higher on measures of anger and irritability than controls.[29, 42] This may be pertinent in the care of women with CPP, because evidence shows that anger intensity contributes to predictions of pain intensity and activity levels.[52]

Difficulties with Sexual Adjustment

In clinical samples, women with a history of abuse, especially sexual abuse, are more prone to dyspareunia, anorgasmia, preoccupation with sex, promiscuity, and even prostitution than are women without a history of abuse.[29, 31] This is particularly likely for women who suffered father-daughter incest or any form of penetration.[28] No community surveys have yet explored these relationships in the general population of abused women.

Revictimization

Women with a childhood history of abuse, especially but not limited to sexual abuse, are more likely to experience rape, battery, and other forms of sexual assault than women without such a history. Most hypotheses offered to explain this emphasize the tendency toward helplessness and hopelessness and an impaired ability to recognize trustworthy people.[28]

Somatic Concerns

Many of the physical symptoms reported by victims of abuse can be attributed to a psychiatric disorder such as depression, generalized anxiety, or posttraumatic stress disorder. Examples include sleep disorders and physical signs of agitation and anxiety such as skin flushing, perspiration, exaggerated startle responses, and restless body movements.[36] However, evidence shows that independent of mood disorders, a history of abuse is associated with increased use of medical services as well as a broad array of somatic concerns, especially gastrointestinal and respiratory disorders, pelvic pain, vaginal and bladder infections, and obesity. This has been demonstrated in clinical populations[19, 22, 44, 46, 53, 54] and in nonclinical populations and community surveys.[36, 55] Women with a history of abuse have been found to have more pelvic and lifetime operations and more physician visits than controls.[21, 22, 53, 54, 56] It is also worth noting that in a large study (n = 2291 women enrolled at a health maintenance organization) of the relationship between being a crime victim and general health perceptions, it was found that victimization was related to lowered health perceptions irrespective of age and other demographic factors and to stressful life events other than the crime, and 93% of the victims saw their physicians in the year after the crime.[57]

Aggravating and Buffering Factors

Why do not all victims of abuse suffer some of the difficulties just described? Several hypotheses have been offered and are supported by some evidence. Certain conditions appear to make it more likely that a victim will suffer long-term consequences: molestation at an early age, ongoing abuse rather than an isolated incident, more than one type of abuse (e.g., physical as well as sexual), use of force or threats, genital contact or penetration, father or stepfather as perpetrator, and multiple perpetrators.[28–30] Family characteristics and response to disclosure also appear to predict subsequent adjustment: In families with greater dysfunction and when disclosure is met with disbelief or accusations, the survivor is more likely to suffer ongoing difficulties.[29, 35, 47] The opposite sort of conditions are hypothesized to serve as buffers, such as having disclosed the information to an adult who believed the child victim and took steps to protect her or him.

Assessment for Women with Chronic Pelvic Pain and an Abuse History

The integrated approach to the treatment and rehabilitation of women with CPP introduced in Chapter 2 and described throughout this text provides the basis for working with women with CPP, regardless of history of abuse. The process of assessment generally begins with taking a thorough history, and in a team approach, this might involve various professionals such as a physician, a mental health worker, and a physical therapist. Each professional approaches a patient with the intention of developing and testing hypotheses about how the chronic pain developed and what variables are contributing to its maintenance.[17] Because of the prevalence of the experience of abuse and because the sequelae of abuse often serve as predisposing vulnerabilities to the development of chronic pain, assessment should always consider abuse and its particular sequelae for each patient. To facilitate this inquiry, a patient's orientation to the doctor's office or pain program should contain an explanation of the multidimensional nature of the assessment process. This explanation can help a patient understand not only why certain questions are asked but why more than one person may seem to ask the same question. The latter is also an opportunity to introduce the patient to the concept of a team and can inform her that the team routinely shares information in order to offer the best help. These suggestions for orienting a patient to the assessment are helpful for all patients, but they communicate several important facts to a patient with an abuse history. First, she will know that all patients are asked about experiences of abuse, and she can decide what and when to disclose. Second, by understanding the reason for apparent duplication of questions, she will be less likely to feel that the team is grilling her about her abuse experiences. Third, by emphasizing the importance of many factors and not just her abuse, the assessment may help to challenge her own beliefs or previous medical interactions that led to assumptions of a psychogenic cause of her pain. Fourth, outlining the limits of confidentiality instructs a patient that the team treats knowledge of an abuse history in the same way it treats other information gathered during the assessment process. If a woman with an abuse history asks that the information not be shared with the team, the clinician should explore her reasons for asking this. Chances are that the request indicates that the patient does not understand or has not yet accepted that the team considers this just one of many variables that might affect her experience of pain. In deciding this issue, team members should remember that complying with a request to withhold information regarding an abuse history from the rest of the team may undermine the ability of the team to function collaboratively.

To assess for history of abuse, ask specific questions about abuse experiences and ask about all forms of abuse: emotional, physical, and sexual. Russell offers a standardized assessment,[10] and Draucker,[56] Gil,[58] and Drossman and colleagues[21, 59] offer suggestions for wording the questions. Because of the sensitive nature of such questions, they should not occur early in the interview but only after a degree of rapport has developed.

Data have indicated a stronger relationship between severe abuse and CPP (and other pains, such as gastrointestinal pain) than "milder" forms of abuse,[22, 60] but this should not lead a clinician to dismiss or underestimate the importance of an abuse event to the individual. For some individuals, less severe forms of abuse also lead to long-term sequelae. Despite the increasing attention paid to the issue of abuse in recent years, many women have not told anyone of their victimization. Because of the sensitive nature of the issue and the possibility that each disclosure is a first disclosure, clinicians must be aware of the importance of their own reactions to a patient. Unhelpful and possibly even harmful responses include statements implying disbelief, questions that are or appear intrusive or voyeuristic, and comments minimizing the importance of the abuse.[56, 58] Helpful responses show sensitivity and calm concern and should include an inquiry about the comfort of the patient after her disclosure. The latter is quite important, because disclosure may unlock strong or unexpected feelings and the woman may require additional support. Of course, if an extremely strong reaction results, such as suicidal thoughts or feelings, a mental health professional should evaluate the woman's safety immediately, and appropriate measures should be taken. After disclosure, survivors benefit from being given a choice about how much to disclose, how often they are asked about the abuse, and whether to accept a psychotherapy referral.[61] Certain aspects of a woman's history should alert the clinician not to press for details: a history of severe mental disorder (e.g., schizophrenia), a recent psychiatric inpatient admission, references to particularly severe or bizarre abuse, and any cognitive deterioration while speaking about the abuse, such as disorganization, psychotic thoughts, or a dissociative reaction.[58] These same circumstances might prevent a woman from engaging in a rehabilitation program.

A psychotherapist takes a very detailed history of abuse experiences, but this is rarely appropriate in a pain management setting. In the latter, the focus is on reduction of pain and its accompanying disability and not on an in-depth exploration of past experiences. Also, although therapeutic relationships will be developed, they will generally not be of sufficient duration or frequency to help abuse survivors deal with the memories. Thus, in the pain management setting, the focus should be on the general parameters of abuse and on identifying the concomitants of the pain problem that might also be sequelae of abuse. The exact questioning might be determined by the discipline of the interviewer. For example, a physician might want to know if any penetration occurred and with what objects and if injuries resulted and if they were treated. A psychologist might be charged with the task of learning enough about the abuse to begin to recognize the sequelae. Issues that might be discussed include the duration of the abuse, use of force or threats, if penetration occurred, the relationship of the perpetrator(s) to the victim, the quality of other family and important relationships, and the woman's beliefs about her own responsibility for the abuse.[28, 35] This information provides an indication of the woman's expectations of assistance from the pain program and her potential willingness to accept a referral if the team should recommend it.

In contrast to women with strong reactions following disclosure, some women may minimize the impact of the abuse on their lives. They are sometimes merely being truthful, because they are in the group of people who, for whatever reasons, are able to survive and move beyond the abuse without long-term negative sequelae. Other times, this represents protective denial. Such minimization may be a means of self-protection developed at the time of the abuse and now habitual even though it is no longer functional.[56, 58] Draucker has advised that clinicians noticing this reaction not address it immediately but merely observe it.[56] Later, if it appears that the patient suffers specific difficulties related to the abuse, it can be addressed. It may also need to be addressed if a denial style of coping prevents a woman from exploring and accepting possible links between her pain and psychosocial factors, such as mood changes or relationship difficulties.

A clinician may sometimes suspect that a patient has suffered abuse, even though she says she has not. Possible explanations are that the woman was abused but does not remember it; the clinician is incorrect; the woman defines abuse differently and the clinician's questions have not elicited the history even though she is willing to acknowledge it; or the woman may have made a conscious decision not to disclose. Clinicians should never challenge a woman's response to questions about abuse. Respecting her answer conveys concern and avoids the invasive and suggestive questioning thought to implant false memories. Importantly, inquiring about abuse in a supportive manner tells each patient that this doctor's office is a setting in which she is allowed to disclose if she wishes.

Sometimes a patient may recover a memory of abuse while in your care. Because examinations and some procedures involve touching the genitals and are performed by a person in a position of authority and control, they can stimulate direct kinesthetic memory or precipitate flashbacks or dissociative episodes.[61] The consensus in the mental health field is that traumatic memories can be suppressed and later recalled;[62] thus, when a woman shares with you that this has occurred, her disclosure needs to be respected and validated. As with disclosure of known memories, take the time to ask how the woman feels after disclosure; if she needs support or crisis intervention, help her get the necessary care.

For survivors of abuse, just seeking health care can be terribly frightening. For a survivor, it implies she is worthy of care—a notion she may have difficulty accepting. It requires trusting a stranger and allowing that person access to her body. Patients may feel afraid of losing control of their bodies or of not being able to protect themselves. Medical examinations that involve previously traumatized body parts can be especially difficult. Medical examinations and tests that restrict movement and freedom can also be retraumatizing.[61]

A comprehensive psychosocial assessment (see Chapters 2, 6, and 9) generally evaluates all or most of the variables that might be sequelae or vulnerabilities linked to an abuse history. For a patient with a known history of abuse, the following factors warrant careful review: ability to regulate affect and self-esteem, especially depression, anxiety, fear, substance abuse, eating disorders, and dissociation; suicidality; sexual adjustment; the nature of interpersonal relationships; experiences of revictimization; and symptoms of physiologic distress other than CPP.[28, 29, 34, 36, 44, 46, 63]

Rehabilitation for Patients with Chronic Pelvic Pain and an Abuse History

Patients with CPP and a history of abuse may require few or many modifications of a typical program of rehabilitation. The following ideas are meant as starting points for creative thinking about how to treat this special population. One modification may be in the order of recommendations. Of course, any medical recommendation that might actually treat an illness or cure pain should generally be offered first. Beyond that, however, the team might first provide medication for the improvement of sleep and reduction in anxiety or depressive symptoms. A woman's pain sensitivity might be lowered as well, but even without that, some early relief in affective distress and fatigue might increase the patient's trust in the team and allow her to feel well enough that she might be able to engage in some self-management activities when they are recommended. Early teaching of strategies such as deep muscle relaxation might be contraindicated, however, because it may lead the woman to feel too relaxed, too out of control.

If withdrawal of narcotic medication is routinely recommended in a pain program, this priority might be altered for women with an abuse history. It may be that the narcotic serves not only to attenuate the pain but also to medicate affective distress related to memories of the abuse. This should be a consideration also when substance abuse is identified and treatment offered. These women might need therapy for the abuse sequelae or just an early focus on self-management strategies such as distraction and self-soothing techniques so that when the narcotics are withdrawn later, they have other ways to manage the distress and the memories.

A third consideration is that a woman with an abuse history might be reactive to the gender of the clinicians working with her. Respect should always be shown for these preferences, and whenever possible, a clinician of the preferred gender should be made available. A fourth issue to consider is that a history of abuse can leave one very concerned about being in control of one's emotions and one's body. Thus, the use of hypnosis may be threatening, especially early in a rehabilitation program. The issue of control also arises if a woman is expected to meet with a team to finalize her treatment plan; this may be overwhelming, and it might be better if she meets with an individual for these discussions.

Treatment groups might be threatening too. For many women with CPP, groups can reduce a patient's feeling that she is suffering alone, and groups are generally a good format for teaching self-management skills.

For a woman with a history of abuse, however, developing trust in a group may be too difficult.

Some modifications might also be made in medical examinations and treatments. Women who have been abused generally benefit from increased explanations, care for their discomfort during examinations, and an opportunity to say what will help them tolerate the planned procedures. The latter might include having a trusted friend or family member present, using a pediatric speculum, and sometimes medication to reduce anxiety and muscle tension (but not to the degree that they will feel out of control).

Women with CPP often report discomfort or pain during sex and say that this has led to withdrawal and sometimes to difficulty in relationships. These women often benefit from suggestions about the use of lubricants and positions that allow them to control the angle and degree of penetration. Women with a history of abuse may especially welcome suggestions that allow them to feel more in control. Keep in mind, however, that past abuse experiences may have resulted in ambivalence about addressing problems in sexual relationships. For example, although a woman may wish to improve sex for the benefit of her relationship, she may also want to avoid it because of the memories it evokes. The possibility of such mixed feelings points to the importance of having such discussions with the patient alone, in the absence of her partner, and allowing her to indicate if she is ready to work on issues in this area.

Women who show significant impairments thought to be related to a history of abuse may benefit from a referral for psychotherapy. This can often occur concurrently with medical and other treatments and may actually facilitate the woman's ability to engage fully in the other therapies. Sometimes it may be apparent that psychotherapy should be a priority, especially in cases of severe depression and active substance abuse. Even when this is the case, however, the woman can still be offered a thorough medical evaluation and any appropriate medical treatment. Further rehabilitation can be offered after the woman's condition has improved and stabilized and her ability to engage in rehabilitation is established.

When making a referral for psychotherapy, offer a rationale related to the woman's pain problem whenever possible. Imagine, for example, a woman whose assessment reveals that her pain predictably increases after she avoids conflict with her husband. Efforts to teach simple assertion have not helped. It might be suggested to her that her childhood history of abuse taught her not to express anger and not to value her own needs and opinions. This was a survival tactic at the time but is no longer functional. Psychotherapy might assist her in exploring her anger and in learning appropriate ways of expressing it.

When a patient is in therapy when she comes to you or when she enters therapy on your recommendation, get her permission to be in touch with the therapist. When you have formed your thoughts about appropriate treatment for the patient, ask the therapist for suggestions about how to offer the treatment in a way that the patient can accept and receive benefit.

Closing Remarks

It does appear to be true that of the women with CPP who seek our help, a history of abuse is disproportionately represented. This has been shown with sexual and physical abuse, and we must investigate if this is true for emotional abuse and neglect. Seen in context, however, it may be that this is not unique to gynecology but rather that women with abuse histories are at greater risk for various health-related concerns and are more likely to turn to physicians for help than nonabused women. From the perspective of the diathesis-stress model, this can be conceptualized as one factor that determines which women with CPP will manage on their own with minimal medical intervention and which ones will seek help repeatedly. Walker and Katon[64] have proposed that we think in terms of direct effects such as injuries or infection as well as indirect effects such as low self-esteem and depression that might result in maladaptive health behaviors. When it is known that a woman has suffered abuse, some accommodations may be made to facilitate her ability to cooperate with evaluations and to participate actively in treatment. These accommodations include attention to the sequential ordering of interventions and the impact of the gender of the team members on the patient, special provisions in medical procedures such as using a pediatric speculum, and an awareness that the sequelae of abuse may interfere with a woman's current ability to participate actively in a self-management approach to chronic pain.

References

1. Gross R, Doerr H, Caldirola G, et al: Borderline syndrome and incest in chronic pelvic pain patients. Int J Psychiatry Med 1980;10:79.
2. Rapkin AJ, Kames LD, Darke LL, et al: History of physical and sexual abuse in women with chronic pelvic pain. Obstet Gynecol 1990;76:92.
3. Reiter RC, Gambone JC: Demographic and historical variables in women with idiopathic chronic pelvic pain. Obstet Gynecol 1990;75:428.
4. Walling MK, O'Hara MW, Reiter RC, et al: Abuse history and chronic pain in women: II. A multivariate analysis of abuse and psychological morbidity. Obstet Gynecol 1994;84:200.
5. Toomey TC, Hernandez JT, Gittelman DF, et al: Relationship of sexual and physical abuse to pain and psychological assessment variables in chronic pelvic pain patients. Pain 1993;53:105.
6. Walker EA, Katon W, Harrop-Griffiths J, et al: Relationship of chronic pelvic pain to psychiatric diagnosis and childhood sexual abuse. Am J Psychiatry 1988;145:75.
7. Walling MK, Reiter RC, O'Hara MW, et al: Abuse history and chronic pain in women: I. Prevalences of sexual abuse and physical abuse. Obstet Gynecol 1994;84:193.
8. Schei B: Psycho-social factors in pelvic pain: A controlled study of women living in physically abusive relationships. Acta Obstet Gynecol Scand 1990;69:67.
9. Finkelhor D: Current information on the scope and nature of child sexual abuse. Future Child 1994; 4:31.
10. Russell DEH: The Secret Trauma: Incest in the Lives of Girls and Women. New York, Basic Books, 1986.
11. Daro D, Mitchel M: Current trends in child abuse reporting and fatalities: The results of the 1989 annual fifty state survey. Report No. 808. Chicago, National Committee for the Prevention of Child Abuse, 1990.
12. Rosenberg DA, Krugman RD: Epidemiology and outcome of child abuse. Annu Rev Med 1991; 42:217.
13. Finkelhor D, Hotaling G, Lewis IA, et al: Sexual abuse in a national survey of adult men and women: Prevalence, characteristics, and risk factors. Child Abuse Negl 1990;14:19.
14. Engel GL: "Psychogenic" pain and the pain-prone patient. Am J Med 1959;26:899.
15. Gidro-Frank L, Gordon T, Taylor HC Jr: Pelvic pain and female identity. Am J Obstet Gynecol 1960;79:1184.
16. Kerns RD, Jacob MC: Toward an integrative diathesis-stress model of chronic pain. In Goreczny AJ (ed): Handbook of Health and Rehabilitation Psychology. New York, Plenum, 1995.
17. Jacob MC: Psychological aspects of chronic pelvic pain in women with endometriosis. In Nezhat CR, Berger GS, Nezhat FR, et al (eds): Endometriosis: Advanced Management and Surgical Techniques. New York, Springer-Verlag, 1995.
18. Kerns RD, Payne A: Treating families of chronic pain patients. In Gatchel RJ, Turk DC (eds): Psychological Approaches to Pain Management: A Practitioner's Handbook. New York, Guilford Press, 1996.
19. Haber JD, Roos C: Effects of spouse abuse and/or sexual abuse in the development and maintenance of chronic pain in women. In Fields HL, Dubner R, Cervaro F (eds): Advances in Pain Research and Therapy. New York, Raven Press, 1985.
20. Domino JV, Haber JD: Prior physical and sexual abuse in women with chronic headache: Clinical correlates. Headache 1987;27:310.
21. Drossman DA, Leserman J, Nachman G, et al: Sexual and physical abuse in women with functional or organic gastrointestinal disorders. Ann Intern Med 1990;113:828.
22. Leserman J, Drossman DA, Li Z, et al: Sexual and physical abuse history in gastroenterology practice: How types of abuse impact health status. Psychosom Med 1996;58:4.
23. Walker EA, Gelfand AN, Gelfand MD, et al: Medical and psychiatric symptoms in female gastroenterology clinic patients with histories of sexual victimization. Gen Hosp Psychiatry 1995;17:85.
24. Drossman DA: Physical and sexual abuse and gastrointestinal illness: What is the link? (editorial). Am J Med 1994;97:105.
25. Karol RL, Micka RG, Kuskowski M: Physical, emotional, and sexual abuse among pain patients and health care providers: Implications for psychologists in multidisciplinary pain treatment centers. Prof Psych Res Pract 1992;23:480.
26. Fry R: Adult physical illness and childhood sexual abuse. J Psychosom Res 1993;37:89.
27. Finkelhor D: Early and long-term effects of child sexual abuse: An update. Prof Psych Res Pract 1990;21:325.
28. Beitchman JH, Zuker KJ, Hood JE, et al: A review of the long-term effects of child sexual abuse. Child Abuse Negl 1992;16:101.
29. Browne A, Finkelhor D: Impact of child sexual abuse: A review of the research. Psychol Bull 1986;99:66.
30. Briere JN, Elliot DM: Intermediate and long-term impacts of child sexual abuse. Future Child 1994;4:54.
31. Briere JN, Runtz M: Differential adult symptomatology associated with three types of child abuse histories. Child Abuse Negl 1990;14:357.
32. Putnam FW: Diagnosis and Treatment of Multiple Personality Disorder. New York, Guilford Press, 1989.
33. Brown GR, Anderson B: Psychiatric morbidity in adult inpatients with childhood histories of sexual and physical abuse. Am J Psychiatry 1991;148:55.

34. Briere JN, Runtz M: Multivariate correlates of childhood psychological and physical maltreatment among university women. Child Abuse Negl 1988;12:331.
35. Gold ER: Long-term effects of sexual victimization in childhood: An attributional approach. J Consult Clin Psychol 1986;54:471.
36. Sedney MA, Brooks B: Factors associated with a history of childhood sexual experience in a nonclinical female population. J Am Acad Child Psychiatry 1984;23:215.
37. Barlow D: Anxiety and its Disorders: The Nature and Treatment of Anxiety and Panic. New York, Guilford Press, 1988.
38. Hibbard S: Personality and object relational pathology in young adult children of alcoholics. Psychother 1989;26:504.
39. Singer MI, Petchers MK, Hussey D: The relationship between sexual abuse and substance abuse among psychiatrically hospitalized adolescents. Child Abuse Negl 1989;13:319.
40. Dembo R, Williams L, LaVoie L, et al: Physical abuse, sexual victimization, and illicit drug use: Replication of a structural analysis among a new sample of high-risk youths. Violence Victims 1989;4:121.
41. Sullivan EJ: Association between chemical dependency and sexual problems in nurses. J Interpersonal Violence 1988;3:326.
42. Briere J, Runtz M: Post sexual abuse trauma: Data and implications for clinical practice. J Interpersonal Violence 1987;2:367.
43. Briere J, Zaidi LY: Sexual abuse histories and sequelae in female psychiatric emergency room patients. Am J Psychiatry 1989;146:1602.
44. Bachman GA, Moeller TP, Benett J: Childhood sexual abuse and the consequences in adult women. Obstet Gynecol 1988;71:631.
45. Cunningham J, Pearce T, Pearce P: Childhood sexual abuse and medical complaints in women. J Interpersonal Violence 1988;3:131.
46. Felitti VJ: Long-term medical consequences of incest, rape, and molestation. South Med J 1991; 84:328.
47. Elliot DM: Impaired object relations in professional women molested as children. Psychother 1994; 31:79.
48. Finkelhor D, Browne A: The traumatic impact of child sexual abuse. Am J Orthopsychiatry 1985; 55:530.
49. Widom C: The cycle of abuse. Science 1989; 244:160.
50. McCord J: A forty year perspective on child abuse and neglect. Child Abuse Negl 1983;7:265.
51. Pollock VE, Briere J, Schneider L, et al: Childhood antecedents of antisocial behavior: Parental alcoholism and physical abusiveness. Am J Psychiatry 1990;147:1290.
52. Kerns RD, Rosenberg R, Jacob MC: Anger expression and chronic pain. J Behav Med 1994;17:57.
53. Lechner ME, Vogel ME, Garcia-Shelton LM, et al: Self-reported medical problems of adult female survivors of childhood sexual abuse. J Fam Pract 1993;36:633.
54. Springs FE, Friedrich WN: Health risk behaviors and medical sequelae of childhood sexual abuse. Mayo Clin Proc 1992;67:527.
55. Golding JM: Sexual assault history and physical health in randomly selected Los Angeles women. Health Psychol 1994;13:130.
56. Draucker CB: Counseling Survivors of Childhood Sexual Abuse. London, Sage, 1992.
57. Koss MP, Woodruff WJ, Koss PG: Relation of criminal victimization to health perceptions among women medical patients. J Consult Clin Psychol 1990;58:147.
58. Gil E: Treatment of Adult Survivors of Childhood Abuse. Walnut Creek, CA, Launch Press, 1988.
59. Leserman J, Drossman DA, Li Z: Obtaining a history of sexual abuse in medical patients: Validity and reliability of a survey instrument (abstract). Psychosom Med 1994;56:147.
60. Walker EA, Katon WJ, Neraas K, et al: Dissociation in women with chronic pelvic pain. Am J Psychiatry 1992;149:534.
61. Courtois CA: Adult survivors of sexual abuse. Primary Care 1993;20:433.
62. Alpert JL, Brown LS, Ceci SJ, et al: Working Group on Investigation of Memories of Childhood Abuse: Final Report. Washington, DC, American Psychological Association, 1996.
63. Wurtele SK, Kaplan GM, Keairnes M: Childhood sexual abuse among chronic pain patients. Clin J Pain 1990;6:110.
64. Walker EA, Katon WJ: Researching the health effects of victimization: The next generation (editorial). Psychosom Med 1996;58:16.

4

One Patient's Experience

Anne Shortliffe, BA, BSN

K.B. is a 38-year-old married white woman, gravida 1, para 0, abortus 1, with a 3 1/2-year history of right lower quadrant pelvic pain. The pain occurred daily and was described as a throbbing ache on the right side. She reported a sense of being so swollen in the pelvis that she could not cross her legs. She also experienced midline low back pain, a general falling out sensation of the pelvis, rectal pain, and shooting radiating pain and numbness down her anterior right thigh. Bowel function alternated between constipation and diarrhea. When she was constipated, her right lower quadrant pain worsened in general and she had rectal pain when trying to pass a stool. She had no difficulties with her bladder function.

Although K.B. continued to work at a full-time desk job, she had stopped nearly every other activity in her life. She did only very light housework, and had ceased getting any regular exercise. Intercourse had become so painful for her that she and her husband had stopped attempts at intimacy for more than 6 months. Her sleep pattern was marked by early morning awakening with an inability to return to sleep. Crying spells pervaded her day-to-day existence. She described herself as anxious and was taking alprazolam (Xanax) 0.5 mg qid, Donnatol for bowel spasms, and naproxen sodium (Anaprox) for pain.

K.B. said that this pain all began within 3 days after her miscarriage in April 1990. After the miscarriage, she had a postabortal infection and reported a 30-pound weight loss, anorexia, and pain so debilitating that it was difficult to walk. She attributed all of these symptoms to the infection, although she readily admitted that since she had tried for years to get pregnant, losing the pregnancy was especially depressing.

In November 1991, she underwent laparoscopy, which revealed a small right anterior lower uterine segment myoma with endometriosis in an adjacent area along with several foci of endometriosis in the posterior cul-de-sac and one focus on the left bladder dome. Omental to anterior pelvic adhesions were present and were lysed. The endometriosis was treated with laser therapy, and symptoms resolved after the surgical treatment and 3 months of leuprolide acetate (Lupron Depot). Pain recurred shortly thereafter. Attempts at a course of depot medroxyprogesterone acetate (Depo-Provera) therapy were abandoned owing to intolerable side effects of headache and nausea. Repeat laser laparoscopy in April 1993 revealed foci of endometriosis on the left ovary near the hilum, on both uterosacral ligaments, on the right posterior broad ligament, and at the vesicouterine junction; adhesions from the omentum to the abdominal wall in the region of the previous incision; and mild midline vesicouterine adhesions. After laser treatment of the pathology, she again took leuprolide acetate for 2 months.

When the pain recurred again by midsummer of 1993, K.B. was referred to an orthopedist who believed she might have endometriosis in the right sciatic nerve. Her physicians thought that the endometriosis was too minimal to warrant a hysterectomy and referred her to the pelvic pain clinic for evaluation. After the records were reviewed, questionnaires were mailed to the patient to be returned before her initial visit.

Her questionnaires revealed severe depression, with a Beck score[1] of 34 (normal ≤ 10), elevations on every scale of the Hopkins Symptom Check List (SCL-90)[2, 3] with particularly high scores on depression and anxiety, and a very high McGill pain rating index[4] of 47.49 (see Chapter 8). Her pain ratings were much higher than could be accounted for on the basis of the degree of organic disease found at her two prior laparoscopies. She did not reveal any episodes of sexual abuse but did acknowledge physical abuse both as a child and as an adult.

At the first pelvic pain clinic visit (September 2, 1993), she and her husband asked for a hysterectomy as the "only solution to the pain." They were very distressed about the demise of their social and sexual relationship and wanted an immediate resolution of her symptoms. At the end of the examination, several problems were identified.

K.B. had significant right pyriformis syndrome, marked pelvic floor tension myalgia (see Chapter 24), a clinically significant depression (see Chapter 27), irritable bowel syndrome (see Chapter 23), and probably some residual endometriosis (see Chapter 14), documented on two prior laparoscopies. We suggested she consult a physical therapist near her home, take a fiber laxative twice a day, and begin the antidepressant sertraline (Zoloft).

The effects of a chronic pain syndrome were explained to the patient and her husband together after that initial examination. They were told that a hysterectomy might ultimately prove to be necessary in the future but that it was not a medical emergency and that, given all the other factors involved, she would probably not recover well from an immediate surgical procedure. All the other problems (i.e., pelvic floor muscle spasm, pyriformis syndrome, irritable bowel syndrome, and her depression) needed to be dealt with first.

K.B. immediately sought out a physical therapist who worked diligently with her one to three times per week for the next year. The bowel symptoms resolved quickly with Citrucel fiber laxative and increased water intake. With reluctance, she did see a psychologist and began to take sertraline 50 mg per day. The decision to begin sertraline was made after many phone conversations to reassure the patient that the recommendation of an antidepressant did *not* mean that we believed the pain was "all in her head." Her general internist of many years also encouraged her to try the medicine.

Four months after her initial visit, K.B. returned to our clinic, showing vast improvement. Her examination, which had been excruciatingly painful at the first visit, was much more comfortable owing to the complete resolution of the pyriformis syndrome and levator spasm. She and her spouse had resumed their sexual relationship without pain and with a full response cycle. Her sleep pattern had normalized, her appetite had improved, and her crying spells had resolved on the sertraline. She had stopped seeing the psychologist because of financial constraints. Some residual right lower quadrant pain remained. At this point, beaming with hope, K.B. chose to continue with sertraline and physical therapy (PT). In a letter that we received not long after this appointment, she wrote:

> *After our visit I began realizing more and more exactly where I was at in my recovery. When you have been sick for a long time, . . . you start living the part of pain. . . . I always believed if I could just get out of pain I would be able to jump back in life where I left off. Well surprise—. . .*
>
> *Slowly I saw pain take away from my life the things I loved and enjoyed doing. When I came to see you all, I was at my worst point—up until two months prior to coming I had not thought of suicide—but at that point, I wanted to die. I couldn't do that to D. and I believe God begins and ends life . . . so . . . I walked my insecurities into your office.*
>
> *I have learned a lot about the body and the mind. It goes hand in hand. It affects the spiritual man also. I feel like I am coming out of the closet (per se). The whole world should know you aren't crazy when the mind gets tired like the body and needs help.*

While continuing work in PT, K.B. began to have flashbacks. When the therapist worked on muscles in the pelvis, memories from her past would be triggered and she often began to cry uncontrollably. When she found herself crying over the abortion her parents had forced her to have at the age of 17, she revealed to us that she had actually had two pregnancies. The physical therapist encouraged these emotional releases in the safety of the office. K.B. remembered that she had to wait for the physician to arrive after she had begun to miscarry the second pregnancy. She tried to hold on to the fetus with all the strength she had, hoping somehow that the inevitable abortion could be stopped. She relived both of these traumatic losses with her physical therapist. Another letter arrived:

I didn't know much about abortions except it was wrong. . . . I could feel the pain and hear the suction. After a couple of hours, we got in the car and left . . . we never spoke of it again. . . . I was lying in the back seat crying silently—always silently.

I remember a feeling of relief that they wouldn't fuss at me any more and it was weird because I also had a feeling as if something was gone. After the miscarriage, Anne, I felt that same feeling, like there was something gone from me. . . . I didn't know all this was there, so I guess I am getting better. I am very tired from crying and fighting but in a weird way, I am beginning to feel relieved.

During her continued phone calls with me (usually about 2 per month), in which she shared these memories, K.B. began to reveal more and more about herself. She had grown up in an emotionally negligent home, was a reformed alcoholic (sober now for 18 years), and had repressed large segments of her past. As the memories surfaced during the PT deep muscle work in the lower right quadrant, she began to experience new levels of emotional pain.

K.B. also had significant present-day stressors. Her employer was getting frustrated by her ill health and her need to leave work to attend PT appointments. K.B. made up for this by coming to work an hour early, working through lunch, and so on, none of which helped her to manage the pain she was having. Her mother-in-law also had Alzheimer's disease and required constant care. K.B. felt she owed her sobriety to this woman who took her in during her worst period of alcoholism and helped her become sober. It was through her mother-in-law that she met her husband. Every morning, K.B. was up early and over to her mother-in-law's house before work to get her up and dressed, give her breakfast, and set up lunch for her. Her husband went every night to take care of her supper and bedtime. There was little time for her and her husband to be together. As present and past stressors accumulated together, K.B. became aware of tightening of the pyriformis muscle on the right side. She began to be able to differentiate the muscle pain from her continued right lower quadrant discomforts.

Six months after the initial visit, her examination showed continued tenderness in the right adnexal area consistent with the right ovary and broad ligament, which we believed might reflect a return of endometriosis. The levator and pyriformis spasms would come and go, depending on her level of stress. Cyclobenzaprine HCl (Flexeril) 10 mg qhs prn was prescribed to help relax the muscles during these times. Her physical therapist sent a letter in to us, saying

She has really come a long way in being able to recognize that some of her family dynamics (primarily relationship with father) are strongly linked to her physical holding patterns.

We are working on breaking this cycle of "holding" when stressful and frustrating situations arise, but her patterns and habits are so ingrained, this is difficult.

One year into working with K.B., we believed that the muscular components of her problem would not get any better if the right lower quadrant pain was not identified and resolved. We decided to perform a laparoscopy under local anesthesia (see Chapter 33) to determine the source of her pain. Mild endometriosis was identified on the right ovary and tube, but her pain was reproduced by probing the uterus rather than the right ovary. Surgery progressed to general anesthesia, and a laparoscopically assisted vaginal hysterectomy and right salpingo-oophorectomy (LAVH/RSO) were performed.

The relief from the right lower quadrant pain was immediate. K.B. called at 1 week postoperatively to discuss her revelation that her body was now open to receiving new sensations since pain was not occupying her mind any more. She felt the "carpet under her feet and the breeze upon her face" for the first time in 3 years. She was aware of some ongoing muscle spasm in the right pyriformis but knew from her work in PT that she could get control over that. She was discharged from PT with a home exercise program approximately 6 weeks after surgery.

Perhaps the most fascinating part of working with this patient has been the year following surgery. When a chronic pain syndrome was first explained to her and her husband, we emphasized that getting over the problem is a rehabilitative process, not an immediate reversal to patterns preceding the onset of pain. K.B. has been amazed at just how difficult it has been to regain her life.

Her first difficulty was returning to work after the postoperative period. She had struggled for years to maintain her job and knew that her supervisor and coworkers expected her to come back at better than 100% now that she had finally had her hysterectomy. The expectations scared her. Requesting to do no overtime for at least the first 2 months enabled her to return to work.

Five months after surgery and 3 months after returning to her job, K.B. came into the clinic for a checkup. Her pain was essentially gone. However, she had begun to see how much chronic pain had changed her life. She explained it this way:

> *I had this friend move in with me 4 years ago. I didn't like this friend much; in fact, it was more like an enemy, but it was there all the time, 24 hours a day and became a part of my life. When this friend moved out, I was changed by it. I could not just go back to who I was before I met this friend. I had become a different person and no longer knew how to act without this friend . . . I have had to relearn who I am.*

She was not the only person who had to relearn and readjust. Family members, particularly her siblings and parents, had come to know her in the sick role and expected her to function in that way. She identified in continued phone calls her insight that they would "not let her get better." They did not want to know what she had learned and did not like her newfound independence. She wrote in a letter to us 4 weeks after surgery:

> *Too bad my problems are ending. Maybe now my family can focus in on their own problems. They will not rob me any longer. . . . I will not be their victim any longer. Sometimes I feel their greatest fear is I will get well and they will no longer have a victim.*

Within the first 6 months after surgery, K.B. suffered two significant losses. The general internist ("Dr. Bob") whom she had seen for years and trusted was diagnosed with cancer and died within just a few weeks. Then, a few months later, her mother-in-law died of a severe cerebrovascular accident. Suddenly, there was the confusion of having more free time since she did not have to be a caregiver anymore. She also had the concomitant need to grieve. Pain had resulted in many losses, and now she had new losses to cope with.

K.B. called about 7 months after her surgery and said, "I think I am overdoing." She was painting walls, installing carpet, hanging curtains, entertaining, and so on. Her right-sided pain was increasing. After talking for a bit, she identified that she was pushing away all grief responses to the deaths of her mother-in-law and Dr. Bob. She thought she had dealt with the surgical loss of fertility, but her mother-in-law's death stirred up guilt about disappointing her husband. He was adopted and loved his mother dearly. She said, "Now, he only has me. . . . He'll never have any more family." She worried that she might not be enough. She attempted to protect her husband by not letting him see her hurt anymore. The harder she worked to prevent sadness, the more her physical pain increased. She was encouraged to talk openly with her husband, cry with him, and work through the loss and the pain.

Eleven months after surgery, K.B. came into the clinic for an annual examination. Her pelvic examination was comfortable, and she had experienced a dramatic change from our first meeting 2 years earlier. She reported that things were better with her husband. She told him to "let me cry, cry with me, or get out and let me do it on my own." They cried together and worked through the loss of his mother. They have had to readjust to spending time together now that they do not have his mother to care for.

Just before this appointment, she had a difficult dental appointment. She had been given an injection to numb her but felt pain anyway as the dentist was working. He became angry and shouted at her, "You couldn't possibly be feeling pain." His shouting was so inappropriate that three waiting patients left the office, choosing to get their care elsewhere. She heard that message as, "Your pain is all in your head—you are making it up." When she attempted to leave in the middle of the visit, he held her in the chair and demanded to finish the procedure. She did not have the assertiveness necessary to get up and leave.

For the next week, she tried to fight the anxiety this stirred up for her. Her pelvic pain on the right came back. Again, she made many phone calls to us. This time, she decided to increase her sertraline to 75 mg and found within a matter of days that she felt better and was sleeping better. Soon thereafter, however, she began to have palpitations and a generalized sense of panic. She reduced her sertraline to 50 mg, but the panic symptoms remained.

With reluctance, she has again accepted the suggestion that she seek psychotherapy, no longer for pain management but for grief work and rehabilitation. She summarized her ongoing rehabilitative process with this remark:

> *You know, when I was sick I felt sure that if I could just get rid of the pain, I would jump back in and start doing everything the way I used to. Now, someone asks me to go to dinner tonight and I say, "tomorrow," even if tonight is just fine—just so I can maintain control. I don't want to commit to anything because for 4 years I couldn't do anything and had no control over it. Now I don't want to say "yes" for fear I will lose control in the other direction. . . . I realize that before I had pain I didn't have control either. I didn't know how to say no to anyone. This is like starting from scratch at the age of 40. I don't know who I am anymore or how to be. . . . In physical therapy, I had to hurt to get better so . . . I guess this (counseling) is another journey.*

After two or three visits in therapy, K.B. had a sudden onset of severe left lower quadrant pain. Ultrasound examination revealed a small hemorrhagic corpus luteum cyst. After consultation, she chose to watch and wait this out just with small doses of propoxyphene (Darvocet-N 100) to help with the pain. Unfortunately, her distress over having pain again resulted in significant muscle spasm, this time on the left side. Her irritable bowel syndrome flared, and her anxiety soared. For the next 5 months, she endured tenderness over the left ovary, intermittent problems with night sweats, and levator spasm. Repeated ultrasound examinations showed small cysts on the left ovary. K.B. was offered either birth control pills or Depo-Provera to suppress her ovarian function. After nearly a month of deliberation, she opted for surgical removal of her remaining ovary. She had had trouble tolerating oral contraceptives in the past and was concerned about further depressive symptoms with hormonal manipulation. Nineteen months after her LAVH/RSO, K.B. underwent laparoscopic left salpingo-oophorectomy. The pathology report revealed several cysts and surface adhesions. No endometriosis was seen at the time of surgery or found on the pathology report.

After the operation, K.B. had an initial struggle adjusting to hormone replacement and some muscle spasm. Two months postoperatively, however, she called in to say that she had no pain at all. She had begun to develop difficulties sleeping and was feeling jittery, however. She felt she was doing very well and could not understand why this was happening now. We decided to taper her off the sertraline. She took 3 weeks to eliminate her minimal dose of 50 mg every morning. She found it difficult to reduce the dose, experiencing heart palpitations, jitters, fluid retention, and weakness. A visit to her local internist was reassuring, and 1 week later, she felt much better. She called the office to say

> *I'm doing so much better. I can concentrate the way I used to before this all started. Remember when I told you I could feel the rug under my feet after my hysterectomy. I feel it even more now. . . . I'm going back to counseling again. Without pain, I think I need to work more on some of the losses I have suffered. I can do it now—I have the strength. . . . My next goal is to quit smoking.*

Our work with K.B. has been rewarding. Although she continues to have some problems, she is no longer a chronic pain patient. She has demonstrated a willingness to take an active role in her own care, responding to interventions with new insight, goal setting, and diligent work toward reaching those goals. She has continued her PT exercises at home throughout the 3 years she has been our patient. K.B. recognizes when she starts to tighten up, gets more anxious, has trouble sleeping, and so on, and she takes appropriate steps to explore the potential causes. While she was in pain, she was very fearful of discussing her negative life experiences, such as her abusive upbringing, alcoholism, and pregnancy loss, for fear that providers would decide that these things caused her pain. When she was given permission to have both pain *and* negative experiences, she was able to work simultaneously on all the contributing factors.

It is important, when working with women with chronic pelvic pain, to explore the *meaning of the pain*, because the *meaning* influences the *impact* of the pain. For K.B., pain meant worsening endometriosis, which meant infertility and more surgery. Feeling the pain then stirred up memories of losses (the forced abortion, the miscarriage) and fear of more losses (i.e., never having her own child). The resultant anxiety contributed to the musculoskeletal components of her pain problem. It is a rare event indeed to find chronic pelvic pain with a single cause and a single cure.

References

1. Beck AT, Ward CH, Mendelson M, et al: An inventory for measuring depression. Arch Gen Psychiatry 1961;4:53.
2. Derogatis LR: SCL-90-R: Administration and Scoring and Procedures Manual—II. Baltimore, Clinical Psychometric Research, 1992.
3. Derogatis LR, Rickels K, Rock A: The SCL-90 and the MMPI: A step in the validation of a new self-report scale. Br J Psychiatry 1976;128:280.
4. Melzack R, Katz J, Jeans ME: The role of compensation in chronic pain: Analysis using a new method of scoring the McGill Pain Questionnaire. Pain 1985;23:101.

5

Basic Pelvic Neuroanatomy

Robert M. Rogers, Jr., M.D.

Chronic pelvic pain (CPP) is a lifestyle-altering, subjective state of the unfortunate patients with this diagnosis. This subjective sensation is the result of complex, poorly understood physiologic interactions among noxious stimuli—clinically explained or idiopathic—in the body wall, skeletal muscles, or viscera; chronic dysfunction within the somatic or visceral nervous systems, both central and peripheral; and inner psychologic and external relationship stress factors.[1] Furthermore, these many confusing interactions are in a dynamic state manifested clinically by different presentations at successive office visits in the same patient. Anatomically, pain instigated by the deeper visceral contents of the abdomen or pelvis characteristically is poorly or even deceptively localized, thus further impeding an accurate and readily treatable diagnosis.[2] The era of telling a patient that her CPP is in her mind has quietly but surely passed away.

This textbook details the personal, physical, psychologic, and financial toll taken by CPP, as well as the varied interpersonal, family, social, and work-related ramifications. This chapter explores the many anatomic and physiologic issues that practitioners must appreciate to understand, diagnose, and treat those women afflicted and tormented by CPP. The information contained here is based mostly on animal research, especially in rats, cats, and monkeys, extrapolated to humans and merged with the relatively few clinical observations and studies performed on humans. Furthermore, the vast majority of this research details findings and theories of *acute* pelvic pain that have been crudely applied to *chronic* pelvic pain in women. Alas, therefore, we all make tremendous assumptions in our present understanding of the neuroanatomy and neurophysiology of *chronic* pelvic pain.

To complicate our understanding of this subject further, each patient has her own unique variations of anatomy and physiology that make her individual symptoms, signs, diagnosis, and treatment slightly or even greatly different from those of other patients with similar complaints. For instance, two young nulliparous women with laparoscopically proven mild endometriosis of the cul-de-sac may present with totally different complaints of pelvic pain. One of these patients may complain of only moderate dysmenorrhea, but the other may complain of only premenstrual dyspareunia. We as clinicians must readily admit our lack of understanding about many of the anatomic issues presented here.

CPP is believed to be visceral or referred to body wall dermatomes. However, CPP in some patients may be due to somatic trigger points within the abdominal wall, pelvic or perineal skeletal musculature, or perivaginal tissues.[3] Such trigger points are completely unrelated to any noxious stimuli from the pelvic viscera. Other more commonly recognized causes of CPP include irritable bowel syndrome, chronic constipation, dysmenorrhea, endometriosis, chronic pelvic infection, urethral syndrome, detrusor instability, and interstitial cystitis. In addition, many patients have coexisting psychologic diagnoses.[4]

True visceral pain is characteristically deep, diffuse, dull, and associated with visceral reflex responses such as nausea, anxiety, tachycardia, and diaphoresis. *Referred visceral pain* is the process by which visceral pain is somewhat localized to the skin and subcutaneous segment innervated by the afferent (sensory) fibers of one spinal nerve. This cutaneous sensory distribution defines a dermatome. The present concept to explain referred visceral pain is *viscerosomatic convergence* at the level of the dorsal horn of the spinal cord.[5] Although this concept is valid for acute visceral pain, some researchers question its validity in chronic pain situations. Dermatomes greatly overlap and interact with adjacent dermatomes; they are not discrete zones. In addition, each dermatome has sensory contributions from as many as four other spinal nerves. Furthermore, as always, individual patients demonstrate significant variations in the sensory distribution of their spinal nerves.[6]

Clinicians interested in understanding pelvic pain must understand the anatomic courses of the sensory nerves to somatic muscles and tissues as well as to the deeper abdominal and pelvic viscera. In addition, clinicians must understand how these nerves may interact physiologically.

General Considerations of the Somatic and Visceral Nervous Systems

Two different nervous systems innervate the female pelvis. One is the somatic nervous system; the other is the visceral nervous system (see Suggested Readings for more information).

Somatic Nervous System

The somatic nervous system has an efferent (motor) division and an afferent (sensory) division. The somatic *efferent* system innervates the skeletal muscles in the body wall and extremities, including the musculature of the pelvic walls and floor and the perineum. The somatic *afferent* system transmits the exteroceptive and proprioceptive sensations from the structures in the body wall and extremities, the pelvic walls and floor, and the perineum to the spinal cord. This also includes important exteroceptive sensory input from the *parietal* peritoneum lining the abdominal and pelvic cavities.

The exteroceptive sensations are elicited by mechanical, thermal, or chemical noxious stimuli from the skin, subcutaneous tissues, skeletal muscles, and parietal peritoneum. The somatic afferent nerves of the *parietal* peritoneum also supply their corresponding segmental areas of skin and subcutaneous tissues (dermatomes) and muscles (myotomes). Thus, when the *parietal* peritoneum is irritated, the corresponding dermatome feels painful (symptom) and tenderness can be elicited (sign). The corresponding myotome, which is spatially located away from the corresponding dermatome owing to embryologic migration, is reflexly contracted, causing rigidity or guarding of the abdominal wall (sign). Proprioceptive sensations originate from the ligaments, tendons, muscles, and joint capsules to give the individual a sense of position of the joints and related limbs and appendages.

Visceral Nervous System

The visceral nervous system consists of the visceral *efferent* system, which is also known as the *autonomic nervous system*, and the visceral *afferent* system, which transmits noxious stimuli and other interoceptive sensations from the abdominal and pelvic viscera, including their covering visceral peritoneum. The viscera and *visceral* peritoneum produce painful sensations when stretched, overdistended, or ischemic or when their visceral muscles are in spasm. The autonomic nervous system is the motor system of the visceral smooth muscles and glands and consists of the sympathetic and parasympathetic divisions. The sympathetic division is further divided into α- and β-adrenergic receptors. The visceral nervous system in females is involved with the pelvic viscera—namely, the urethra, bladder, ureters, vagina, cervix, uterus, tubes, ovaries, sigmoid colon, rectum, and anal canal, as well as their supplying vasculature and *visceral* peritoneum. In addition, the sympathetic nervous system, but not the parasympathetic, provides innervation to the smooth muscles of the arteries and arterioles and to the veins and venules in the pelvic basin and perineal musculature, as well as to the sweat glands, arrector pili muscles, and vasculature in the body wall and extremities.

Muscular Pelvic Basin

The *muscular pelvic basin* (Fig. 5–1) is composed of skeletal muscles forming two sidewalls, a back wall, and the floor.[7] The front wall is simply the back of the pubic bone. Each sidewall is formed by the obturator internus muscle on that side. The back wall is formed by the sacrum centrally and the two piriformis muscles laterally. Lying on each piriformis muscle is the sacral plexus of nerves (somatic). The floor is formed by the almost horizontal arrangement of the levator ani muscles and the coccygeus muscles. These muscles are covered by a continuous parietal fascia that is derived from the transversalis fascia. All visceral arteries and veins, lymph channels and nodes, and visceral nerves travel within a network of sheaths of endopelvic (visceral) fascia found between the parietal peritoneum and the parietal fascia of the muscular pelvic basin.

Each psoas muscle travels over the arcuate line of the ilium at the base of the iliac fossa and is not part of the pelvic basin. The perineal musculature consists of voluntary muscles that span the space between the ischiopubic rami. These muscles are involved in urethral function and urinary continence; support to the anus, lower one third of the vagina, and perineal body; and sexual responses.

Spinal Cord and Nerves

Observation of the cross section of the spinal cord (Fig. 5–2) discloses white matter and gray matter. The white matter simply represents the tracks of dendrites and axons (peripheral processes) that travel up and down the spinal cord. Dendrites carry nerve impulses toward the cell body. Axons carry nerve impulses away from the cell body. The gray matter represents the collection of cell bodies of these neurons. The configuration of the butterfly gray matter in the spinal cord is such that the dorsal, or posterior,

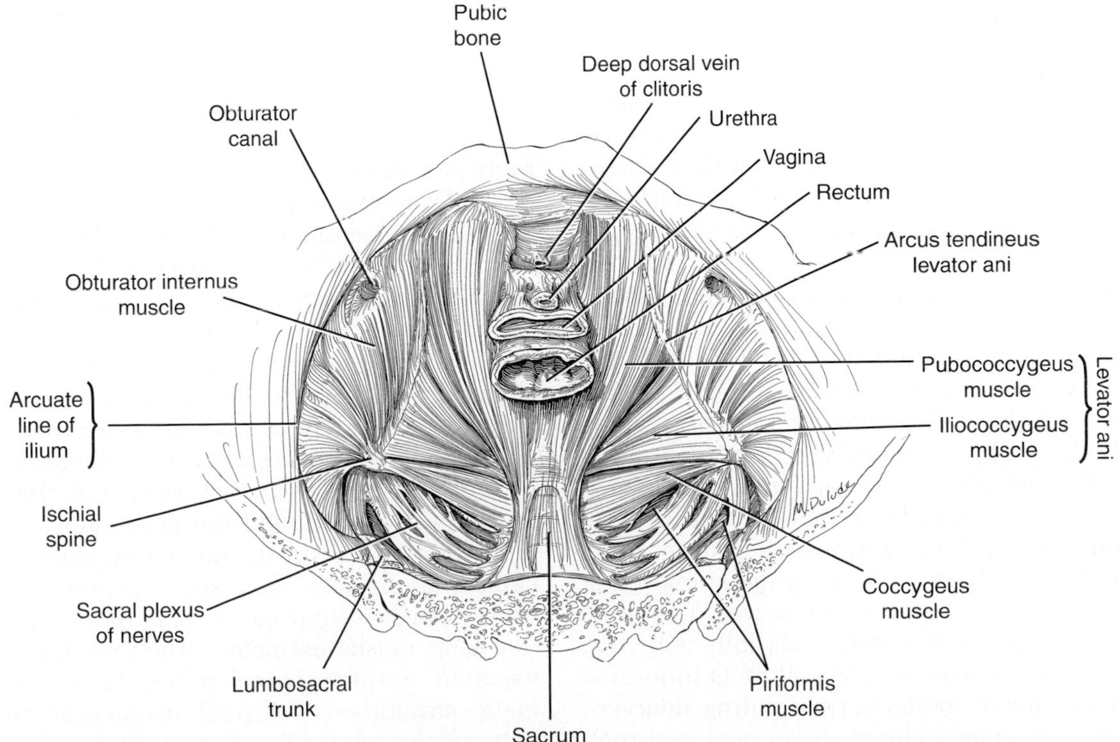

Figure 5–1. The muscular pelvic basin.

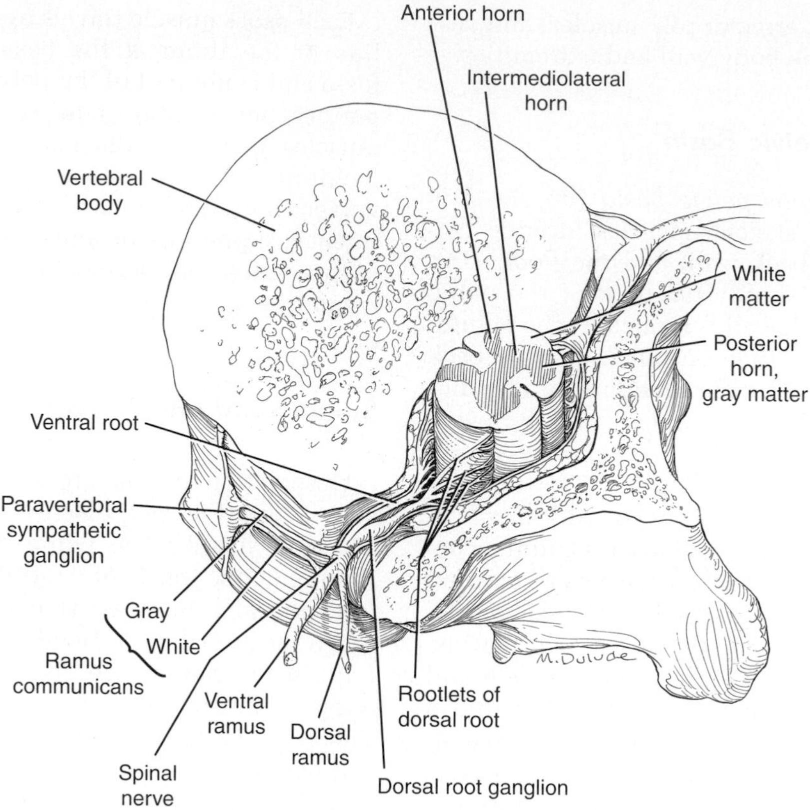

Figure 5–2. Spinal cord and spinal nerve.

horn represents cell bodies that receive the afferent fibers and their impulses from *both* the visceral and the somatosensory nervous systems. The ventral, or anterior, horn is the location of the motor neurons of the somatic nervous system. The intermediolateral horn of the gray matter contains the cell bodies of the autonomic nervous system (efferent or motor visceral nervous system). From T1 to L2, these latter represent sympathetic cell bodies. In the intermediolateral cell column of the spinal cord from S2 through S4 are located the cell bodies for the parasympathetic system of the pelvis.

The peripheral processes from these many cell bodies from both somatic and visceral nervous systems form rootlets and then roots, which emanate from the spinal cord to join and form the spinal nerves. The anterior or motor (ventral) roots join with the posterior or sensory (dorsal) roots to form a spinal nerve in the corresponding intervertebral foramen. The posterior or dorsal root ganglion contains cell bodies from the peripheral afferent (sensory) nerves, *both* somatic and visceral. Because these cells have only one peripheral process, they are named *unipolar neurons.* Immediately after the two roots join to form a spinal nerve, a posterior or dorsal ramus is given off. The dorsal ramus innervates the musculature, subcutaneous areas, and skin of the back and accompanying vasculature for that particular nerve segment or dermatome.

The anterior or ventral rami innervate the skeletal musculature, subcutaneous areas and skin of the lateral and anterior aspects of the body wall and extremities; the skeletal muscles that form the walls and floor of the pelvic basin; and the perineum. The *dermatomes* are those transverse sensory bands on the skin that share innervation from a single spinal nerve. *Sclerotomes* are the deep musculoskeletal structures innervated by a single spinal nerve. "Deep somatic structures refer pain in sclerotomic patterns that are similar, but not identical, to dermatomes. The spinal segment supplying innervation to painful sites should be identified in the clinical evaluation of pain patterns, and all musculoskeletal, visceral, and superficial structures receiving innervation from that same segment should be considered as possible sources of referred pain."[8]

Also, immediately after each spinal nerve is formed, all the sympathetic nerves leave the spinal nerve via the white ramus communicans to join the sympathetic ganglion that is located just lateral to each vertebra. White rami communicantes are found only from the spinal nerves T1 to L2. Some synapses are formed here. From the sympathetic ganglion, sympathetic fibers have only two choices—either rejoin a spinal nerve to travel to the body wall or an extremity *or* form a *splanchnic nerve* to innervate abdominal or pelvic viscera and their corresponding visceral vasculature (Fig. 5–3).

Concerning *sympathetic innervation to the body wall and extremities,* the preganglionic fibers synapse in a paravertebral sympathetic ganglion, and the postganglionic fibers reach the spinal nerve through the gray ramus communicans. In addition to a direct synapse in the sympathetic ganglion, the preganglionic fibers (from the intermediolateral horn of the gray matter) may also travel up or down the anastomosing connections between the sympathetic chain ganglia and synapse at a higher or lower level. These postganglionic fibers then join the corresponding spinal nerve via the gray ramus communicans. Gray rami communi-

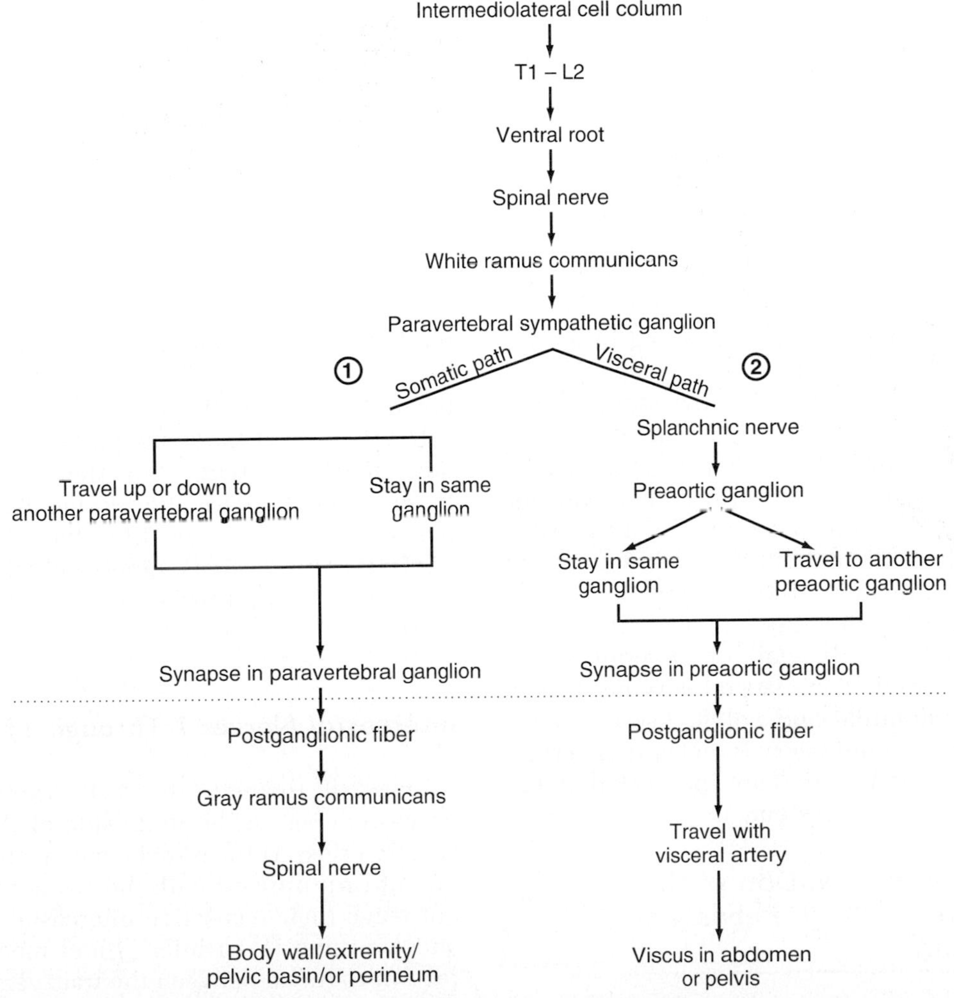

Figure 5–3. Sympathetic fibers have only two choices, to go to the body wall/extremity or to the viscus in the abdomen/pelvis.

cantes connect paravertebral sympathetic ganglia to all spinal nerves, including the lower lumbar and sacral, which descend into the pelvic area.

The postganglionic sympathetic nerves then travel with a spinal nerve to innervate the smooth muscle surrounding the parietal vasculature of the body wall and extremities, muscular basin of the pelvis, perineum, and sweat glands and arrector pili of the skin. The preganglionic fibers use acetylcholine as a neurotransmitter, whereas the postganglionic fibers give off norepinephrine, except for the postganglionic fibers of the sweat glands, which give off acetylcholine. In the sympathetic nervous system, the synapse of the preganglionic and postganglionic fibers is anatomically far away from the viscus to be innervated.

Any *spinal nerve*, whether it services the body wall, an extremity, the pelvis, or perineum, contains the following nervous system elements: (1) general somatic afferent (sensory) fibers for exteroceptive and proprioceptive sensation; (2) general somatic efferent (motor) fibers for innervation of skeletal muscles, including those in the pelvis and perineum; (3) general visceral afferent (sensory) fibers from parietal blood vessels in the body wall or extremity, muscular pelvic basin, or perineum, traveling backward along the same routes as the postganglionic sympathetic fibers from the sympathetic chain of ganglia; and (4) general visceral efferent (motor) fibers from the sympathetic nervous system to the parietal blood vessels, sweat glands and arrector pili muscles of the body wall, extremities, perineum, and skeletal muscles of the pelvic basin. No parasympathetic innervation of any structures in the body wall or extremities has been reported. The visceral nervous system of the abdominal and pelvic viscera travels via the splanchnic nerves, not spinal nerves. Visceral blood vessels are innervated by the visceral nervous system.

Somatic Innervation of the Abdominal Wall, Pelvis, and Perineum

The anterior abdominal wall is recognized today as an important site of CPP.[3, 9] The concept of trigger points in the skin, subcutaneous tissues, ligaments, or bone and myofascial trigger points in or around skeletal muscle is poorly understood, but these are becoming more commonly identified as causes of abdominopelvic pain. Trigger points have also been associated with the vaginal and sacral areas. This section traces the somatic innervation to the anterior abdominal wall, the muscles of the pelvic floor and walls, the perineum, and the lower extremities.

The somatic nerves that innervate the anterior and lateral abdominal wall down to the mons pubis are the 7th to 11th intercostal nerves (the anterior rami of spinal nerves T7 to T11), the subcostal nerve (T12), and the iliohypogastric and ilioinguinal nerves from the L1 branch of the lumbar plexus (Fig. 5–4). These all are ventral or anterior rami of their respective spinal nerves. At each midaxillary line, a lateral cutaneous branch is given off. The lateral cutaneous branches of the subcostal and iliohypogastric nerves innervate the gluteal region posteriorly. An anterior cutaneous branch from each of these spinal nerves is given off near the midline. As a general guideline to cutaneous innervation, the nerve from T7 innervates a transverse anterior body wall strip at the level of the xiphoid process, the nerves from T10 innervate the strip that includes the umbilicus, and the nerves from L1 innervate the level of the mons pubis. A tremendous amount of sensory overlap is noted in these segmental dermatomes (Fig. 5–5). The dorsal or posterior rami from the T10, T11, and L1 spinal nerves innervate the lower lumbar region and the upper portion of the sacrum.

Intercostal Nerves 7 Through 11

The 7th through the 11th intercostal nerves course on the underside of their respective ribs. At the midclavicular line, they do not turn upward with the costocartilages but leave their respective intercostal spaces and continue in an inferior and medial direction to travel between the transversus abdominis muscle and the internal oblique muscle until they reach the lateral edge of

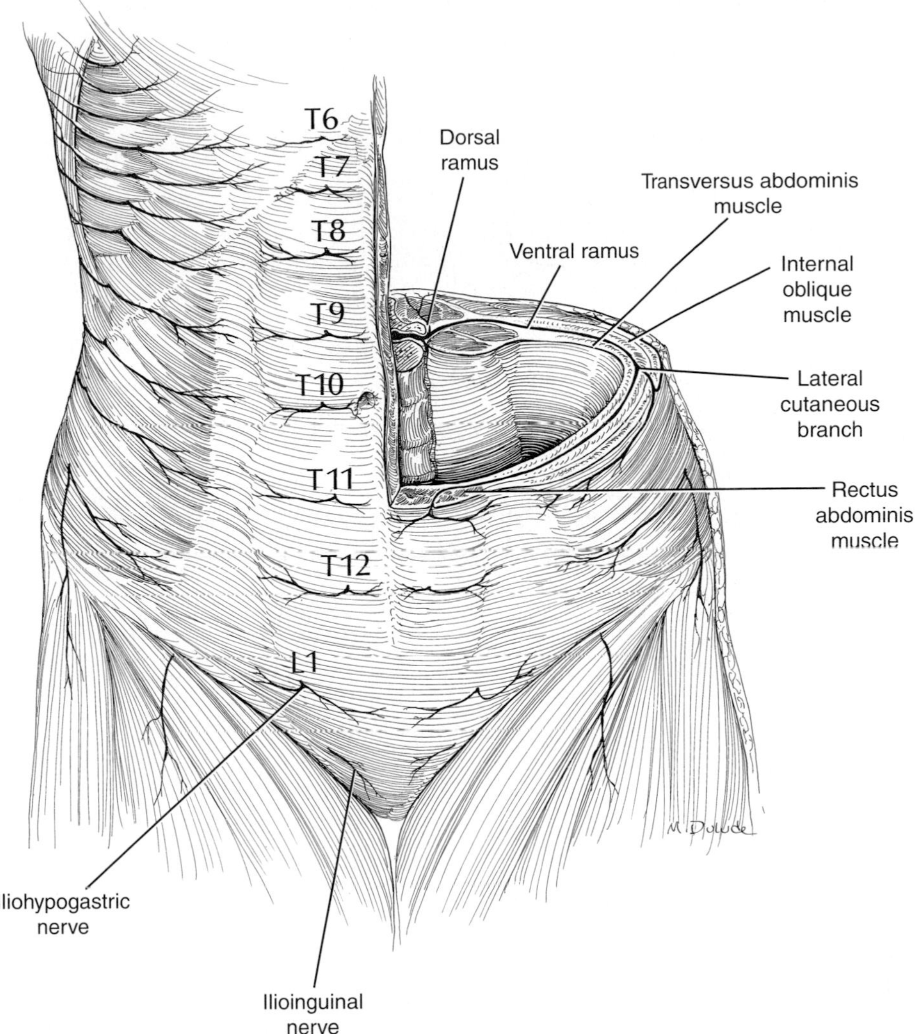

Figure 5–4. Somatic innervation of the abdominal wall.

the rectus abdominis muscle. Each nerve then traverses the posterior rectus sheath to course through the rectus muscle itself and pierce the anterior rectus sheath to branch as the anterior cutaneous nerves. Each of these anterior rami gives innervation to the abdominal muscles surrounding it (myotome), as well as to the dermatome segment.

Subcostal Nerve

The subcostal nerve (anterior ramus of T12) travels in the same layers in the same direction as the intercostal nerves but does so below the 12th rib. This nerve descends inferiorly and medially in the same manner as the intercostal nerves to innervate the cutaneous area just above the mons pubis.

Lumbar Plexus of Nerves

The lumbar plexus of nerves consists of the anterior rami of L1 to L4 and supplies somatic innervation to the lower abdominal wall and thighs. In addition, the lumbosacral trunk, from part of the anterior ramus of spinal nerve L4 and all of the anterior ramus of spinal nerve L5, feeds into the sacral plexus of nerves, found over the piriformis muscle in the pelvis. The lumbar plexus of nerves supplies motor innervation to the voluntary skeletal muscles in these

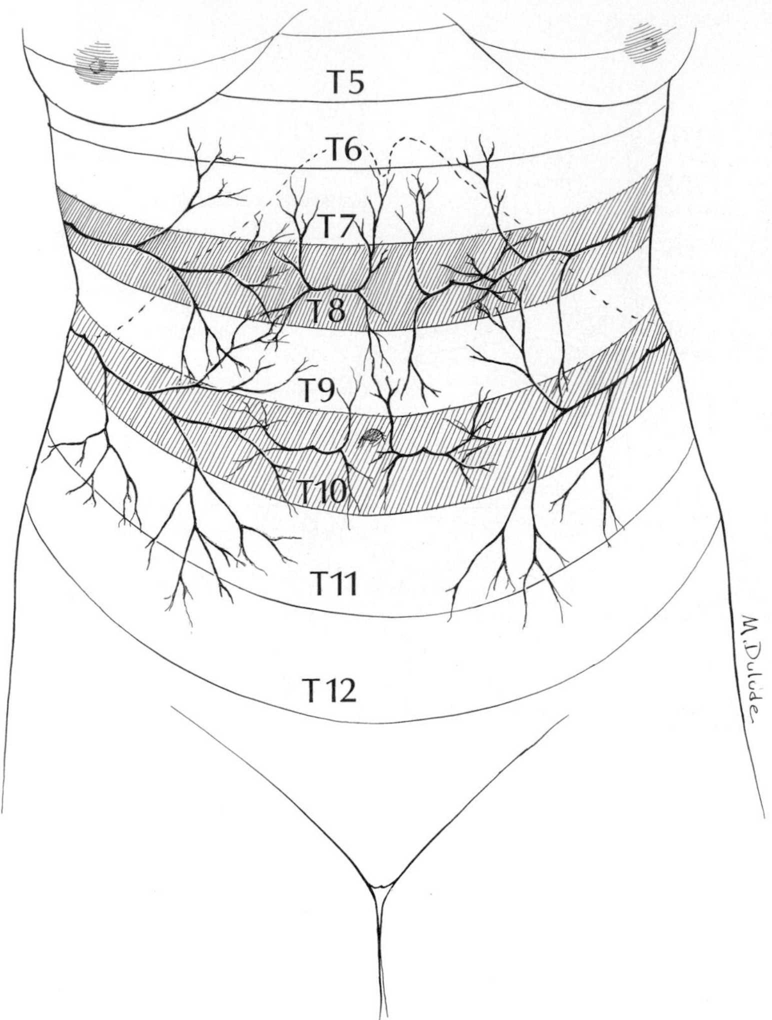

Figure 5–5. Anterior abdominal dermatomes.

areas, as well as sympathetic efferents to the vasculature smooth muscle surrounding the arteries, arterioles, veins, and venules in the muscles and skin of these areas. These nerves also supply sympathetic efferents to the arrector pili muscles and sweat glands in the cutaneous areas.

The nerves of the lumbar plexus (Fig. 5–6) are just anterior to the quadratus lumborum muscle in the posterior body wall but travel within or posterior to the psoas muscle. These nerves are the iliohypogastric, ilioinguinal, lateral femoral cutaneous, femoral, genitofemoral, and obturator.

The *iliohypogastric* and *ilioinguinal* nerves, both from L1, travel in parallel above the iliac crest, pierce the transversus abdominis muscle at different locations, and course between that muscle and the internal oblique muscle to the level of the anterior superior iliac spine. The *iliohypogastric* nerve pierces the internal oblique muscle approximately 2 to 3 cm *superior* to the spine and travels between the internal oblique and external oblique muscles. Approximately 2 to 3 cm superior to the superficial inguinal ring, the iliohypogastric nerve pierces the external oblique muscle to innervate the skin above the pubic bone in the area of the mons pubis. This nerve also innervates the surrounding musculature along its course. A lateral cutaneous branch travels to the posterolateral gluteal region.

The *ilioinguinal* nerve, traveling in the same muscle planes but just inferior to the course of the iliohypogastric nerve, continues between the transversus abdominis and internal oblique muscles. At approximately

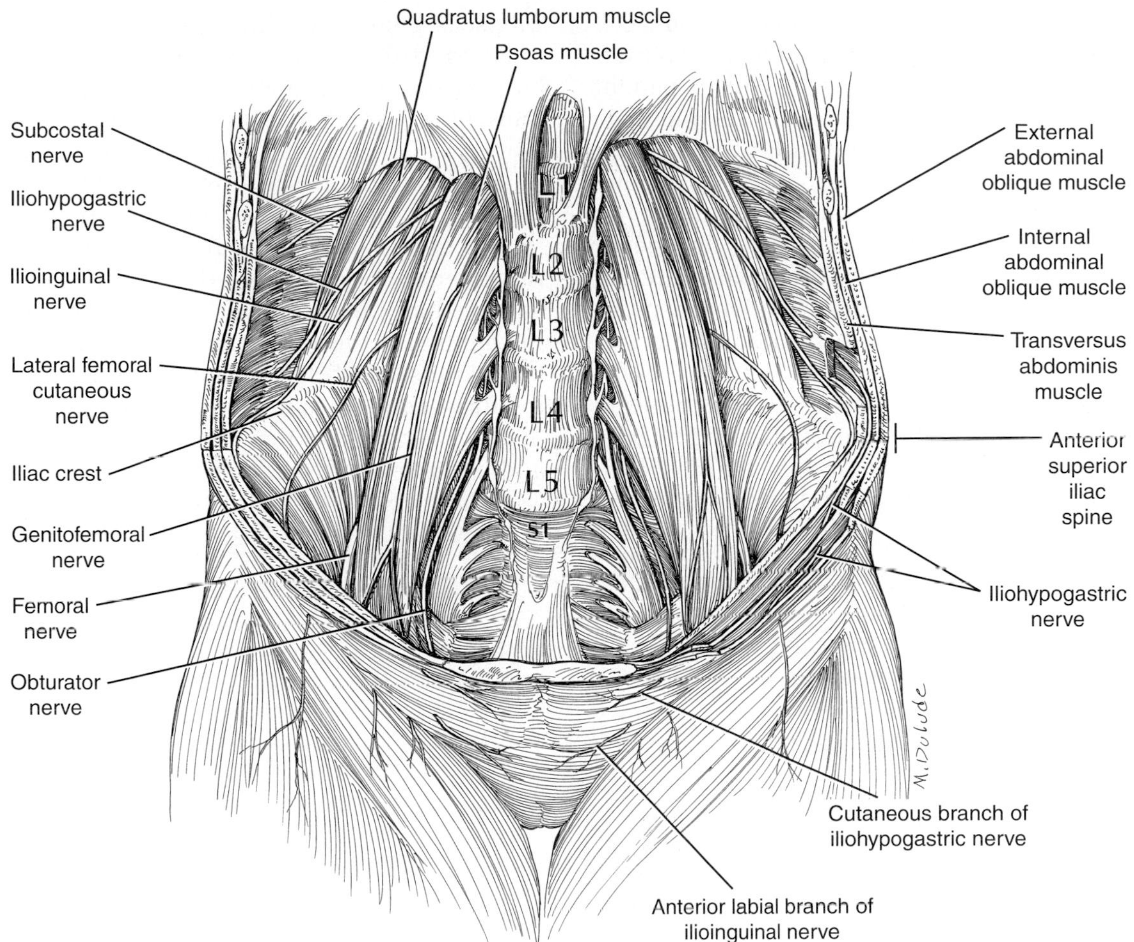

Figure 5–6. Lumbar plexus of nerves.

2 to 3 cm *medial* to the anterior superior iliac spine, this nerve pierces the internal oblique muscle to pass between that muscle and the external oblique muscle. It then enters and continues through the inguinal canal, exiting via the external inguinal ring approximately 2 cm lateral and superior to the pubic tubercle. The ilioinguinal nerve innervates the mons pubis and the anterior aspect of the labia majora, as well as a cutaneous area in the upper medial thigh area. It also innervates its surrounding musculature. There is no lateral branch.

Clinically, injury to the iliohypogastric and ilioinguinal nerves may occur in transverse incisions owing to excessive retraction during the surgical procedure, or it may occur during closure of the fascia as a result of suture entrapment of these nerves.[10] In addition, in placement of sutures for vaginal needle urethropexies, these nerves may also be entrapped by the suture in the anterior rectus fascia near the pubic tubercle.[11] Such injuries cause very sharp and constant pain in the area of cutaneous distribution.

The *lateral femoral cutaneous nerve* (see Fig. 5–6), from the anterior rami of L2 and L3, is purely a cutaneous innervating nerve. It courses behind the psoas muscle just anterior to the quadratus lumborum muscle and then travels laterally on top of the iliacus muscle to pass just underneath the inguinal ligament, approximately 1 cm medial to the anterior superior iliac spine. It passes anterior to the sartorius muscle and divides into branches. The lateral femoral cutaneous nerve innervates the lateral cutaneous region of the thigh from the buttocks, down the anterior and lateral thigh, to the knee. It also innervates the parietal peritoneum of the iliac fossa. This nerve may be damaged during positioning for gynecologic or obstetric procedures, particularly with a patient in the position of hip hyperflexion. Meralgia paresthetica is the condition of the lateral femoral cutaneous nerve that gives paresthesias to the lateral aspect of the thigh.

The *femoral nerve* (Fig. 5–7) is one of the largest nerves in the body and actually courses through the substance of the psoas muscle. This nerve is derived from branches of the anterior rami of L2, L3, and L4. It exits from the psoas muscle and appears on its lateral border approximately half-way between the iliac crest and the inguinal ligament. The femoral nerve then travels in the iliopsoas groove and innervates both these muscles. It then courses underneath the inguinal ligament, where it immediately separates into several muscular and cutaneous branches. The femoral nerve innervates the quadriceps femoris muscles, the sartorius muscle, and the pectineus muscle, in addition to giving extensive cutaneous innervation medially and anteriorly on the thigh and medially in the lower leg. Branches of the femoral nerve also innervate the hip and knee joints. In obstetrics, for example, during the second stage of labor, when a patient may be repeatedly hyperflexed at the hip and hyperflexed at the knee for pushing, the attendant must be careful that the femoral

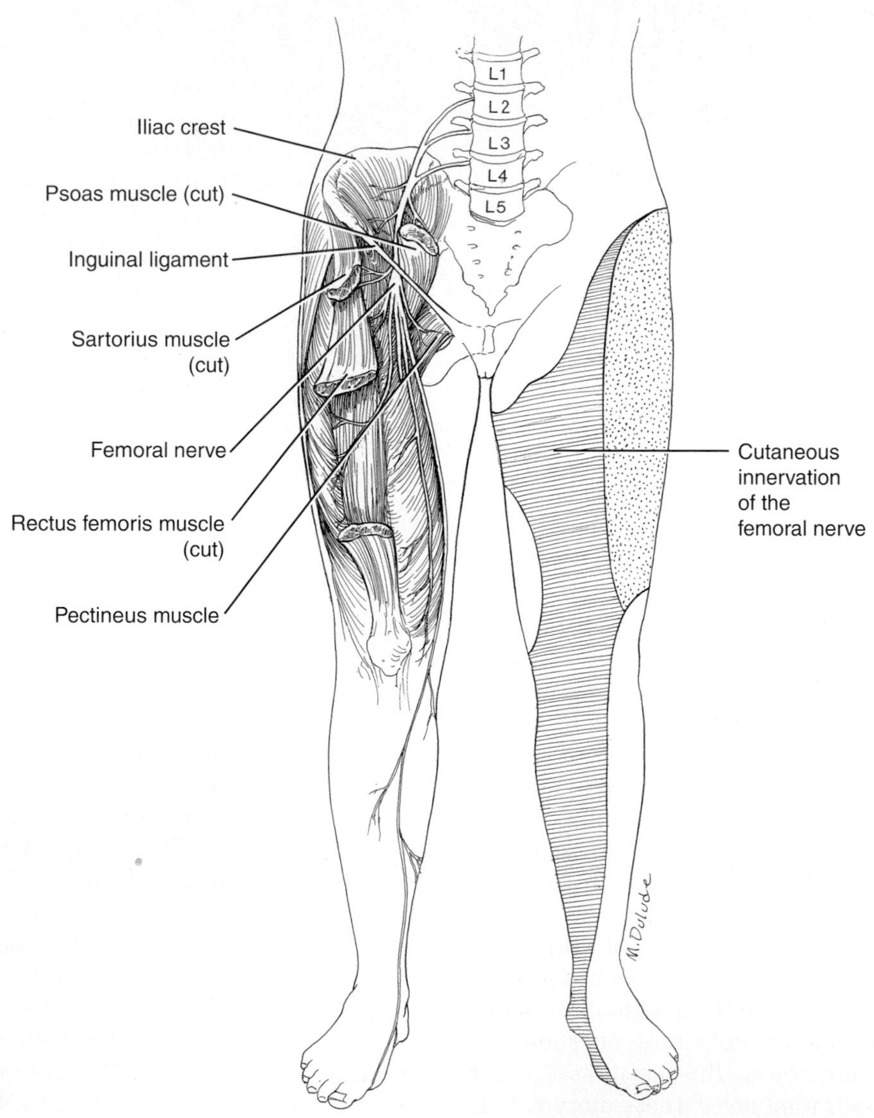

Figure 5–7. The femoral nerve.

nerve is not impinged under the inguinal ligament.[12] Such compression occurs primarily in primigravid patients with successful epidural anesthesia in place and with the second stage of labor lasting more than 2 hours.

The femoral nerve is a rather large nerve with, unfortunately, a relatively poor blood supply. Therefore, the femoral nerve is very susceptible to compression hypoxia. Also, this nerve is one of the first nerves affected by diabetic vasculopathies. Compression and relative hypoxia of this nerve can result from the previously mentioned hip hyperflexion during the second stage of labor, as well as deep lateral retraction in lower transverse abdominal incisions.[13] These lateral retractors should be placed so that the tips of the lateral blades are above the psoas muscle and not resting on it. Lateral pressure on the psoas muscle squeezes the femoral nerve between the psoas muscle and the iliacus muscle, which lies on the bony backstop of the iliac fossa. Retroperitoneal and psoas muscle hematomas and abscesses can also cause such pressure. Femoral nerve injury is manifested by numbness or paresthesias of the anterior and medial aspect of the thigh and medial aspect of the lower leg. Pain and discomfort may be felt in the hip and knee areas. Also, a patient has trouble extending her lower leg and may experience instability of her knee and hip when walking.

The signs are numbness in the cutaneous areas mentioned earlier, a very poor patellar reflex, and a patient's inability to voluntarily raise her lower leg in a straight manner. Injury of the femoral nerve within the pelvis itself also decreases the power of hip flexion owing to compromise of the innervation to the psoas and iliacus muscles. This of course depends on where the injury occurred and at what level on the nerve.

The *genitofemoral nerve* (see Fig. 5–6) from L1 and L2 gives cutaneous innervation only to the upper anterior aspect of the thigh from its femoral branch and to a portion of the mons pubis from its genital branch. The genitofemoral nerve courses on the anterior surface of the psoas muscle and may be damaged or compressed during lateral retraction in a transverse gynecologic incision or injured during the harvesting of external iliac lymph nodes.

This nerve travels through the substance of the psoas muscle and then appears on the anterior surface of that muscle above the iliac crest. It may branch anywhere along its course. The genital branch courses through the inguinal canal, whereas the femoral branch travels lateral to the external iliac artery and underneath the inguinal ligament.

The *obturator nerve* (Fig. 5–8), like the femoral nerve, is derived from the anterior rami of L2, L3, and L4. It travels within the substance of the psoas muscle and exits that muscle on its medial aspect, appearing in the pelvis underneath the iliac vessels just superficial to the sacroiliac joint at the pelvic brim. The *lumbosacral trunk* is found in the same plane just medial to this area. The obturator nerve then passes underneath the arcuate line of the ilium (linea terminalis) on the anterior and superior border of the obturator internus muscle. This nerve then travels through the obturator notch along with the obturator artery and vein into the obturator canal to innervate the adductor muscles and a cutaneous area on the medial aspect of the thigh.

The obturator nerve along with the obturator vasculature is contained within a loose, fatty endopelvic fascial sheath that easily is bluntly dissected away to reveal the obturator nerve, vein, and artery, all traveling together. The obturator nerve may be damaged by surgical transection during pelvic lymph node dissection or by a deep pelvic retractor placed below the level of the arcuate line of the ilium. Such injuries may occur during surgery in either the obturator space of the pelvis or in the space of Retzius, via either laparotomy or laparoscopy.

Injury to the obturator nerve may lead to weakness in adductor function of the thigh. A patient may develop a wide-based gait owing to the inability to pull her leg medially while walking. Also, she may have instability of her hip and knee because fibers from this nerve are found coursing to these areas. If the nerve supply is compressed, not cut, these injuries can be self-limited, and fortunately they are rare.

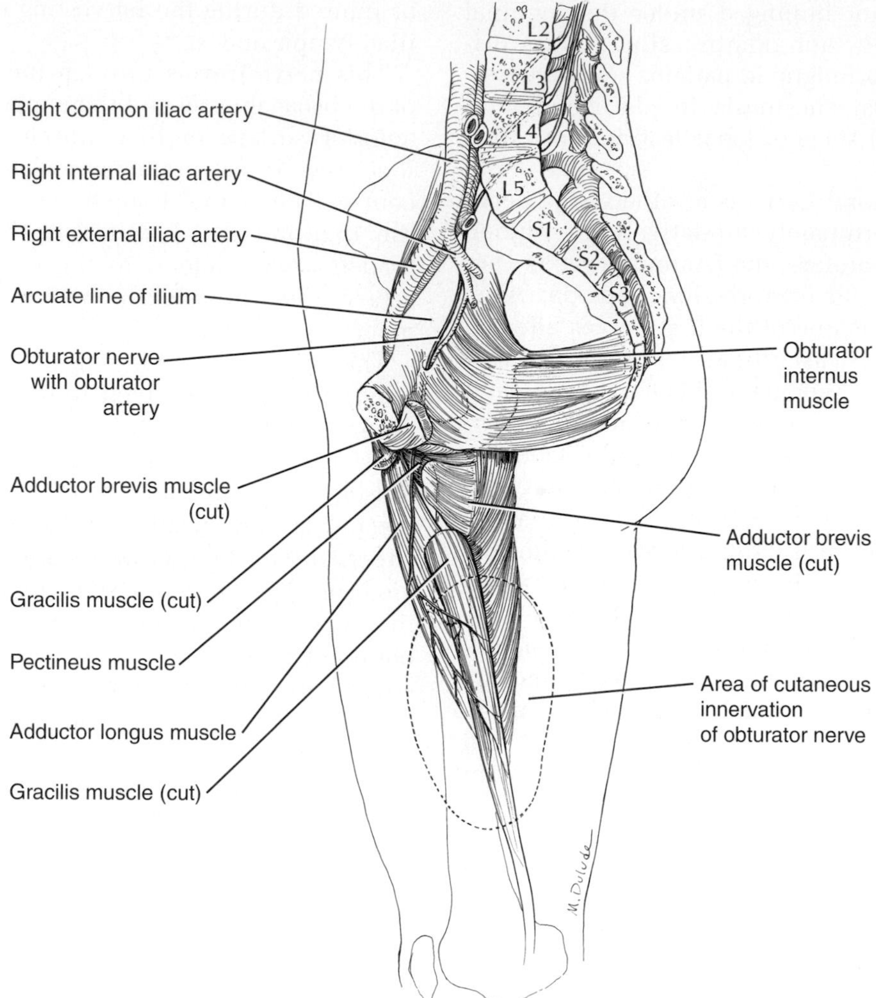

Figure 5–8. The obturator nerve.

Sacral Plexus of Nerves

Each sacral plexus of nerves (Fig. 5–9) is a substantial junction of many somatic nerves on top of each piriformis muscle in the pelvis. This plexus is formed from the lumbosacral trunk, L4 and L5, of the lumbar plexus and the anterior rami of S1 through S4, which course into the pelvis through the anterior sacral foramina. It is encased in its own envelope of parietal fascia and is adjacent to the posterior edge of the coccygeus muscle and sacrospinous ligament complex. Because many major and important nerves originate from the sacral plexus, a surgeon should not put any sutures or instruments above or posterior to the sacrospinous ligament during any surgical procedure. Injury to this plexus of nerves may cause severe, prolonged gluteal or lower extremity pain or loss of function.

The *sacral plexus of nerves innervates the following muscles*: levator ani, obturator internus, coccygeus, piriformis, gemelli, and quadratus femoris. All these voluntary skeletal muscles are innervated directly from branches of the sacral plexus.

The sacral plexus of nerves also gives off the *superior and inferior gluteal nerves*, which innervate the gluteal muscles. These nerves are so named because they travel either superior or inferior to the piriformis muscle when leaving the pelvis. The superior gluteal nerve innervates the gluteus medius, the gluteus minimus, and the tensor fasciae latae muscles. The inferior gluteal

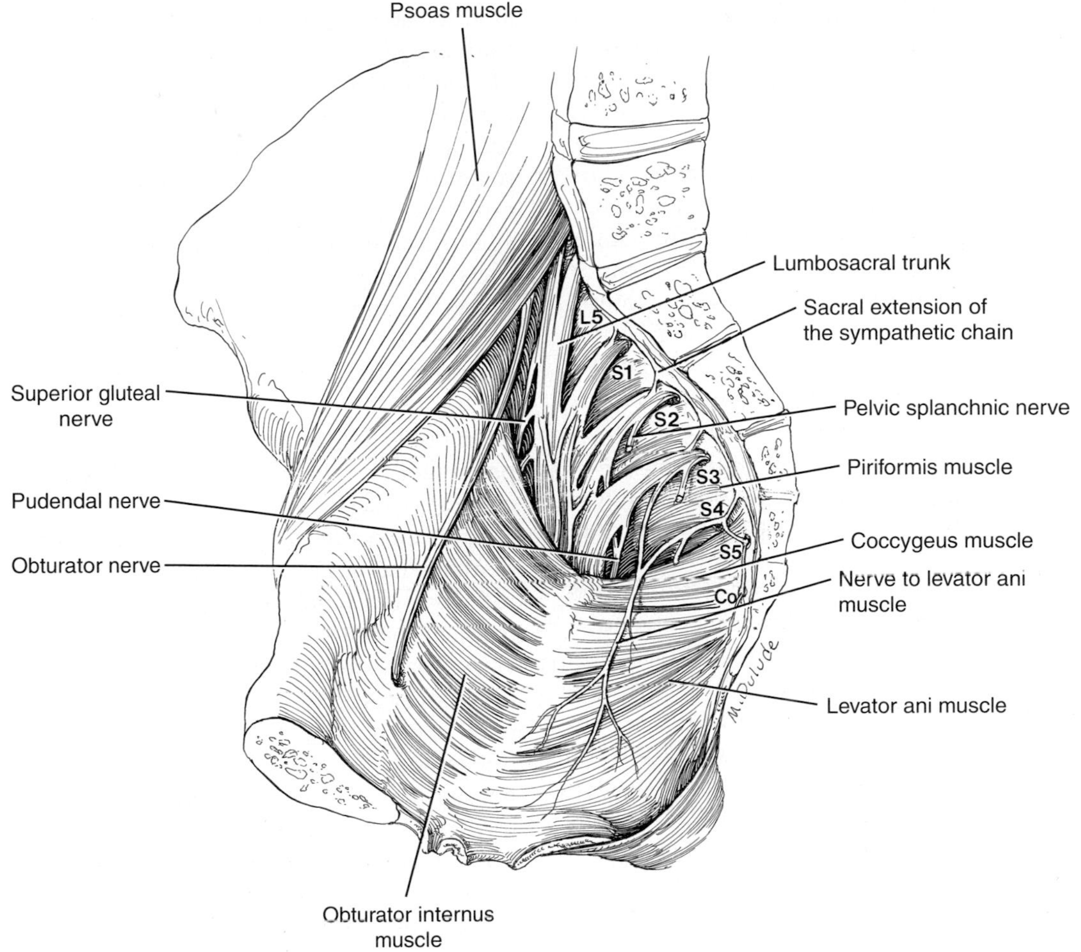

Figure 5–9. The sacral plexus of nerves.

nerve services the gluteus maximus muscle. In addition, the sacral plexus of nerves gives off the *pudendal nerve*, the *posterior femoral cutaneous nerve*, and a *branch from the fourth sacral nerve*, which innervates the posterior aspect of the external anal sphincter muscle.

The sacral plexus is also the origin of the *sciatic nerve*, which is actually a combination of the *tibial nerve* and the *common peroneal nerve*. The sciatic nerve, from the anterior rami of L4, L5, S1, S2, and S3, is by far the largest nerve in the body. It courses through the gluteal region. This nerve appears on the inferior border of the piriformis muscle, just posterior to the obturator internus muscle tendon. This area is several centimeters lateral to the ischial spine, between the spine and the greater trochanter of the femur. This is well away from the sacrospinous ligament, which courses medially from the ischial spine to the lower sacrum. The sciatic nerve has limited stretchability in the gluteal region. It is important to be careful that a patient is not hyperflexed at the hip. Not only can the femoral nerve be compressed under the inguinal ligament, but the sciatic nerve can also be relatively compressed in stretching. This stretching can actually injure some of the nerve fibers and even compromise crucial blood supply to this large nerve.

Stretching the sciatic nerve is usually manifested as a peroneal nerve injury, particularly footdrop. For reasons that are not well understood, the peroneal nerve is more sensitive than the tibial nerve to such injury. Footdrop is manifested by numbness in the lateral aspect of the lower leg, weakness in dorsiflexion and eversion of the foot, and the inability to extend the toes. The tibial nerve component of the sciatic nerve mainly gives muscular innervation to the hamstring muscles of the back of the thigh and gastrocnemius muscles.

The peroneal nerve gives cutaneous innervation to the lateral aspect of the lower leg and innervates the muscles of the lateral compartment of the lower leg. The *common peroneal nerve* courses across the lateral head of the fibula to enter the anterior surface of the leg. During vaginal or laparoscopic procedures with a patient in the dorsolithotomy position, an assistant can inadvertently lean against the patient's leg and compress the common peroneal nerve against the fibula, causing a footdrop problem.

The cutaneous innervation of the *posterior femoral cutaneous nerve*, from the anterior rami of S1, S2, and S3, primarily involves the lower posterior gluteal region down the back of the upper thigh to the skin behind the knee. It travels directly from the sacral plexus, inferior to the piriformis muscle, medial and posterior to the sciatic nerve, deep to the fascia lata. A perineal branch innervates a portion of the perineum.

Another major nerve originating from the sacral plexus of nerves is the *pudendal nerve*. The pudendal nerve (Fig. 5–10) leaves the pelvis through the greater sciatic foramen and then immediately wraps behind the ischial spine (the origin of the sacrospinous ligament), thereby entering the perineal region through the lesser sciatic foramen. This nerve is accompanied by the internal pudendal artery and vein. This neurovascular complex is right behind the sacrospinous ligament, at times as much as 2 cm medial to the ischial spine. In addition to somatic efferent and afferent fibers, the pudendal nerve also contains sympathetic and parasympathetic efferents as well as visceral afferents. Remember that the anatomic definition of the perineum is those structures inferior to the pelvic diaphragm (consisting of the levator ani and coccygeus muscles), laterally to the sidewalls formed by the obturator internus muscles, and inferiorly down to the musculature and skin of the urogenital and anal triangles.

Once into the perineal area in the ischioanal fossa, the pudendal nerve travels in the pudendal (Alcock's) canal, which is a tunnel of fascia formed of parietal fascial layers from the obturator internus muscle and the sacrotuberous ligament. Continuous stretching and compression of the pudendal nerve rarely may be responsible for nerve and tissue injury, edema, and scarring in or around the pudendal canal. Such injury may compress the pudendal nerve and compromise pudendal nerve function or cause chronic pain sensations from this area. This pudendal canal syndrome may result when a patient consistently strains at stool, suffers a prolonged and difficult labor and delivery,[14] or receives a deep mediolateral episiotomy.

After entering the pudendal canal, the pudendal nerve gives rise to one or several inferior rectal nerves, which course across the ischioanal fossa within the fat pad toward the external anal sphincter. Some of these nerves may be cut during the performance of a large mediolateral episiotomy. Subsequent injury to and scarring of these nerves may result in decreased function of the external anal sphincter, as well as neuroma formation, which may cause chronic pain in this area. Clinical studies of the neurologic and functional effects of the various types of episiotomies are sorely needed.

The pudendal nerve also gives a branch to the underside of the levator ani muscles to assist in their innervation. In a standing woman, the pudendal nerve in the pudendal canal travels in an inferior and anterior oblique direction. As the pudendal nerve approaches the posterior edge of the perineal membrane, two branches are formed, one superficial and the other deep (Fig. 5–11). Superficially, the perineal nerve enters the superficial space of the urogenital triangle to innervate the musculature there, as well as the cutaneous areas medially and posteriorly via the posterior labial branches. As the perineal nerve enters the superficial space, it also gives off branches that pierce the perineal membrane to innervate the muscles of the deep perineal compartment. More deeply, the dorsal nerve of the clitoris enters the deep space of the urogenital triangle at the posterior edge of the perineal membrane and courses in the deep space in

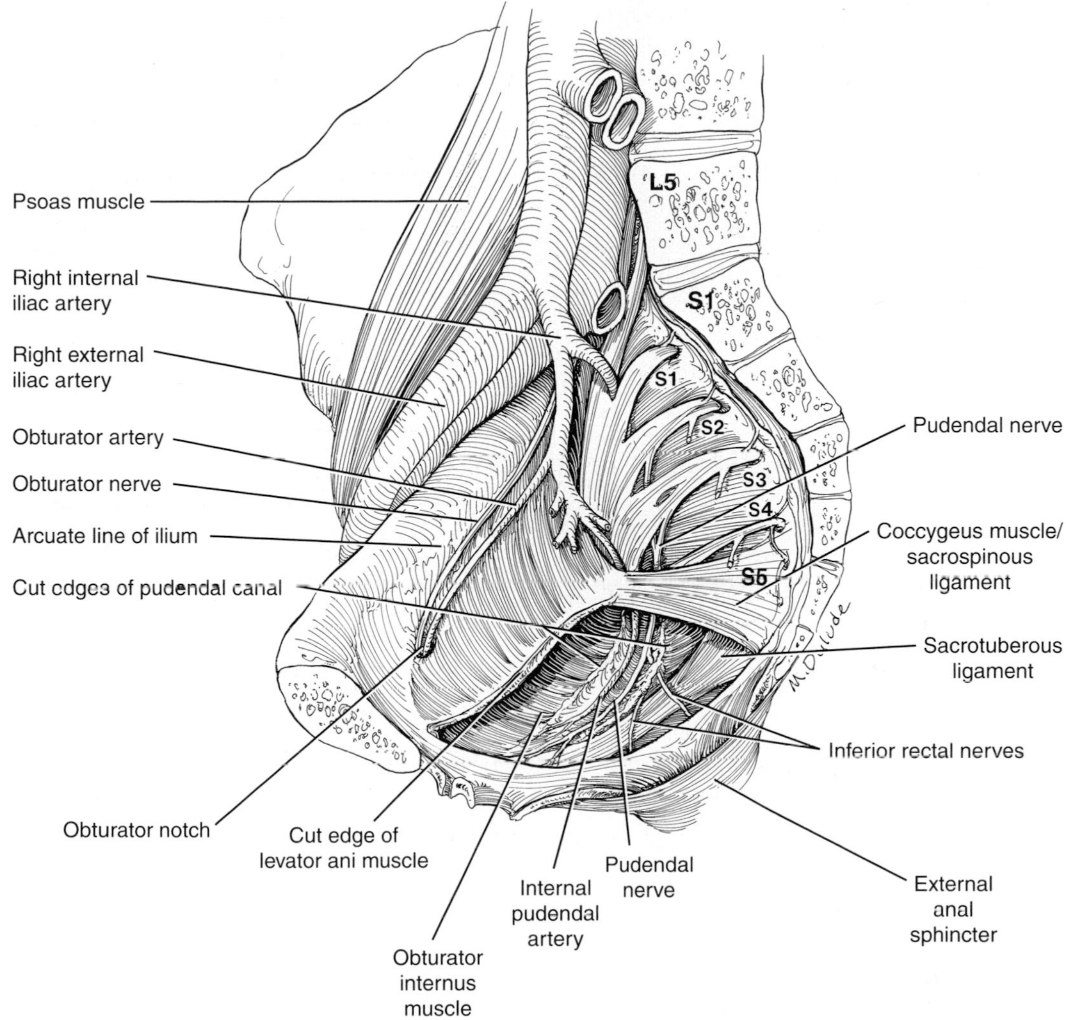

Figure 5–10. The pudendal nerve.

an anterior direction to reach the dorsum of the clitoris.

Coccygeal Plexus

The coccygeal plexus is formed by a small branch from the fourth sacral anterior ramus and by the fifth sacral and coccygeal anterior rami. The anococcygeal nerves arise from this plexus and pierce the sacrotuberous ligaments to supply the cutaneous area over the coccyx and between the coccyx and anus.

Cutaneous Innervation of the Perineum

The skin covering the perineum is innervated as follows from posterior to anterior (see Fig. 5–11): The anococcygeal nerves innervate the area between the coccyx and anus; the cutaneous branches of the inferior rectal nerves give sensation to the anus and the areas lateral to the anus; the perineal branch of the posterior femoral cutaneous nerve innervates the lateral aspects of the labia majora, and the posterior labial branches of the perineal nerves innervate the medial aspects of the labia; the ilioinguinal nerve innervates the anterior portion of the labia majora, and the genital branch of the genitofemoral nerve innervates an area similar to this. The mons pubis is innervated by the iliohypogastric nerve, overlapping with the ilioinguinal nerve. The innervation of the perineum primarily involves dermatomes L1, S2, S3, and S4 (Fig. 5–12).

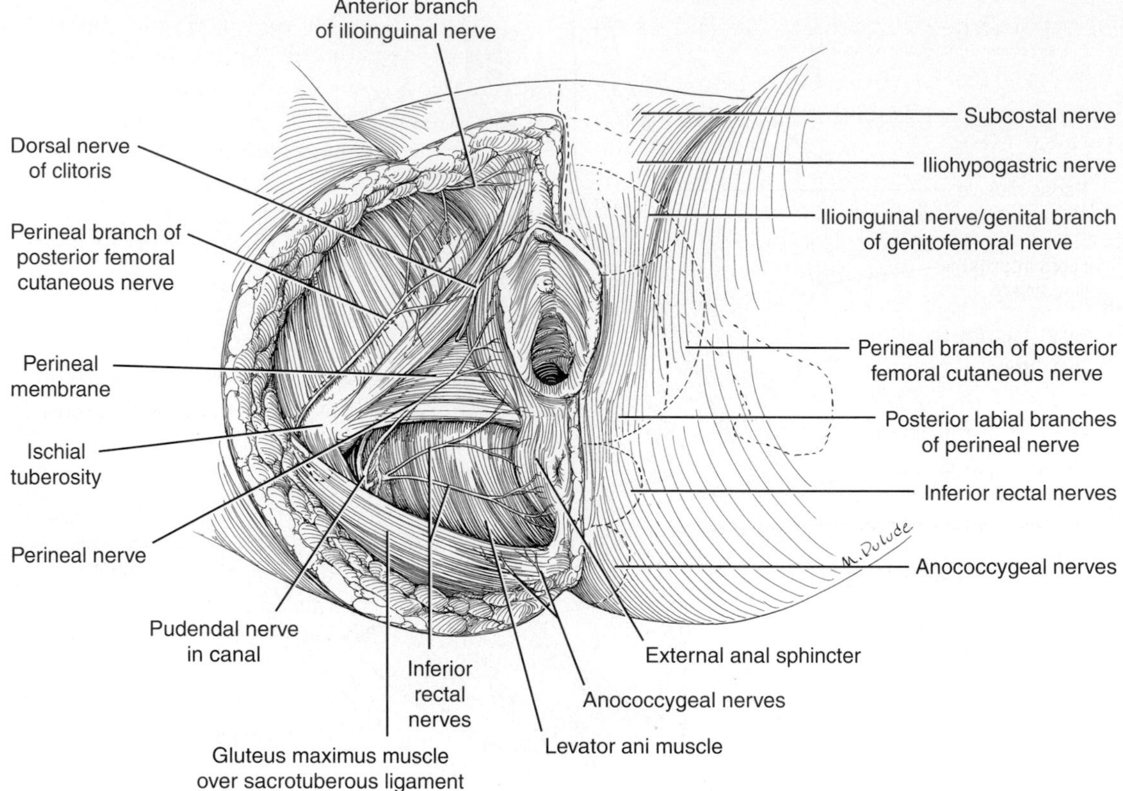

Figure 5–11. The nerves and cutaneous innervation of the perineum.

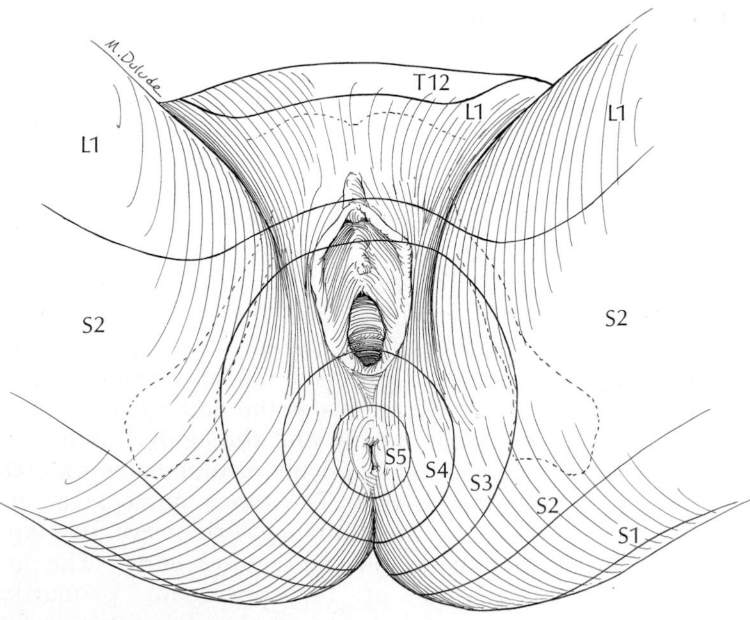

Figure 5–12. The approximate dermatomes of the perineum.

Visceral Innervation to the Pelvis

The afferent (sensory) fibers from the abdominal and pelvic viscera, including their visceral peritoneum and visceral vasculature, follow the same routes out of the pelvis to the dorsal root ganglia and to the dorsal horns of the spinal cord as the efferent (motor) routes of the sympathetic and parasympathetic nervous systems. There are at least five pathways to transmit nociceptive stimuli *out of* the pelvis. Three of these pathways travel through the inferior hypogastric plexus. Once through this plexus, the nociceptive signals can travel upward with the hypogastric nerve; or with the pelvic splanchnic nerves (parasympathetic) to S2, S3, S4; or with the sacral splanchnic nerves (sympathetic) to the sacral extension of the paravertebral sympathetic chain of ganglia. An additional route is with the ovarian vessels in the infundibulopelvic ligament. Another courses with the superior rectal artery to the inferior mesenteric plexus. To understand the many areas of overlapping afferent fibers and the complexities of their courses out of the pelvis, readers *must* take the time to understand the sympathetic and parasympathetic efferent routes *into* the pelvis.

The visceral efferent neurons of the sympathetic nervous system originate in the interomediolateral cell column of the spinal cord from T1 to approximately L2. The parasympathetic efferent neurons originate in the intermediolateral cell column of the S2, S3, and S4 regions of the spinal cord. These parasympathetic efferent neurons innervate all the pelvic viscera, mediate perineal sexual function through the pudendal nerve, and innervate the terminal aspects of the colon including the left colonic flexure, descending colon, sigmoid colon, rectum, and anal canal. The proximal portion of the colon and all abdominal viscera receive their parasympathetic innervation from the vagus nerve, which is the 10th cranial nerve.

Efferent (Motor) Visceral Innervation (Autonomic)

Sympathetic System in the Pelvis

For visceral sympathetic innervation of the abdominal and pelvic viscera, the preganglionic sympathetic fibers enter the paravertebral ganglion via the white ramus communicans and without synapsing continue through that ganglion in a splanchnic (visceral) nerve to enter one of the preaortic ganglia. Therefore, each splanchnic nerve bypasses the gray ramus communicans that would rejoin the particular spinal nerve. The preaortic ganglia have a multitude of interconnections among them. The *splanchnic nerves*, therefore, transport preganglionic sympathetic fibers that synapse in a preaortic ganglion with postganglionic sympathetic fibers. The postganglionic sympathetic fibers then travel with a visceral artery originating from the aorta to reach the particular viscus to be innervated. In addition, the splanchnic nerves contain visceral afferent (sensory) fibers from the particular abdominal or pelvic organ thus innervated.

The preaortic ganglia of the splanchnic nerves are located around the root of the artery from the aorta after which the ganglion is named (Fig. 5–13). These are the celiac, the superior mesenteric, the aorticorenal, and the inferior mesenteric. Many individual variations in the shape, size, location, and number of these preaortic ganglia are noted. The greater splanchnic nerve is traditionally composed of the preganglionic sympathetic efferent fibers from T5 to T9 and travels to the celiac ganglion. The lesser splanchnic nerve, from T10 and T11, travels to the superior mesenteric ganglion. The least splanchnic nerve, from T12, travels to the aorticorenal ganglion. The inferior mesenteric ganglion receives preganglionic fibers that pass through the more superior preaortic ganglia, as well as preganglionic fibers through lumbar splanchnic nerves from L1 and L2.

These splanchnic fibers can either synapse in an individual preaortic ganglion or may continue through a particular ganglion to synapse in another preaortic ganglion (see Fig. 5–3). Sympathetic fibers, whether preganglionic or postganglionic from these preaortic ganglia, then feed into the superior hypogastric plexus of nerves. The superior hypogastric plexus of nerves lies on the anterior surface of the lower portion of the aorta, the left common iliac vein, the pre-

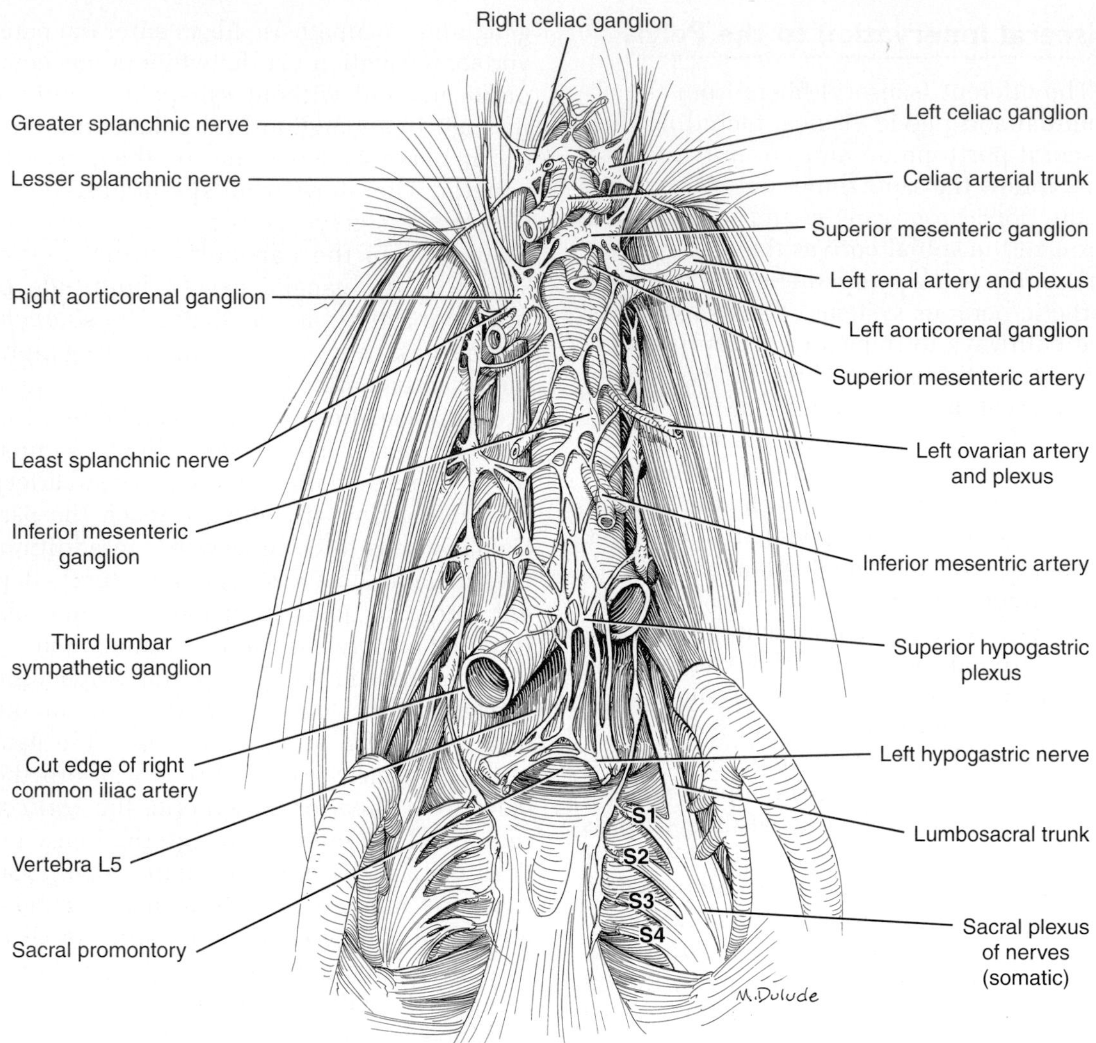

Figure 5–13. The visceral nerves in the abdomen.

lumbar area over L4 and L5, and the promontory of the sacrum.

The *superior hypogastric plexus* (Fig. 5–14) is a lacy, variable network of visceral nerve fibers that may be difficult to see at the time of a presacral neurectomy. This plexus can be physically distributed widely in the presacral space or occasionally fused into one or several presacral nerves (Fig. 5–15). This plexus also communicates with the lumbar splanchnic nerves emanating from the lumbar sympathetic chain of paravertebral ganglia. These fine communications course behind the common iliac vessels. Most of the fibers in the superior hypogastric plexus of nerves are normally found to the left of the midline and are contained in the subperitoneal visceral fascia. This visceral fascia also envelops the arteries, veins, lymph nodes and channels, and ureter found within the retroperitoneum between the peritoneum and the *parietal* fascia, which covers the skeletal muscles of the posterior abdominal wall and the pelvic basin.

The presacral space is important to gynecologic surgeons performing a presacral neurectomy. *Presacral* is actually a misnomer, because this area is just in front of the fourth and fifth lumbar vertebrae. The correct terminology should be the *lower prelumbar* space. Posteriorly, this space is bounded by the parietal fascia, which fuses with the periosteum and anterior longitudi-

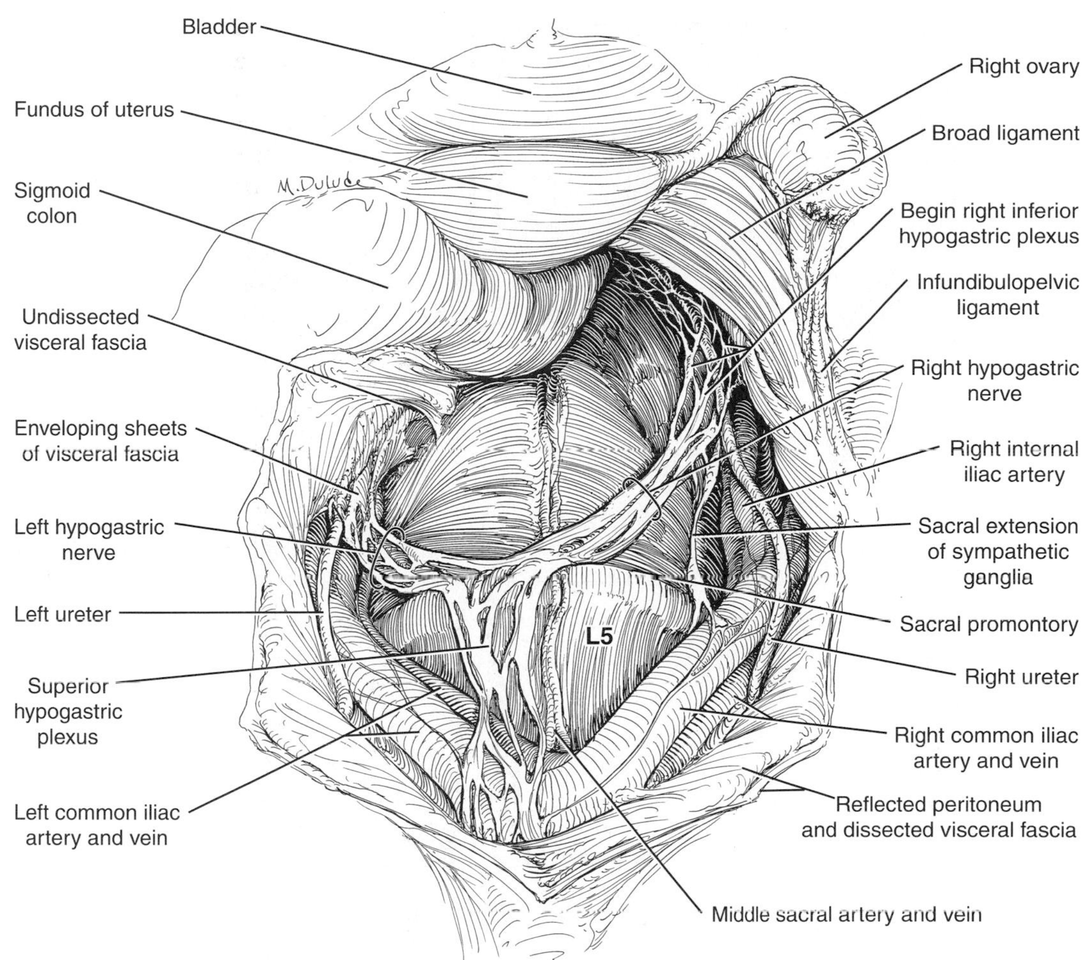

Figure 5–14. The superior hypogastric plexus.

nal ligament over the last two lumbar vertebrae and the promontory of the sacrum. The middle sacral artery and a plexus of veins are adherent to the parietal fascia in the posterior boundary of the presacral space.

The right lateral boundary of the presacral space is the right common iliac artery and the right ureter. The left lateral border is the left common iliac vein and left ureter, as well as the inferior mesenteric artery and vein traversing the mesentery of the sigmoid colon. The roof is simply the peritoneum over the fourth and fifth lumbar vertebrae and the promontory of the sacrum. Injuries to any or all of these structures are possible during a dissection in this area.

One reason why a presacral neurectomy may fail to relieve central pelvic pain is inadequate dissection and excision of the visceral nervous tissue in this area.[15] In addition, the various physical combinations of the presacral nerves may even bypass the presacral space and subsequent surgical dissections here, by traveling over the more lateral iliac vessels, especially to the left (see Fig. 5–15*A*).[16, 17] A third reason for continued central visceral pelvic pain after this procedure is the extensive intermingling of visceral afferent fibers in various areas of the pelvis and the several different paths these fibers can travel to leave the pelvis, bypassing the superior hypogastric plexus, as explained later.

To emphasize, all the visceral nerve fibers, both efferent and afferent, are contained within the thin, fused sheets of visceral endogastric fascia beneath the posterior abdominal peritoneum and the endopelvic fascia beneath the pelvic parietal peritoneum.[7] This endogastric and endopelvic fascia also

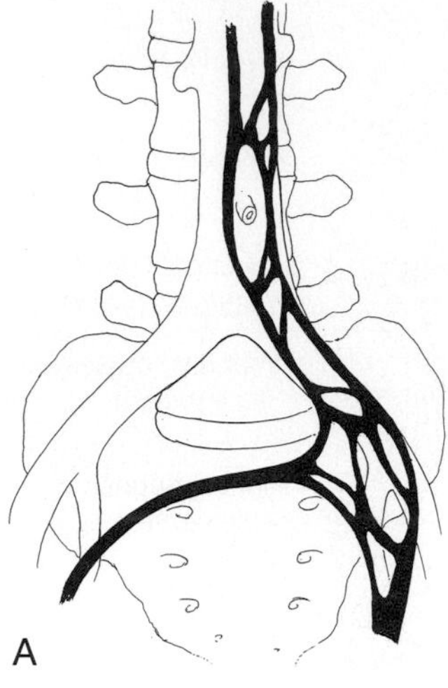

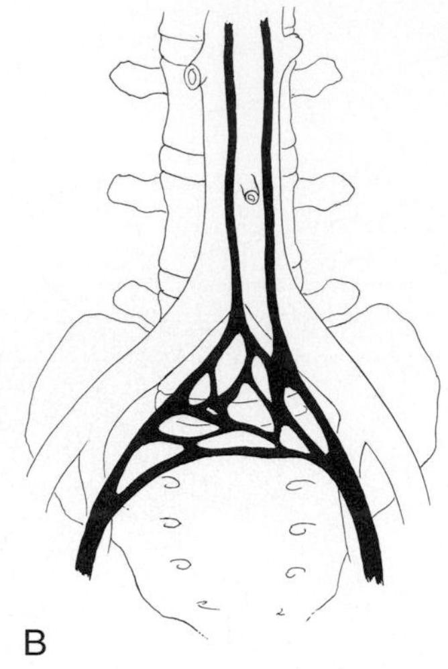

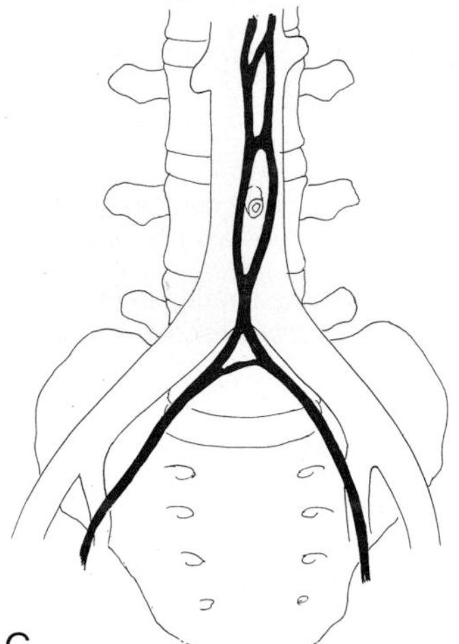

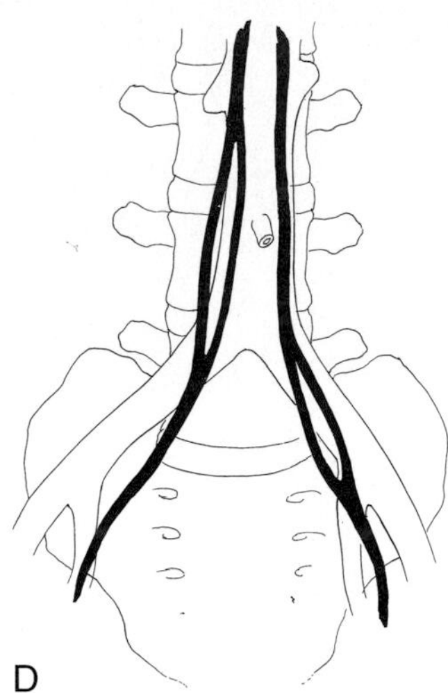

Figure 5–15. Anatomic variations of the superior hypogastric plexus.

envelops the visceral arteries, veins, and lymph nodes and channels within the retroperitoneum. This visceral fascia in the abdomen is called the *endogastric fascia.* The same fascia is continued in the subperitoneal regions of the pelvis as the *endopelvic fascia* (see Fig. 5–14).

The superior hypogastric plexus of nerves then divides into the right and left *hypogastric nerves.* These nerves travel just posterior to and then with the ureters and feed into the *inferior hypogastric plexuses* (Fig. 5–16). Each inferior hypogastric plexus spreads over an area 2 to 3 cm by 3 to 5 cm within the endopelvic fascial sheaths accompanying and surrounding the ureter and the internal iliac vessels, lateral to the rectum and upper vagina at the base of the broad ligament.[18] This area is just lateral to each uterosacral ligament. This plexus forms a dense web that contains many small ganglia, primarily sympathetic with some parasympathetic. In addition, many afferent fibers from the bladder, uterus, and middle and lower rectum pass through this region, following various routes to their respective dorsal root ganglia.

The sympathetic nerve supply to the inferior hypogastric plexus is derived from several sources. The first is simply the downward continuation of the superior hypogastric plexus via each hypogastric nerve. The second is from preganglionic fibers from the *sacral* splanchnic nerves from the downward or sacral extension of the sympathetic chain of paravertebral ganglia.

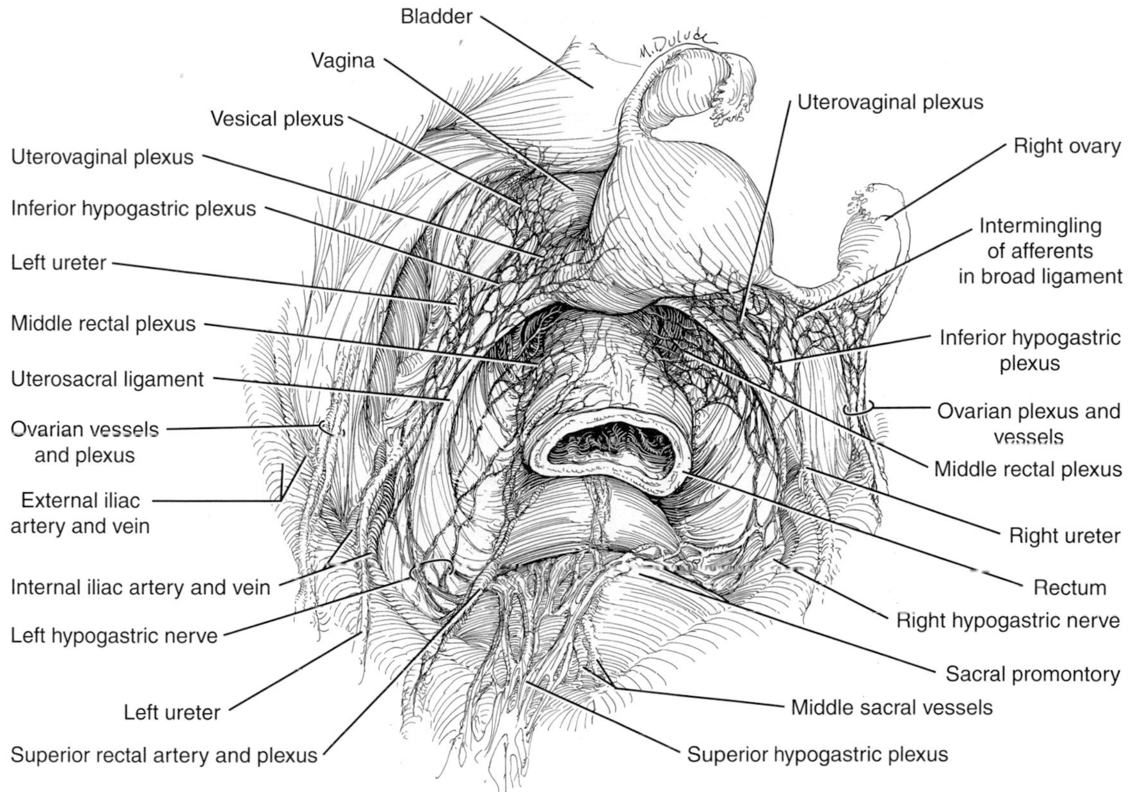

Figure 5–16. The visceral nerves of the pelvis.

The third source is postganglionic sympathetic fibers, having synapsed in the sacral sympathetic ganglia chain, that innervate the smooth muscle in the somatic blood vessels—both arterial and venous—in the pelvis. The accompanying visceral afferent fibers from these vessels probably have little input into visceral pain per se but may give pain sensation from perhaps a pelvic congestion syndrome. This has not yet been fully investigated.

The inferior hypogastric plexus then immediately gives rise to three other plexuses. These contain preganglionic and postganglionic sympathetic fibers, preganglionic parasympathetic fibers, and many afferent fibers. The first is the *middle rectal plexus*, which travels to the rectum via the middle rectal blood vessels. The visceral afferent fibers from the middle rectal plexus intermingle with the visceral afferent fibers from the superior rectal plexus in the wall of the rectum (Fig. 5–17). The superior rectal plexus is derived from the inferior mesenteric plexus and travels to the rectum along the superior rectal blood vessels.

The second is the *uterovaginal plexus* (Frankenhäuser's plexus) to the uterus, cervix, and vagina. The third is the *vesical plexus*, which travels to the bladder via the vesical blood vessels, especially the inferior vesical artery.

The uterovaginal plexus (Frankenhäuser's plexus) is contained within the endopelvic fascia surrounding the ureter and uterine vessels, just lateral to the uterosacral ligaments as they insert into the uterus. This is the reason for the placement of a paracervical block just lateral to the insertion of each uterosacral ligament into the cervix. However, many of these nerve fibers enter the lower uterine segment with the uterine vessels and *not* through the uterosacral ligaments. This is one reason why procedures that transect the uterosacral ligaments have a relatively high failure rate for the relief of uterine pain.[19] Also, too lateral a transection of the uterosacral ligaments may damage the

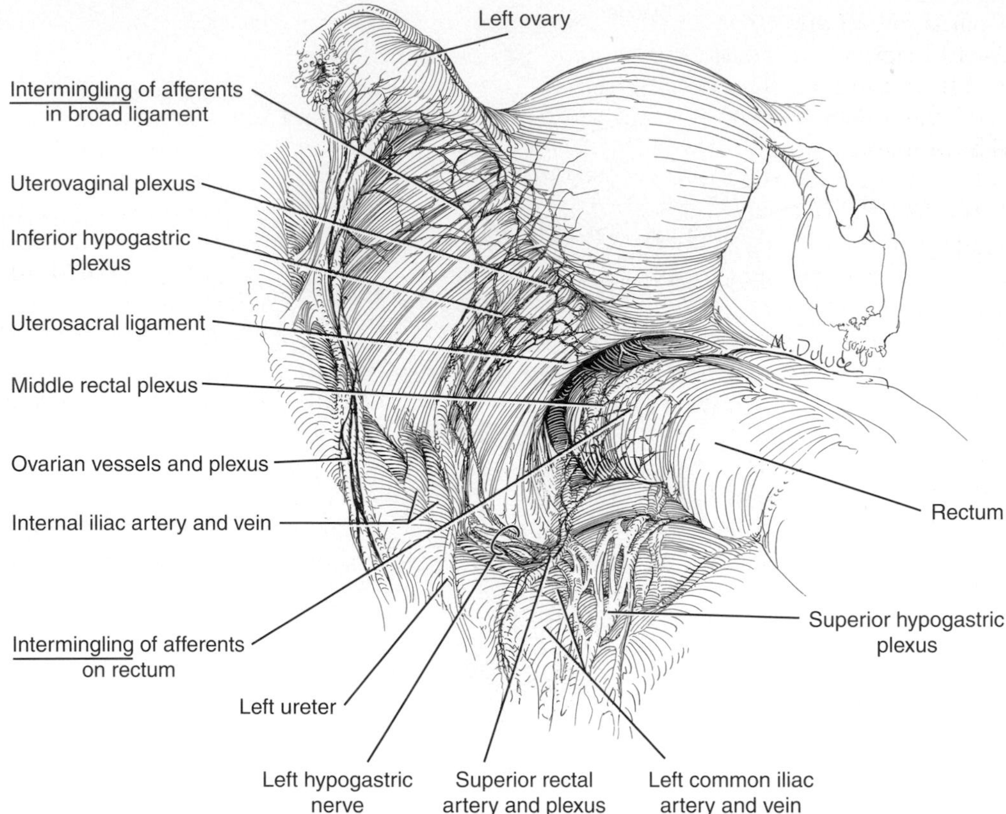

Figure 5–17. Intermingling of visceral nerves on pelvic viscera.

ureters by producing subsequent scarring and fixation of the ureters in these areas. This may make subsequent performance of a hysterectomy very dangerous, and injury to the ureter may be a threat.

The uterovaginal plexus sends fibers to the vagina via the vaginal artery and vein, to the cervix via the uterine artery and vein, and to the lower uterine segment and fundus of the uterus via the ascending uterine arteries and veins. These visceral nerves also supply the upper part of the broad ligament and the uterine tube and intermingle in the broad ligament with the visceral nerves from the ovarian plexus, as well as other nerves directly from the inferior hypogastric plexus (see Fig. 5–17).

The *ovary* has its own visceral innervation. The parasympathetic supply is derived from the vagus nerve, and the sympathetic supply is derived from the preaortic plexuses. The ovarian plexus is a fine network of visceral nerves from the 10th and 11th thoracic segments of the spinal cord. These enter the paravertebral sympathetic ganglia at the level of the fourth lumbar vertebra and accompany the ovarian vessels to the ovaries, tubes, and broad ligaments. Therefore, visceral afferent (sensory) fibers that transmit nociceptive impulses in the broad ligament and in the tubes intermingle here before exiting via the inferior hypogastric plexus, the uterovaginal plexus, and the ovarian plexus (see Figs. 5–16 and 5–17). Pain from the ovary is traditionally referred to the T10 and T11 dermatomes.

Parasympathetic System in the Pelvis

The parasympathetic supply to the abdominal viscera and ovaries is from the vagus nerve to the level of the left colonic flexure. The parasympathetic innervation to the pelvic viscera and descending colon, sigmoid colon, rectum, and anal canal is through the *pelvic splanchnic nerves* from the anterior rami of spinal nerves S2, S3, and S4.

The parasympathetic fibers in the pelvis (Fig. 5–18) originate from the interomediolateral cell column of the S2, S3, and S4 region of the lower portion of the spinal cord. These fibers then travel with the ventral roots to help form the anterior rami of S2, S3, and S4. The parasympathetic preganglionic fibers then exit these anterior rami and form the *pelvic splanchnic nerves* (nervi erigentes). The parasympathetic fibers do not pass through the sympathetic chain of ganglia but course directly from the anterior rami. These preganglionic parasympathetic fibers then enter the endopelvic fascia and travel with the appropriate visceral artery to the wall of the viscus to be innervated. In doing so, many of these fibers pass through the inferior hypogastric plexus. The preganglionic parasympathetic fibers synapse in ganglia contained within the endopelvic fascial capsule of the target viscus. Therefore, the postganglionic parasympathetic fibers are microscopic in length.

The superior hypogastric plexus and the inferior mesenteric plexus also contain parasympathetic fibers from the pelvic splanchnic nerves coursing through the inferior hypogastric plexuses. These parasympathetic fibers extend up alongside the sympathetic fibers of the hypogastric nerve or may pass independently to the left of the superior hypogastric plexus and then cross the sigmoid vessels to reach the inferior mesenteric plexus. In this manner, parasympathetic supply to that part of the colon supplied by the inferior mesenteric artery is provided.

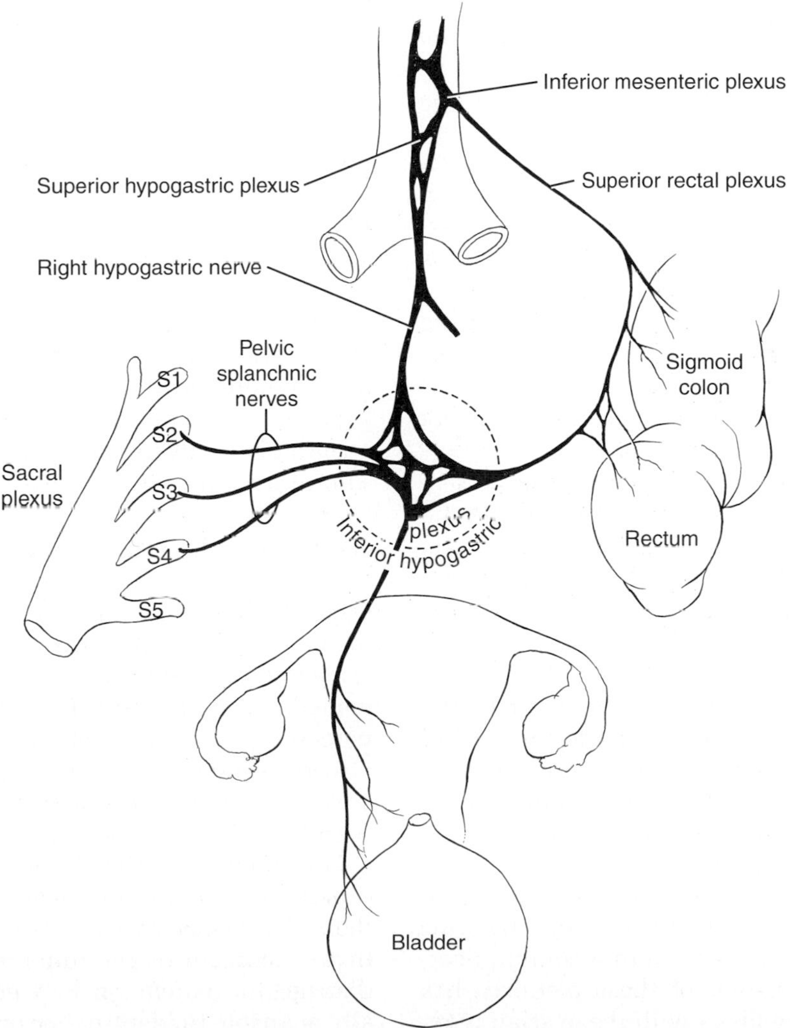

Figure 5–18. Schema—parasympathetic fibers in the pelvis.

Afferent (Sensory) Visceral Innervation of the Female Pelvis

The *visceral afferent fibers* travel the same routes with the preganglionic and postganglionic fibers of both the sympathetic and parasympathetic divisions. The peripheral process (dendrite) of a visceral afferent fiber is very long and does not synapse in any autonomic ganglia. This process travels uninterrupted to its cell body in a dorsal sensory root ganglion. The afferent fiber begins its journey in the wall of a viscus—epithelial lining, muscularis, or serosal covering—or in the wall of a blood vessel. These various fibers transmit visceral sensation such as nausea, pressure, diffuse pain, and distention from the abdominal or pelvic viscera. The visceral afferents also transmit sexual sensations from the perineum, vulva, and clitoris via their presence within the pudendal nerves.

Deviations from traditional descriptions of pelvic sensation are explained by the extensive intermingling of the various sympathetic and parasympathetic afferent fibers in the various visceral nerve plexuses. For example, a noxious stimulus from the fundus of the uterus is normally referred to dermatomes T11, T12, L1, and L2. Pain from the cervix is traditionally felt in the sacral dermatomes of S2, S3, and S4. However, original work by Bonica has demonstrated that visceral afferent fibers from the upper portion of the cervix and the lower uterine segment do not travel with the parasympathetic pelvic splanchnic nerves (nervi erigentes) but follow routes through the inferior hypogastric plexus, superior hypogastric plexus, and aortic plexuses to leave with the spinal nerves from T10, T11, T12, and L1.[20] Because of the embryologic migration of the cutaneous branches of the posterior rami of these lower thoracic and upper lumbar nerves in the back, these dermatomes overlie the lower three lumbar vertebrae and the upper half of the sacrum.

To confuse pelvic sensations further, the superior hypogastric plexus and inferior mesenteric plexuses have intercommunicating fibers, and each of these plexuses has communicating fibers with the ovarian plexuses, as well as the ureteric plexuses, as the ureter courses through these areas. Other examples of afferent fibers from different nerve plexuses intermingling occur in the middle rectum, broad ligament and inferior hypogastric plexus (see Figs. 5–16 and 5–17). Nociceptive stimuli from the middle rectal region are relayed via both the middle rectal plexus and the superior rectal plexus. The middle rectal plexus relays visceral information along the middle rectal blood vessels back to the inferior hypogastric plexus at the base of the broad ligament. The superior rectal plexus transmits the same information from the same overlapping rectal region along the superior rectal vessels to the inferior mesenteric artery to the inferior mesenteric plexus of nerves over the lower aorta. The inferior mesenteric plexus also communicates with the superior hypogastric plexus.

In the broad ligament, afferent fibers from the uterovaginal plexus, as well as directly from the inferior hypogastric plexus, intermingle with afferent fibers from the ovarian plexus. The ovarian plexus travels out of the pelvis with the ovarian artery and vein and likewise has some communication with the superior hypogastric plexus.

The inferior hypogastric plexus is a relatively widespread junction of sympathetic ganglia, a few parasympathetic ganglia, but multiple efferent (motor) and afferent (sensory) nerve fibers. These sensory fibers are essentially unmyelinated—poorly insulated. Therefore, electric action potentials from some of these afferents can instigate message activity in adjacent afferent nerves. These adjacent nerves may very well anatomically originate from other viscera different from the specific visceral source that initiated the nociceptive stimulus. This concept is named *crosstalk*.[21] In this manner, a patient perceives nociceptive signals from a specific visceral source as pain from a much wider area, such as the left side of the pelvis or even the whole pelvis.

For example, irritable bowel syndrome causes smooth muscle spasms in the wall of the colon, especially the left side, and patients complain of pelvic pain and possibly diarrhea. A patient on first encounter usually is unable to identify her pain perception specifically as a spastic colon. She frequently complains of "pain in my lower abdomen" or "pelvic cramps that stay and occasionally ease up." Many women consider their obstetricians and gynecologists to be their primary physicians. Therefore, they first report any pain in or around their lower abdominal and pelvic region to their gynecologist.

Because of such examples of intermingling of visceral nerve fibers—both efferent and afferent—*visceral nociceptive signals can be transmitted out of the pelvis in at least five distinct ways* (Fig. 5–19): via (1) the inferior hypogastric plexus to the hypogastric nerves to the superior hypogastric plexus of nerves; (2) the pelvic (parasympathetic) splanchnic nerves (nervi erigentes), many of which pass through the inferior hypogastric plexus; (3) the sacral (sympathetic) splanchnic nerves from the inferior hypogastric plexus back to the sacral extension of the paravertebral sympathetic chain; (4) the superior rectal nerves leading to the inferior mesenteric plexus of nerves; and (5) the ovarian plexus of nerves. This helps explain why visceropelvic pain is typically vague and ill defined and may result in abdominal malaise and nausea. Stronger stimuli are referred to the anterior or lateral abdominal wall dermatomes in *general* cutaneous areas—not sharp or specific.

Therefore, reasoning gynecologists need to realize that one simple operation such as a presacral neurectomy or uterosacral nerve ablation may not necessarily address the pain route that is causing a patient's deep visceral pain. More academic study and understanding of CPP, both somatosensory and visceral, is being pursued.

Concerning *specific visceral sensations*,[22] the *parietal* peritoneum is sensitive to mechanical trauma and to thermal and chemical stimuli. The *visceral* peritoneum and mesentery are insensitive to cutting, burn-

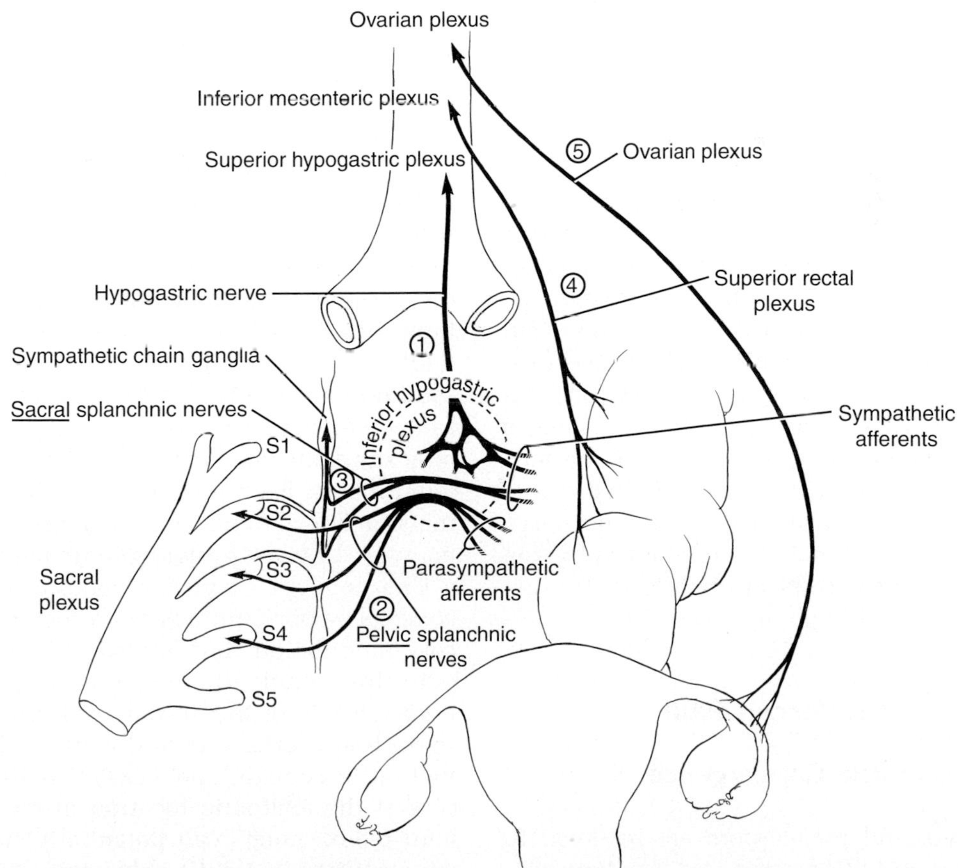

Figure 5–19. Transmission of nociceptive signals out of the pelvis.

ing, and chemical irritation but react to traction, rapid distention, visceral muscle spasm, and ischemia. The gastrointestinal tract is also insensitive to cut, crush, and burn but reacts to give painful sensations with traction, rapid distention, and strong contractions or spasm. Inflammation, particularly of the mucosa, significantly increases the sensitivity of these tissues to touch, pressure, and chemical stimuli.

The fundus of the uterus is relatively insensitive to mechanical stimuli but is very sensitive to myometrial contractions. The fallopian tubes and ovaries are primarily sensitive to traction and distention. Electric stimulation or rapid distention of the cervix gives rise to painful sensations referred to the lower abdomen, although pinching the cervix evokes little pain sensation. The normal vaginal mucosa is relatively insensitive to mechanical stimuli yet is very sensitive when inflamed. The female external genitalia are considered moderately pain sensitive to various electric and mechanical stimuli.

Noxious stimuli from the pelvis can result from irritation to the afferent fibers from scar tissue or adhesions, neuroma formation, and inflammatory processes such as infection and endometriosis externa. In addition, benign and malignant pelvic tumors, vascular congestion, uterine prolapse and pelvic floor dysfunction, spasm of the muscular pelvic floor, and vulvovaginal disorders can also cause CPP. Specific mechanisms that cause such pain are not always well established but can involve mechanical irritation as well as chemical irritation due to substances such as prostaglandins and other substances released from damaged tissues in the surrounding area such as potassium, histamine, serotonin, and substance P from the nerve itself. These substances can activate free nerve endings, thus contributing to sustained states of hyperalgesia.

Patterns of Referred Pain

Viscerosomatic Convergence

The visceral nociceptors are believed to be free, unmodified nerve endings. Pain sensations travel to the spinal cord from peripheral nerve fibers that are very poorly myelinated or completely unmyelinated, known as A-δ and C fibers, respectively. These fibers mediate both somatic and visceral noxious stimuli. Surprisingly, only 2% to 7% of all afferent fibers passing through each dorsal root ganglion are visceral afferents.[5, 23] Thus, the spinal interneurons in the spinal cord that receive visceral afferent input are overwhelmingly influenced by somatic input. Some spinal interneurons receive only somatic afferent influence. This is the neuroanatomic conception of *viscerosomatic convergence*.[5] Such a diffuse input of sensory information does not allow for fine discrimination and precise localization. This also helps explain the diffuse nature of visceral pain.

In addition, because of the poorly myelinated and unmyelinated fibers that constitute these afferent fibers, visceral noxious stimuli may be able to stimulate somatic afferent fibers via the phenomenon of crosstalk.[21] These poorly insulated nerves allow electric action potentials to excite adjacent fibers. Remember that these afferent fibers converge at the dorsal root ganglion as well as in the dorsal horn of the spinal cord. In this manner, strong noxious visceral stimuli may stimulate and irritate many somatic afferent fibers. These irritated afferents then relay in the dorsal horn of the spinal cord onto interneurons to be eventually distributed to the various dermatomes of the lower back, lateral sidewall, and anterior abdominal wall, as well as to the dermatomes surrounding and within the female perineum. Likewise, strong noxious somatic stimuli may stimulate and irritate many visceral afferent fibers. Each preganglionic fiber entering the dorsal horn may synapse with as many as 15 to 20 postganglionic neurons.

The concept of viscerosomatic convergence is a poorly understood process of sensory modulation that is also influenced by conscious and unconscious centers in higher levels of the spinal cord, as well as in the brain cortex and midbrain.[5] This modulation of somatic and visceral pain sensation at the anatomic location of the spinal cord reflex centers can potentially suppress or magnify a patient's subjective sensation of pain. This mechanism applies to acute pain situations but may have some validity in chronic pain modulation. This latter point is still under study.

Dermatomes

Each spinal nerve traditionally courses laterally around the flank of the abdomen to the anterior abdominal wall and gives off sensory fibers in a transverse narrow band to innervate the skin and subcutaneous areas of that particular dermatome. Interestingly, because of embryonic distribution, the afferent (sensory) and efferent (motor) fibers do not coincide. In other words, from the same spinal nerve, the innervation of muscles (myotome) may be spatially removed from the cutaneous sensory innervation (dermatome). Knowledge of the approximate distribution of the *dermatomes* and relevant nerves is very important in understanding and treating patients with CPP.[6]

Studies by several investigators have shown a tremendous overlap among neighboring dermatomes, particularly in the limbs. Each dermatome is supplied by one primary spinal nerve segment but can also contain secondary sensory fibers from as many as four other spinal nerves (see Fig. 5–5). Therefore, one dermatome cannot be rendered insensitive by cutting only one dorsal root.

Many other variable and complex interactions also influence referred pain. Although these dermatomes overlap, the threshold for various stimuli apparently is lowest in the central portion of the field. In addition to the considerable secondary overlap of sensory nerves from several spinal nerves in each dermatome, significant variation in the location of these dermatomes is found in each individual patient.

Moreover, each abdominal or pelvic organ or tissue is supplied by afferents that travel through dorsal roots of a number of spinal nerves. The nociceptive stimulation then converges on the involved posterior horn areas in the spinal cord. These are the localized reflex areas of the spinal cord where noxious stimuli are transmitted through the afferent fibers to the spinal interneurons to bring about an efferent response. Nociceptive stimulation from these various tissues produce reflex responses that may include cutaneous hyperalgesia in the same dermatome segments whose nerves service the particular tissue in question. In CPP, receptors seem to be hypersensitized peripherally, so that nociceptive thresholds are reduced, making even minor stimuli magnified significantly. In addition, each visceral afferent fiber extending to one dorsal root ganglion supplies a much larger area within abdominal or pelvic visceral tissues than a corresponding somatic afferent fiber does in somatic tissue such as skin or skeletal muscle.

Spinal Paths

At the level of the posterior horn of the spinal cord, a number of influences from higher up in the spinal cord, as well as from supraspinal areas within the midbrain and cortex, can modulate the noxious stimuli being reported to this area.[24] The primary ascending spinal routes for nociceptive information are the spinothalamic tracts. These tracts travel from the dorsal horn areas up one to two segments and then cross in the midline to join the contralateral tract. These tracts travel in the anterolateral quadrants of the spinal cord and eventually connect with neurons within the midbrain. The spinothalamic afferents interface with the neospinothalamic tract, which gives sensory discriminative information directly to the thalamus. Within the thalamus, some of the painful sensations are brought to conscious perception and allow sensory discrimination of pain—namely, location, nature, and intensity. Other painful sensations remain in the unconscious and take part in mediating autonomic as well as emotional reactions to pain, such as arousal, fear, and general orientation to pain.

From other centers in the cortex and midbrain, powerful circuits are initiated, and some of these descend in various analgesic pathways to modify the noxious stimuli at the level of the dorsal horn. These descending systems are part of the complex modulation that converges on the dorsal horn of the spinal cord and modulates pain sensation at the level of viscerosomatic convergence.

Dorsal Horn Substances

In addition to the spinal tracts, various receptors in the dorsal horn have also been found to modulate the perception of pain. For example, serotonin release seems to enhance the release of endogenous opiates in this area, and these opiates help suppress the subjective perception of pain from various noxious stimuli. Tricyclic agents seem to enhance release of serotonin in these areas and indeed may have a role in pain management. Opiate receptors also have been found in the dorsal horns of the spinal column.

Afterword

These examples are only part of our present, incomplete knowledge of the many mechanisms involved in the perception of CPP. The explanations of CPP are much more complex and much less understood than those of acute pelvic pain. The purpose of this chapter is to allow clinicians an opportunity to delve into the complex details and incompletely understood interactions of both the somatic and visceral nervous systems so that they can begin to understand the pathways, causes, and possible treatments of CPP and, just as important, can avoid those practices and surgical procedures that may cause more harm than help.

References

1. Bonica JJ: Cause and mechanisms of chronic pain. In Bonica JJ (ed): The Management of Pain, 2nd ed, vol 1. Philadelphia, Lea & Febiger, 1990, p 183.
2. Wall PD: On the relation of injury to pain. Pain 1979;6:255.
3. Slocumb JC: Chronic somatic, myofascial, and neurogenic abdominal pelvic pain. Clin Obstet Gynecol 1990;33:145.
4. Reiter RC, Milburn A: Management of chronic pelvic pain. Postgrad Obstet Gynecol 1992;12:3.
5. Cervero F, Tattersall JEH: Somatic and visceral sensory integration in the thoracic spinal cord. Prog Brain Res 1986;67:189.
6. Bonica JJ: Applied anatomy relevant to pain. In Bonica JJ (ed): The Management of Pain, 2nd ed, vol 1. Philadelphia, Lea & Febiger, 1990, pp 133–140.
7. Retzky SS, Rogers RM, Richardson AC: Anatomy of female pelvic support. In Brubaker LT, Saclarides TJ (eds): The Female Pelvic Floor: Disorders of Function and Support. Philadelphia, FA Davis, 1996, pp 9–16.
8. Baker PK: Musculoskeletal origins of chronic pelvic pain. Obstet Gynecol Clin North Am 1993;20:722.
9. Baker PK: Musculoskeletal origins of chronic pelvic pain. Obstet Gynecol Clin North Am 1993;20:719.
10. Sippo WC, Burghardt A, Gomez AC: Nerve entrapment after Pfannenstiel incision. Am J Obstet Gynecol 1987;157:420.
11. Miyazaki F, Shook G: Ilioinguinal nerve entrapment during needle suspension for stress incontinence. Obstet Gynecol 1992;80:246.
12. Vargo MM, Robinson LR, Nicholas JJ, et al: Postpartum femoral neuropathy: Relic of an earlier era? Arch Phys Med Rehabil 1990;71:591.
13. Kvist-Poulsen H, Borel J: Iatrogenic femoral neuropathy subsequent to abdominal hysterectomy: Incidence and prevention. Obstet Gynecol 1982;60:516.
14. Shafik A: Pudendal canal syndrome. Description of a new syndrome and its treatment. Report of seven cases. Coloproctology 1991;13:102.
15. Tjaden B, Schlaff WD, Kimball A, et al: The efficacy of presacral neurectomy for the relief of midline dysmenorrhea. Obstet Gynecol 1990;76:89.
16. Curtis AH, Anson BJ, Ashley FL, et al: The anatomy of the pelvic autonomic nerves in relation to gynecology. Surg Gynecol Obstet 1942;75:743.
17. Lierse W: Applied Anatomy of the Pelvis. New York, Springer-Verlag, 1987, pp 70–72.
18. Hollinshead WH: Textbook of Anatomy, 3rd ed. Hagerstown, MD, Harper & Row, 1974, p 712.
19. Papasakelariou C: Long-term results of laparoscopic uterosacral nerve ablation. Gynecol Endosc 1996;5:177.
20. Bonica JJ: The pain of childbirth. In Bonica JJ (ed): The Management of Pain, 2nd ed, vol 2. Philadelphia, Lea & Febiger, 1990, p 1327.
21. Maciewicz R, Sandrew BB: Physiology of pain. In Aronoff GM (ed): Evaluation and Treatment of Chronic Pain. Baltimore, Urban & Schwarzenberg, 1985, pp 19–20.
22. Bonica JJ: Applied anatomy relevant to pain. In Bonica JJ (ed): The Management of Pain, 2nd ed, vol 1. Philadelphia, Lea & Febiger, 1990, pp 141–146.
23. Janig W, Morrison JFB: Functional properties of spinal visceral afferents supplying abdominal and pelvic organs, with special emphasis on visceral nociception. Prog Brain Res 1986;67:91.
24. Maciewicz R, Sandrew BB: Physiology of pain. In Aronoff GM (ed): Evaluation and Treatment of Chronic Pain. Baltimore, Urban & Schwarzenberg, 1985, pp 21–30.

Suggested Readings

Crafts RC: A Textbook of Human Anatomy, 3rd ed. New York, Churchill Livingstone, 1985.

Williams PL, Bannister LH, Berry MM, Collins P, Dyson M, Dussek JE, Ferguson MWJ (eds): Gray's Anatomy, 38th ed. New York, Churchill Livingstone, 1995.

6

History

Barbara S. Levy, MD

There are two purposes for taking a complete medical history. The first is to gather information, searching for clues to establish a diagnosis. The second is equally important and often more difficult to accomplish: to establish a physician-patient relationship that creates a partnership in healing. Trust and confidence are not easily won from patients with chronic long-standing conditions. A physician's desire to establish a diagnosis quickly and efficiently may interfere with the creation of an atmosphere that demonstrates compassion and caring. The initial encounter with a patient with chronic pain offers the best opportunity to collect information and observe her demeanor. These visits are often time consuming, and sufficient time must be allocated in the physician's schedule to evaluate these patients. Alternately, a series of shorter visits may be set up initially when consultation is requested for a chronic pain problem.

The setting for the initial interview of the patient is critical for establishing the rules of the physician-patient relationship. The patient is at a disadvantage in a strange and often hostile-appearing environment. Make an effort to greet the patient as an equal human being. Introduce yourself and any other staff members who will be participating in the patient's care. Attempt to make the patient as comfortable as possible. The history should be taken with the patient fully clothed and in an office setting rather than in the examination room. The mere presence of an examination table, instruments, and stirrups is intimidating. It is useful to have the basic demographic information as well as a superficial medical history completed by the patient and reviewed with a nurse or medical assistant before the interview with the physician. This permits a patient some time to review and consider her complaints and serves to alert the physician to specific areas of concern. Sexual complaints are particularly difficult for a patient to verbalize, and a questionnaire may allow her to express elements of her social or medical history which she would not otherwise disclose (Table 6–1). Similarly, patients often write down their questions, concerns, and goals for treatment when they may have difficulty expressing them verbally to the physician or the staff. Allowing time and opportunity for a patient to express herself initiates the concept that physician and patient are partners together in healing. This message must be continually reinforced during the entire treatment process. A patient's empowerment and a sense of control over her situation may be as therapeutic as any medical or surgical intervention.

When the specifics of a patient's medical history have been established either by questionnaire or by the office staff, the physician is freed from the need to gather the immediate details of the history. By listening to a patient's own description of her problem and its impact on her life, the physician may discover not only something about the disease process but also a great deal about the patient. Body language, facial expressions, and inflections of the voice provide clues to the meaning of the symptoms to the patient. Fear is a significant factor for many people with chronic pain. As a patient talks about her situation, pertinent events in her life may become clear to an astute clinician. For example, a young woman whose mother died of ovarian cancer at a young age may present with a host of confusing complaints. Her underlying goal is to be reassured that she does not have ovarian cancer. However, unless the clinician cues

Table 6–1. **PATIENT QUESTIONNAIRE**

Name_________________________DOB_______________Marital status______No. of pregnancies______
No. of children______Ages_______________

Within the past year, have you taken any prescription or nonprescription medications for pain? If so, please list them:____

List all other medications:____

Do any of the following help decrease your pain?

Lying down	( ) yes	( ) no
Heating pad	( )	( )
Hot bath	( )	( )
Relaxation	( )	( )
Exercise	( )	( )
Cold	( )	( )
Other_______________		

Treatments that have been tried in the past:
( ) Surgery ( ) Physical therapy ( ) Acupuncture ( ) Antidepressant medications
( ) Chiropractic ( ) Birth control pills ( ) TENS unit ( ) Hormone shots or sprays
( ) Biofeedback ( ) Danazol ( ) Naturopathic remedies ( ) Psychotherapy
( ) Trigger point injections ( ) Nonsteroidal antiinflammatory drugs (like ibuprofen)
( ) Narcotics (pain killers) ( ) Other

Is your pain constant in location? ( ) Yes ( ) No
Is your pain always present? ( ) Yes ( ) No
When is the pain worst? Check all that apply:
( ) Morning ( ) Midday ( ) Evening ( ) Night ( ) All the time ( ) With menses
( ) During intercourse ( ) After intercourse ( ) During exercise ( ) Before menses
( ) After menses ( ) Standing for long periods of time ( ) Riding in a car
( ) Other____________

What do you think is responsible for the pain you are experiencing?______________
How do you feel you are currently coping with the pain?______________________________
What are your expectations about the outcome of treatment?____________________________
Have you been hurt either physically or emotionally or sexually at any time?
( ) Yes ( ) No
Have you experienced depression or anxiety related to pain or medical treatment?
( ) Yes ( ) No
If so, have you received psychologic treatment for it? ( ) Yes ( ) No
Who are the people you talk to about pain or during stressful times?
( ) Partner ( ) Friend ( ) Doctor/health care professional
( ) Support group ( ) Other

For each of the symptoms listed below, please circle the one number that most accurately reflects its severity in the past month, according to the following descriptions:

5 = Excruciating, incapacitating, intense, severe
4 = Horrible, pain severe, but undemanding tasks possible, concentration difficult
3 = Distressing, painful but able to continue job
2 = Uncomfortable, pain can be ignored at times
1 = Mild, low-level pain
0 = None, no pain

Pelvic pain before menses	0	1	2	3	4	5
Uterine cramps with menstruation	0	1	2	3	4	5
Pelvic pain (not cramps) during flow	0	1	2	3	4	5
Pelvic pain with exercise	0	1	2	3	4	5
Deep pain with intercourse	0	1	2	3	4	5
Burning vaginal pain with intercourse	0	1	2	3	4	5
Pelvic pain after intercourse	0	1	2	3	4	5
Pain with urination	0	1	2	3	4	5
Urinary frequency/urgency	0	1	2	3	4	5
Pain with bowel movements	0	1	2	3	4	5
Urgency with bowel movements	0	1	2	3	4	5
Diarrhea	0	1	2	3	4	5
Constipation	0	1	2	3	4	5
Intestinal cramping	0	1	2	3	4	5
Bloating	0	1	2	3	4	5
Nausea/vomiting	0	1	2	3	4	5
Backache	0	1	2	3	4	5
Muscle/joint pain	0	1	2	3	4	5
Hot flashes	0	1	2	3	4	5
Decreased sex drive	0	1	2	3	4	5
PMS symptoms (i.e., pain, irritability, headaches, etc.)	0	1	2	3	4	5
Fatigue	0	1	2	3	4	5
Chronic yeast/vaginal infections	0	1	2	3	4	5
High stress	0	1	2	3	4	5
Pain with movements/activities	0	1	2	3	4	5
Symptoms of depression	0	1	2	3	4	5
Trouble sleeping	0	1	2	3	4	5

in to this situation, a great deal of time, effort, and money may be spent chasing the cause of her symptoms. Asking a patient what her goals are in seeking treatment and what specific expectations she has of the encounter often helps guide the first visit.

As much as practical, a patient should be permitted to disclose her chief complaint and her current symptoms without interruption. The physician can provide encouragement and demonstrate active listening by occasionally validating a point or asking for clarification. Avoid the tendency to control the interview. A great deal of valuable information may be lost, but more importantly, this reinforces a power dichotomy between physician and patient and destroys any sense of partnership.

It may be necessary to begin the discussion with a question or comment from the physician, giving the patient permission to tell her story. Establishing why she came to consult the physician at this particular time may be especially revealing. For example, records or videotapes may have been transferred from another physician. These should be reviewed with the patient, treating her as a collaborator in discovering the critical information contained within them and using them as a springboard for establishing the essential elements of the history.

The current status of a patient's symptoms must be established. The character, location, duration, and intensity of pain are outlined (Table 6–2). The relationship of the pain to physical activity and other bodily functions is sought. It is important to ascertain which actions and behaviors are associated with exacerbation or relief of the pain. Does the pain radiate to surrounding areas or organ systems? Does the pain awaken the patient at night? What is the pattern of pain throughout the day and the menstrual cycle? Has the character of the pain changed over time? Searching diligently for postural changes as well as mechanical and position effects on the character, initiation, and radiation of the pain may help to focus attention on musculoskeletal factors that may be integral to the patient's pain syndrome. Not infrequently, old and adequately treated intraperitoneal processes have created compensatory posture and mechanical changes that perpetuate painful stimuli.

Table 6–2. **CHARACTERISTICS OF PAIN**

Character
Sharp, shooting, lancinating, knifelike
Dull, cramping, aching, constricting
Intensity
Causes doubling over, abruptly halts activity
Constant, wearing
Location
Dermatomal distribution
Superficial versus deep
Focal versus diffuse
Radiation
Direction and character of radiated discomfort
Duration
Overall time frame
Relationship to life events
Duration and frequency of individual episodes
Changes after prior operations
Associated events
Menses
Sexual intercourse
Orgasm
Urination/defecation
Relationship to exercise, position, meals, and so on
Define exacerbating and relieving events
Responses to medication or therapy

Once these issues are clarified, the impact of the pain on a patient's daily life must be understood. Alterations in daily activities due to the pain are outlined. Specifically, it is important to determine if sleep patterns have been disrupted, if appetite and exercise have been affected, or if the patient's ability to accomplish tasks of daily living has been hampered. Impact of the pain on sexuality, social and family relationships, and mood must also be determined.

Pain may be described as excruciating, and yet the patient may report that she continues working, caring for her children, and functioning at a normal level. Alternatively, another patient may reveal that she has been unable to function at work or at home for some time because of her symptoms. Clearly, intervention is required to return the second patient to an acceptable quality of life, whereas the first patient may be seeking reassurance that nothing serious or life threatening is causing her pain. The approach to these patients is quite different.

It is important to understand clearly what diagnostic studies have been performed in the past and the patient's interpretation of the results of these studies. Wherever possible, these studies must be obtained directly and reviewed with the patient. An inadvertent remark by a prior caregiver sometimes will have left the patient with an inaccurate assessment of her diagnosis. She may visualize a catastrophic, destructive process going on inside her pelvis, and this apprehension may exacerbate even mild symptoms. Fear of infertility or of future disability may color her interpretation of her pain.

Query which therapeutic interventions have been attempted and their success in controlling the patient's symptoms. What things has she herself tried to improve her pain, and which of them were helpful? It is important to know what medications have been used as well as their specific dosing regimens. Side effects and therapeutic success are noted. A history of narcotic or substance abuse is established. Have surgical procedures been performed in an effort to either diagnose or treat the pain? Beware of a history of many surgical procedures. Patients with a history of sexual or physical abuse may present with a series of acute abdominal emergencies prompting surgical intervention by an unsuspecting physician. A useful rule of thumb is that any patient who has had three operations within a year is depressed until proven otherwise. Such a patient may be eager for any procedure that can "cut out the pain." A history of frequent surgical procedures should prompt a careful investigation of the patient's current and past social situation. If her partner accompanies her to the office, it may be necessary to separate them in order to safely and accurately obtain this information. The patient may be unable or unwilling to share this history in the presence of her partner. Watch for her body language when the issue is addressed. If she appears anxious or upset, consider bringing the issue up again under other circumstances.

It is especially worthwhile to follow the course of the pain from its beginnings, finding out the chronology of spread to other organ systems. What was the first time the patient can remember feeling this pain? What was its character in the beginning, and how has it changed over time? Was it localized initially, and what circumstances have been associated with improvement or exacerbation of the pain? Specifically search for associated life stresses, relationship changes, moves, job changes, and deaths of family members or friends, which may be associated with episodes of increased disability. If the patient has undergone repeated surgical procedures, the impact of *each* operation on the overall experience of pain should be ascertained.

Finally, the patient's current and past state of mental health must be evaluated. This is essential information, but it must be obtained in a nonjudgmental and careful manner. Many of these patients have come to the conclusion that physicians think their pain is "in their head," and therefore they are sensitive about disclosing psychiatric illness or treatment. Validating their current situation by explaining that all people experiencing chronic pain must have some element of depression just because of the chronicity and frustration of their disability may help alleviate concerns about the physician's attitude toward depression and its relationship to patients' physical status.

Past Medical History

In addition to a detailed surgical history, a pattern of other pain syndromes may be elicited. People with chronic constipation as a child may develop irritable bowel symptoms and chronic pelvic pain as teenagers and adults. Inquire about childhood school absences due to illness or menstrual disturbances. A detailed menstrual history must be obtained to determine the relationship of menses to the onset of the pain. Childhood history of frequent urinary tract infections or vaginal bleeding and irritation may be clues to sexual abuse. The recollection of a traumatic hospitalization or examination may be helpful in explaining reactions to current and past interactions with the medical profession. Patients' emotional response to these queries should also be noted. They may not trust the physician sufficiently to disclose details of abuse at the initial encounter; if the physician detects unusual emotional overlay to any issues, these should be highlighted in the chart.

Returning to these questions at a future time may be useful and rewarding.

Social and Family History

A detailed social and family history is essential to understanding a patient and her illness. In particular, a family history of alcoholism or substance abuse may be a clue to physical and emotional abuse as a child. Adult children of alcoholics may develop specific coping mechanisms, burying stresses and avoiding confrontation. They are prone to many stress-related illnesses. A family history of depression, anxiety disorders, and institutionalization is sought. Health habits including diet and exercise are discussed. Does the patient use nicotine or alcohol to help her cope with stressors? Have there been significant changes in weight over time? Employment outside the home and its impact on the patient's family responsibilities should be determined. Is chronic pain the only acceptable mechanism available to the patient to escape from overwhelming social, economic, and family duties? This is a good opportunity to gain some insight into a patient's value systems and her responses to circumstances within the family. A significant illness in a sibling or child may at times create substantial guilt in the patient. Coping with a child with attention deficit disorder can be particularly challenging and frustrating for a working parent. Parents' inability to control the behavior of their child or to help him or her succeed in school may contribute to low self-esteem. Each of these factors has an impact on the perception and interpretation of pain.

It is important to determine the impact of a patient's current level of pain on her personal and sexual relationships. Is the pain problem *the family's* most important problem? How has family life changed in relationship to the patient's problem and treatments for pain? What would change in the family structure and function if the pain went away? Are there any secondary gains from the pain problem? At the same time, a detailed sexual history should be elicited, outlining the evolution of the current level of sexual adjustment or compromise. In particular, search for any events that heralded the onset of pain and sexual dysfunction. Was there any time in the patient's past when sexual activities were pleasurable? Look for specific religious or cultural biases that may affect the patient's interpretation of life events.

Expectations

The interview phase of the evaluation should conclude with a discussion of the patient's hopes and fears. What does she hope to gain from consultation with the clinician, and what are the concerns that she can express? What does she think is causing the pain, and what does she want/hope/expect the outcome of her visit to be? A successful outcome to the encounter can only be achieved if the patient's needs are addressed. It is possible that her goal is to be reassured that she does not have a life-threatening illness, rather than to undergo an exhaustive search for the cause of her pain.

Once her concerns are expressed, it will be possible for the physician to educate her appropriately and tailor the work-up, evaluation, and treatment to the patient's specific goals. This is a true therapeutic partnership and will be most successful in approaching the patient's problem.

7

Physical Examination

Barbara S. Levy, MD

Skill in physical diagnosis reflects a way of thinking more than a way of doing.
Harrison's Textbook of Internal Medicine

The physical examination of a patient with chronic pelvic pain, especially someone with a history of sexual or physical abuse, requires patience, trust, and skill. Nowhere is the attitude of the examiner more important or more obvious than in his or her demeanor. The examination should follow a complete and thorough medical and social history obtained by the examiner. The patient must be permitted to control the situation by choosing to undergo a physical examination. At times, it may be worthwhile to delay the physical examination until a second visit if the patient appears distressed after detailing her history. Reviewing circumstances of prior abuse and previous medical evaluations may be stressful and uncomfortable. Removing one's clothing and submitting to a physical examination may further a sense of vulnerability and lack of control. It is vital to convey to the patient that the physician works for her and will accommodate her wishes with respect to the timing of an examination.

The examination actually begins with observation of the patient while she is still clothed in the consultation room. The general body habitus, posture, and tension level may be assessed while the interview is in progress. Watching the patient as she describes her pain also provides valuable insight. Musculoskeletal factors are assessed as the patient walks from the consultation area to the examination room. Allow a patient time to empty her bladder. Provide a comfortable environment for the examination. Be sure that the temperature is appropriate for someone dressed in a light gown and that the facilities permit privacy. Make every effort to keep the patient waiting as briefly as possible while she is undressed. This situation is stressful for all patients. A chaperone should be available; give the patient the option and record her preference in the chart for the future.

Begin the examination by reassuring the patient that she will not be hurt and that she is in control of the situation. If she elects to terminate the examination, she may do so at any time. This reinforces the concept of a partnership in healing and helps alleviate any sense of vulnerability the patient is experiencing. A systematic approach to the examination progresses from superficial to deep structures. The amount of information gathered is directly proportional to the gentleness and thoroughness of the examiner. As a general rule, specialists begin a physical examination by searching for pathology in the organ system of their specialty. In order to be successful in evaluating and treating patients with chronic pain, it is important to approach the patient as an integrated whole, recognizing that disruption in one organ system may trigger a reaction in adjacent systems.

The sequence of the examination is critical. The bimanual pelvic examination is the most threatening and least useful part of the evaluation because it incorporates many tissue levels. It should be reserved as the final step in the examination.

Examination Sequence

1. Observe the posture and carriage of the patient. Be aware of guarding and careful positioning.
2. *Back.* With the patient seated, look at

her back. Evaluate the symmetry of her paraspinous muscles. Look for scoliosis. Palpate the sacroiliac joints. Gently examine the trapezius and deltoid muscles and their attachments, looking for overall tone and potential trigger points.

3. *Skin.* Hypersensitivity of the abdominal skin is evaluated. Have the patient shift to the supine position. Have her locate the area of maximal discomfort on the abdominal wall. Pinch the skin lightly in each dermatome, comparing the right with the left side to identify the distribution of any hypersensitivity. Skin lesions or scars may be present in a dermatomal distribution, suggesting herpes zoster.
4. *Abdominal wall.* Abdominal wall trigger points are identified by gentle finger pressure. Areas of tenderness are localized and mapped. Scars are gently explored for hernias or nerve entrapment. The ilioinguinal nerve is not uncommonly incorporated into the angle of a Pfannenstiel's incision. Evaluation of the abdominal wall with the patient's head raised off the table and the rectus muscles tense distinguishes abdominal wall from intraabdominal pathology. The tense rectus muscles protect the peritoneum from stretch. Therefore, tenderness that is diminished when the head is raised is likely to be intraperitoneal in origin. Discomfort that is not relieved with this maneuver originates in the abdominal wall and superficial structures or in the neural pathways.
5. *Vulva.* The patient is now guided into the lithotomy position and may be offered a mirror to participate in the examination if she chooses. A sensory examination is performed using light touch with a cotton swab. Observation of the anal wink documents an intact pudendal nerve and functional levator ani. The cotton swab is used to explore the entire introitus, searching for point tenderness. If an area of point tenderness is identified and the structures appear normal to the naked eye, colposcopic examination may be helpful in recognizing vulvar vestibulitis. A single digit is then used to palpate the muscular attachments along the pubic arch and the insertion of the levator ani and coccygeus muscles. Any areas of previous trauma or scar such as episiotomies are also explored for pinpoint tenderness. Have the patient contract and relax the perineal floor around the examiner's finger to assess the general tone of the muscles and the patient's ability to isolate the levators and bulbocavernosus muscles voluntarily.
6. *Vagina, cervix, and paracervical tissues.* Gently continuing into the vaginal canal with a single digit, palpate the lateral vaginal sidewalls. Tenderness in this region may correspond to the sympathetic fibers traveling with the vaginal artery and may identify reflex sympathetic hypersensitivity. Use a cotton swab or a single digit to palpate the paracervical tissues superficially. Vigorous motion stretches the peritoneum and confuses the examination. Palpate the levators (at 4:30 and 7:30) and ask if that reproduces any of the patient's usual discomfort.
7. *Visceral examination.* Continue with a unimanual examination of the genitalia with a single- or double-digit vaginal examination. The abdominal hand should be kept behind the back to remind the examiner not to use it. Begin with palpation of the urethra and the bladder base. Continue cephalad to the cervix and touch it gently. Proceed to the uterosacral ligament region, searching for nodularity and pinpoint tenderness. The lower uterine segment and the lateral vaginal fornices are then examined, noting the position and mobility of the uterus with deliberate, gentle motions. Abnormalities in the shape, size, position, and character of the uterus and ovaries are noted.
8. *Bimanual examination.* Finally, the abdominal hand is added to the examination to clearly define the uterus and adnexal structures. Leave the vaginal digits in place but remove any pressure. Gently place the other hand on the abdomen and again begin a systematic examination of the superficial structures. Note areas of abdominal wall versus visceral discomfort. Avoid trigger points and areas previously identified as significantly uncomfortable for the patient. Finally, a repeat survey of the pelvic viscera including the

cervix, uterus, adnexae, sigmoid colon, cecum, uterosacral ligaments, and the pelvic floor musculature is completed. A rectovaginal examination with a well-lubricated glove facilitates evaluation of the cul-de-sac, the uterosacral ligaments, and rectal disease, including nodularity and polyps. A test for occult blood should be prepared from any stool present on the examining glove.

9. *Speculum examination.* At the conclusion of the bimanual examination, a speculum may be introduced into the vagina for visualization of the cervix, vaginal walls, and fornices. If significant levator spasm is appreciated with the unimanual or bimanual examination, it may not be possible to place a medium speculum comfortably for the patient. A pediatric speculum may be used, or this portion of the examination may be deferred until the levator spasm has been addressed and relaxation of the muscle can be accomplished. During the speculum examination, mucosal lesions, infections, and cervical abnormalities can be visually appreciated. Endometriosis implants may be observed in some patients.

The examination may afford an opportunity for the clinician to begin the educational process. Anatomy should be defined for the patient, and specific areas of tenderness are identified for her as they are found. The relationship, if any, between the areas of pain and recognized pathologic syndromes should be addressed. Many people have only a vague concept of anatomy and the location of structures within the abdomen and pelvis. It is reassuring to patients to be included in the clinician's assessment as painful foci are found. Dictating a note to the referring physician or for the chart in the patient's presence may be educational.

Selected Readings

Braunwald E, Isselbacher K, Petersdorf R, et al (eds): Harrison's Principles of Internal Medicine, 11th ed. New York, McGraw-Hill, 1987, pp 1–25.

Slocumb J: Neurological factors in chronic pelvic pain: Trigger points and the abdominal pelvic pain syndrome. Am J Obstet Gynecol 1984;149:536.

Slocumb JC: Chronic somatic, myofascial, and neurogenic abdominal pelvic pain. Clin Obstet Gynecol 1990;33:145.

8

Pain Intensity, Psychiatric Diagnoses, and Psychosocial Factors: Assessment Rationale and Procedures

Mary Casey Jacob, PhD

Physicians who come to understand the value of managing chronic pelvic pain from a broad, multivariable, interdisciplinary perspective can be bewildered by all the different approaches, perhaps especially by all the different measures of pain and pain-relevant variables. Contributions can be made by many fields, including psychology and psychiatry, physiology, physical and occupational therapy, and even economics. These disciplines may contribute to assessment, prediction of treatment success, treatment planning, and treatment itself. This chapter focuses on the contributions to measurement and evaluation made by psychology. Although psychologic counseling is offered by many types of mental health workers, psychologists are routinely trained in instrument development and psychometrics.

What Psychometric Instruments Do

Psychometric instruments can gather information about many important variables including pain intensity, the experience of pain, psychiatric diagnoses, and psychosocial variables relevant to a person's experience of pain. This information can be useful in a number of ways. First, it can help you to understand a patient's experience of pain and therefore to develop a treatment plan specific to and appropriate for her. Second, the very act of participating in a multivariate assessment is often illuminating to a patient. She may discover that her pain waxes and wanes in ways she did not realize or that her mood and her pain reciprocally influence each other. Third, pretreatment measures can serve as a baseline against which later measures can be compared to determine the patient's progress in her rehabilita tion. Because she may continue to have pain, determining when and where progress is being made can be quite difficult. Thus, specific measures conducted before, during, and after treatment can help you and your patient determine what is helpful in her case. Fourth, data collected with psychometric instruments allow an initial evaluation to be more efficient: Rather than ask each question yourself, you can use the results of a questionnaire battery to focus your own interview with the patient. Importantly, however, one must "distinguish between the role of psychological factors as causal agents in pain and the role of psychological factors in the maintenance and exacerbation of pain. Regardless of the initial cause of nociception . . . a range of cognitive and affective factors can modulate the experience."[1]

Psychometric instruments can be completed by the patient (self-report), by significant others (corroborative reports), or by the clinician. All can be useful, but it is especially important to allow the patient a significant amount of self-reporting and then for her to be given feedback on the records and instruments she completes so that she knows what is being done with the information.

Many attempts have been made to examine psychologic factors associated with pain. Many early attempts relied on traditional psychologic tests, including personality tests, that had been developed and standardized on mentally ill populations. More recently, attempts have been made to develop instruments specifically for pain populations, to explore the use of instruments developed for medical patients generally, and to develop norms for chronic pain populations for instruments developed using other populations.

Validity of Psychometrics

Pain is a perception, and as such can be measured only indirectly. This is also true of many other variables pertinent to the care of a patient with chronic pain, including mood and coping variables. Because many of these constructs can be measured only indirectly (behavioral observations of pain behaviors are an exception), the validity and reliability of the instruments are critical.

Validity is a crucial consideration in selecting an assessment instrument for use. It refers to the "appropriateness, meaningfulness, and usefulness *of the specific inferences made from test scores*"[2] (italics added). In other words, does the instrument give you information that is appropriate for the inferences you wish to make? There are several different kinds of validity-related evidence. Two are especially important in this context. *Construct-related validity* refers to evidence that a test or instrument does in fact measure a specific theoretic construct. Examples of theoretic constructs are pain, depression, hypochondriasis, and extroversion. Construct-related validity is established by collecting information in a number of ways and then looking at the relationship of that information to the test score of interest. Does the information correlate with the test score in the predicted fashion? *Criterion-related validity* refers to evidence that test scores are systematically and predictably related to one or more outcome criteria. The key question is, How accurately can performance (e.g., participation in a rehabilitation program) be predicted from the test results? *Standardization* refers to the development of norms for specific populations. An instrument standardized on patients in a psychiatric day hospital, for example, is not necessarily valid for use with people in pain.

When a person takes a test or completes a measurement instrument on two different occasions, different scores may result. When this happens, the variations could be due to different test-taking conditions, fatigue or anxiety, true changes (from interventions or maturation) in the individual such that different scores *should* result, or flaws in the test itself called *errors of measurement*. *Reliability* "refers to the degree to which test scores are free from errors of measurement."[2] Several kinds of reliability are important, and each is determined statistically. *Internal consistency* refers to the degree to which items purporting to measure one construct "hang together" statistically; this form of reliability is generally reported with a statistic called *Chronbach's alpha*.[3] Stability is measured with *test-retest reliability*. This refers to the likelihood that the same score will result if a person retakes the test several weeks or so after the first administration, under the same conditions. Take marital satisfaction as an example. Although a woman may feel somewhat differently about her marriage from day to day, a reliable marital satisfaction instrument does not pick up those tiny fluctuations, and if she completed the instrument twice, several weeks apart, she should have very similar scores. If, on the other hand, a year passes, change might well have occurred, for better or worse. Thus, test-retest reliability is important when we select instruments that might show treatment effects: We want to be able to assume that changes are due to treatment and not to instability in the measure. A third form of reliability is *parallel-form reliability*. An instrument is sometimes administered more than once, and a concern is that memory for the first administration might influence answers on the second administration. To avoid this, two or more different forms of an instrument are developed. Parallel-form reliability refers to the degree to which the forms are truly comparable, so that if a person took both of them, one right after the other, similar scores would be obtained on each.

Many reliable and valid measures are available to clinicians. Some are developed specifically to measure pain variables, and others are used more widely to measure pain-relevant variables such as mood, marital/relationship satisfaction, and tendency to somatize. Knowledgeable and ethical developers of tests make their validity and reliability information available to all potential test users so that informed judgments can be made about when and how a test might be appropriately used. I recommend operating primarily from the perspective of what might be helpful to you and the patient in planning treatment, unless you are researching theoretic questions. For this reason, I do not discuss a number of instruments about which much has been written, such as the Minnesota Multiphasic Personality Inventory (MMPI)[4] and the MMPI-2,[5] because their results require extensive training and expertise to interpret but rarely contribute significantly to treatment planning.

Table 8–1 and the following paragraphs describe some commonly used measures, but this is not by any means an exhaustive list. Note that all the instruments in Table 8–1 can be administered and scored after minimal training. Interpretation of the results, however, is more complex. Some of the instruments, such as those that measure pain intensity or a history of abuse, have obvious face validity, and any experienced pain clinician can make use of the results after some training and experience. If you wish to use these instruments, you should at least read the published reports of their development, including their purpose and appropriate uses. Other instruments, such as the Beck Depression Inventory, target constructs and can be purchased and interpreted only by someone with specific training in the use and interpretation of psychometric instruments. Instruments that fall into the latter group are noted with an asterisk.

Pain Measures

Turk and Melzack have written that pain intensity is the "most salient" feature of pain.[1] (Other salient features are its related affective dimension and its location.[6] I focus on intensity here.) Patient recall of past pain intensity is influenced by present pain intensity,[7] and retrospective reports are generally overestimates.[8] Pain ratings are also known to be influenced by gender, exposure to role models tolerating painful stimuli (or not), setting, and time of day.[6] Pain does fluctuate in most cases, although patients are often unaware of this or unaware that the fluctuations may be predictable. An accurate clinical picture can be formed only with pain ratings gathered in real time and with summaries of ratings gathered over days or weeks.[9] These summary ratings are also more sensitive to treatment effects than single ratings.[10]

It is important to understand that many patients have, over time and unconsciously, escalated their reports of pain severity in their efforts to be believed and to get help. One important step to take then is to let patients know that you understand this, ask that they attempt to report their pain accurately to you, and request that they follow your instructions for rating pain in a routine way.[6] This is a good way of introducing the need for methodic pain ratings for a period of time.

The most common methods of pain intensity evaluation are verbal rating scales, visual analogue scales (VASs), and numeric rating scales.

Verbal rating scales consist of lists of adjectives describing different levels of pain, and the patient is asked to pick the word that best describes her pain. Benefits of this approach include good compliance rates (probably because the directions are easy to understand),[11] established validity, and sensitivity to treatments known to influence pain intensity.[6, 12] Drawbacks include the need for a relatively high rate of literacy, the need to be sure that patients read the whole list of adjectives before selecting one, and inherent difficulties in the assumption that the words are equidistant in terms of pain intensity.[6]

Table 8–1. **COMMONLY USED INSTRUMENTS**

Instrument	Description	Pros and Cons	Source
Pain and the Pain Experience			
McGill Pain Questionnaire[14]	Measures subjective pain experience	Widely used. Short form available.[30] May aid in differential diagnosis of various pain syndromes.	Melzack, 1975[14]
West Haven–Yale Multidimensional Pain Inventory (WHYMPI)[17, 31]	52 items, 12 scales. Evaluates varied dimensions of the pain experience	Helps identify targets for treatment. Widely used.	Kerns and Jacob, 1992[31]
Significant-Other WHYMPI[19]	17 items; solicitous, distracting, and punishing scales corresponding to the WHYMPI scales	Significant-other data are a useful addition to patient self-reports, but it can be difficult to involve family members. Can help indicate if intervention in the relationship is needed.	Kerns and Rosenberg, 1995[19]
Illness Behavior Inventory[20]	20 items; measure of illness behaviors on work and social dimensions	Easily used with pain patients. Assists in educating patients about the role of pain behaviors in the maintenance of pain.	Loyd S. Pettegrew, Dept. of Communication, University of South Florida, Tampa, FL 33620
Pain Behavior Check List[21]	17 items, 4 scales to measure frequency of pain behaviors	Allows evaluation of low-frequency behaviors not easily observed; points to areas for clinical intervention.	Kerns et al, 1991[21]
Daily Sleep Diary[18]	Nightly monitoring of 7 sleep variables found to be more related to mood disorders than to pain	Allows assessment of need for sleep interventions and may be valuable in monitoring treatment gains.	Haythornthwaite et al, 1991[18]
Mood Measures: State and Trait			
*Beck Depression Inventory[32]	21 items to assess the severity of depression	Widely used with pain populations. Caution required because some items are somatic and not easily interpreted in the presence of pain.	Copyrighted. Must be purchased from The Psychological Corp., 555 Academic Court, San Antonio, TX 78204
*Hamilton Rating Scale for Depression[33]	17 or 21 item *interview* for use with persons known to be suffering an affective disorder	Not meant to be used as a self-rating scale; requires skilled interviewers and raters for reliability; self-report forms have not been validated.	Hamilton, 1960[33]
Zung Self-Rating Depression Scale[34]	20 items to measure severity of depression	Does not distinguish depression well in persons who are also anxious.[35]	Zung, 1965[34]
Center for Epidemiologic Studies Depression Scale[36]	20 items to screen for presence of depression	Designed to assess point prevalence depressive symptoms in a general population for research purposes (not clinical screening); too many items are not specific to depression; high rate of false positives.[35]	Markush and Favero, 1974[36]

Table 8–1. **COMMONLY USED INSTRUMENTS** *(Continued)*

Instrument	Description	Pros and Cons	Source
*State-Trait Anxiety Inventory[37, 38]	Separate state and trait anxiety scales each of 20 items	Widely used in clinical settings; has published norms for medical and surgical patients.	Copyrighted. Must be purchased from Mind Garden, 3803 East Bayshore Rd, Palo Alto, CA 94303
*State-Trait Anger Expression Inventory[39–41]	44 items total, 5 clinical scales: state anger, trait anger, anger in, anger out, anger control	Published medical and surgical norms	Copyrighted. Must be purchased from Psychological Assessment Resources, Inc., P.O. Box 998, Odessa, FL 33556-9901
Marriage and Relationships			
Dyadic Adjustment Scale[42]	32 items to assess quality of relationship	Written for any dyad, married or not. Behaviorally specific.	Spanier, 1976[42]
Locke-Wallace Marital Adjustment Test[43]	15 items to assess marital adjustment	Worded for married couples only. Global measure; won't target areas for treatment.	Locke and Wallace, 1959[43]
Miscellaneous			
Abuse history[44]	12 items eliciting history of sexual and physical abuse in childhood and in adulthood	Coming into common use. Describes specific experiences rather than asking about abuse generally. Easily adapted to include history of emotional abuse. No published reliability data.	Drossman et al, 1990[44]; Leserman et al, 1995[45]

*Cannot be purchased and/or should not be interpreted without specific training in psychology and/or testing; see catalogs for details.

A VAS uses a line, generally 10 cm long (Fig. 8–1). The line is labeled at each end by either words (e.g., *no pain* to *the worst pain possible*) or numbers (e.g., 0 to 10 or 0 to 100). Some VASs also have intermediate words or numbers, and these are called *graphic rating scales.* In either case, the patient rates her pain by marking the line at the point most representative of the pain for her. VASs are scored by measuring the distance from the no-pain end of the line to the point marked by the patient. The scale of measurement generally is the millimeter, and thus the VAS has 101 points. VASs are valid and reliable and are sensitive to treatment effects. They are easy to administer, but some patients have difficulty understanding them. Scoring can be time consuming and influenced by measurement error. It is not clear that the VAS offers advantages over verbal or numeric rating scales in a clinical setting, and it probably should not be used as the only measure of pain intensity.[6]

Numeric rating scales ask patients to assign a number to their pain, generally on a scale of 0 to 10 or 0 to 100, where 0 = no pain and the high end of the scale equals the worst pain possible. Numeric scales are commonly used and are appealing for their simplicity, but it is not clear whether they are responsive to treatment changes.[6, 13]

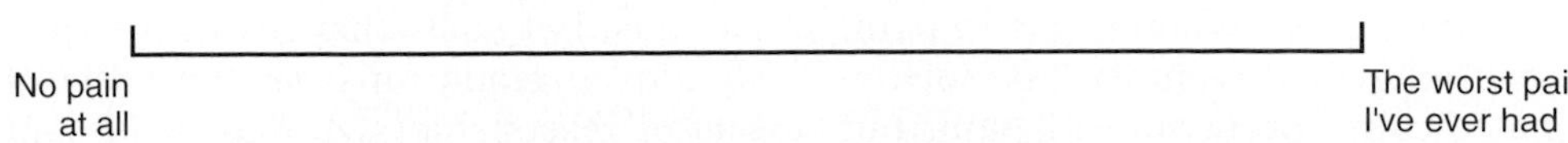

Figure 8–1. Visual analogue scale.

These scales can be combined in some instances. For example, the McGill Pain Questionnaire,[14] part 4, uses a 1 to 5 scale in which each number is verbally anchored: 1 = mild, 2 = discomforting, 3 = distressing, 4 = horrible, and 5 = excruciating. If you add a zero point anchored by the words *no pain*, you have a combined verbal and numeric rating scale.[15] This verbal/numeric scale can be further enhanced by adding the components of a behavioral rating scale such as that of Budzynski and colleagues.[16] They have definitions for all six points on the scale. Two examples are 1 = mild = pain that "enters awareness only at times when attention is devoted to it" and 5 = excruciating = "intense, incapacitating." I have found that the use of behavioral anchors helps patients use the scales more deliberately, and they are frequently surprised by the relatively low ratings they use.

The Pain Experience

In addition to measuring pain intensity in some way, it is important to evaluate other aspects of a patient's experience of pain. Variables commonly assessed include

- Pain beliefs
- Pain intrusion
- Pain behaviors
- Common responses of others to the patient when she expresses her pain
- Amount of disability
- The reciprocal relationship between pain intensity and depression, anxiety, and anger
- Marital/relationship satisfaction
- General somatic vigilance
- Sleep

The WHYMPI (pronounced why-em-pee-eye)[17, 18] is an example of an instrument designed to assess a number of the variables listed earlier. The Significant-Other WHYMPI[19] is intended to be completed by the patient's most significant relation, asking for that person's self-report of how he or she responds to the patient when she is in pain. The Illness Behavior Inventory[20] is not designed specifically for people in pain, but its general evaluation of illness behaviors is applicable to them. The Pain Behavior Check List[21] asks for patient self-reports on frequency of behaviors that communicate pain in four areas: distorted ambulation, affective distress, facial and audible expressions, and seeking help. The Daily Sleep Diary[18] describes one approach to monitoring changes in sleep patterns. All these instruments are available for use in general clinical practice, but because their utility is enhanced by familiarity with their details, they are most often used in specialty pain clinics.

Mood Measures

Mood *disorders* are common sequelae of chronic pain, are related to perceived pain intensity,[22] can influence a patient's readiness and ability to participate in rehabilitation,[23] and are among the most treatable of psychiatric conditions. Mood *dispositions* can also influence a person's response to the experience of pain and her readiness to take a self-management perspective. In psychologic parlance, measures of current mood disorders are often referred to as *state* measures and those of disposition are referred to as *trait* measures. For patients with chronic pain, the most useful mood measures are ones of depression, anxiety, and anger (see Table 8–1). Be cautioned, however, that these instruments should never be used as the sole method of diagnosis. Additional confirmatory information should always be acquired (e.g., by interview) before judging the patient to have a psychiatric diagnosis. This is especially true in evaluating patients with medical conditions, because a condition such as pain often directly causes a number of symptoms, such as fatigue or worry, that might be counted by an instrument as part of a mood problem when in fact it is present purely because of the pain and is not generalized. This is why instruments designed for general or psychiatric populations are sometimes used with different diagnostic cutoff scores for medical patients, but such changes in interpretation should be made only on the basis of data sets of reasonable size and good statistical analyses.

Marital/Relationship Variables

Measures of marital/relationship satisfaction and functioning can be useful in several ways. Numerous publications testify to a relationship between depression and marital satisfaction independent of pain intensity or duration.[23–28] It may be that people with strong relationships are buffered from developing depression in response to chronic pain. Also, some ways that partners/spouses respond to a woman in pain are helpful in coping and some ways are not and may even contribute to the maintenance of the pain.[26, 28]

Interpretation

The results of psychometric measures are preliminarily interpreted by comparing them with the means and standard deviations of those of other, similar individuals. For patients with chronic pain, that ideally means comparing them with other patients with chronic pain. Some instruments have norms for pain or medical patients, but many do not. After making initial interpretations based on the instruments, all other data from interviews and observations should be incorporated into your thinking about the variables having a role in any one patient's pain.

Interview Data

Almost certainly it is already your practice to interview each of your patients to ascertain her history and her concerns. In working with patients with chronic pain, it is important to have a fairly routine way of doing so, in order to collect complete data for each person. Without an outline of sorts, you run the risk of pursuing your first hypothesis to the exclusion of others. Because we know that chronic pain is virtually always multifactorial, any one hypothesis is almost sure to be incomplete. A single hypothesis might lead you to the patient's original, organic source of pain, but it does not help you understand all the ways in which her pain has now altered her life and all the areas in which she might need help to recover or adapt.

Structured interviews are ones in which a script is followed and each answer is coded on a scale, for example a scale of 1 to 4. Few reliability data are available for the published structured interviews, and most clinicians rely on semistructured interviews or guides for the interview in which notes are taken rather than answers coded. Bradley and colleagues[29] suggest that any semistructured interview have at least the following goals:

- Obtain a pain history
- Identify events that reliably precede or follow pain exacerbations
- Identify predictable responses from the patient's significant others when she expresses her pain
- Evaluate the patient's activities and the ways that they have changed since the onset of the pain
- Determine if the patient has other relatives or friends with chronic pain and what her exposure to them has been or currently is
- Inquire about a history of abuse
- Evaluate the current degree of affective distress

In general clinical practice, once you recognize that a patient is presenting a chronic pain problem, it may be practical to break up the evaluation into several visits. This communicates to the patient that you are taking a deliberate, thoughtful approach to her condition, which is not an emergency. It also allows the mental health evaluation to be integrated with the medical evaluation, and you avoid the pitfall of referring to a mental health worker only when an organic cause is not identified.

Talking to Patients About Psychometric Instruments

Used with tact and honesty, psychometric instruments can be immensely helpful. Introducing them to a patient who may already wonder if you believe that her pain is real must be done with care. Your introduction should include the following topics and statements:

- A conversation that addresses the common concomitants of pain such as mood changes, insomnia, missed time from work, feeling that others don't understand, and changes in primary relationships.
- A statement that your work with the patient will have two goals: (1) to diagnose and treat her medical condition to the best of your ability and (2) to help her reclaim her life from the pain.
- To work toward these two goals, it is important that you have as much information as possible about all the ways in which the pain has affected her life. You could ask her a million questions and charge her for your time, or you could ask her to complete some questionnaires and self-monitoring tasks and let you have a look at them before you meet the next time.
- The information she provides will be used in two ways: first, to help plan her treatment, and later, to see what kind of progress is being made in what areas.
- After you receive the questionnaires from her, you (or your consultant) will discuss with her what they suggest, and she will have a chance to say, "I don't think that is really accurate about me."

Using this approach, I have never had a patient refuse or even demonstrate reluctance to complete these instruments.

Collaboration with Mental Health Specialists

Most physicians choose to team up with other specialists to develop a comprehensive interdisciplinary assessment and treatment approach—but where to start? A number of mental health disciplines have something to offer. You might want to bring someone directly into your practice, you might want to refer as needed, or you might want to have one person in your office manage the assessment process and then perform much of the treatment with outside referrals as appropriate.

What individual disciplines are allowed to do varies greatly from state to state, with few exceptions. One exception is that only psychologists (and some educators) are routinely trained in psychometric development and standardized testing and are licensed to conduct personality assessments. In some states, only doctoral level psychologists and psychiatrists are licensed to conduct therapy. In other states, master's level psychologists, social workers, and nurses are legally able to provide these services. Unfortunately, even where these professionals can legally practice, they may be shut out of participation in managed care plans.

Ordinary clinical training for most mental health professionals does not include exposure to normal and abnormal responses to health and illness or to the issues around coping with chronic illness. A *health* or *medical* psychologist is a person with ordinary clinical training but also with extensive training in working with medical patients and working in a medical setting. I recommend that you use a Ph.D. or Psy.D. Health or Medical Psychologist licensed for clinical practice to help you plan your assessment and to train you in the consumption of the resulting information. Depending on the complexity of the assessment, you might not need a Ph.D. to carry out the assessments or offer treatment. A master's level clinician might carry out the assessments, or you might develop an assessment battery that can be managed by physicians and nurses. Even so, however, it is a good idea to have a Ph.D. consultant who can advise on complex cases or cases in which serious mental illness coexists with the chronic pain problem. This consultant can also offer treatment.

Collaboration Issues

Mental health professionals are trained to observe confidentiality strictly except when a patient is believed to be an imminent danger to herself or others. This doctrine is interpreted literally, and thus we do not even acknowledge a person to be a patient unless we have been given permission to do so. What this means when mental health professionals collaborate with physicians is that we must take the step of explaining to the patient how the team works and that the team does share information, and we should obtain written consent for this. The consent should outline the limits of confidentiality very clearly. This step protects the team from a liability perspective, and importantly, it is another way the patient is educated about this team approach.

During the course of evaluation and treatment, it is common for a patient to ask one professional to keep a secret from the team. It is generally not advisable to agree to this, although the patient should also understand that medical records and team conversations focus only on what is pertinent to her care.

Collaboration also means that a patient may feel she is being repeatedly asked the same questions. In some cases this is true, and she can be prepared for this by educating her about each person's role and by explaining that the questions are asked for different reasons by each discipline. For example, a physician may ask about a patient's current narcotic use from a medical perspective and to consider what the patient expects now. A psychologist may ask because this has a bearing on depression and on willingness to undertake self-management tasks. A physical therapist may ask because the patient appears sedated. Keep in mind that just as interdisciplinary collaboration may be new to you, it is probably new to the patient too.

Closing Thoughts

Patients with chronic pain generally pose quite a challenge: They can puzzle you and they can frustrate you. Patients feel frustrated too, and they benefit from an evaluation and treatment plan that takes into account not just medical status but all the other variables that affect pain or are a result of pain. A wealth of clinical experience is available to you through the use of psychometric instruments. Used appropriately and judiciously, they will help you feel more able to care for the whole patient.

References

1. Turk DC, Melzack R: The measurement of pain and the assessment of people experiencing pain. In Turk DC, Melzack R (eds): Handbook of Pain Assessment. New York, Guilford Press, 1992, p 3.
2. American Educational Research Association, American Psychological Association, National Council on Measurement in Education: Standards for Educational and Psychological Testing. Washington, DC, American Psychological Association, 1985, pp. 9, 19.
3. Chronbach LJ: Coefficient alpha and the internal structure of tests. Psychometrika 1951;16:297.
4. Hathaway S, McKinley JC: MMPI Manual. Minneapolis, University of Minnesota Press, 1970.
5. MMPI Restandardization Committee: MMPI-2 Manual for Administration and Scoring. Minneapolis, University of Minnesota Press, 1989.
6. Jensen MP, Karoly P: Self-report scales and procedures for assessing pain in adults. In Turk DC, Melzack R (eds): Handbook of Pain Assessment. New York, Guilford Press, 1992, p 135.
7. Eich E, Reeves J, Jaeger B, et al: Memory for pain: Relation between past and present pain intensity. Pain 1985;23:375.
8. Linton SJ, Gotestam KG: A clinical comparison of two pain scales: Correlation, remembering chronic pain and a measure of compliance. Pain 1983; 17:57.
9. Jensen MP, McFarland CA: Increasing the reliability and validity of pain intensity measurement in chronic pain patients. Pain 1993;55:195.
10. Max MB: Neuropathic pain syndromes. In Max MB, Portenoy R, Laska E (eds): Advances in Pain Research and Therapy. New York, Springer, 1991, p 193.
11. Jensen MP, Karoly P, Braver S: The measurement of clinical pain intensity: A comparison of six methods. Pain 1986;27:117.
12. Fox EJ, Melzack R: Transcutaneous electrical stimulation and acupuncture: Comparison of treatment for low-back pain. Pain 1976;2:141.
13. Turner JA: Comparison of group progressive-relaxation training and cognitive-behavioral group therapy for chronic low back pain. J Consult Clin Psychol 1982;50:757.
14. Melzack R: The McGill Pain Questionnaire: Major properties and scoring methods. Pain 1975;1:277.
15. Kerns RD, Finn P, Haythornthwaite J: Self-monitored pain intensity: Psychometric properties and clinical utility. J Behav Med 1988;11:71.
16. Budzynski TH, Stoyva JM, Adler CS, et al: EMG biofeedback and tension headache: A controlled outcome study. Psychosom Med 1973;35:484.
17. Kerns RD, Turk DC, Rudy TE: The West Haven–Yale Multidimensional Pain Inventory (WHYMPI). Pain 1985;23:345.
18. Haythornthwaite JA, Hegel MT, Kerns RD: Development of a sleep diary for chronic pain patients. J Pain Symptom Manage 1991;6:65.
19. Kerns RD, Rosenberg R: Pain relevant responses from significant others: Development of a significant-other version of the WHYMPI scales. Pain 1995;61:245.
20. Turkat ID, Pettegrew LS: Development and validation of the Illness Behavior Inventory. J Behav Assess 1983;5:35.
21. Kerns RD, Haythornthwaite J, Rosenberg R, et al: The Pain Behavior Check List (PBCL): Factor structure and psychometric properties. J Behav Med 1991;14:155.
22. Haythornthwaite JA, Sieber WJ, Kerns RD: Depression and the chronic pain experience. Pain 1991;46:177.

23. Kerns RD, Haythornthwaite JA: Depression among chronic pain patients: Cognitive-behavioral analysis and effect on rehabilitation outcome. J Consult Clin Psychol 1988;56:870.
24. Thomas M, Roy R: Pain patients and marital relations. Clin J Pain 1989;5:255.
25. Kerns RD, Turk DC: Depression and chronic pain: The mediating role of the spouse. J Marriage Fam 1984;46:845.
26. Kerns RD, Haythornthwaite J, Southwick S, et al: The role of marital interaction in chronic pain and depressive symptom severity. J Psychosom Res 1990;34:401.
27. Kerns RD, Haythornthwaite J: Marital support as a buffer from depression among chronic pain patients. Paper presented at the annual meeting of the Association for the Advancement of Behavior Therapy, Boston, November 1987.
28. Kerns RD, Haythornthwaite J: The differential roles of global marital support and specific spouse response to chronic pain behavior. Paper presented at the annual meeting of the Association for the Advancement of Behavior Therapy, Boston, November 1987.
29. Bradley LA, Haile JM, Jaworski TM: Assessment of psychological status using interviews and self-report instruments. In Turk DC, Melzack R (eds): Handbook of Pain Assessment. New York, Guilford Press, 1992, p 193.
30. Melzack R: The short-form McGill Pain Questionnaire. Pain 1987;30:191.
31. Kerns RD, Jacob MC: Assessment of the psychosocial context of the experience of chronic pain. In Turk DC, Melzack R (eds): Handbook of Pain Assessment. New York, Guilford Press, 1992, p 235.
32. Beck AT, Ward CH, Mendelson M, et al: An inventory for measuring depression. Arch Gen Psychiatry 1961;4:561.
33. Hamilton M: A rating scale for depression. J Neurol Neurosurg Psychiatry 1960;23:56.
34. Zung WWK: A self-rating depression scale. Arch Gen Psychiatry 1965;12:63.
35. Rabkin JG, Klein DF: The clinical measurement of depressive disorders. In Marsella AJ, Hirschfeld RMA, Katz MM (eds): The Measurement of Depression. New York, Guilford Press, 1987, p 30.
36. Markush RE, Favero RV: Epidemiologic assessment of stressful life events, depressed mood, and psychophysiological symptoms: A preliminary report. In Dohrenwend BS, Dohrenwend BP (eds): Stressful Life Events: Their Nature and Effects. New York City, John Wiley, 1974, p 171.
37. Speilberger CD: Manual for the State-Trait Anxiety Inventory: STAI (Form Y). Palo Alto, Consulting Psychologists Press, 1983.
38. Spielberger CD, Vagg PR, Barker LR, et al: The factor structure of the State-Trait Anxiety Inventory. In Sarason IG, Spielberger CD (eds): Stress and Anxiety. New York, Hemisphere/Wiley, 1980.
39. Speilberger CD: State-Trait Anger Expression Inventory. Odessa, FL, Psychological Assessment Resources, 1991.
40. Spielberger CD, Jacobs G, Russell S, et al: Assessment of anger: The state-trait anger scale. In Butcher JN, Spielberger CD (eds): Advances in Personality Assessment. Hillsdale, NJ, Lawrence Erlbaum Associates, 1983, p 161.
41. Spielberger CD, Johnson EH, Russell SF, et al: The experience and expression of anger: Construction and validation of an anger expression scale. In Chesney MA, Rosenman RH (eds): Anger and Hostility in Cardiovascular and Behavioral Disorders. New York, Hemisphere/McGraw-Hill, 1985, p 5.
42. Spanier GB: Measuring dyadic adjustment: New scales for assessing the quality of marriage and similar dyads. J Marriage Fam 1976;38:15.
43. Locke HJ, Wallace KM: Short marital-adjustment and prediction tests: Their reliability and validity. Marriage Fam Living 1959;21:251.
44. Drossman DA, Leserman J, Nachman G, et al: Sexual and physical abuse in women with functional or organic gastrointestinal disorders. Ann Intern Med 1990;113:828.
45. Leserman, J, Drossman DA, Li Z: The reliability and validity of a sexual and physical abuse history questionnaire in female patients with gastrointestinal disorders. Behav Med 1995;21:141.

9

Sexual Dysfunction

Gloria A. Bachmann, MD, and Nancy A. Phillips, MD

Human sexual activity is a complex process requiring precise coordination between neurologic, vascular, and endocrine systems. The sexual development and expressions of both men and women also incorporate personal, cultural, religious, and societal attitudes. Additionally, the sexuality of an individual is significantly influenced by the interpersonal relationship between the partners, each of whom brings unique psychologic needs and responses into the union. A breakdown in any of these areas, which often occurs in patients with chronic pelvic pain (CPP), may result in either sexual difficulties or in some instances sexual dysfunctions.

CPP, whether organic or psychosocial, is generated through organ systems and neural pathways in a manner similar to the sexual response, and thus the two may be interrelated. A history of past or current sexual abuse or trauma may have a role in the development or CPP or sexual dysfunction. Conversely, CPP may be the cause of unpleasant sexual encounters, creating an environment that contributes to or facilitates the development of sexual dysfunction through both psychologic and physical mechanisms.

Primary health care providers should be especially attentive to patients with CPP and should inquire about sexual difficulties because pelvic pain and sexual problems often coexist. An understanding of the basic sexual response and treatment of common sexual dysfunctions helps practitioners provide comprehensive care to patients with CPP.

The Sexual Response

Masters and Johnson first described the sexual response in four phases: excitement, plateau, orgasm, and resolution.[1] Since then, the sexual response cycle has usually been described as desire, arousal (excitement), orgasm, and resolution. The plateau period, which is defined as the bridge between arousal and orgasm, is included in the arousal (or excitement) phase.[2, 3]

The desire phase encompasses sex drive and interest, the feelings that commence the sexual response cycle. Various psychosocial factors such as self-esteem and relationship status and organic factors such as health and medication use influence this sexual phase. Neurologic and endocrine factors probably contribute as well, but few studies have explored these areas. Of all endocrine factors, androgens appear to be most directly related to sexual motivational thoughts, feelings, and desires.

The arousal phase is physiologically a preparation for orgasm. Psychologically, it can be a potent reinforcer (either positive or negative) for sexual behavior and is initiated by both physical and emotional stimuli. Arousal results in pronounced vasodilatation, causing penile erection in males and vaginal lubrication and clitoral engorgement in females. Erection, primarily a parasympathetic response, results from dilatation of the arteries of the penis, causing vasocongestion in the erectile tissue of the corpus cavernosum and spongiosum located within the shaft. The erectile tissue, which is embedded in fibrous sheaths, consists of many arterioles and venules that form cavernous venous sinuses. Smooth muscle bundles at the base of the arterioles and venules relax with excitement, facilitating blood flow, and the fibrous sheaths aid in the buildup of hydrostatic pressure. Venous closure, which may be sympathetically mediated, also aids in this process.

In females, sexual arousal is also a parasympathetically mediated response, resulting in vasodilatation of the genital vasculature. Vaginal lubrication is mainly a transudate from the engorged capillary beds of the vaginal epithelium, although mucoid secretions from the Bartholin's glands and the endocervical glands of the cervix contribute a small amount. Erectile tissue similar to that in males is found around the introitus and in the clitoris and is responsible for clitoral tumescence and the formation of the *orgasmic platform*, an area at the distal one third of the vagina where blood becomes sequestered.[2] The smooth muscle of the internal vaginal vault relaxes, with a resultant increase in vaginal depth and length and elevation of the uterus (Fig. 9–1).

Orgasm, the third phase of the sexual cycle, is a series of 0.8-second contractions of the pelvic musculature resulting in a feeling of release from the progressive engorgement of the genitalia in both sexes. It is a predominantly sympathetic response, thought to be the culmination of neural recruitment, although the mechanism is not clearly understood.[4] In males, orgasm consists of emission and ejaculation, followed by a refractive period, whereas the female orgasm has no corresponding emission or refractive period.

In males, emission is the simultaneous movement of sperm from the vas deferens and the expulsion of prostatic and seminal fluid to the internal urethra, where they mix together with mucus from the bulbourethral glands to become semen. The semen remains in the internal urethra under pressure, creating a sense of fullness known as *ejaculatory inevitability*. This feeling is first relative (because it can be controlled by decreasing stimulation); then it becomes absolute. At the point where it becomes absolute, sensory signals trigger sympathetic impulses

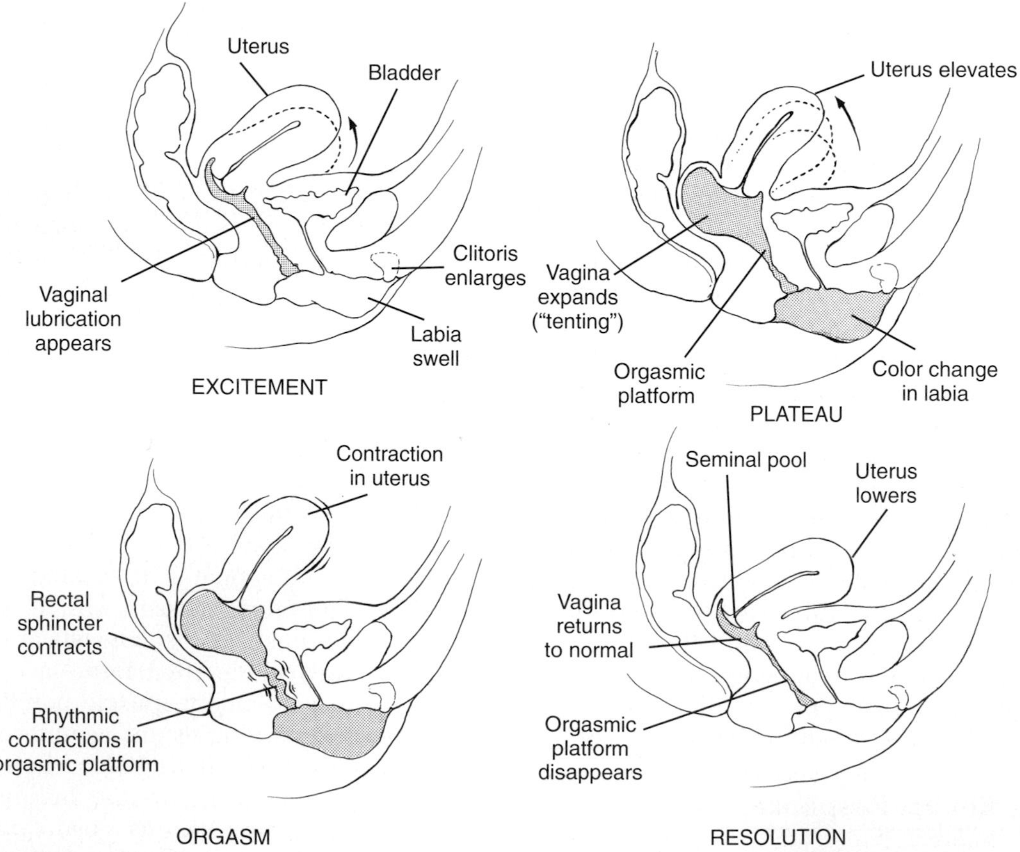

Figure 9–1. Female genital organs' adaptation to the sexual response cycle. (From Masters W, Johnson V: Sex and Human Loving. Boston, Little, Brown & Co, 1985.)

resulting in rhythmic contractions of the striated muscles of the bulbocavernosus and ischiocavernosus muscles, causing ejaculation. The resolution phase in males has a refractory period during which no further orgasm is possible. The length of time of the refractory period is variable among individuals and is also age dependent.

The female orgasm, which is still not clearly defined, probably results from neuronal recruitment from clitoral and anterior vaginal wall stimulation with a sympathetically mediated component. Orgasm results in recurrent 0.8-second contractions of the bulbocavernosus and ischiocavernosus muscles and the uterus. No refractory period follows female orgasm, and thus women can experience many orgasms in quick succession.

In both men and women, tachycardia (110 to 180 beats per minute), an increased respiratory rate (as high as 40 per minute), and blood pressure elevation (systolic from 30 to 80 mm Hg and diastolic from 20 to 40 mm Hg) occurs during arousal and orgasm.

The resolution phase is the period during which the physiologic changes of excitement and orgasm revert to resting levels. Although the arousal and orgasm phase may resolve in minutes and most vasocongestion within seconds, complete resolution may take as long as 1 hour.

Neurologically, the phases of the sexual response cycle are incompletely defined, although animal studies and human pathologic conditions show that the limbic system and hypothalamus are intimately involved not only in sexual behavior but also in other emotional responses such as rage, fear, and motivation. Autonomic responses (e.g., blood pressure and respiration) are also tied to the limbic system and hypothalamus.[5] Dopamine is thought to promote the sexual response, whereas serotonin inhibits it.[4]

Neural pathways may be stimulated by physical and nonphysical (visual, imagined) stimuli. The former involve an afferent arc from the genitals by way of the pudendal nerve and sacral reflex center in the spinal cord and from nongenital areas by way of their afferent pathways to the spinal cord, with both ascending to the cerebral cortex. The efferent loop travels through the spinal

Table 9–1. **ENDOCRINOPATHIES CAUSING DISORDERS OF DESIRE (DIMINISHED LIBIDO)**

Acromegaly
Addison's disease
Cushing's disease*
Diabetes mellitus†
Hyperprolactinemia
Hypothyroidism or hyperthyroidism
Hypopituitarism

*May cause diminished or increased desire.
†Also causes arousal disorders.
Adapted from Munjack D: The recognition and management of desire phase sexual dysfunction. In Sciarra JJ (ed): Obstetrics and Gynecology, vol 6. 1986[39]; *and* Ganong WF (ed): Review of Medical Physiology, 17th ed. Norwalk, CT, Appleton & Lange, 1995, pp 233–236.[5]

cord to its sacral portion, where parasympathetic impulses are activated in the arousal phase, and to its lumbar and sacral portion, where sympathetic impulses are activated in the hypogastric and pelvic plexus for the orgasm phase.[4] Penile erection ability following spinal cord injury suggests that the cerebrum and spinal reflex center may also act independently.

Data on the effects of gonadal hormones on sexual behavior are accumulating. Both androgens and estrogen appear to affect sexual behavior in both men and women. Androgens seem to be the more significant hormone for sexual motivational responses in both males and females, whereas in females, estrogen is needed for maintenance of vaginal vault anatomy and physiology. The absence of gonadal hormones before puberty and after menopause does not, however, negate the sexual response: Prepubertal boys experience erection, and postmenopausal women report orgasm.

Various nongonadal endocrinopathies also affect libido and the sexual response, as in thyroid and adrenal disease, suggesting a more complex relationship than currently defined (Table 9–1).

Sexual Dysfunction in the Presence of Pelvic Pathology

Sexual dysfunctions can be found in each stage of the sexual response cycle. When CPP is also present, the sexual dysfunction may be exacerbated. Diminished or absent sexual desire in both sexes may lead to decreased sexual exchange or abstinence. Loss of sexual arousal is marked by impotence in men and vaginal lubrication problems in women. Orgasmic dysfunctions include premature or retarded ejaculation in men and infrequency of orgasm or nonorgasmic response in women. Also included are dyspareunia and vaginismus in women.

Sexual dysfunction is further categorized as primary if it has been present from the first sexual encounter or secondary if it occurs after prior successful encounters. Finally, a sexual dysfunction may be situational if present only with a specific partner or situation, or it may be global if present in all circumstances.

The prevalence of each of these sexual dysfunctions is uncertain. Even more unclear is the prevalence of sexual dysfunctions in the presence of pelvic pathology. Masters and Johnson, who have devoted a significant portion of their research to the study of human sexual response, estimate that 50% of married couples experience sexual difficulties at some point in their marriage.[4] Various other studies report a wide range of estimates (e.g., 33% in a community survey of women age 33 to 45,[6] 63% of women and 40% of men in a group of "normal couples" surveyed, who otherwise claimed an 83% rating of happy to very happy marriages,[7] and 19% of consecutive female patients who were seen in a gynecology office and were directly questioned about sexual problems[8]).

The distribution of sexual dysfunctions in these prior studies was inhibited sexual desire, 17% to 48%; dyspareunia, 8% to 48%; and orgasmic problems, 4% to 35%.[6, 8, 9] When explored, contributory physical factors, such as atrophic vaginitis, pelvic adhesions, lower and upper genital infection, or endometriosis, were found in 32% to 47% of patients with sexual complaints (whether volunteered or elicited). Psychosocial factors could be found in 33% to 58%.[8, 10]

Although these studies did not examine sexual dysfunction specifically in the context of pelvic pathology, the common organic and psychogenic causes would suggest a high degree of correlation. Conversely, it could be expected that a surveyed population of CPP sufferers would have a higher prevalence of sexual dysfunctions or difficulties than a randomly surveyed population.

To consider pelvic pathology and sexual dysfunction, two pathways need to be explored, direct and indirect. Direct pathways involve mechanical barriers to sexual functioning, such as an atrophic vagina or endometriotic implants that elicit pain on deep thrusting. Indirect pathways can contribute to the psychosomatic development of a sexual dysfunction—for instance, a sexual encounter that results in dyspareunia, even if isolated, can result in anticipation of pain during future encounters. This in turn may lead to impaired sexual desire and arousal with decreased vaginal expansion (see Fig 9–1), which propagates and reinforces the pain, or impaired orgasm, which may lead to further decreases in desire and arousal.

Thus, a pain-dysfunction-pain cycle is created in which even a treatable contributing factor such as lack of lubrication or a urinary tract infection may be resolved but the learned dysfunctional behavior exists. This is demonstrated in Figure 9–2.[11]

Vaginismus

Vaginismus is the involuntary contraction of the perineal muscles (bulbocavernosus)

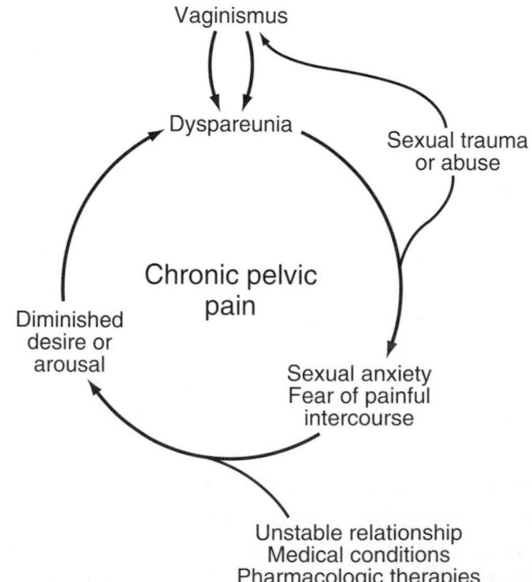

Figure 9–2. Pelvic pain/sexual dysfunction cycle. (Adapted from Lamont JA: Vaginismus. Am J Obstet Gynecol 1978;131:632[11]; *and* Steege JF: Dyspareunia and vaginismus. Clin Obstet Gynecol 1984;27:750.[37])

and often the levator sling; it can make vaginal penetration difficult or impossible.[2, 11, 12] The spasm is likely a conditioned response to a painful stimulus, which most often is appropriate and associated with a current or prior physical discomfort. In its milder forms, vaginismus is quite common and very likely underdiagnosed. It can present even when a complete sexual response cycle is experienced during intercourse. However, vaginismus in its more severe forms may also be a result of an unresolved psychologic conflict or prior sexual trauma or assault.[12, 13]

Secondary vaginismus that precludes intercourse may be an extreme outcome of the pain-dysfunction-pain cycle.

A history of an unconsummated marriage, entry dyspareunia, or inability to tolerate a pelvic examination or to insert a tampon or diaphragm should alert the physician to the possibility of vaginismus. Physical demonstration of the involuntary muscle spasm makes the definitive diagnosis; however, its absence does not rule out the disorder. Reproduction of the discomfort on palpation of the perineal muscles is also a strong diagnostic sign, especially when combined with a suggestive history. Vaginismus may be situational such that the woman can tolerate a pelvic examination but cannot engage in vaginal intercourse because of extreme pain.

Treatment is aimed at reconditioning the learned response. Ongoing physical causes should be evaluated and treated. The originating stimulus can be explored, but in the absence of persistent physical processes or significant psychologic issues, therapy is highly successful even without its recognition.

A combination of patient education and counseling, muscle awareness exercises, and vaginal dilatation is the recommended treatment.

The initial pelvic examination should familiarize a patient with her vulvar anatomy (the use of a hand-held mirror is helpful) and should help her to understand vaginismus as a learned involuntary response. It should be emphasized to a patient that she can unlearn this behavior and begin to control the muscle response. When her partner sits by her side and witnesses the involuntary contraction through the mirror, he may better understand that her painful vaginal contraction is not a reaction to (or rejection of) him.

Muscle awareness is subsequently taught. The patient is asked to squeeze the examiner's gloved finger after it is placed in her vagina. She is then instructed to perform this exercise with her own finger at home, when she is alone and in a relaxed setting. This home exercise can be attempted even if vaginal penetration by the examiner or patient cannot be performed at the initial examination. The patient is told to focus first on the finger being squeezed, then on the contraction and relaxation of the muscle itself.

The other key component of therapy, vaginal dilatation, should begin once the patient is comfortable with the previous exercise. The phrase *vaginal dilatation* should be carefully explained to avoid the misunderstanding that the vagina is actually being stretched, because actual stretching occurs only in cases of strictures or scar tissue.[2] Rather, dilatation is gradual and progressive muscle relaxation occurs as the patient recognizes that nonpainful penetration is possible. She may use her fingers, tampons, or graduated dilator sets.

Once a patient feels comfortable with this exercise, she is instructed to involve her partner, who may at first observe, then insert his finger or the dilating object she has used. Throughout these exercises, it is important that the woman have the sense of remaining in control of anything that happens in her vagina. The couple must agree beforehand that no penile penetration is to occur until the woman is comfortable and gives her permission to do so. The first penile penetration should involve no thrusting motion. Once penile penetration is tolerated, rapid progression to intercourse usually occurs.

Success rates range from 68% to 98%.[9, 11] Any patient with significant psychologic disorders or issues or an unstable relationship should be referred for appropriate psychologic counseling. Even when these exercises are not initially successful, the feelings that emerge from both partners may give clues to emotional issues that may benefit from counseling.

Vaginal Lubrication

For CPP sufferers, decreased vaginal lubrication probably begins the initial path into the pain-dysfunction-pain cycle, with possible subsequent progression to sexual dysfunction. However, there are many other reasons for absent or diminished vaginal lubrication in females.

Vaginal lubrication is a result of arousal and is dependent on vaginal health and intact vascular and parasympathetic function. It also requires sexual desire, and more than in any other phase of sexual response, estrogen plays an important part.

In the majority of patients who report a lack of vaginal lubrication, the cause can usually be traced to estrogen deficiency. Estrogen-deficient vaginal mucosa is thinner, drier, and more susceptible to trauma, which can cause pain and increased anxiety. Perimenopausal and postmenopausal as well as postpartum (especially breast-feeding) women are at risk for hypoestrogenism.

Lack of arousal may result from insufficient foreplay or interest or a woman's feelings of fear, guilt, or anger.[3] Mood disorders such as depression may be responsible for decreased arousal, as are the medications used to treat them. Tricyclic antidepressants, fluoxetine, and monoamine oxidase inhibitors have been found to affect vaginal lubrication.[2, 9, 14, 15]

From the very first drink, alcohol decreases the ability to lubricate. At higher blood levels it also produces a longer latency to orgasm. Use of narcotics and sedatives also contributes to the problem of vaginal lubrication.[2, 9, 16] Chronic pain sufferers often use one of these medications, whether prescribed or self-treated, thus contributing to the sexual dysfunction.

Anticholinergics, antihistamines, and antihypertensives are frequently used medications with similar results (Table 9–2). Diabetes, peripheral neuropathies, and other chronic diseases that affect small vessels may also lead to insufficient vasocongestion and lubrication. Selective serotonin reuptake inhibitors such as fluoxetine may increase the time needed to reach orgasm, although in some cases this change reverts to normal over time even though the antidepressant efficacy of the medication is maintained.

Table 9–2. **COMMON DRUGS THAT INHIBIT FEMALE AROUSAL OR ORGASM**

Arousal
Alcohol
Anticholinergics (e.g., propantheline bromide [Pro-Banthine])
Antihistamines (e.g., terfenadine [Seldane], diphenhydramine [Benadryl])
Antihypertensives (e.g., clonidine, methyldopa [Aldomet])
Benzodiazepines (e.g., diazepam [Valium], lorazepam [Ativan])
Monoamine oxidase inhibitors
Selective serotonin reuptake inhibitors (e.g., fluoxetine [Prozac], sertraline [Zoloft])
Tricyclic antidepressants (e.g., amitriptyline [Elavil], clomipramine [Anafranil])
Orgasm
Aldomet
Amphetamines and related anorexic drugs
Antipsychotics (e.g., thioridazine [Mellaril], chlorpromazine [Thorazine])
Benzodiazepines (e.g., diazepam, alprazolam [Xanax], lorazepam)
Fluoxetine
Narcotics (e.g., methadone)
Trazodone
Tricyclic antidepressants (e.g., amitriptyline, clomipramine)*

*Also associated with painful orgasm.
Adapted from Abramowicz M (ed): Drugs that cause sexual dysfunction: An update. Med Lett 1992 Aug;876(34):73.

Treatment regimens may include hormone replacement therapy when indicated, which increases vaginal cornification and rugal folds, leading to strengthened tissue and decreased trauma as well as increased lubrication. Nonhormonal bioadhesive lubricants used regularly also work to increase vaginal fluid volume and elasticity significantly.[17] Lubricants may be used alternatively at the time of sexual activity or added to the regimen. Investigation into relationship problems and past traumatic or painful sexual encounters should also be explored.

Educating a patient and her partner about the physiologic need for foreplay and the adverse effects of alcohol often yields excellent results. Medication changes or decreased doses may lead to significant improvement. Sensate focus exercises to increase arousal in a nonsexually demanding and therefore less threatening way should be taught, especially to patients with CPP. Sensate focus exercises are designed to encourage communication between partners, minimize anxiety, and allow patients to focus on pleasurable sensations rather than painful ones. Intercourse and orgasm are avoided during these exercises. The partners take turns being the giver or the receiver of nondemanding pleasuring during sensate focus exercises. For example, the woman may first lie prone while her partner gently massages and caresses her, beginning at her head and continuing down her back, over her buttocks, and down her legs to her feet. The woman is not to think about the partner's being bored or fatigued and is to focus only on the pleasure experienced. Conversation is limited to affirmations of pleasurable sensations and descriptions of how to increase pleasure (e.g., caress more firmly, softly, and so on). When both agree, the woman turns to the supine position, and massage by the man is again started at her head and continued downward, initially avoiding her breasts and genitals. The man and woman then switch places and repeat the exercise. At subsequent sessions, the breasts and genital areas are caressed, still avoiding intercourse and orgasm. Intimacy and sexual communication skills should improve, and they can then be applied to other sexual activities and intercourse.

Investigation into relationship problems should be undertaken and past traumatic or painful sexual encounters explored. Individual or marriage counseling should be recommended as needed.

Nonorgasmic Response

Nonorgasmic response may be divided into primary or secondary. Women who never consciously experienced orgasm by any means have the primary form, and women who are currently unable to achieve orgasm despite their ability to do so in the past have the secondary form. As with other sexual dysfunctions, situational or absolute conditions exist as well. Inability to achieve coital orgasm should not be considered a sexual dysfunction, in that only 30% to 40% of women are able to achieve orgasm through intercourse alone.[3] Rather, inability to experience coital orgasm should be considered a problem only if it affects the relationship or the woman's self-image.

Primary nonorgasmic response affects 8% to 15% of American women.[4, 6] The secondary form, more difficult to define because of its inconsistent expression, has been described in 4% to 46% of patients identified as having sexual dysfunctions.[6, 8, 9]

A nonorgasmic response may result from inadequate stimulation, inadequate sexual information, or general sexual inhibition. Performance anxiety, distraction, or relationship discourse are also etiologic factors. Pelvic pain may contribute to any of these factors through a learned inhibition based on prior painful encounters or lack of adequate stimulation from a partner because of fear of inflicting worsening pelvic pain. Medications (see Table 9–2), alcohol, and drugs may also delay or impede orgasm. Just as pelvic pain can cause thrusting dyspareunia and can subsequently lead to vaginismus, patients with pelvic pain may eventually describe anorgasmy because pelvic pain may be exacerbated after orgasm. Postorgasmic pain has been described by patients with endometriosis, interstitial cystitis, and atrophic vaginitis.

Diagnosis of orgasmic dysfunction requires a careful exploration of prior sexual experiences and basic knowledge about the sexual response. For instance, inadequate stimulation may be identified as the etiologic factor in some women, whereas other women who think of themselves as nonorgasmic may actually not be so when they learn what an orgasm is.

The mainstay of therapy of nonorgasmic patients is education and self-exploration. Some gynecologists and other primary care providers may feel comfortable with providing counseling for this problem, but others prefer to send the couple to a therapist trained and experienced in the treatment of sexual dysfunctions. For patients with CPP and anorgasmy, education should include detailed information on the cause (or possible cause) of the pelvic pain, explaining ways to ameliorate the pain during episodes of sexual encounters and suggesting to the couple that they attempt to have sexual activity at times when the pelvic pain is absent or less intense. It is important to reinforce to the woman that orgasm will not exacerbate the pelvic pain, although some patients may note pelvic discomfort after orgasm.

Initial therapy uses self-stimulation by the patient when she is alone and in an environment free from interruption, to minimize performance anxiety and eliminate her partner's anxiety. The exercise should start with self-exploration of the external genitalia, using a mirror or anatomy guide for increased success. The patient should be instructed to identify the areas of maximal pleasure and gradually increase stimulation over these areas. Three basic principles of this exercise—genital stimulation, sexual fantasy to distract from pelvic pain (when present), and muscular control of sexual tension—should be discussed with the patient.

Tactile stimulation should be continuous (women lose the orgasmic platform quickly), directed to the areas of maximum pleasurable sensation, and progressively increased in intensity and duration. Stimulation up to 1 hour initially to achieve orgasm is not unusual.

Fantasy should be used to distract the patient from fear of pain or loss of control and from *spectatoring*, or observing herself from a third-person position. Fantasy may include not only mental pictures but books, films, and so on.

Patients should be taught to contract and relax the pelvic and vaginal muscles at high levels of sexual tension. This often facilitates orgasm and may also provide distraction from the pelvic pain or coexisting anxiety.

If an orgasm is not achieved with these methods, addition of an externally applied vibrator may be helpful. Once the woman experiences an orgasm, many preexisting fears, such as unbearable or renewed pelvic pain, are eliminated. As the exercise is subsequently repeated, orgasm usually occurs regardless of decreasing stimulation, fantasy, and time.

At this point, the orgasmic ability is transferred to a joint session with the woman's partner. Initial encounters may include the patient's masturbating in her partner's presence or sensate focus (as described in the previous section) to maximize communication and relaxation. Distraction techniques, muscle exercises, and a vibrator may still be used by the patient.

The exercise gradually moves to the partner's manually stimulating the patient to orgasm. If coital orgasm is desired and cannot be achieved spontaneously, the bridge technique, in which the clitoris is manually stimulated by either partner during vaginal intercourse, may be used.

A success rate of 85% to 90% is usually achieved by this protocol. Secondary nonorgasmic response generally has a better success rate. Individual sessions with the patient are needed to explore conflicts, give permission for self-exploration, and allow discussion that may be inhibited in the presence of her partner. Joint sessions with the patient and her partner are necessary at some point during therapy to explore relationship issues and interactions, to educate about the physiology of orgasm and CPP, and to involve the partner in what may be a time-intensive exercise protocol.

For positively motivated couples with a generally strong relationship, office counseling by the primary care provider may serve well, whereas more complicated relationships should be referred to an appropriately trained therapist.

Deep Dyspareunia

Deep dyspareunia is pain on penile penetration, especially with thrusting, in heterosexual couples and digital or other sexual methods of vaginal penetration in homosexual couples. Patients may describe a feeling of diffuse or localized tenderness or the sensation that their partner is bumping into something when thrusting. Deep dyspareunia is probably the sexual dysfunction most associated with the presence of pelvic pathology and frequently coexists with CPP.

Myriad overlapping causes of deep dyspareunia and CPP exist, including endometriosis, adhesions, and vaginal, bladder, or bowel disease. Uterine retroversion may be a cause of deep dyspareunia, although infrequently and usually in the presence of coexisting pathology. Some studies, however, show relief of deep dyspareunia with uterine suspension procedures.[18, 19] Pelvic congestion syndrome remains a controversial entity but is still cited in the literature as a cause of either dyspareunia or pelvic pain (see Chapter 17). Acute processes such as salpingitis, ovarian pathology, or ectopic pregnancy may also present as deep dyspareunia associated with pelvic pain.

Endometriosis remains the most well-defined cause of deep dyspareunia, so much so that the presence of two or more symptoms of pain, dysmenorrhea, or deep dyspareunia carries a relative risk of 3.1 that endometriosis will be confirmed on diagnostic laparoscopy.[20] The extent of endometriosis generally is poorly correlated with the severity of symptoms; however, some evidence suggests worsening dyspareunia with increasing depth and volume of black-brown and stellate scarred implants.[20, 21]

Pelvic adhesions are a disputed source of both deep dyspareunia and CPP. Some studies report a high incidence of pelvic adhesions in asymptomatic populations. However, supportive evidence of a cause-and-effect relationship is the increased incidence of both CPP and deep dyspareunia in patients with a history of salpingitis, because adhesive disease is the most likely organic long-term sequela of previous pelvic infection.[22, 23] Possible mechanisms for pain include restriction of pelvic organs, resulting in stretching of the peritoneum,[23] or acute or chronic inflammation by the infectious disease or subsequently from the adhesions that develop. Nerve fibers have been identified within adhesions themselves, suggesting that pain may be conducted directly from adhesions in response to stretching.[24] The thrusting movement with vaginal penetration and intercourse would result in stretching of the adhesions, thereby initiating pain. Laparoscopic lysis of adhesions also offers various degrees of relief of symptoms, ranging from no change to improvement of CPP in 40% of those with a psychologically and behaviorally defined chronic pain syndrome and improvement in 75% of cases of deep dyspareunia (in the absence of chronic pain syndrome).[23, 25]

Vaginal apex intrinsic pain is a source of deep dyspareunia described as midline pain on penetration, with or without the presence of a uterus. Vaginal apex pain in the absence of pelvic pathology may be a consequence of insufficient arousal, especially in postmenopausal patients. A woman with normal anatomy may feel tactile contact with the cervix, and this may be described as a painful or unpleasant sensation. In the presence of pelvic pathology such as adenomyosis, cervicitis, or vaginitis, this sensation may be even further intensified. Uterine immobilization such as occurs with severe endometriosis or adhesive disease is another potential source of pain. Studies of sexuality in posthysterectomy patients yield conflicting results. Some show increased rates of sexual difficulties (10% to 37%), and others report decreased rates (31% to 50%).[26–28] These studies often fail to differentiate between indications for surgery, deep or superficial dyspareunia, or whether concomitant oophorectomy was performed. The data[26–29] also suggest that psychologic factors, especially preoperative concerns about sexuality and expectations of decreased sexual function, correlated with a significantly increased incidence of postoperative sexual dysfunction. Studies of sexuality in patients having undergone gynecologic oncology procedures, with or without chemotherapy or radiation therapy, also show variable results for deep dyspareunia, from slight to 40%.[30–32] These populations, however, would seem especially at risk for vaginal apex intrinsic pain, as well as arousal and sexual desire disorders. An occasional woman may have organically based vaginal apex pain after hysterectomy (see Chapter 15).

The bladder represents a frequently overlooked source of CPP and dyspareunia. The intimate relationship between the urinary tract and reproductive tract, starting even in the embryologic period, would suggest a likely source for coexisting disorders. Postcoital voiding difficulties and dyspareunia are frequently associated complaints of urethral syndrome (frequency, urgency, and dysuria in the absence of bacteriuria). In one study, interstitial cystitis sufferers reported a 57% incidence of dyspareunia.[33] Dyspareunia in these patients may be associated with arousal or orgasm. Theories for this phenomenon suggest that vasodilatation is the main pathologic etiology in interstitial cystitis; therefore, sexual arousal acutely worsens the pain. Other data suggest that the pain may be directly related to bladder wall trauma by thrusting during intercourse or to intercoital release of neurotransmitters that are locally irritating to the bladder.[33] Increased pelvic musculature tone and spasm are also thought to be contributing factors in dyspareunia (and CPP) associated with bladder and urethral disorders.

Treatment of deep dyspareunia includes medical or surgical treatment of endometriosis, lysis of adhesions (variable results, as discussed), and treatment of associated pathologic conditions of the bladder, vagina, and urethra.

Sex therapy counseling should advocate limiting deep thrusting until sufficient levels of arousal are achieved to allow for maximal vaginal apex expansion and movement of the uterus upward (see Fig. 9–1). Sexual positions such as the woman astride or the man and woman side by side (Fig. 9–3) or cross-wise (Fig. 9–4) may minimize discomfort. Vaginal entry from behind may further help displace the pelvic organs upward. Preoperative hysterectomy candidates should have their sexual concerns addressed openly and honestly. Postoperatively, these concerns should again be explored and any new difficulties discussed. This may best be accomplished by scheduling a routine follow-up visit 3 to 4 months after surgery.

Patients with interstitial cystitis form a more challenging therapy group. Stress reduction techniques may be implemented. Pelvic vasocongestion symptoms may be decreased with use of these techniques during arousal. Hastening arousal by placing a heating pad over the pubis and rapid stimulation to orgasm (such as from a vibrator) may also decrease pain from vasocongestion. Patients describe postcoital relief with both hot and cold packs placed on the perineum.[33]

Time-Limited Office Counseling

The introduction of basic sexual counseling into a gynecologic practice may seem overwhelming to busy practitioners, especially with the already time-intensive patients with CPP. Brief inquiries into sexual functioning followed by counseling sessions may, however, significantly improve quality of life of these patients and overall decreased office time demands from this population.

Sex therapy, as first introduced by Masters and Johnson[38] and in its subsequent evolution,[4, 13, 35] is based primarily on behavior modification. Psychoanalytic therapy and marriage counseling are not attempted. The goal is to treat the dysfunction, not to uncover unconscious drives and motivations. Therefore, the office sessions are instructional and the emphasis and time demands are placed on home sexual exercises. Sex

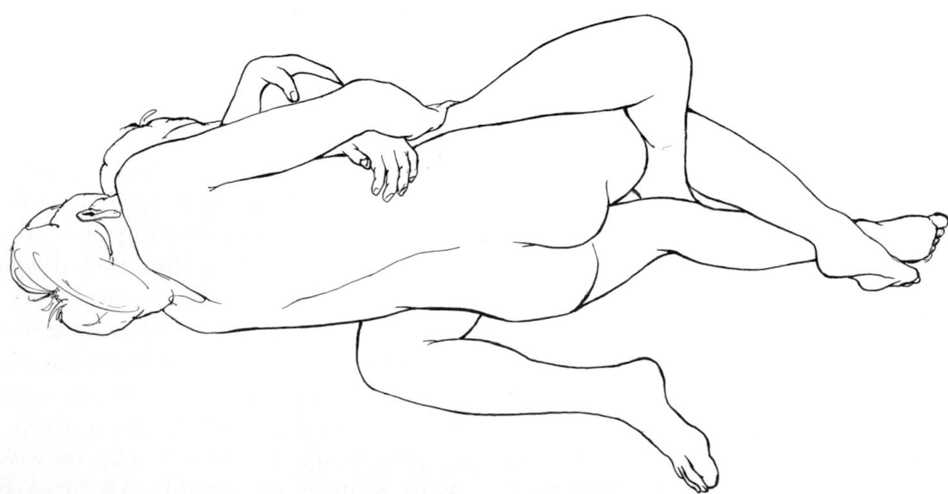

Figure 9–3. Side-by-side position.

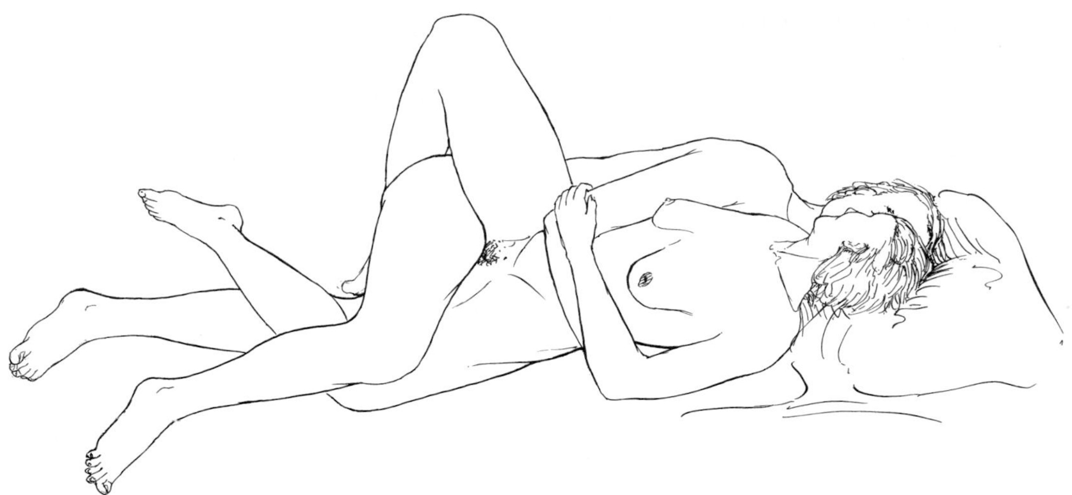

Figure 9–4. Cross-wise position.

therapy in this fashion can resolve as much as 80% of sexual dysfunction.[34]

Annon[40] coined the mnemonic PLISSIT for office counseling. P stands for the permission that needs to be given to patients to explore their sexuality and abandon unhealthy beliefs and taboos in order to change behavior. Masturbation is an example, because this often conjures up negative memories and feelings of a forbidden action. LI stands for limited information, which gives the necessary facts to the couple to explore new sexual scripts and activities. Anatomy, pelvic pain causes, and physiology should be explained as needed. SS stands for the specific suggestions and instructions that should be given for home exercise. IT stands for intensive therapy, which is reserved for patients who do not respond to the first three stages.

For example, vaginismus, as previously described, is highly responsive to sex therapy in the practitioner's office. Office counseling, as well as home exercises, such as advising a patient to perform vaginal exercises with her fingers, a familiar object, is very successful.[37] For patients who find using their fingers distasteful, a sample of dilators, kept in the office, expedites teaching and enhances patients' comfort and understanding.

However, a patient with nonorgasmic response may require several sessions, in both individual and couple meetings. Available illustrations of anatomy, including take-home material, can help improve a patient's understanding and compliance, as well as decrease subsequent visits for questions and repeated information. Dividing sessions for specific purposes, such as CPP or sexual dysfunction, with the later eliminating any physical examination (except the initial instructional one), helps to limit time needed for each session.

Practitioners can often provide sexual counseling and therapy for a patient's male partner. Impotence problems are often medication induced (Table 9–3), and a history of the husband's medications may be all that is needed to uncover the cause of the impotence.[36] Consultation with his primary care physician and medication changes, if possible, or referral for other therapies should be undertaken if desired by the couple. Another example of a male sexual dysfunction for which gynecologists can provide counseling is premature ejaculation, a sexual dysfunction that is readily corrected in most cases by sex education. The dysfunction lies in the man's inability to exert voluntary control over ejaculation, resulting in too rapid a climax.

Therapy is aimed at increasing his conscious perception of the sensations leading to orgasm. Two main techniques are used: Seman's start-stop method and Masters and Johnson's squeeze technique.[38]

The start-stop method begins with normal sex play, leading to erection. The woman then manually stimulates the man until he

Table 9–3. **COMMON DRUGS THAT CAUSE MALE IMPOTENCE**

Amphetamines and related anorectics
Anticholinergics
Antipsychotics (chlorpromazine [Thorazine], thiothixene [Navane], haloperidol [Haldol], fluphenazine [Prolixin])
Antiseizure medications (carbamazepine [Tegretol], phenytoin [Dilantin], primidone)
Barbiturates
β-Blockers (propranolol [Inderal], metoprolol [Lopressor], atenolol [Tenormin])
Calcium channel blockers (verapamil [Calan])
Clonidine (Catapres)
Digoxin
Diuretics (thiazides, spironolactone [Aldactone])
Histamine$_2$ blockers and antireflux agents (ranitidine [Zantac], cimetidine [Tagamet], metoclopramide [Reglan])
Hypolipidemic agents (gemfibrozil [Lopid], clofibrate)
Ketoconazole
Lithium
Naproxen (Anaprox, Naprosyn)
Methadone
Reserpine
Sulfasalazine
Tricyclic antidepressants (amitriptyline [Elavil], clomipramine [Anafranil])

Adapted from Abramowicz M (ed): Drugs that cause sexual dysfunction: An update. Med Lett 1992;34:73.

feels near orgasm, at which time he signals his partner and she stops stimulation until the ejaculatory urge diminishes. She then resumes stimulation until the ejaculatory urge recurs, then stops again. This is repeated four times, and on the last stimulation he is allowed to ejaculate. He is to focus on the sensations he feels and should not use fantasy or other distraction methods. After two successful sessions, a lubricant (e.g., Astroglide or Replens) is used to increase arousal. Finally, coitus is undertaken with the woman astride the man and with all movement at first done by the woman, without any thrusting from the man. Movement is to stop when the man approaches orgasm and to resume once the ejaculatory urge diminishes. The man is not to thrust until the fourth time, when he is allowed to ejaculate. With successive sessions, his thrusting should increase gradually, until he obtains control. The side-to-side position (see Fig. 9–3) is the next step, and the man astride is the final step because this is the most difficult position for control.

The Masters and Johnson squeeze technique is essentially the same process except that instead of just stopping stimulation, the woman then also grasps the penis between her thumb and forefinger just below the glans until the erection decreases by about one third, then resumes stimulation.

Good control usually ensues within 2 to 10 weeks, but absolute control may take months longer. A maintenance stop-start or squeeze exercise should be used approximately once per week during this period. Either of these methods has a 95% success rate.[34]

Position changes, as previously described, can be discussed for deep dyspareunia or in general for arousal, desire, or sexual boredom. Pictures may complement the descriptions, and the couple should be encouraged to experiment and use trial and error. Already inhibited or frustrated couples should be encouraged to try new things, and they should be advised to expect occasional failure.

Either in the initial session or after attempted home exercises, a deeper marital or psychologic problem occasionally becomes evident. This is an appropriate time to refer the patient to a marriage counselor, experienced sex therapist, or psychiatrist. Resistance to home exercises or lack of response despite understanding of the process may also signal underlying pathology. Examples include a patient with vaginismus who harbors a deep mistrust of her current (or any) partner and cannot transfer her successful self-penetration to a joint session with her partner, or a CPP sufferer who, despite adequate treatment of the pain process and sexual counseling, continues to have an arousal phase dysfunction.

Desire phase disorders are a complex array of dysfunctions in which desire is absent or diminished or is not at a satisfactory level within the relationship.[39] Psychologic pathology, such as depression, and marital discord are common in these disorders. Inherent individual desire differences and the wide variation of normal desire make diagnosis and management of these disorders difficult. Once medical causes, medication effects (Table 9–4), and vaginal and pelvic pathology have been ruled out, referral of these patients is appropriate.

Finally, patients with long-standing or

Table 9–4. **COMMON DRUGS THAT DECREASE SEXUAL DESIRE IN MEN AND WOMEN**

Antilipid medications (e.g., clofibrate [Atromid], gemfibrozil [Lopid])
Antipsychotics (e.g., fluphenazine [Prolixin], chlorpromazine [Thorazine])
Barbiturates
Benzodiazepines (e.g., lorazepam [Ativan], diazepam [Valium], alprazolam [Xanax])
β-Blockers (e.g., propranolol [Inderal])
Clonidine (Catapres)
Danazol
Digoxin
Fenfluramine (Pondimin)
Fluoxetine (Prozac)
Gonadotropin-releasing hormone agonists (leuprolide [Lupron], nafarelin [Synarel])
Histamine$_2$ blockers and antireflux agents (e.g., cimetidine [Tagamet], ranitidine [Zantac], metoclopramide [Reglan])
Indomethacin (Indocin)
Ketoconazole (Nizoral)
Lithium
Phenytoin (Dilantin)
Spironolactone (Aldactone)
Tricyclic antidepressants (e.g., amitriptyline [Elavil], clomipramine [Anafranil])

Adapted from Abramowicz M (ed): Drugs that cause sexual dysfunction: An update. Med Lett 1992;34:73.

compound problems—such as one or more sexual dysfunctions, a history of past abuse with obvious residual psychologic issues, current abuse, or concomitant dysfunction in a spouse—should be referred for more specialized and time-intensive therapy.

In summary, the medical history of patients with CPP should include questions about their sexual functions and perceived or actual dysfunctions because these problems often exist concomitantly in this subset of women. Therapy should include education and counseling about the impact that CPP has on their sexuality and ways to improve sexual function despite chronic discomfort. In addition, patients should be made aware that a sexual dysfunction such as dyspareunia secondary to atrophic vaginitis or interstitial cystitis can exacerbate pelvic pain. In either case, the primary objective of treatment is to break the pain-dysfunction-pain cycle by addressing the pathophysiologic causes as well as the psychosocial ones that are contributing to its perpetuation. Office management and counseling often provide definitive treatment or amelioration of symptoms, making referral to a sex therapist necessary for only a small percentage of patients.

References

1. Masters W, Johnson V: Human Sexual Response. Boston, Little, Brown & Co, 1966.
2. Sexual Dysfunction. ACOG Technical Bulletin No 211, American College of Obstetrics and Gynecology (ACOG), Washington, DC, September 1995.
3. Droegemueller W: Sexuality and sexual dysfunction. In Visscher H (ed): Precis V—An Update in Obstetrics and Gynecology. American College of Obstetrics and Gynecology (ACOG), Washington, DC, 1994, pp 97–103.
4. Bjorksten O: The physiology of sexual response and classification of sexual dysfunction. In Sciarra JJ (ed): Obstetrics and Gynecology, vol 6. Philadelphia, JB Lippincott, 1986.
5. Ganong WF (ed): Review of Medical Physiology, 17th ed. Norwalk, CT, Appleton & Lange, 1995, pp 233–236.
6. Osborne M, Hawton K, Gath D: Sexual dysfunction among middle aged women in the community. BMJ 1988;296:959.
7. Frank E, Anderson C, Rubinstein D: Frequency of sexual dysfunction in normal couples. N Engl J Med 1978;299:111.
8. Bachmann G, Leiblum S, Grill J: Brief sexual inquiry in gynecologic practice. Obstet Gynecol 1989;73:425.
9. Hammond DC: Screening for sexual dysfunction. Clin Obstet Gynecol 1984;27:732.
10. Glatt AE, Zinner SH, McCormack WM: The prevalence of dyspareunia. Obstet Gynecol 1990;75:433.
11. Lamont JA: Vaginismus. Am J Obstet Gynecol 1978;131:632.
12. Steege JF, Ling FW: Dyspareunia: A special type of pelvic pain. Obstet Gynecol Clin North Am 1993;20:779.
13. Kaplan HS: The Illustrated Manual of Sex Therapy, 2nd ed. New York, Brunner/Mazel, 1987.
14. Silverglat MJ, Hopkins HS, Gelenberg AJ: Fluoxetine and sexual dysfunction (letter). JAMA 1995;273:1489.
15. Sarazin SK, Seymour SF. Causes and treatment options for women with dyspareunia. Nurse Pract 1991;16:30.
16. Hoon PW: Physiological assessment of sexual response in women. The unfulfilled promise. Clin Obstet Gynecol 1984;27:767.
17. Nachtigall LE: Comparative study: Replens versus local estrogen in menopausal women. Fertil Steril 1994;61:178.
18. Perry CP, Sarria C: Minimal incision Pereyra needle uterine suspension. J Laparoendosc Surg 1991;1:151.
19. Gordon SF: Laparoscopic uterine suspension. J Reprod Med 1992;37:615.
20. Ripps BA, Martin DC: Endometriosis and chronic pelvic pain. Obstet Gynecol Clin North Am 1993;20:709.
21. Koninckx PR, Meuleman C, Demeyere S, et al: Suggestive evidence that pelvic endometriosis is a progressive disease, whereas deeply infiltrative endometriosis is associated with pelvic pain. Fertil Steril 1991;55:759.
22. Heisterberg L: Factors influencing spontaneous

abortion, dyspareunia, dysmenorrhea, and pelvic pain. Obstet Gynecol 1993;81:594.
23. Lipscomb GH, Ling FW: Relationship of infection and chronic pelvic pain. Obstet Gynecol Clin North Am 1993;20:699.
24. Kligman I, Drachenberg C, Papadimitriou J, Katz E: Immunohistochemical demonstration of nerve fibers in pelvic adhesions. Obstet Gynecol 1993;82:566.
25. Steege J, Stout AL: Resolution of chronic pelvic pain after laparoscopic lysis of adhesions. Am J Obstet Gynecol 1991;165:278.
26. Virtanen H, Makinen J, Tenho T, et al: Effects of abdominal hysterectomy on urinary and sexual symptoms. Br J Urol 1993;72:868.
27. Dennerstein L, Wood C, Burrows G: Sexual response following hysterectomy and oophorectomy. Obstet Gynecol 1977;49:92.
28. Poad D, Arnold EP: Sexual function after pelvic surgery in women. Aust N Z J Obstet Gynecol 1994; 34:471.
29. Sloan D: The emotional and psychosocial aspects of hysterectomy. Am J Obstet Gynecol 1978; 131:598.
30. Thranov I, Klee M: Sexuality among gynecologic cancer patients—a cross-sectional study. Gynecol Oncol 1994;52:14.
31. Mitchell MF, Gershenson DM, Soeters RP, et al: The long term effects of radiation therapy on patients with ovarian dysgerminoma. Cancer 1991;67:1084.
32. Cull A, Cowie VJ, Farquharson DI, et al: Early stage cervical cancer: psychosocial and sexual outcomes of treatment. Br J Cancer 1993;68:1216.
33. Webster DC: Sex and interstitial cystitis: Explaining the pain and planning self-care. Urol Nurs 1993;13:4.
34. Kaplan HS: The New Sex Therapy. Active Treatment of Sexual Dysfunctions. New York, Random House, 1974.
35. Reamy K: Sexual counseling for the nontherapist. Clin Obstet Gynecol 1984;27:781.
36. Annon JS: The Behavioral Treatment of Sexual Problems: Brief Therapy. New York: Harper & Row, 1976.
37. Steege JF: Dyspareunia and Vaginismus. Clin Obstet Gynecol 1984;27:750.
38. Masters W, Johnson V: Sex and Human Loving. Boston, Little Brown & Co, 1985.
39. Munjack D: The recognition and management of desire phase sexual dysfunction: In Sciarra JJ (ed): Obstetrics and Gynecology, vol 6. Philadelphia, JB Lippincott, 1986.
40. Annon JS: The Behavioral Treatment of Sexual Problems: Brief Therapy. New York, Harper & Row, 1976.

Selected Readings

Barbach L: For Yourself: The Fulfillment of Female Sexuality. New York, Signet, 1975.

Barbach L: For Each Other: Sharing Sexual Intimacy. New York, Anchor Books, 1983.

Kaplan HS: How to Overcome Premature Ejaculation. New York, Brunner/Mazel, 1984.

Kaplan HS: The Illustrated Manual of Sex Therapy, 2nd ed. New York, Brunner/Mazel, 1987.

Zilbergeld B: Male Sexuality, a Guide to Sexual Fulfillment. Boston, Little, Brown & Co, 1978.

Zilbergeld B: Sex and serious illness. In Garfield CA (ed): Stress and Survival. St. Louis, CV Mosby, 1979.

10

Pelvic Pain in the Adolescent

Ellen S. Rome, MD, MPH, and Gita P. Gidwani, MD

Chronic pelvic pain (CPP) in adolescents occurs relatively commonly and can be a frustrating problem for patients, families, and clinicians. In primary care settings alone, approximately 3% to 5% of all visits by adolescents are precipitated by a chief complaint of chronic abdominal pain.[1, 2] Adolescent patients with CPP pose an interesting challenge to clinicians for various reasons. First and foremost, knowledge of adolescent development is a prerequisite for the provision of adolescent-specific care; a discussion of long-term consequences can be perceived as meaningless or irrelevant to a young person in early or middle adolescence who lacks the ability for abstract thought. Moreover, the clinician often is faced with at least two patients: the adolescent herself and the parent(s). This chapter presents the psychology of persons in early, middle, and late adolescence and addresses the issues of confidentiality, the doctor-patient relationship, and the doctor-parent relationship. Specific interviewing techniques that can be useful in working with these teenagers and aspects of physical examination of the adolescent are discussed. The last section covers specific disease processes in which care may differ between teens and adults, including adolescent endometriosis, pelvic inflammatory disease (PID), other sexually transmitted diseases (STDs), and vaginitis.

The Adolescent Mindset

Adolescence is a time of physical, emotional, and cognitive changes, each of which occurs in a fairly predictable sequence across the population. Timing of these changes can vary, and a particular teenager may be moving from early to middle adolescence physically, while emotional or cognitive skills may lag behind. In the transition from childhood to adulthood, a teenager must come to terms with growing independence, a rapidly changing body image, sexuality and relationships, and eventual decision-making on career and long-term goals that require more abstract thought processes. Although adolescence was originally construed as a time of storm and stress,[3] most teens survive with no lasting difficulties and remain unperturbed by the process.[4] Overall, 80% of teens cope well with the developmental process. Thirty percent of adolescents have an easy, continual growth process, 40% have periods of stress intermixed with periods of relative calm, and another 30% manifest a rather tumultuous course marked by bouts of intense emotional upheavals.[4]

Early Adolescence

This psychosocial phase usually occurs between the ages of 11 and 14 years, corresponding with rapid bodily changes that can make a teenager feel like Alice in Wonderland, at one minute too big and out of proportion and at another minute treated like a child. The key question for early adolescents is, Am I normal? This preoccupation can become apparent as a teenager begins to spend more time comparing her own body with other girls' physiques. Normal physiologic changes can be misinterpreted as pain or abnormality. Curiosity about menstruation and body changes increases at this age.

At this same time, adolescents begin to shift from full dependence on parents to a more independent stance, preferring the company of friends to parents. They may show more reluctance to accept advice or criticism and may forgo family events to be alone or to be out with peers. The unisex peer group predominates. Young adolescents have crushes on adults, rock stars, or other figures. The early sexual curiosity may be manifested by thought/fantasy with some experimentation. They begin to test their parents' values in an attempt to define themselves more clearly. At the same time, these teenagers continue to feel unique and have a self-centered world view. Their convenient use of denial and lack of impulse control at this age can lead to a feeling of invulnerability that can result in pregnancy before a first period in those initiating sexual activity. Young teenagers may become aware of their pregnancy at a relatively late stage and either may attribute quickening of a fetus to intestinal gas or may be seemingly oblivious to body changes naturally occurring in pregnancy.

Middle Adolescence

Encompassing ages 15 to 17 years for most teenagers, middle adolescence becomes a time of increasing focus on the all-important peer group. The main question shifts from Am I normal? to Am I liked? and to be liked, teenagers (including boys) begin to spend inordinate amounts of time, energy, and finances (if available) on cosmetics, clothes, and other means of achieving a certain look to make themselves feel more attractive. Teenagers try out different images, often much to the parents' great dismay. Although a teenager in middle adolescence may feel ambivalent about the growing separation between parent and child, reliance on peers predominates and parental conflicts are usually at their peak.

The now heterosexual peer group has a role in much of the risk-taking behavior and sexual experimentation characteristic of this stage. Youths with low self-esteem may lack the ability to negotiate condom use with a partner or to feel capable of choosing abstinence; those rebelling against authority may choose sexuality as an expression of defiance or as a means of acting out their feelings. The sense of invulnerability predominates, worsened by many early and middle adolescents' inability to foresee consequences. Thus, the United States averages 1.2 million teenage pregnancies annually, with more than one third of these pregnancies resulting in abortion.[5] Although parents' words may be heard but not followed, many youths seek out other adults as role models or for advice, and an astute clinician can use this receptivity to foster healthy decision-making in teens with a developing moral stance of their own.

Cognitively, midadolescents may show a new ability to examine the feelings of others, with intensifying feelings of their own. Career aspirations may become more realistic, and teenagers with average or below average intellectual abilities or school performance may identify their own limitations at this time, with subsequent lowered self-esteem and depression. In particular, teenagers with school failure are at risk for substance abuse, sexual activity with resultant pregnancies or STDs, or avoidance of life indirectly with a problem such as CPP.

Late Adolescence

During late adolescence, which typically ranges from 17 to 21 years, an adolescent ideally has developed a strong sense of self, a satisfying body image, and a distinct set of his or her own values and beliefs. Parents' advice may now be acceptable and welcome to the teenagers, although many teenagers may lag behind in tolerating parents' views. Peers become less important than an intimate relationship, and friends may be forsaken on Saturday night in favor of a date. Relationships tend to involve less exploitation and more sharing, and partner selection depends more on mutual understanding than on peer acceptance. If teenagers do not yet feel comfortable with their sexual identity, they may experience much anxiety or depression.

The ability to think abstractly occurs at this stage. These teenagers develop a sense of perspective combined with a rational, realistic conscience. They have a heightened ability to delay gratification, to set limits for themselves or for friends, and to reach compromises. Although many teenagers reach financial independence at this stage, others may be hesitant to accept the responsibilities of adulthood and may remain both emotionally and economically dependent on family or peers.

Interviewing the Adolescent

A successful medical interview with an adolescent both collects information and sets the tone for future interactions. Clinicians caring for adolescents need to develop or fine-tune skills and techniques that take into consideration a teenager's development, beliefs, values, unique personality traits, and lifestyle. Ideally, the primary care clinician has had the opportunity to develop a relationship with an adolescent patient before a visit for pelvic pain. A subspecialist may be meeting the teenager and family for the first time. In either case, each visit presents an opportunity for the clinician to make the teenager feel that she has priority; questions are addressed first to her, allowing her the right to defer to a parent if she wishes. In those cases in which the mother automatically answers for the teenager, insight into the mother-daughter relationship can be gained. For instance, the mother may have a very different agenda from the teenager or may not have allowed her daughter to develop autonomy and responsibility with respect to choices about her body. Setting limits and redirecting questions to the teenager herself convey a sense of respect for the teenager's views while teaching the teenager to be a better health care consumer. At this point in the interview, it is also wise to tell both the mother and daughter that you will give each some time alone with you to address their respective concerns confidentially (examples of this discussion are given later).

Confidentiality

Teenagers may or may not bring a family member to a medical appointment; in both cases, confidentiality must be clearly explained initially, with reiteration at subsequent interviews. Adolescents with CPP frequently are accompanied by their mothers, many of whom have preconceived notions or fears of pain etiology. In such instances, the clinician has two patients and must treat each with sensitivity. In initiating the conversation, the health care provider defines the context for care, reassuring the teenager that care can occur in an atmosphere of trust and reassuring the parent that life-threatening situations will be revealed and treated accordingly. Most providers for adolescents state at the outset that they will try to give both the parent and teen time alone to address their respective concerns. In our practice, we state, "Everything we talk about when your parent is out of the room is confidential, which means I won't tell your parents what you tell me confidentially, and I won't tell you what your parents say confidentially, unless there is something going on that is life-threatening or dangerous, in which case I'll tell you that I think we need to talk with your parents." Different clinicians may prefer their own styles, but content should be similar. If possible, confidential questioning of the parent should precede that of the daughter so that the teenager does not feel that you are tattling to her parent.

When a teenager is accompanied by her mother, the clinician can choose to interview both together initially or to have the teenager alone in the room. In the latter case, care must be taken to allow the mother to voice her concerns and to bring her in at the end of the interview/examination to discuss the treatment plan. In issues of sexuality, a teenager's right to confidentiality should be maintained in all areas that are not life threatening; however, all efforts should be made to help open the lines of communication between parent and child. A clinician can often use discussions individually with patient and parent to highlight areas of concern as well as to provide positive feedback to both parties. For instance, a sexually active teenager with dysmenorrhea may desire to start oral contraceptives both for contraception and to treat her menstrual cramps. In discussion alone with the teenager, the clinician should ask her whether she has discussed the issue of sexuality with her mother; compliance with oral contraceptives has been shown to be improved in suburban girls whose mothers are actively involved in the decision.[6] For those who have not had such a discussion, the clinician can ask if he or she can help start communication with the parent. Some teenagers welcome the opportunity for the health care provider to supply the vocabulary and to facilitate communication; others state that they prefer to have the discussion with the mother in private or wish to maintain confidentiality.

Office tools and a friendly staff versed in the meaning of confidentiality can also create an atmosphere of adolescent-sensitive care. Many teenagers express concern about accessing health care when neighbors or friends work at or frequent the site. Reassurance that visits and records can be kept confidentially can be useful; for those seeking contraception, the clinician can offer the teenager the chance to pay a bill herself if necessary, with payments in low monthly increments if desired. The presence of adolescent-specific literature in the waiting room or examination rooms can help put teenagers at ease; examination tables should be positioned so that the teen's bottom half does not face the door.

Legally, the constitutional right to privacy, the physician-patient relationship, and federal and state statutes explicitly require confidentiality to be maintained, and many cases confirm minors' rights to privacy with respect to reproductive health care.[7–10] Virtually every health care profession maintains a code of ethics that mandates confidential care and record keeping[9]; most organizations involved in the care of adolescents have created policy statements promoting confidentiality for teenagers except under life-threatening conditions.[11] In some states, a teenager's authorization is required for parental access to information (e.g., in family planning or substance abuse treatment). Ethically, whenever possible, the provider should request the teenager's permission to disclose confidential information and should explain the limits of confidentiality. Specific legal provisions vary from state to state with respect to mandatory disclosures—for example, to child welfare authorities in the case of sexual abuse of a minor or to a law enforcement agency with respect to gunshot or stab wounds.

Taking a History in the Teenagers with Chronic Pelvic Pain

The history for the teenagers with CPP should contain many of the same questions that would be asked of adult patients (see Chapter 6), including the nature and timing of the pain, intensity, location and radiation, and relationship to food, the menstrual cycle, and other factors. CPP can be a source of immense frustration for patients and their parents, and many may seek opinions from several sources in the medical community. Therefore, the clinician should elicit information on prior treatments tried, with a focus on what has and has not worked for a particular patient. Parents and teenagers who feel that their complaints have not been heard will continue to search for a sympathetic physician. A careful dietary history, bowel and bladder history, and musculoskeletal pain history can be key, especially because spondylolysis, slipped capital femoral epiphysis, lactose intolerance, irritable bowel syndrome, constipation, and other gastrointestinal problems can appear at this age. Stress fractures of the pubic ramis and ischium can occur in runners; they present with groin or hip pain worsened by activity, with bone tenderness.[12]

All psychosocial questions should be asked with the parent out of the room; otherwise, the teenager may feel unable to disclose issues of sexuality, abuse, or other events. When a provider privately repeats questions that had initially been asked with a parent present, he or she sends a perhaps unintended message that "it is okay to lie to the parent, but I expect the whole truth." A more sensitive clinician will have explained confidentiality and does not give the teenager the occasion to deceive the parent actively. The acronym HEADS is commonly used to recall the key aspects of the adolescent psychosocial history[13, 14] (Table 10–1). Parental stress or recent divorce can be manifested in a teenager as CPP. In this case, the

Table 10–1. **THE HEADS EXAMINATION**

Home: Who lives at home? What happens when there is an argument at home?
Education: Grade level, school failure/success
Activities/attitude: Peer influence, gangs, guns/weapon carrying, sports/protective influences
Drugs/depression: Cigarettes/drugs/alcohol. How much, how often? Suicidal ideation/plan?
Sex: Sexually active in the past? Method(s) of contraception used? Attitudes about contraceptive options, including abstinence

patient and parent must understand that the pain is real and is being physiologically experienced by the patient. Many families seek care elsewhere if they feel that the patient is being told that the pain is "all in her head." After medical causes have been precluded by a detailed history and physical examination plus judicious use of any necessary laboratory tests, a careful explanation should focus on the use of certain techniques, including biofeedback, relaxation training, or ongoing counseling, to help train the teenager to ameliorate or control the pain completely, using mind over body. Spending inadequate time for explanations can result in performance of further unnecessary laboratory tests and perpetuated pain in this case.

Declining school performance can promote the chronicity of abdominal or pelvic pain. A teenager may miss school for an initial illness and fall behind in homework. Fear of being too far behind adds to her ongoing pain, with subsequent increased pain and school avoidance. Short-term tutoring can be encouraged as a means of helping a teenager catch up and resume activities. Teenagers who are overstressed by commitment to a plethora of activities may have irritable bowel syndrome or another manifestation of chronic stress.

With the HEADS interview (see Table 10–1), the youth's developmental stage can be used to modify the interview. For instance, those in early and middle adolescence respond more to the influence of peers. Thus, eliciting a history of smoking should start with questions on peers' use, followed by questions on the teenager's use. For instance, a smoking history could ask, "Do your friends smoke? Do you smoke?" If a teen answers yes to the first question and no to the second question, the provider can ask what the teenager does when she is asked to smoke by peers. If she can think of no appropriate response, alternative answers ("I'm an athlete"; "I'd rather live longer"; "I have asthma", if applicable) can be shared, providing an informal opportunity for role playing to build a teenager's refusal skills.

Similarly, questions on sexual activity should be made adolescent specific. Teens who are still concrete thinkers may not understand the meaning of "sexual activity," and assumptions of their understanding can prove misleading. Asking, "Have you had sex? Vaginal, oral, anal?" can be more useful with an adolescent. Whenever possible, ask open-ended questions to allow the teenager the opportunity to speak, with questions solicited in a nonjudgmental manner. Runaway teens should be asked if they have traded sex for food, clothing, shelter, or drugs; such teens do not view their activity as prostitution but as "survival sex." When asking about contraception, the provider should inquire if the teenager uses condoms and other methods sometimes, most of the time, always, or never. All teens should be asked if they have been sexually abused or have ever been forced to do something sexually that made them uncomfortable.

We often tell teenagers that we will ask them these same questions on repeat visits, that we ask all teens these questions, and that they should not feel singled out. Such reassurance can help establish the provider as a safe, receptive person for future disclosures. Many teens "check out" a clinician before disclosing confidential or distressing information. Clinicians should also search for a hidden agenda, often revealed by a teenager's comment, "Oh, by the way . . . " at the end of the interview. If time is limited, the clinician should make the teenager feel that her questions are important and relevant to her pain and that you need to see her back in the fairly immediate future to get more history and check on her pain.

Physical Examination

The adolescent should be asked if she prefers the parent in the room for the examination; this empowers the teenager to consider herself an active participant in her own health care. In the case of emergent lower abdominal pain, if a mother refuses to leave the room for the examination, all confidential questions should still be elicited in private, telling the mother that you will ask both her and her daughter a few questions alone and then you will bring her back in the room with her daughter for the examination. A complete physical examination including abdominal palpation, musculoskeletal assessment, rectal examination, and pelvic examination should be performed. Asking the teenager to point with one finger to areas of pain can be most useful, especially if combined with questions on activities that make the pain worse (defecation, urination, certain movements including intercourse). The smaller Huffman's speculum should be used with virginal girls; if sexual activity is suspected, tests for *Chlamydia trachomatis* and *Neisseria gonorrhoeae* should be performed, along with a Papanicolaou smear. Should suspicions of genital anomaly exist or an adequate examination proves difficult, a pelvic ultrasound study can be a useful tool. Further details of the adolescent examination are discussed in the later sections on various disease processes.

Role for Laparoscopy

Gynecologic pathology was traditionally taught to be an uncommon cause of CPP in very young women. Adolescent girls' complaints were often dismissed as functional or as an expected part of menstruation. The high incidence of organic pathology in adolescent patients who were selected for laparoscopy has changed this view. Advances in laparoscopy and endoscopic techniques offer the opportunity for early definitive diagnosis and therapy for such patients.

Selecting the right patient for laparoscopy in the evaluation of CPP requires careful attention to the patient's complaints. Adequate assessment with a thorough history and physical examination emphasizing the duration, location, and pattern of pain as well as its association with the menstrual cycle must be obtained. Other associated pathology in the gastrointestinal or urinary tract as well as the history of surgical procedures and past therapies must be documented.

If the physical examination and sonogram give no clue to the cause and the patient does not respond to simple medical treatment including use of oral contraceptives, stool softeners, or antispasmodics, the physician should consider laparoscopy. Youngsters with a chaotic family history or with a history of psychosexual trauma have traditionally been equated with absence of organic pathology, but our experience shows that these patients definitely merit laparoscopy when organic pathologies cannot be ruled out. Candidates for laparoscopy with simultaneous treatment include young women who have had significant alterations in their lifestyle and are unable to participate in school or sports. Similarly, an adolescent with disabling dysmenorrhea not responding to ovulation suppression drugs and nonsteroidal agents must be further evaluated with diagnostic laparoscopy. We use the laparoscope aggressively in the evaluation of recurrent abdominal pain in adolescents for the following reasons:

1. To reassure patients and their parents
2. To differentiate gynecologic and nongynecologic causes
3. To rule out serious pathology that may jeopardize the future reproductive potential of the adolescent
4. To detect early endometriosis and congenital anomalies
5. To avoid laparotomy and the resulting adhesion formation, thus minimizing iatrogenic compromise of fertility

Endometriosis in Adolescents

In teenagers, the most common symptom requiring diagnostic laparoscopy is cyclic pain.

Before the early 1970s, cases of endometriosis in adolescents were reported in the gynecologic literature so rarely that the disease was believed not to occur in teenagers. The advent of the laparoscope and the later description of nonpigmented disease (see

Chapter 14) prompted greater recognition of the importance of endometriosis in adolescents. Cases of endometriosis were reported very sporadically in the literature at that time and were usually related to obstructive anomalies. However, one review of teenage patients did identify a patient as young as 11 years,[15] with another study documenting the disease in a 13-year-old who had no obstruction of the reproductive outflow tract.[16] Both reviews noted the obvious limitation: Endometriosis was identified only at laparotomy, suggesting that other youngsters may have had undiagnosed endometriosis. The first report of adolescent endometriosis identified with endoscopy appeared in 1973. In the retrospective study by Goldstein and colleagues,[17] CPP was the chief complaint in 43% of the adolescent patients who were diagnosed as having endometriosis. In a study at the Cleveland Clinic Foundation, endometriosis was found in 61.2% of 178 patients undergoing laparoscopy before 20 years of age.[18]

Another study by Chatman and Ward[19] showed that 42% of the patients complained primarily of pelvic pain. The pain is usually severe enough that patients miss a number of days at school and may have scant localizing signs. On the other hand, some tenderness in the uterosacral ligaments, nodularity, or masses may be palpated. Menorrhagia and other abnormal findings (e.g., dyspareunia) have also been described in this series of patients. The abnormal bleeding in teenagers with endometriosis is usually not the typical anovulatory bleeding of adolescents but rather heavy bleeding accompanied by a major component of pain that can be cyclic or acyclic. Prostaglandin formation most likely accounts for patients' cramping and bleeding, and younger endometriosis implants are usually associated with more symptoms than are the burned-out, older implants. When no clear implants are seen, a biopsy of the pelvic peritoneum in the cul-de-sac may occasionally help in the diagnosis.

In 1980, Malinak and colleagues also described inheritable aspects of endometriosis, and it became quite apparent that the chances of a young person having endometriosis would be higher if she had a first-degree relative (mother or sister) with the disease. Moreover, if the relatives' endometriosis was severe, the girl's risk for such severe endometriosis increased significantly.[20] Goldstein and associates[17] found 10 congenital anomalies in 109 patients with CPP, and Schifrin and coworkers[15] found that menstrual outflow tract anomalies were common in adolescents with endometriosis. Sanfilippo and Yussman[21] have described endometriosis with outflow tract obstruction, noting that endometriosis disappears after the obstruction has been released. In performing a laparoscopy, the clinician must visualize the appendix as well as all sides of both ovaries. Indigo carmine may be injected to determine the patency and architecture of the tubes, and the upper quadrants must be examined to rule out perihepatic adhesions indicative of past pelvic infection.

At present, no prospective study data on the management of adolescent endometriosis are available to allow any conclusions about the benefit of early diagnosis and intervention. Therefore, most of the information is obtained from experience with the pathophysiology of endometriosis in adult patients.[22]

Medical treatment, including use of gonadotropin-releasing hormone agonists and continuous oral contraceptives (not allowing menstruation) is effective in the care of adolescent patients with endometriosis. Both agents have been found to be equally effective, although symptoms recurred in most subjects within 6 months of drug discontinuation.[23] Oral contraceptives are significantly less expensive and have fewer side effects than depot leuprolide acetate (Lupron Depot). This agent and danazol are similarly efficacious in decreasing the pain and extent of endometriosis.[24] The former is better tolerated in teenagers because of the androgenizing side effects of the latter. Finally, repeated laparoscopies with an idea of "clearing out the endometriosis that may have developed again" and attempts at presacral neurectomy or laser ablation of the uterosacral nerves must be avoided at all costs.

It is a challenge to take care of these patients. A multidisciplinary approach in which nonsurgical methods of pain reduction are used extensively (see Chapter 28) tends to complement the treatment and management of these patients with minimal endometriosis. In our series, fertility has never been a problem, and patients need repeated reassurance in this regard.

Pelvic Inflammatory Disease

PID causes more morbidity in 15- to 25-year-old women than all other major infections combined.[25, 26] Major sequelae include tubal occlusion, increased risk of ectopic pregnancy, infertility, and CPP, with adolescents being most at risk because they have their reproductive years still ahead.[27, 28] Prevention, early detection, and immediate treatment remain the mainstays in averting the serious sequelae of PID. In fact, the 1993 sexually transmitted diseases treatment guidelines from the Centers For Disease Control and Prevention recommend *inpatient admission* for *all* adolescents with PID due to the risk of noncompliance with outpatient use of antibiotics.[29] Antibiotic regimens are similar to those used in hospitalized adults, with hospitalization until substantial clinical improvement is displayed.

Risk factors for PID in teenagers are both physiologic and behavioral. Teenagers physiologically are at increased risk because of low levels of protective antibody in the local immune system due to lack of previous exposure to the various pathogens, estrogenic dominance with cervical ectopy in postpubertal girls, and the higher prevalence of *N. gonorrhoeae* and *C. trachomatis* in youths ages 15 to 19 years.[28] Behavioral risks include the clustering of risk behaviors characteristic of teenagers, reflecting the lack of abstract thought and sense of omnipotence that many teenagers display. Younger age of first sexual contact has been clearly associated with greater numbers of partners and less consistent condom use.[30, 31] Vaginal douching has been associated with an increased risk of PID. Possible mechanisms of action include upward spread of lower genital tract pathogens by mechanical pressure or creation of a more hospitable environment for infectious agents via alterations of vaginal pH.[32–34] Adolescents who have multiple partners, who practice serial monogamy, and who have more frequent exposures to STDs should not use intrauterine devices because of increased association with PID.[28]

The diagnosis of PID has traditionally proved problematic. Bevan and colleagues[35] reported on 147 women presenting with acute abdominal pain and clinical evidence of acute salpingitis. Although 70.7% had acute salpingitis at laparoscopy, other pathologic conditions were found in 13.6% and no pathology was found in 15.6%. A similar study by Kleinhaus and associates[36] of 50 girls ages 12 to 15 years revealed comparable results. Thus, it is important to use the laparoscope aggressively in adolescent patients presenting with recurrent episodes of PID in which positive cultures are not obtained. Laparoscopy in these cases can help identify adhesions, tubal blockage, or other pathology; perihepatic adhesions also suggest gonococcal PID as a cause of a patient's pain. Complete evaluation for *Chlamydia* may require culturing directly from the fallopian tubes at laparoscopy.

Do pelvic adhesions cause pain or not? In the series by Goldstein and coworkers, pelvic adhesions were found in 12.8%.[17] The entire relationship of adhesions without organ restrictions in patients with pelvic pain is being questioned. The severity and extent of these adhesions should be documented and in discussion with the patient and family should be interpreted in the context of all the contributing factors discovered in your evaluation (see Chapter 28). Laparotomy in adolescents should be avoided because adhesions formation can take place more commonly than after laparoscopy.

Sexually Transmitted Diseases and Vaginitis

STDs and vulvovaginitis are fairly common complaints in adolescent girls. Adequate cultures in the case of sexual abuse and other tests (DNA probes, polymerase chain reaction, immunoassays) in the remainder of the population remain critical, and when results of these tests are negative, we need to reassure patients that all is well. After a positive culture, teenagers need to be rechecked in 4 to 6 weeks after treatment because of the increased risk of reinfection and to prevent doctor shopping if pain recurs. In many of these patients, with adequate examination and timely reassurance that cultures are negative, the pain dissipates. Thus, it is important that we consider the patient as a whole and define her anxieties and fears as well as educate her about vaginal discharge and STDs.

Ovarian Cysts

A multifollicular ovary with preovulatory follicles measuring 2 cm can be found commonly in an adolescent. The patient and family need to understand that functional cysts of the ovary can be up to 3 cm and are nonneoplastic. Unfortunately, the use of pelvic ultrasonography has resulted in patients' attributing their pain to a cyst, creating fears of cancer and undue anxiety in both the patient and family. If the mass is palpated and feels fixed or solid, tumor markers must be sought preoperatively, and the patient requires definitive surgery with a gynecologic oncologist. Mature teratomas are the most common ovarian tumors in young women, and 40% of these tumors have teeth. An abdominal flat plate would show a calcification, making the diagnosis certain. A cystic mass 5 to 7 cm in size is usually mobile and can be managed conservatively with observation and return to the emergency room if the patient has acute pain. Torsion of the ovary is the greatest hazard, because delay in treatment can lead to ovarian necrosis. Torsion usually presents as severe unremitting pain of sudden onset and is a surgical emergency.

Conclusions

Some problems and solutions are unique to the treatment of adolescents with CPP. These can be defined as follows:

1. Evaluation of an adolescent patient with CPP should be fairly aggressive, because certain pathologies can compromise a girl's future fertility if the proper diagnosis is not made.
2. The possibility of pregnancy and its complications must always be considered in the evaluation of a teenager with acute or chronic pelvic pain. Repeat urine pregnancy tests at different times can be a useful adjunct to the history.
3. The presentation of acute and chronic causes of abdominal pain in adolescents may be confusing—for example, one teenager with severe dysmenorrhea may present in the emergency room whereas another with intermittent ovarian torsion may come to an outpatient clinic with CPP.
4. The adult pathologic model of endometriosis and pelvic ovarian disease may not apply to adolescents. Further prospective research is needed in this age group.
5. Most patients, regardless of the cause of their CPP, need assistance in dealing with the discomfort and associated disability. Stress reduction, muscle strengthening exercises, and relaxation techniques can be useful. The patient as a whole needs to be addressed, not just the illness or the gynecologic condition.
6. Confidentiality for non–life-threatening conditions improves adolescent compliance with treatment regimens and can foster a teenager's growing sense of responsibility for her own health. With adolescents, both the family and patient often need ample explanations, reassurance, and guidance, especially with the difficult issue of sexuality in teenagers with PID and other problems. The clinician can help open the lines of communication between parent and child while helping the teenager to take an active role in her own care.
7. Extirpative surgery (e.g., salpingo-oophorectomy, ovarian cystectomy, hysterectomy, cutting of uterosacral or presacral nerves) must be avoided as much as possible.

Caring for teenagers and their families can be a rewarding experience, especially because most teenagers feel better with appropriate attention to psychosocial as well as physical factors.

References

1. Poole SR, Morrison ID: Adolescent health care in family practice. J Fam Pract 1983;16:103.
2. Smith MS, Tyler DC, Womack WM, Chen AC: Assessment and management of recurrent pain in adolescence. Pediatrician 1989;16:85.
3. Hall GS: Adolescence: Its Psychology and Its Relationship to Physiology, Anthropology, Sociology, Sex, Crime, Religion and Education. New York, D Appleton & Co, 1904.
4. Neinstein LS: Psychosocial development in normal adolescents. In Neinstein LS (ed): Adolescent Health Care: A Practice Guide. Baltimore, Urban & Schwarzenberg, 1991, pp 39–44.
5. Greydanus DE, Shearin RP: Adolescent Sexuality and Gynecology. Philadelphia, Lea & Febiger, 1990, pp 1–16.
6. Emans SJ, Grace E, Woods ER, et al: Adolescents' compliance with the use of oral contraceptives. JAMA 1987;257:3377.
7. English A: Legal aspects of care. In McAnarney ER, Kreipe RE, Orr DP, Comerci GD (eds): Textbook of Adolescent Medicine. Philadelphia, WB Saunders, 1992, pp 164–171.
8. Morrissey JM, Hofmann AD, Thrope JC: Consent and Confidentiality in the Health Care of Children and Adolescents: A Legal Guide. New York, Free Press, 1986.
9. English A: Treating adolescents: Legal and ethical considerations. Pediatr Clin North Am 1990; 74:1097.
10. English A, Matthews M, Extarar K, et al: State minor consent statutes: A summary. Cincinnati, Center for Continuing Education in Adolescent Health, and San Francisco, National Center for Youth Law, April 1995.
11. Policy Statement: Confidentiality in Adolescent Health Care. In The American Academy of Pediatrics News, Chicago, April 1989, p 9. Also endorsed by the American Academy of Family Physicians; the American College of Obstetricians and Gynecologists; NAACOG—The Organization for Obstetric, Gynecologic, and Neonatal Nurses; and the National Medical Associations.
12. Emans SJ, and Goldstein DH: Pelvic pain, dysmenorrhea, and the premenstrual syndrome. In Emans SJ, Goldstein DP (eds): Pediatric and Adolescent Gynecology, 3rd ed. Boston, Little, Brown & Co, 1990, pp 277–284.
13. Cohen E, Mackenzie RG, Yates GL: HEADS, a psychosocial risk assessment instrument: Implications for designing effective intervention programs for runaway youth. J Adolesc Health 1991;12:539.
14. Goldenring JM, Cohen E: Getting into adolescent heads. Contemp Pediatr 1988;5:75.
15. Schifrin JB, Erez S, Moore J: Teenage endometriosis in young women. Can Med Assoc J 1995;72:190.
16. Fallon J: Endometriosis in youth. JAMA 1946;131:1405.
17. Goldstein D, Decholnoky C, Leventhal J, et al: American Fertility Society classification of endometriosis. Fertil Steril 1979;32:633.
18. Gidwani GP: Treating endometriosis in the adolescent. Contemp Ob/Gyn 1989;33:75.
19. Chatman D, Ward A: Endometriosis in adolescents. J Reprod Med 1982;27:156.
20. Malinak LR, Buttram VC, Elias S, et al: Heritable aspects of endometriosis: II. Clinical characteristics of familial endometriosis. Am J Obstet Gynecol 1980;137:332.
21. Sanfilippo J, Yussman M: Gynecological problems of adolescence. In Lavery J, Sanfilippo J (eds): Pediatric and Adolescent Obstetrics and Gynecology. New York, Springer-Verlag, 1985, pp 74–79.
22. Durinzi KL, DeLeon FD: Endometriosis in the adolescent and teenage female. Adolesc Pediatr Gynecol 1993;6:3.
23. Vercellini P, Trespidi L, Colombo A, et al: A gonadotropin-releasing hormone agonist versus a low-dose oral contraceptive for pelvic pain associated with endometriosis. Fertil Steril 1993;60:75.
24. Wheeler JM, Knittle JD, Miller JD: Depot leuprolide versus danazol in treatment of women with symptomatic endometriosis. Am J Obstet Gynecol 1992;167:1367.
25. Burnakis TG, Hildebrandt NB: Pelvic inflammatory disease: A review with emphasis on antimicrobial therapy. Rev Infect Dis 186;8:86.
26. Washington AE, Katz P: Cost of and payment source for pelvic inflammatory disease: Trends and projections, 1983–2000. JAMA 1991;226:2565.
27. Westrom L, Joesoef R, Reynolds G, et al: Pelvic inflammatory disease and fertility: A cohort study of 1,844 women with laparoscopically verified disease and 657 control women with normal laparoscopic results. Sex Transm Dis 1992;19:185.
28. Rome ES: Pelvic inflammatory disease in the adolescent. Curr Opin Pediatr 1994;6:383.
29. Centers for Disease Control and Prevention: 1993 Sexually transmitted diseases treatment guidelines. MMWR Morb Mortal Wkly Rep 1993;42(RR-14):75.
30. DiClimente RJ, Durbin M, Siegel D, et al: Determinants of condom use among junior high school students in a minority, inner-city school district. Pediatrics 1992;89:197.
31. Hingson RW, Strunin L, Erlin BM, Heeren T: Beliefs about AIDS, use of alcohol and drugs, and unprotected sex among Massachusetts adolescents. Am J Public Health 1990;80:295.
32. Scholes D, Daling JR, Stergachis A, et al: Vaginal douching as a risk factor for acute pelvic inflammatory disease. Obstet Gynecol 1993;81:601.
33. Forrest KA, Washington AE, Daling JR, Sweet RL: Vaginal douching as a possible risk factor for PID. J Natl Med Assoc 1989;81:159.
34. Wolner-Hanssen P, Eschenbach DA, Paavonen J, et al: Association between vaginal douching and acute pelvic inflammatory disease. JAMA 1990;263:1936.
35. Bevan CD, Johal BJ, Mumtaz G, et al: Clinical, laparoscopic and microbiological findings in acute salpingitis: Report on a United Kingdom cohort. Br J Obstet Gynecol 1995;102:407.
36. Kleinhus S, Hein K, Sheran M: Laparoscopy for diagnosis and treatment of abdominal pain in adolescent girls. Arch Surg 1977;112:1178.

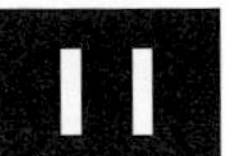

Diagnostic Studies

Barbara S. Levy, MD

The modern age in medicine has endowed us with fantastic tools with which to investigate and manage disease. The challenge created by this vast array of modern technology is to discriminate between that information that is essential to the care and treatment of patients and that information that allows us to place labels on a process but does not contribute substantially to the outcome of care. Clinical diagnosis requires analysis of a problem and synthesis of information. The more challenging the clinical problem, the more important is a logical approach to it. Appropriate tests are invaluable to clinicians, whereas indiscriminate testing increases the cost of care, the investment of time and energy, and the suffering of patients while contributing little or nothing to the treatment plan. It is possible to legitimize patients' symptoms without subjecting them to myriad tests in order to arrive at a definitive diagnosis. Indeed, it may be argued that many of the diagnoses we use to explain a patient's chronic pelvic pain (CPP) may have little if anything to do with her actual symptoms. Just because two things coexist, they do not have a cause-and-effect relationship. It is common knowledge that the degree of pain associated with pelvic endometriosis is unrelated to the surgically determined stage of disease. In fact, at the time of infertility evaluation, it is not uncommon to discover severe endometriosis in asymptomatic patients. Similarly, the relationship between pelvic adhesions and CPP has been questioned.[1, 2]

The goal of diagnostic testing for patients with CPP must be to identify correctable causes of persistent pain and to rule out life-threatening illness. Secondarily, tests may be used to reassure patients about their prognosis. Unfortunately, many patients interpret a physician's report of a normal test result as a statement that their anatomy is normal and therefore the pain must be in their mind. Patients, as collaborators in their own care, should be informed ahead of time about the goal of each diagnostic test and the potential for the results to influence their care and treatment. Only then may patients determine for themselves whether the expense and discomfort of the evaluation are worthwhile for them. This partnership in healing leads to a therapeutic relationship with the care provider, and this in itself contributes to a successful outcome.

It is useful to recall the physiology of pain before embarking on a discussion of appropriate diagnostic testing. A symptom is an abnormal sensation perceived by a patient. Acute pain is most often a result of direct tissue injury. A noxious stimulus is received by peripheral nerves, carried to the dorsal root ganglion in the spinal cord, and then transmitted via the spinothalamic tract to the thalamus and the cerebral cortex, where the message is interpreted. Substances are released at the site of tissue injury in response to chemical messengers that increase the area of sensitivity and create hyperesthesia. A response to the noxious stimulus is then generated by the organism to protect itself from further injury. This response to acute injury with muscle spasm and guarding may begin to establish conditions for chronic pain to develop.

Fear of the inciting agent of pain is often what directs a patient to medical attention. The amount of discomfort experienced may generate significant concern about the cause of the pain. Patients may envision large tumors, cancer, or endometriosis eating away at their tissues. The efforts by many groups to educate the public about cancer awareness, diagnosis and treatment of endometriosis, and other medical conditions are laudable but often serve to confuse and alarm patients who have chronic pain and who search the lay press constantly for answers to their dilemma. One of the functions of diagnostic testing therefore must be to reassure patients without invalidating their pain. In cases of acute pelvic pain, diagnosis can be established readily in most circumstances. Success is not so easily achieved in patients with CPP.

"Functional" diseases are not those confined to a patient's mind but those related to aberrant function of structurally normal organs—the intestines, the bladder, the uterus, or indeed the brain. The premise of this text is that there is no distinction between the mind and the body. Therefore, the ability to demonstrate normal anatomy should be a reason for celebration for both the physician and the patient. It does not relegate the disease to the mind but rather allows us to focus on appropriate mechanisms to permit reanalysis and reinterpretation of nociceptive signals. Our goals of therapy are to simplify and minimize drug treatment, increase functional ability, and educate patients about the causes and factors that exacerbate the pain. Diagnostic tests that help us accomplish those goals must be performed. Those that specify a diagnosis without altering our treatment approach must be avoided. Therefore, to determine whether a test is useful, a clinician must decide how the results of that specific study will alter the course of therapy. If no therapeutic alteration would be contemplated on the basis of the results, then the test is of no real value to a patient. Diagnostic studies do at times serve a purpose in reassuring both a patient and a physician that no life-threatening disease is present. If a patient is at significant risk for carcinoma, for example, then diagnostic studies must be performed to rule out a curable lesion.

Diagnostic testing is generally most useful in evaluating patients with acute episodes of pelvic pain. Under these circumstances, a diagnosis is critical to effect appropriate surgical or medical intervention. In patients with chronic pain, however, the testing should serve an identifiable purpose. It is not beneficial to patients to repeat a multitude of tests that were performed previously—including diagnostic laparoscopy. Only if the circumstances have changed and the treatment would be altered should additional tests be performed. Tests should progress from least expensive and invasive to most expensive and invasive in a logical and thoughtful manner.

Imaging Studies

Ultrasonography

It is tempting to order transabdominal or transvaginal ultrasonography for most patients with gynecologic or pelvic complaints. Rarely, however, does this study shed any light on the etiology of chronic pain. A thorough physical examination in combination with a complete medical and social history is more likely to yield useful information. If a patient is concerned about her symptoms and requires visual reassurance that she does not have significant organic pathology, an ultrasound examination may be appropriate. Unfortunately, transvaginal ultrasound is sensitive enough to identify normal cystic structures within the ovary, and these may be misinterpreted by technicians, referring physicians, and patients as pathologic. Care must therefore be taken to educate patients in advance about normal pelvic anatomy and what structures and findings are expected. Many patients and families have spent anxious days awaiting consultation for benign physiologic cysts. In the setting of an inadequate pelvic examination due to abdominal rigidity or a patient's preference, an ultrasound examination is useful to confirm the anatomy. Transvaginal ultrasonography is more sensitive than transabdominal scanning but may have limited use in patients who will not permit a pelvic examination.

X-Ray Studies

Intravenous pyelogram, barium enema, and upper gastrointestinal series may be appropriate examinations under specific clinical conditions, but they serve no purpose in the general evaluation of CPP. Colicky flank and groin pain may raise the question of renal calculi, and under those circumstances intravenous pyelography is required for assessment. Renal ultrasonography may also be useful in establishing this diagnosis. Barium enema is of limited usefulness because of incomplete visualization of the rectosigmoid area and should be performed in conjunction with flexible sigmoidoscopy. In the diagnosis of lower gastrointestinal disorders, colonoscopy is the most sensitive and specific study available. Upper gastrointestinal series with small bowel follow-through is helpful in establishing the diagnosis of Crohn's disease. Once again, however, other modalities including sedimentation rate and endoscopy may also be used. Plain films of the abdomen are essential in evaluating patients with acute pelvic and abdominal pain but serve little purpose in the work-up of chronic pain. Ultrasound examination of the upper abdomen, specifically the right upper quadrant, establishes a diagnosis of gallstones. Although sensitive (90% to 95%) for detection of gallstones, ultrasound examination can give a false-negative result.

Other Imaging Studies

Before considering more sensitive and expensive testing, a clinician must be clear about what disease processes remain in the differential diagnosis. It is inappropriate to order these studies in the absence of significant clinical suspicion. Systemic symptoms such as weight loss, night sweats, or unexplained fever in addition to the patient's pain complaints should prompt a search for occult malignancy. Under these circumstances, computed tomography or magnetic resonance imaging is appropriate. No other modality effectively visualizes the retroperitoneal structures including the lymph nodes. Which technique is used is determined by local availability and expense. In general, either method adequately views the abdomen and pelvis, but neither is required to confirm findings identified on examination. When a mass is found in the pelvis, transvaginal ultrasonography is the most sensitive study for distinguishing solid from cystic lesions and determining the vascular characteristics of the tumor by using color Doppler flow analysis. Small nodules, suspicious for endometriosis, which are palpable in the rectovaginal septum or at the vaginal apex may be visualized with magnetic resonance scanning; however, the presence of this physical abnormality prompts surgical evaluation without the additional expense.

Endoscopic Studies

Cystoscopy. Direct visualization of the bladder is essential when symptoms are referable to the lower urinary tract and infection has been ruled out. Interstitial cystitis may be suspected when pain symptoms are associated with urinary frequency or dysuria and when they increase with a full bladder. Although cystoscopy may usually be accomplished in women in an office setting, evaluation for interstitial cystitis requires an anesthetic for adequate evaluation. The typical petechial hemorrhages in the bladder wall are seen only after full distention of the bladder, which is intolerable to patients with this condition without proper anesthesia.

Colonoscopy. Bowel symptoms are not uncommon in patients with CPP. Alternating constipation and diarrhea are most likely due to irritable bowel syndrome, but patients who have predominantly diarrhea with blood and mucus in their stool must be evaluated for lesions of the colonic mucosa. In the absence of inflammatory symptoms, colonoscopy is of limited usefulness. Although a colon polyp may be a serendipitous finding, it is unlikely that such lesions contribute to the CPP. Endoscopic evaluation of the gastrointestinal tract should be reserved for those patients with specific indications.

Office Laparoscopy. With the development of new, small-caliber fiberoptic endoscopic equipment, it is now feasible to perform diagnostic laparoscopy in an office setting under local anesthesia. Tiny "needle" scopes have markedly improved optics and permit access to the abdominal cavity with minimal trauma. These laparoscopes provide excellent visualization of the pelvis despite their small size. This invasive technique must be reserved for those patients whose treatment is dependent on the information sought by the study. For patients with areas of specific and reproducible pain on examination, endometriosis or pelvic adhesive disease is quite likely. Under these circumstances, it may be more appropriate to perform laparoscopy in a hospital setting, where extensive resection and adhesiolysis may be accomplished at the same time. For patients with diffuse pain and no clear findings on examination, the clinician must determine what treatment plan would be altered by information gained at laparoscopy. If it is determined that a specific diagnosis will alter therapy, then office laparoscopy is an excellent tool. Specifically, the procedure may be performed with patients consciously sedated and therefore available to confirm areas of specific discomfort as they are examined laparoscopically. If it can be documented that specific adhesions are the source of a patient's pain, it may not be unreasonable to proceed with adhesiolysis. It may frequently be the case that the pain is not reproduced with traction on the adhesion, and a more extensive operative endeavor may be avoided. Photodocumentation of the laparoscopic procedure may prove therapeutic as well. Visualization of normal anatomy may allow a patient to begin to overcome her fear about the cause of the pain and to concentrate on mechanisms to deal with it effectively.

Other Modalities

Slocomb[1] found that injection of abdominal wall and pelvic trigger points with local anesthetic agents is especially helpful in distinguishing visceral from musculoskeletal discomfort. When regions of muscular pain are eliminated, the pelvic organs may be palpated in a more isolated situation, permitting the clinician to distinguish true visceral painful stimuli from those of the surrounding musculature.

Psychologic evaluation with the Minnesota Multiphasic Personality Inventory may be useful in evaluating patients with chronic pain (see Chapter 8). It is important to emphasize to a patient in advance, however, that most people with chronic pain suffer from depression as a result of their pain and that you, as her care provider, do not plan to use the results of the test to determine whether or not the pain is psychogenic in origin. Rather, the test may be useful in determining an appropriate care plan and in establishing a baseline for future analysis. As managed care becomes a reality everywhere, we will be challenged to document that our treatment of patients with chronic pain is efficacious. Only with baseline evaluations of their functional and emotional status will we be able to assess the impact of our therapeutic regimen on the quality of life.

Conclusion

The diagnostic evaluation of patients with chronic pain is challenging. It is most critical to establish rapport with patients and obtain a complete medical, social, and family history. This process may be time consuming and may occur over several visits. Once a trusting relationship has been established, a thorough physical examination is the most useful diagnostic tool available. This in combination with the history establishes a reasonable diagnosis and determines an appropriate course of treatment in most circumstances. When nongynecologic disease is suspected, consultation with other specialists with a specific interest in chronic pain is appropriate. Clear communication with the consultant is important. Patients must be reassured that referral does not mean that you are giving up on their care. The consultant should be informed of significant items in a patient's history and physical examination and guided about the question you would like addressed. For example, for a patient with suspected interstitial cystitis, a urologist may be consulted. The specialist should be given copies of any prior testing as well as a summary of your evaluation to date. The referral, then, would specifically ask the urologist to perform cystoscopy on the patient under anesthesia to rule out interstitial cystitis and to communicate with you if any further testing is contemplated. This allows the gynecologist to remain the primary caregiver for the patient and to solidify the partnership relationship with her. Diagnostic testing can therefore be limited by the working diagnosis and treatment strategies, and expensive, invasive, and unnecessary studies may be avoided.

References

1. Slocomb JC: Neurological factors in chronic pelvic pain: Trigger points and the abdominal pelvic pain syndrome. Am J Obstet. Gynecol 1984;149:536.
2. Rapkin AJ: Adhesions and pelvic pain: A retrospective study. Obstet Gynecol 1986;68:13.

12

Laparoscopy in Diagnosis

Deborah A. Metzger, PhD, MD

Since the first recorded optical inspection of the abdominal cavity by a culdotomy incision in 1901,[1] the concept of visualization of the pelvic cavity for both diagnosis and operative procedures has expanded dramatically, especially during the past few years. The growth of laparoscopy as a diagnostic tool and as a means of minimally invasive surgery has led gynecologists to consider laparoscopy an integral part of the evaluation of chronic pelvic pain (CPP).

Although the actual prevalence is not known, it has been estimated that 10% of all office visits to a gynecologist are for CPP[2] and that more than 40% of all laparoscopies are performed for the evaluation of CPP.[3–5] In women with CPP, findings on physical examination are not a reliable predictor of laparoscopic findings. Although abnormal examination findings are highly predictive of abnormal laparoscopic findings (70% to 90%) in the primary care setting,[6, 7] more than half of women with normal results from preoperative pelvic examination have abnormal laparoscopic findings.[4, 7] Thus, the use of laparoscopy allows detection of potentially treatable pathology not detected or detectable by other types of evaluation such as ultrasonography, imaging studies, endoscopy, and laboratory studies.

Not all investigators agree with the importance of laparoscopy in the management of CPP. In a randomized trial of a traditional gynecologic approach to CPP, which routinely included a laparoscopy, compared with an integrated approach, which included attention to somatic, psychologic, dietary, environmental, and physiotherapeutic components, Peters and colleagues[8] found that laparoscopy had no important role in the treatment of CPP when patients were assessed 1 year after the beginning of treatment. The researchers concluded that an individual woman usually has more than one factor that can be responsible for the complaint of CPP, although this is not always recognized by those providing care. Equal attention to both organic and other causative factors from the beginning of therapy is more likely to result in a reduction of pelvic pain than is an approach based solely on somatic symptoms.

When to Perform Laparoscopy

The indications for a laparoscopic examination in the presence of acute pain are generally obvious. In contrast, CPP, by most definitions, does not even exist until the symptoms have been present for 6 months.[9–12] Furthermore, duration alone is not the only criterion for defining CPP. Various researchers have included different modifiers such as noncyclic, cyclic, dysmenorrhea, deep dysparunia, intermenstrual pain, consistent location, and not relieved by nonnarcotic analgesics as part of their definitions.[2, 7, 9–11]

These definitions do not provide a gynecologist with very much guidance about when to perform a laparoscopy on a patient who has nonacute pain. One concern is that laparoscopy may fail to reveal any pathology if performed too early. On the other hand, waiting arbitrary periods such as 3 or 6 months may delay appropriate treatment in the early stages of pain-causing disease and may lead to permanent tissue damage, with a subsequent poor response to any treatment.[13] Thus, timely intervention may limit the development of chronic pain syndrome (see Chapter 2).

The goal of laparoscopy is to find and

appropriately treat any underlying or contributing somatic or visceral pathology.[14] However, it should be recognized that this addresses only a portion of the patient's pelvic pain, which may have many components: medical, psychosocial, and dysfunction of pain perception. Before a laparoscopy is contemplated, the data obtained from the initial evaluation should be used to develop a list of contributing factors. Only when the physician is convinced that the results of the laparoscopic examination would contribute materially to the overall treatment of the patient should a laparoscopy be scheduled. It is not sufficient to perform a diagnostic laparoscopy merely to document whether or not visual abnormalities exist. The most valuable information is obtained when the physical examination guides the laparoscopic examination. Finally, the physician should arrange for the appropriate surgical consultants so that the suspected pathology can be diagnosed or treated as a multidisciplinary team.

Preoperative Counseling

Before any surgical procedure, the surgeon is required by law and bound by moral and ethical standards to discuss the nature of the procedure and its risks. Although this step is generally viewed as an attempt to avoid malpractice suits, little attention has been directed to patients information needs, particularly given the relative recent development of laparoscopic techniques and the special needs of women with CPP.

A woman with CPP may have other issues to consider besides the technical aspects of her upcoming operation, the possible outcome and results, possible complications, and the surgeon's experience in performing these procedures. Because laparoscopic surgery is often performed in conjunction with a diagnostic laparoscopy, the preoperative diagnosis is often undetermined with pelvic pain. Therefore, the preoperative discussion should include a list of possible findings and their potential surgical treatments. For example, despite having no clear-cut clinical signs of adhesions, endometriosis, or other pathology, patients with CPP may have completely normal laparoscopic findings or may have significant pathology that requires extensive surgery. To outline the surgical options, the physician needs a clear understanding of the patient's wishes concerning preservation of fertility.

It is incumbent on the surgeon to describe the chances of success of the procedure along with possible treatments should surgery be unsuccessful. Special care should be exercised not to give any guarantees of success or false assurance that the procedure has no risk or minimal risk. Particularly for patients with chronic pain, any surgical procedure is viewed with an overblown sense of optimism. It is not unusual for these patients to feel disappointed after surgery when they realize that they still have some degree of pain. These patients require extensive evaluation and counseling preoperatively, sometimes in conjunction with a psychotherapist familiar with chronic pain. Along with discussing the possible surgical outcomes, the physician needs to describe the outlook if the proposed surgical procedure is declined. This is an appropriate time to discuss a rehabilitation plan.

Other treatment alternatives should be discussed, including medical therapy, laparotomy (either as planned treatment or to deal with a complication of laparoscopy), and no treatment at all. The precise nature of the problem may not be apparent before laparoscopic assessment, and the range of surgical options may be wide. For example, endometriosis may be treated either with ablation of implants or with hysterectomy and bilateral salpino-oophorectomy. It may be difficult for a patient and her family to prepare emotionally for such a range of options. A patient may choose a diagnostic laparoscopy alone, leaving discussion of further treatment until to the postoperative discussion.

All possible complications including bleeding, organ perforation, infection, incisional hernia, shock, and even death must be mentioned. Some laparoscopic procedures carry an increased risk of complications; for example, severe endometriosis with cul-de-sac obliteration may be associated with a higher risk of bowel injuries.

The informed consent discussion should

not be rushed and may require more than one session. Charts, anatomic models, videos, and pamphlets can help increase a patient's understanding of the procedure. Patients should be given ample time to ask questions and have them thoroughly answered.

Preoperative Instructions and Preparation for Surgery

To be able to interpret the findings of the laparoscopic examination relative to a patient's pain, it is necessary to identify those areas of the pelvis that when palpated reproduce the patient's pain. This preoperative pelvic mapping examination can be performed at the preoperative visit or can be deferred until the patient is positioned on the operating room table. It is essential that decisions that guide the laparoscopic examination be based on reproducible physical findings. This generally requires more than one pelvic examination.

The examination should be a careful stepwise combination of unimanual and bimanual palpation of the pelvic organs while the examiner asks the patient what reproduces different components of her pain. The examination should not be rushed. The structures that should be palpated individually include the urethra, bladder, cervix, uterine fundus, ovaries, broad ligaments, uterosacral ligaments, cul-de-sac, rectum (see Chapter 7), coccyx, levator and piriformis muscles, and inguinal areas (see Chapter 32). A more detailed examination such as this facilitates the interpretation of laparoscopic findings.

Laparoscopic Evaluation of the Pelvis

Clear documentation of the laparoscopic findings allows the operator to plan the surgical procedures to be performed. Photographic and written documentation in the operative record allows the surgeon to review the procedure when planning additional treatment or if another laparoscopic procedure is performed subsequently.

It is important that the examination be conducted in a standardized and thorough manner. Soon after the laparoscope and accessory trocar are inserted, the omentum and bowel directly beneath the trocar should be inspected for Veress' needle and trocar injury. First, a general survey of the pelvis is undertaken so that all of the pelvic structures are in view of the laparoscope. The blunt probe is gently used to manipulate the organs of interest, in particular areas with scarring or areas that correlate with pelvic tenderness. The laparoscope is then moved closer to the left adnexa, and the ovary is lifted, if possible, and the pelvic sidewall is carefully inspected. The ovary is then released, and the laparoscope is then directed over the anterior cul-de-sac and swept over to the right adnexa. Again the right ovary is elevated, and the pelvic sidewall is carefully inspected. The posterior broad ligaments and cul-de-sac are then carefully evaluated. The surface of the bowel should be examined next, followed by an inspection of the appendix, liver, and diaphragm.

The examiner's efforts should be concentrated primarily in the region of the patient's pain. For example, when a pelvic examination suggests tenderness in the right adnexa, most of the laparoscopic effort should be concentrated there. However, the examiner should also be receptive to other possible abnormalities that could contribute to the pain or that may be one of several pain sources for the patient.

Visual records via still photographs or video aid your postoperative discussion with the family. Patients often benefit immensely when they can see what was responsible for their pain or, alternatively, may be reassured if their pelvis is normal. Many surgeons give the patient a copy of the photographic and written record.

Specific conditions commonly found in women with CPP are reviewed next.

Endometriosis (see Chapter 14)

Although typical endometriosis implants appear as blue-black powder-burn implants often surrounded by stellate scarring, the atypical lesions are less apparent visually but more active physiologically, as determined by their production of prostaglandins.[15] Atypical implants may appear as reddish vesicles, clear vesicles, slight irregularities on the surface of the peritoneum, or white patches. Detection of subtle nonpigmented lesions requires laparoscopic inspection at close range (1 to 2 cm) or inspection of the surface at moderately close range using different lighting angles.

Teenagers are more likely to have atypical implants, particularly the nonpigmented type.[16] An extraordinary effort may sometimes be required to make a diagnosis, including reperformance of peritoneal biopsies that are nondiagnostic of endometriosis at first glance. Early detection of endometriosis has an important impact on treatment selection.

Endometriosis implants are sometimes buried under scar tissue that develops as a result of the natural progress of the disease or from previous superficial attempts at ablation. Palpation of these areas with the manipulating probe allows detection of occult nodules. Resection of the overlying scar tissue may be necessary to discover and remove underlying implants and fibrosis.

Bowel endometriosis may be difficult to diagnose preoperatively even in the presence of rectal bleeding, dyschezia, or deep dysparunia. Only 20% of women with bowel endometriosis can be identified by either colonoscopy or barium enema (Redwine, Sharpe: Unpublished data). However, if a patient has suspected bowel involvement, several techniques may be helpful in improving the diagnostic yield. Because most bowel endometriosis is associated with the rectosigmoid, a careful examination may yield evidence of scarring and distortion of the serosa of the bowel. Palpation of any abnormalities with the manipulating probe allows assessment of the extent of the lesion. Inserting ring forceps or a rectal probe into the rectum and gradually withdrawing it may disclose retroperitoneal nodules that would otherwise remain undetected. Similarly, the pelvic floor tissues can be palpated in detail using a rectovaginal examination with a blunt laparoscopic probe (see Fig. 15–1). Finally, the diagnosis of significant bowel endometriosis may require a laparotomy in order to visualize the entire bowel.

Adhesions (see Chapter 13)

Not all adhesions that are found at the time of a laparoscopy for CPP are responsible for the patient's pain. In general, filmy adhesions are not associated with CPP, although it is tempting to use their presence as an explanation. In contrast, dense adhesions that distort anatomy or function *may* be a significant source of pain. Careful pelvic mapping before the laparoscopy as well as correlation of laparoscopic findings with a description of the patient's pain characteristics may allow a certain degree of discrimination. When a patient has localized pain and the only findings are adhesions limited to the anatomic location of the pain, it is highly probable that the adhesions contribute significantly to the pain. In other patients, the judicious use of laparoscopy under conscious sedation allows a more definitive diagnosis (see Chapter 33).

Hernias (see Chapter 32)

Direct inguinal, indirect inguinal, and femoral hernias are seldom visible in women at the time of laparoscopy as indentations or defects of the peritoneum. Moreover, hernias may be difficult to palpate externally, making diagnosis in women problematic.[17] The presence of hernias is suspected on the basis of a vaginal examination associated with inguinal tenderness that reproduces the patient's pain. A retroperitoneal laparoscopic examination by an experienced general surgeon confirms the diagnosis and allows treatment at the same time.

Pelvic Congestion (see Chapter 17)

Dilated ovarian and pelvic veins, when present in a patient with ovarian tenderness and postcoital ache, are diagnostic of pelvic congestion. However, laparoscopy is not a definitive method of diagnosing pelvic varicosities, because Trendelenburg's positioning enhances venous drainage and minimizes the size of the veins. Transvaginal ultrasound examination and transcervical venography are less invasive and more definitive means of diagnosing this condition. Testing should preferably be performed before the laparoscopy so that appropriate treatment can be instituted.

Pathology That Is Rarely Associated with Chronic Pelvic Pain

Some pathology is often encountered during laparoscopic examinations for CPP but is only rarely responsible for CPP. Findings such as functional ovarian cysts, cysts of Morgagni, filmy adhesions, and peritoneal windows (Allen-Masters syndrome) should be viewed as red herrings, which may distract attention from the real reason for pain. More widespread use of laparoscopy under conscious sedation (see Chapter 33) provides additional information about the spectrum of sources of pelvic pain.

Postoperative Care

It is useful to provide patients with postoperative instructions before the day of surgery. In this way they will be maximally prepared for what to experience postoperatively. Although this advises patients about what to do and not to do and when to call, it is not unusual for patients with CPP to become discouraged or anxious. Thus, regular calls from the physician or staff and regular postoperative visits are important to provide reassurance. Because anxiety and a complication of surgery may be difficult to distinguish over the phone, it is important to see patients with postoperative complaints in a timely way.

Patients with CPP are seen for a routine postoperative visit 5 to 7 days after surgery. Most women return to work 3 to 21 days after surgery. This interval depends on a number of factors, such as the length of time under anesthesia, the surgical procedure performed, the nature of the patient's job, and the individual patient's constitution.

A most important aspect of the postoperative visits is a review of the findings and the surgical management, postoperative treatment, and the patient's expectations. This discussion may be facilitated immensely by the use of videotapes or photographs of the patient's operation and should also include the anticipated course of recovery, proposed adjunctive treatments, and the possible options should unacceptable pain relief result. A physician's offer of reassurance of continued support is a significant factor in alleviating patients' fear of abandonment.

Laparoscopy-Negative Patients

Diagnosis of the underlying cause of CPP can be difficult: A combination of history, physical examination, laboratory findings, and imaging techniques leads to incorrect diagnoses in 20% to 70% of women.[4, 14, 18, 19] Even with laparoscopy, the causes of CPP can be identified in only about 60% of women.[14] Thus, it is not surprising that a significant proportion of laparoscopic examinations for CPP fail to reveal any obvious pathology.

Treatment of Laparoscopy-Negative Patients

For the 30% to 40% of women with nondiagnostic laparoscopy, many outcomes are possible. Some patients may be reassured by the negative findings, with resulting improvement or resolution in their symptoms.[20] Others may assume or are led to believe that the laparoscopy is a definitive diagnostic procedure and that if no pathology is found, then the pain is all in their head. However, a nondiagnostic laparoscopy does not mean that these women have no physical basis for their pain. Reiter and Gambone found that with thorough evaluation, occult somatic pathology was diagnosed in 47% of women with nondiagnostic laparoscopies.[10] In addition, Beard's group found that 80% of these patients had pelvic congestion on venography.[21] These very high percentages may be due to a referral bias. In fact, for many causes of CPP, laparos-

Table 12–1. **VISUALIZATION OF COMMON LAPAROSCOPIC FINDINGS**

Reliably seen
Adhesions
Endometriosis (powder-burn type)
Usually visible but may be missed
Endometriosis (atypical appearances)
Intermittent partial small bowel obstruction
Diverticulosis
Often not visible
Hernias
Pelvic congestion
Not visible
Piriformis muscle spasm
Ilioinguinal nerve entrapment
Interstitial cystitis
Myofascial pain (abdominal wall trigger points)
Levator spasm
Adenomyosis
Rectocele

copy is not the optimal method of diagnosis (Table 12–1). Therefore, if a patient continues to have significant pain after a nondiagnostic laparoscopy, other causes of the pain should be pursued. In my experience, the most common diagnoses are abdominal wall trigger points (see Chapter 26), hernias (see Chapter 32), and pelvic congestion (see Chapter 17). Other tips for treating laparoscopy-negative patients are summarized in Table 12–2.

For the physician who is evaluating a patient with a previous nondiagnostic laparoscopy, what is the probability of detecting treatable pathology with a second laparoscopy? If a single-puncture laparoscopic examination was performed previously, the probability of finding previously undetected pathology is significant. If findings on pelvic examination indicate a source of pain that was not previously considered, laparoscopy may be helpful. In general, if a second laparoscopy is contemplated in previously laparoscopy-negative patients, it should be performed by someone knowledgeable about CPP. Laparoscopy under conscious sedation with pelvic mapping may also have a role in selected patients (see Chapter 33).

Table 12–2. **TIPS FOR TREATING LAPAROSCOPY-NEGATIVE PATIENTS WITH CONTINUED PAIN**

Reassurance of a normal pelvis may help decrease anxiety, with a proportion of the patients having subsequent resolution of their pain.
Reevaluate patients every 2 to 3 months (review history, pain characteristics, and physical examination).
Reevaluate patients for causes that are generally not visible on laparoscopy (see Table 12–1), particularly hernias, pelvic congestion, and trigger points.
Obtain a second opinion from someone who specializes in chronic pelvic pain or chronic pain management.
Reinforce supportive therapy—antidepressants, physical therapy, chiropractic, nutrition, and so on (see Chapter 28).
Continue to see patients on a regular basis for support and coordination of services.

Women who continue to have pain after a nondiagnostic laparoscopy require continued emotional support and regularly scheduled visits. They should be reassured that the pain is real but that the reason for the pain eludes our ability to diagnose it at this time. Different options should be offered to the patient, including a second opinion from someone knowledgeable about CPP. This is a time for attention to adjunctive treatments such as antidepressants, relaxation/meditation therapy, biofeedback, physical therapy, attention to diet and nutrition and environmental factors, and so on (see Chapter 28). Controlled studies show that these interventions are associated with diminished impairment by pain and improved functioning.[22–24] It is important that the patient's physician (gynecologist, primary care physician, internist, other) serve as the coordinator of this care.

Hysterectomy for the Treatment of Laparoscopy-Negative Patients

Although medical therapy for CPP has been demonstrated to produce significant improvements in symptoms and quality of life,[8, 23, 24] half of women treated medically for CPP still rate symptoms as a medium or big problem after 1 year of follow-up.[23] In contrast, hysterectomy is associated with more marked improvement in symptoms and quality of life than nonsurgical therapy (odds ratio 10.45) despite the fact that on average, those undergoing hysterectomy had more severe symptoms and more long-standing conditions than those treated medically.[23] Thus, hysterectomy remains an important alternative when conservative treatment fails.

CPP is the most common indication for hysterectomy in the United States.[25] Hysterectomy has been found to be highly effective in ameliorating CPP but less effective in resolving it. Although 95% of women undergoing hysterectomy for CPP experience long-term improvement, about 25% of women report persistent pain 1 year after surgery.[26] The probability of persistent pain was even higher among women who were younger than 30 years, those who had no identified pelvic disease, those who were on public assistance, and those who had a history of pelvic inflammatory disease.[26]

The observation that approximately 25% of women continue to experience pelvic pain after hysterectomy is of concern because it reflects our limited ability specifically to diagnose and treat sources of CPP unrelated to the female reproductive organs. As discussed earlier, occult somatic pathology unrelated to the female reproductive organs accounts for a significant proportion of pain in laparoscopy-negative women with CPP. Although pain due to pelvic congestion would be expected to improve after a hysterectomy, pain from abdominal wall trigger points (see Chapter 26), hernias (see Chapter 32), or interstitial cystitis (see Chapter 22) would continue unabated. Thus, the 25% who continue who have CPP after hysterectomy may have occult somatic pathology, although this has not yet been studied (see Chapter 31). In my practice, the most common diagnoses in women with continued CPP after hysterectomy are retained ovaries with or without ovarian vein varicosities, abdominal wall trigger points, ovarian remnant(s), vaginal cuff trigger points, hernias, and adhesions. Some of these pain sources were present before the hysterectomy, and some developed as a result of the hysterectomy.

Denervation Procedures and Uterine Suspension

In the absence of gross pathology or specific indications, denervation procedures and uterine suspension should be considered only when the perceived benefits outweigh the risks (see Chapters 18 and 19). The use of unproven denervation procedures as a last resort in response to a patient's desperation is to be condemned because of the limited experience with these procedures.

Conclusions

Laparoscopy can be a powerful diagnostic tool for assessing CPP, particularly when preceded by careful evaluation. Although the identification of pathology is reassuring that the pain has a physical basis, the lack of findings can have several implications. Although some women may be reassured that no serious abnormalities exist, the lack of visible findings is not indicative of a lack of pathology. Indeed, numerous conditions are associated with CPP but may not be apparent on laparoscopic examination, thus emphasizing that laparoscopy is important but not definitive in the diagnosis of CPP.

References

1. von Ott D: Die direkte Beleuchtung der Bauchhohle, der Harnblase, des Dickdarms und des Uterus zu diagnostischen Zwecken. Rev Med Tcheque (Prague) 1901;2:27.
2. Reiter RC: A profile of women with chronic pelvic pain. Clin Obstet Gynecol 1990;33:130.
3. Renaer M: Chronic Pelvic Pain in Women. New York, Springer-Verlag, 1981, p 3.
4. Cunanan RG, Courey NG, Lippes J: Laparoscopic findings in patients with pelvic pain. Am J Obstet Gynecol 1983;146:587.
5. Bahary CM, Gorodeski IG: The diagnostic value of laparoscopy in women with chronic pelvic pain. Ann Surg 1987;11:672.
6. Ripps BA, Martin DC: Focal pelvic tenderness, pelvic pain and dysmenorrhea in endometriosis. J Reprod Med 1991;36:470.
7. Kresch AJ, Seifer DB, Sachs LB, et al: Laparoscopy in the evaluation of 100 women with chronic pelvic pain. Obstet Gynecol 1984;64:672.
8. Peters AAW, vanDorst E, Jellis B, et al: A randomized clinical trial to compare two different approaches in women with chronic pelvic pain. Obstet Gynecol 1991;77:740.
9. Vercellini P, Fedele L, Arcaini L, et al: Laparoscopy in the diagnosis of chronic pelvic pain in adolescent women. J Reprod Med 1989;34:827.
10. Reiter RC, Gambone JC: Nongynecologic somatic pathology in women with chronic pelvic pain and negative laparoscopy. J Reprod Med 1991;36:253.
11. Steege JF, Stout AL: Resolution of chronic pelvic

pain after laparoscopic lysis of adhesions. Am J Obstet Gynecol 1991;165:278.
12. Rapkin AJ: Adhesions and pelvic pain: A retrospective study. Obstet Gynecol 1986;68:13.
13. Bonica JJ: The Management of Pain. Philadelphia, Lea & Febiger, 1989, p 180.
14. Howard FM: The role of laparoscopy in chronic pelvic pain: Promise and pitfalls. Obstet Gynecol Surv 1993;48:357.
15. Venturini PL, Semino A, DeCecco L: The biological basis of medical treatment of endometriosis. Gynecol Endocrinol 1995;9:259.
16. Redwine D: Age-related evolution on color appearance of endometriosis. Fertil Steril 1987;48:1062.
17. Spangen L: Nonpalpable inguinal hernia in women. In Nyhus LM, Condon RE (eds): Hernia. Philadelphia, JB Lippincott, 1995, p 87.
18. Steege JF, Stout AL, Somkuti SG: Chronic pelvic pain in women: Toward an integrative model. Obstet Gynecol Surv 1993;48:95.
19. Farquhar CM, Rogers V, Granks S, et al: A randomized controlled trial of medroxyprogesterone acetate and psychotherapy for the treatment of pelvic congestion. Br J Obstet Gynecol 1989;96:1153.
20. Baker PN, Symonds EN: The resolution of chronic pelvic pain after normal laparoscopic findings. Am J Obstet Gynecol 1992;166:835.
21. Beard RW, Reginald PW, Wadsworth J: Clinical features of women with chronic lower abdominal pain and pelvic congestion. Br J Obstet Gynecol 1988;95:153.
22. Peters AAW, van Dorst E, Jellis B, et al: A randomized clinical trial to compare two different approaches in women with chronic pelvic pain. Obstet Gynecol 1991;77:740.
23. Carlson KJ, Miller BA, Fowler FJ: The Maine Women's Health Study: II. Outcomes of nonsurgical management of leiomyomas, abnormal bleeding and chronic pelvic pain. Obstet Gynecol 1994;83:566.
24. Reginald PW, Adams J, Franks, et al: Medroxyprogesterone acetate in the treatment of pelvic pain due to venous congestion. Br J Obstet Gynecol 1989;96:1148.
25. Wilcox LS, Koonin LM, Podras R, et al: Hysterectomy in the United States, 1988–1990. Obstet Gynecol 1994;83:549.
26. Hillis SD, Marchbanks PA, Peterson HB: The effectiveness of hysterectomy for chronic pelvic pain. Obstet Gynecol 1995;86:941.

13

Adhesions and Pelvic Pain

John F. Steege, MD

Adhesions are among the most common organic findings noted at the time of diagnostic laparoscopy performed for the evaluation of chronic pelvic pain (CPP). Adhesions have been noted to be more prevalent in women with chronic pain,[1, 2] although they are frequently present, sometimes to an extensive degree, without being associated with pain. This chapter reviews the role of adhesions in pelvic nociception, the impact of adhesiolysis on the relief of pain, the biology of adhesion formation and peritoneal healing, and the various methods for preventing adhesion formation. New diagnostic techniques that will undoubtedly further clarify the role of adhesions in the causation of chronic pain are reviewed.

Clinical Observations About Adhesions

Approximately 60% to 90% of women who have had a previous laparotomy have some form of pelvic adhesions, most of which involve adherence of the omentum to the anterior abdominal wall.[3] Few of the adhesions cause acute problems, but intestinal obstruction is encountered after 0.3% of benign adnexal gynecologic surgeries, 2% to 3% of hysterectomies and about 5% of radical hysterectomies,[3] and 1% of general surgical laparotomies.[4] The economic cost of the treatment of adhesive disease is substantial, amounting to approximately 1.2 billion dollars annually in the United States, according to some estimates.[5]

Although adhesions very often are a result of previous surgical intervention, they also may occur after subclinical inflammatory processes such as pelvic inflammatory disease, ruptured cysts, and postpartum infection. Autopsy studies reveal about a 30% prevalence of some adhesions in women who have never had pelvic surgery.[6] Most of the subjects in that study were older than 60 years; hence, the prevalence of adhesions in younger, reproductive-age women may be significantly lower. Kresch and colleagues[1] found a 12% incidence of adhesions in women undergoing laparoscopy for tubal sterilization. In contrast, adhesions are more prevalent in women with pelvic pain. These researchers found pathologic changes in 89% of women undergoing laparoscopy for pelvic pain and formed the subjective impression that adhesions that tightly adhered adjacent organs together were more likely to be associated with pain. A subsequent study[7] demonstrated that adhesions were most commonly present on the side of the pelvis that was most symptomatic. The development of minilaparoscopy under local anesthesia will doubtless allow the development of far more specific data defining the role of adhesions in pelvic pain (see Chapter 33). With a patient awake and able to report pain intensity on a 1 to 10 scale, traction on the adhesions and probing of involved organs allow the surgeon to estimate the benefit of potential adhesiolysis.

Treatment of Adhesion-Related Pain

Surgical approaches to adhesiolysis for the relief of pain have yielded variable but encouraging results. Sutton and MacDonald[8] reported 85% relief of CPP after laparoscopic lysis of adhesions. Steege and Stout[7] reported that 67% of women experienced significant relief of pain after laparoscopic adhesiolysis. However, relief was found in

75% of those without the psychologic and behavioral hallmarks of a chronic pain syndrome (see Chapter 2), but only 40% of women who did have a chronic pain syndrome profile improved. Only one controlled study has been performed: Peters and colleagues[9] performed laparoscopy on 48 women and graded their adhesions. Half the women subsequently underwent laparotomy for lysis of adhesions, and half had only the diagnostic procedure. At 9 to 12 months postoperatively, no difference in pain level was found in the two groups, except for those who were noted to have had severe bowel adhesions at the time of the initial procedure. In this group, eight of the nine who had laparotomy had improvement, compared with one of six who improved after the diagnostic laparoscopy only. A second-look laparoscopy to evaluate the effectiveness of the adhesiolysis was not performed; this is important because of the high rate of adhesion re-formation after laparotomy.

Many observers have noted that the formation of adhesions follows the chronology of the healing process after peritoneal injury. That is, adhesions begin to be seen within 1 to 2 weeks after peritoneal insult. Despite this early regrowth of adhesions, pain associated with adhesion re-formation often does not begin until 1 to 3 months after surgery or later. The reasons for this delay are rather unclear. Contraction and mechanical shortening of the adhesions may play a part. The role of the possible ingrowth of nerves into the adhesions has been preliminarily explored in only one study, with inconclusive results.[10]

Diagnosis of Adhesions

Despite a number of attempts, nonsurgical methods of diagnosing adhesions have been largely unsuccessful. Stovall and colleagues[11] found the physical examination to be a poor predictor of the presence and location of adhesions visualized during subsequent laparoscopy. Early investigators attempted such techniques as creating a pneumoperitoneum just before obtaining an abdominal radiograph.[12, 13] The technique was not evaluated statistically. Maroulis and coworkers[14] developed the procedure of hydrogynecography by instilling sterile saline via the uterus and fallopian tubes in 28 infertile patients and 10 patients with CPP. They described the technique as 100% sensitive for detecting adhesions in the lower pelvis. It did not accurately predict periovarian adhesions.

Standard vaginal ultrasound examination has been used as well, with the observation that ovarian mobility relative to surrounding structures (slide-by) noted during transvaginal ultrasonography usually means that periovarian adhesions are not present. Although this may be a reasonable generalization, it has quite low sensitivity and specificity in my view. In a pilot study of eight patients, my colleagues and I attempted to compare standard vaginal sonography with minilaparoscopy and transvaginal ultrasonography with the presence of 150 ml of fluid in the lower pelvis. Vaginal sonography with or without a fluid contrast medium was found to be substantially inferior to either minilaparoscopy or a standard operating room laparoscopy.

Clinical Assessment of Patients with Pelvic Adhesions

Surgically oriented gynecologists must be aware of a seductive trap: Women with pain tend to be operated on, and operations tend to cause adhesions; subsequently, the postoperative adhesions may incorrectly be held responsible for continued pain. The challenging task is to take a mental step backward and reevaluate all possible components of the pain before advocating yet another surgical procedure. This includes taking a detailed history of the chronology of the pain and a history designed to elicit potential musculoskeletal, gastrointestinal, urinary tract, and emotional contributions. All reasonable and cost-effective treatments for these components should be brought to bear as first measures, before proceeding to the operating room.

At some point in this process, minilaparoscopy under local anesthesia can be very informative (see Chapter 33). However, I have found it is often useful to attempt to diminish some of the other contributing factors, especially musculoskeletal factors, before performing minilaparoscopy. This approach results in a more informative procedure that is better tolerated. Including the laparoscopy as one treatment measure among several also puts proper emphasis on it from a patient's perspective.

Adhesion Formation and Re-formation

The peritoneum heals with remarkable speed and with minimal scarring. Indeed, it is far more forgiving of surgical or pathologic trespass than are most other layers of the body, especially the skin. Clinical impressions often lead one to believe that some patients are much more prone to adhesion formation than others.

The peritoneum is so forgiving because it heals from the depths of the injured area, not from the edges.[15] The integrity of the parietal peritoneum is complete within 3 to 4 days, but visceral peritoneal injury takes 5 to 8 days to heal.[16] A study performed on mice[17] implies that adhesions are much more likely to form if two adjacent peritoneal surfaces are denuded; denudation of one surface is much less likely to result in adhesions.

The stages in the reperitonealization process are relatively well defined (Fig. 13–1). The area of peritoneal injury is first coated by a fibrin matrix. Peritoneal macrophages secrete mitogens that suppress the activity of tissue repair cells during the first 2 days after peritoneal injury.[18] On the third to fourth days after peritoneal injury, tissue repair cells (mesothelial cells) start to migrate outward from the depths of the wound and begin to repave the injured area. Plasminogen activator produced by macrophages begins to appear during this time, initiating the process of fibrinolysis. If fibrin is deposited in excessive amounts or persists for too long, it becomes infiltrated with fibroblasts that begin to lay down a collagen matrix. Vascularization of this matrix begins 5 to 6 days after injury, and collagen is deposited during postinjury days 5 through 10.

By 2 weeks after injury, the cellular elements are far less obvious, with fibroblasts predominating. Two to 3 months after peritoneal injury, the collagen matrix is covered with mesothelium and is fully infiltrated with blood vessels. Neural ingrowth has not been fully evaluated but probably occurs much later, because nerve cells grow much more slowly.

Extensive animal work as well as clinical observations of humans have demonstrated that a host of factors can increase the tendency of adhesions to form (Fig. 13–2).

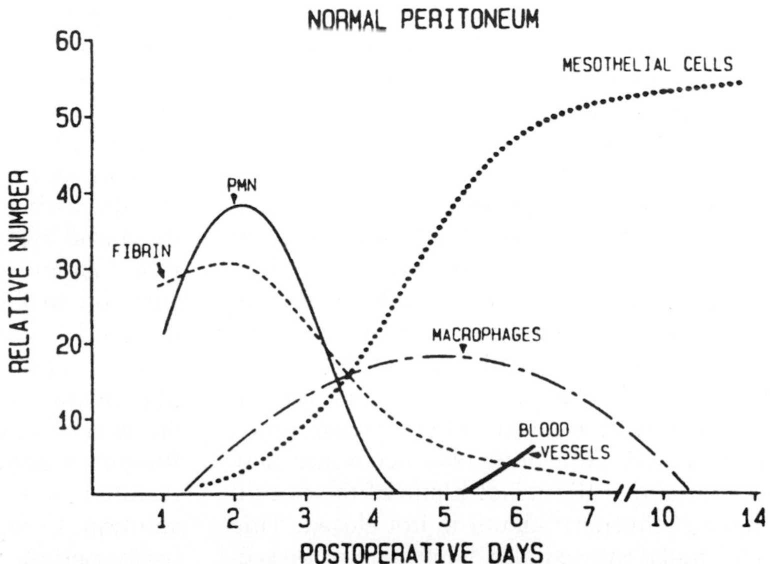

Figure 13–1. Change in the relative number of cellular elements and fibrinolysis (fibrin) at the site of peritoneal injury in mature rats during the course of reepithelialization. The principal cellular elements in control of peritoneal healing are macrophages, which appear in large numbers 1 to 2 days after surgery. Macrophages are involved in regulating fibroblast and mesothelial cell functions. Approximately 2 days after surgery, mesothelial cells appear in large numbers over the damaged peritoneum. By day 6 or 7 after surgical injury, virtually all of the peritoneal injury is covered by at least one layer of mesothelial cells. (From diZerega GS, Rodgers KE: The Peritoneum. New York, Springer-Verlag, 1992.)

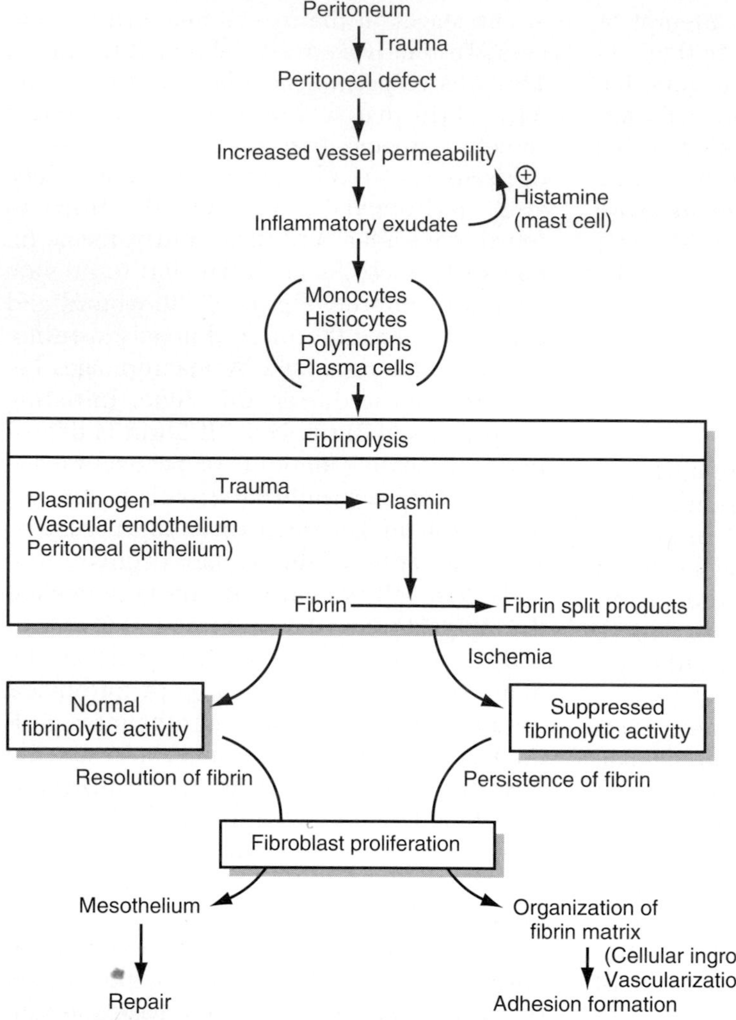

Figure 13–2. Summary of normal tissue repair and adhesion formation after surgical trauma.

These include the presence of any factors that increase inflammatory response (e.g., sutures), increase the quantity of devitalized tissue (e.g., tissue crushing), tissue drying, and the presence of infection. In some animal models, adhesion formation is increased when a peritoneal incision is sutured closed rather than left open to repair itself.[19, 20] In humans, suturing the abdominal wall peritoneum closed after a laparotomy seems to make no difference in the subsequent rate of adhesion to this area.[21] However, if adhesions to the anterior abdominal wall do form after a laparotomy, small bowel adhesions may occur and may extend above the usual plane of the peritoneum if the peritoneum is not closed. This may make subsequent laparoscopic dissection in this area more likely to result in bowel injury.

The nature of irrigant fluids used during abdominal and laparoscopic surgery may influence postoperative adhesion formation. Kappas and colleagues[22] demonstrated that in rats, saline irrigation above 45°C caused increased rates of adhesion formation. In a rabbit laparoscopy model, irrigation with saline led to more postoperative adhesions than did irrigation with lactated Ringer's solution.[23] This was attributed to the tendency of ambient carbon dioxide (CO_2) to form carbonic acid when exposed to saline. Lactated Ringer's solution, being a buffered solution, resulted in a less acidic pH of the irrigant solution. Comparable studies have not been performed on humans.

Laparoscopy Versus Laparotomy

In an animal model, Luciano and coworkers[24] clearly demonstrated that laparoscopy is more successful than laparotomy in treating postoperative adhesions. In multicenter studies of adhesion formation after microsurgery for infertility, postoperative adhesion formation is reported in approximately 50% of women, regardless of whether laser or standard microsurgical techniques were used.[25, 26] Pregnancy rates after surgery for infertility have been comparable in some series that randomized patients to laparotomy versus laparoscopy,[27] whereas microsurgery at laparotomy has been superior to laparoscopic salpingostomy in others.[28]

After laparoscopic adhesiolysis, the total adhesion score is reduced approximately 50%,[29] although some adhesions re-form in almost all patients. When no adhesion barriers are used, 45% of filmy, 62% of dense, and 80% of cohesive adhesions reform. *De novo* adhesions can form to some degree after laparoscopy;[29] hence, laparoscopic lysis of adhesions may not be an entirely innocuous procedure, although it appears to result in improvement more often than does laparotomy.

In one study that randomized patients with ectopic pregnancy to laparoscopy versus laparotomy, second-look laparoscopy revealed adhesions to be much less severe in the laparoscopy group, causing "tubal impairment" less often (16% versus 52%).[30] The two techniques have never been directly compared in the treatment of chronically painful gynecologic conditions.

Adhesion Prevention

Virtually all authorities in the field of adhesions agree that correct surgical technique is of paramount importance in minimizing the tendency of adhesions to reform. This means careful atraumatic handling of tissues and avoidance of drying or crushing of tissue, suturing, and infection. The laparoscopic approach follows all of these recommendations. Further, considerable controversy has surrounded the relative merits of different energy sources for dividing tissue: electrocautery versus CO_2 laser versus neodymium:yttrium-aluminum-garnet (Nd:YAG) laser versus sharp dissection. When applied by the same surgical approach (i.e., laparotomy[28] or laparoscopy[31]) and when power density is controlled, electrocautery, CO_2 laser, and KTP laser cause equivalent amounts of tissue damage. Even with the inherent advantages of laparoscopy, careful technique and gentle dissection of tissues are still of substantial importance in minimizing tissue damage during the course of adhesiolysis.

The prevention of adhesion *de novo* formation and adhesion re-formation has been the subject of much study in the past 75 years. The long list of medications, solutions, and barriers used is testimony to the difficulty of the problem and to the incomplete efficacy of all known methods. The improvements in barriers and topical gels currently under investigation, together with the advent of lower-cost options for repeated laparoscopic adhesiolysis (see Chapter 33), raises the hope that substantial progress may at last be made in dealing with this difficult clinical problem.

Medications

Perhaps the earliest pharmacologic interventions used dealt with systemic or intraperitoneal steroids. The early studies with Horne's regimen used steroids in combination with antihistamines and other agents.[32] The regimen was never tested in a controlled trial but was compared with historical controls. Its use diminished with the development of alternative measures. The use of steroids has always carried with it the fear that wound strength would be impaired to the same degree that adhesions were prevented. This same general concern applies to virtually all medications that are aimed at somehow impeding the physiologic healing process described earlier, for it appears that the process of healing is very similar to the process of adhesion formation, an exaggerated and unbalanced form of healing.

Nonsteroidal antiinflammatory drugs have shown promising effects in animals and are currently being tested in humans. Montz and associates[33] demonstrated very effective adhesion prevention in a pig laparotomy model, using ketorolac 4 mg/kg 45 minutes before incision and 2 mg/kg IM every 8 hours for 3 days postoperatively. Similarly, Marcovici and colleagues,[34] using a rabbit model, found that colchicine was more effective than an antibiotic in preventing postoperative adhesions. Golan and associates[35] found that intraperitoneal instillation of prostaglandin E_2 promoted adhesions and that prophylactic use of aspirin reduced adhesion formation in a rat model.

More recent work has used recombinant tissue plasminogen activator (rt-PA) in rabbits[36, 37] and dogs.[38] The impact of rt-PA on wound strength has been variably reported as none[36] or adverse.[39, 40]

Heparin may facilitate fibrinolysis by enhancing macrophage activation.[41] It also may facilitate the generation of plasmin from plasminogen and tissue plasminogen activator.[42] However, adding heparin to lactated Ringer's solution did not contribute to adhesion prevention,[43] although it may augment the effect of the oxidized cellulose adhesion barrier.[44]

Progesterone, which has some antiinflammatory properties, prevents postoperative adhesions in a guinea pig model,[45] whereas medroxyprogesterone inhibits adhesion formation in a rat model.[46] The approach may merit clinical trials.

Several studies have used multidrug protocols. Gehlbach and coworkers[47] showed that rt-PA plus carboxymethylcellulose was no more effective than carboxymethylcellulose alone, saline, or dextran in a rabbit model and was associated with an increased risk of hemorrhage. Wiseman and associates[48] investigated the problem of blood's interfering with the effectiveness of oxidized cellulose. They applied heparin-soaked Interceed to surgically damaged rabbit uterine horns with or without prior application of thrombin to accomplish complete hemostasis. Bleeding nullified the effect of the oxidized cellulose barrier; prior application of thrombin preserved Interceed's effectiveness.

Barrier Methods

Barrier methods of adhesion prevention have perhaps received the greatest attention in recent years. Although a whole host of mechanical barriers have been used in the past, the two with the greatest experimental and human experience are oxidized cellulose (Interceed) and polytetrafluoroethylene (PTFE; Gore-Tex).

DiZerega reviewed both animal and human studies using oxidized cellulose.[49] When comparing Interceed with no treatment in animal adhesion models, eight studies yielded results favoring oxidized cellulose but five showed no efficacy. Haney and Doty,[50] using a mouse model, demonstrated that Interceed itself causes injury to the intact peritoneum, as well as a mild inflammatory response.

In human research, in six studies in which Interceed was applied to one pelvic sidewall and compared with no treatment on the other sidewall when adhesions were lysed or endometriosis treated at the time of laparotomy, the Interceed-treated side when examined at second-look laparoscopy had diminished severity and area involved with adhesions in all cases. The degree of difference seen varied significantly from study to study. Although the proportion of adhesion-free sidewalls was improved in all studies, substantial numbers still had some adhesions on the Interceed side in all of the studies cited.[51–56] In one study of eight women undergoing laparoscopic ovarian cautery for polycystic ovarian disease refractory to medical therapy, Interceed was applied to one ovary and second-look laparoscopy performed 3 to 4 weeks later. The barrier did not reduce adhesion formation, but the degree of adhesions did not affect fertility, and seven of the eight ultimately conceived.[57]

The PTFE surgical membrane has also been extensively evaluated in both animals and humans. Early work by Fowler and colleagues[58] in dogs revealed that if wrinkles were allowed to persist after suturing PTFE membrane in place, adhesions formed to the wrinkles. Adhesions to the edges of the membrane also formed when absorbable sutures were used to secure it in place. In further work using a porcine model in which radical hysterectomy was performed, PTFE substantially reduced adhesions when compared with no treatment,[59] but oxidized cellulose performed slightly better than PTFE.[60] Haney and Doty[61] compared PTFE with Interceed in an animal model and found PTFE to be clearly superior.

The PTFE membrane has been studied extensively in humans as well. An early uncontrolled study[62] demonstrated by second-look laparoscopy that PTFE dramatically reduced adhesion formation after myomectomy and after lysis of pelvic sidewall adhesions. In a controlled study comparing PTFE with no treatment after myomectomy by laparotomy, PTFE-treated patients had dramatically reduced adhesion formation at second-look laparoscopy 2 to 6 weeks after surgery.[63] The membrane was removed at the time of the second-look laparoscopy. PTFE was then compared with Interceed by another group,[64] and the membrane then removed at the time of laparoscopy 1 to 6 weeks later. In PTFE-treated sidewalls, 73% had no adhesions versus 24% of Interceed-treated sidewalls.

The accumulated evidence comparing oxidized cellulose with PTFE might be best summarized as follows: Oxidized cellulose has the advantage of being an absorbable substance and hence does not require the surgeon to make a decision about whether to leave the membrane in place or remove it. PTFE does require such a clinical decision, and in most instances surgeons are still removing the membrane at second-look laparoscopy. However, PTFE is approved for permanent implantation and might certainly be left in place indefinitely in many clinical situations. The oxidized cellulose membrane seems to have substantial impact in diminishing the densest adhesions but is less effective than PTFE in eliminating them completely. Understanding that activated macrophages are required for reabsorption of Interceed would help make sense of this phenomenon: It would appear that Interceed may diminish the more severe types of adhesions, but the inflammatory response required for its reabsorption may leave some patients with mild adhesions in their place.

Solutions

Perhaps the most common method used to prevent postoperative adhesions after laparoscopic surgery has been placing a variable volume of lactated Ringer's solution in the pelvis and leaving it there. In one study using a rat model, lactated Ringer's performed better than either Interceed or PTFE in preventing postoperative adhesions.[65] The same result was obtained by Tulandi and coworkers,[66] even when the oxidized cellulose was saturated with heparin. Four studies of humans using maximum volumes of 200 ml have not demonstrated any efficacy in preventing re-formation of adhesions after laparoscopic surgery (summarized by DiZerega[49]); however, most laparoscopic surgeons now leave as much as 1000 ml of the lactated Ringer's solution in the pelvis. In patients on dialysis, the peritoneal dialysate is absorbed at about 35 ml per hour, suggesting that a larger volume is likely to be present for at least several days after surgery, allowing a greater length of time for tissue repair cells to form a new surface over the treated areas. Theoretically, one might be concerned that a large volume of fluid left in the peritoneal cavity would dilute opsonic proteins that help fight intraperitoneal infection,[49] but in clinical practice, infections following laparoscopic surgery have proved to be extremely rare, despite the widespread use of lactated Ringer's solution.

Other nonmembrane barriers have been explored, such as a hydrogel barrier,[67] poloxamer materials that convert from a liquid to a gel form when heated from room temperature to body temperature, hyaluronic acid,[68] polyvinylpyrrolidone,[69] and fibrin glue.[70] To date, all of the gel methods have been promising in animal models but disappointing when used in pilot human studies. Further modifications of these materials are under way, and they may yet prove promising for human use.

Finally, other treatments that have been aimed at modifying the inflammatory response have been tested on animals. These include cytokine inhibitors (e.g., interleukin-1 and -10) and the use of protease peptone placed intraperitoneally 3 days before surgery to develop a population of induced peritoneal macrophages that contain increased levels of plasminogen activator.[71]

Second-Look Laparoscopy

Repeated laparoscopy has been advocated for some time as a means of further reducing the adhesion burden before the adhesion re-formation process is complete. Raj and Hulka[72] advocated a second-look laparoscopy 4 to 8 weeks after laparotomy for infertility surgery. Trimbos-Kemper and colleagues[73] performed second-look laparoscopy 8 days after laparotomy for infertility surgery in 188 patients. In those who did not become pregnant, third-look laparoscopy demonstrated that the second-look laparoscopy had accomplished a 50% reduction in pelvic adhesions. The ectopic pregnancy rate was also lower in those who received the second-look laparoscopy. The study was not a randomized trial of second-look laparoscopy.

Jansen[43] also performed second-look laparoscopy within 12 days of laparotomy for infertility surgery. In 38 cases, third-look laparoscopy was performed, demonstrating a dramatic reduction in adhesion scores on average and improvement in adhesions in 33 of the 38 patients thus treated. Malinak[52] reported that the timing of the second-look laparoscopy (between 14 days and 3 months) did not correlate with the amount of adhesions observed. This would suggest that whatever adhesions are going to form develop within the first 2 weeks after a surgical procedure.

Although controlled studies have not yet been carried out, it would thus appear that early second-look laparoscopy can substantially reduce pelvic adhesion re-formation after either laparoscopy or laparotomy. This adhesion reduction has not been demonstrated to improve pregnancy rates after infertility surgery, but it may demonstrate significant potential for reducing CPP and thus demands systematic study.

Summary

In summary, let me offer the approach that I have applied in my own practice. I routinely attempt to perform all adhesiolysis procedures via laparoscopy. On rare occasion this proves impossible, and laparotomy is then performed, followed by second-look laparoscopy within 1 week of the first surgery. If extensive adhesions are lysed at the time of the first laparoscopy, then a second-look laparoscopy is offered to the patient, again to occur within 1 week after the first surgery.

At the first laparoscopy, a 1-L volume of lactated Ringer's solution is left in place. In selected circumstances involving adhesions limited to the area between the ovary and the broad ligament, Interceed is placed as long as hemostasis is excellent (Ringer's solution is omitted). If hemostasis is less than perfect, a PTFE membrane is sutured in place with PTFE suture and then removed at the time of second-look laparoscopy 1 week later. If tubal ligation or hysterectomy was performed previously, thus eliminating the potential for subsequent pregnancy, then either a lactated Ringer's solution or PTFE is used, depending on whether or not a second-look laparoscopy is planned.

At present, structured clinical trials and randomized trials are being initiated to evaluate these approaches further. It is my opinion that a most effective adhesion reduction protocol has several components: optimum laparoscopic technique at the first surgery with placement of an adhesion prevention barrier over the involved operated areas, followed by second- and perhaps third-look laparoscopies at very short intervals (such as 5 to 7 days). The cost-effectiveness of this approach may be dramatically improved as the techniques of laparoscopy under local anesthesia are further developed.

In the days before laparoscopy, one resorted to laparotomy for the treatment of adhesions only in the most desperate of circumstances. Medical and psychobehavioral treatments for adhesion-related pain were the only therapies available. Now, ironically, ready availability of laparoscopy may lead to the unfortunate deemphasis of the complexity of pain and the utility of nonsurgical pain management techniques. Our best surgical tool can become our worst enemy. Throughout the process of attempting to reduce the adhesion burden, a clinician must ever remain aware that even when adhesions are present, their role in producing a patient's pain must be constantly reevaluated. Clinicians need to be watchful for the emergence of other components, such as those attributed to musculoskeletal problems and functional bowel disorders and so on. Undue emphasis on surgery in the overall management plan may serve only to divert a patient's and her physician's attention away from other significant components of the pain problem.

References

1. Kresch AJ, Seifer DB, Sachs LB, et al: Laparoscopy in the evaluation of pelvic pain. Obstet Gynecol 1973;64:672.
2. Stout AL, Steege JF, Dodson WC, et al: Relationship of laparoscopic findings to self-report of pelvic pain. Am J Obstet Gynecol 1991;164:73.
3. Monk BJ, Berman ML, Montz FI: Adhesions after extensive gynecologic surgery: Clinical significance, etiology, and prevention. Am J Obstet Gynecol 1994;170:1396.
4. Menzies D, Ellis H: Intestinal obstruction from adhesions—How big is the problem? Ann R Coll Surg Engl 1990;72:60.
5. Ray NF, Larsen JW, Stillman RJ, Jacobs RJ: Economic impact of hospitalizations for lower abdominal adhesiolysis in the United States in 1988. Surg Gynecol Obstet 1993;176:271.
6. Weibel MA, Majno G: Peritoneal adhesions and their relation to abdominal surgery. Am J Surg 1973;126:345.
7. Steege JF, Stout AL: Resolution of chronic pelvic pain after laparoscopic lysis of adhesions. Am J Obstet Gynecol 1991;165:278.
8. Sutton C, MacDonald R: Laser laparoscopic adhesiolysis. J Gynecol Surg 1990;6:155.
9. Peters AAW, Trimbos-Kemper GCM, Admiraal C, Trimbos JB: A randomized clinical trial on the benefit of adhesiolysis in patients with intraperitoneal adhesions and chronic pelvic pain. Br J Obstet Gynecol 1992;99:59.
10. Kligman I, Drachenberg C, Papadimitriou J, Katz E: Immunohistochemical demonstration of nerve fibers in pelvic adhesions. Obstet Gynecol 1993;82:566.
11. Stovall TG, Elder RF, Ling FW: Predictors of pelvic adhesions. J Reprod Med 1989;34:345.
12. Yung M: Radiographie des organes du petit bassin de la femme apres pneumoperitoine. Gynecol Obstet 1923;8:329.
13. Stein IF: Gynecography: X-ray diagnosis in gynecology. Surg Clin North Am 1943;23:165.
14. Maroulis GB, Parsons AK, Yeko TR: Hydrogynecography: A new technique enables vaginal sonography to visualize pelvic adhesions and other pelvic structures. Fertil Steril 1992;58:1073.
15. Ellis H, Harrison W, Hugh TB: The healing of peritoneum under normal and pathological conditions. Br J Surg 1965;52:471.
16. diZerega GS: Contemporary adhesion prevention. Fertil Steril 1994;61:219.
17. Haney AF, Doty E: The formation of coalescing peritoneal adhesions requires injury to both contacting peritoneal surfaces. Fertil Steril 1994; 61:767.
18. Rogers KE, diZerega GS: Modulation of peritoneal reepithelialization by postsurgical macrophages. J Surg Res 1992;53:542.
19. O'Leary DP, Coakley JB: The influence of suturing and sepsis on the development of postoperative peritoneal adhesions. Ann R Coll Surg Engl 1992;74:134.
20. Buckman RF, Buckman PD, Hufnagel HV, Gervin AS: A physiologic basis for the adhesion-free healing of deperitonealized surfaces. J Surg Res 1976;21:67.
21. Tulandi T, Hum GS, Gelfand MM: Closure of laparotomy incisions with or without peritoneal suturing and second look laparoscopy. Am J Obstet Gynecol 1988;158:536.
22. Kappas AM, Fatouros M, Papadimitriou K, et al: Effect of intraperitoneal saline irrigation at different temperatures on adhesion formation. Br J Surg 1988;75:854.
23. Sahakian V, Rogers RG, Halme J, Hulka J: Effects of carbon dioxide–saturated normal saline and Ringer's lactate on postsurgical adhesion formation in the rabbit. Obstet Gynecol 1993;82:851.
24. Luciano AA, Maier DB, Koch EL, et al: A comparative study of postoperative adhesions following laser surgery by laparoscopy versus laparotomy in the rabbit model. Obstet Gynecol 1989;74:220.
25. Diamond MP, Daniell JF, Feste J, et al: Adhesion reformation and *de novo* adhesion formation after reproductive pelvic surgery. Fertil Steril 1987;47:864.
26. Diamond MP, Daniell JF, Martin DC, et al: Tubal patency and pelvic adhesions at early second-look laparoscopy following intraabdominal use of the carbon dioxide laser: Initial report of the intraabdominal laser study group. Fertil Steril 1984;42:717.
27. Bruhat MA, Mage G, Chapron C, et al: Present day endoscopic surgery in gynecology. Eur J Obstet Gynecol 1991;41:4.
28. Audebert F, Hedon B, Arnal F, et al: Therapeutic strategies in tubal infertility with distal pathology. Hum Reprod 1991;6:439.
29. Operative Laparoscopy Study Group: Postoperative adhesion development after operative laparoscopy: Evaluation at early second look procedures. Fertil Steril 1991;55:700.
30. Lundorff P, Thorburn J, Hahlin M, et al: Adhesion formation after laparoscopic surgery in tubal pregnancy: A randomized trial versus laparotomy. Fertil Steril 1991;55:911.
31. Luciano AA, Randolph J, Whitman G, et al: A comparison of thermal injury, healing patterns, and postoperative adhesion formation following CO_2 laser and electromicrosurgery. Fertil Steril 1987;48:1025.
32. Horne HW Jr, Clyman M, Debrovner C, Griggs G: The prevention of postoperative pelvic adhesions following conservative operative treatment for human infertility. Int J Fertil 1973;18:109.
33. Montz FJ, Monk BJ, Lacy SM, Fowler JM: Ketorolac tromethamine, a nonsteroidal anti-inflammatory drug: Ability to inhibit postradical pelvic surgery adhesions in a porcine model. Gynecol Oncol 1993;48:76.
34. Marcovici I, Brill AI, Scommegna A: Effects of colchicine on pelvic adhesions associated with the intrauterine innoculation of *Neisseria gonorrhoeae* in rabbits. Obstet Gynecol 1993;81:118.

35. Golan A, Bernstein T, Wexler S, et al: The effect of prostaglandins and aspirin—an inhibitor of prostaglandin synthesis—on adhesion formation in rats. Hum Reprod 1991;6:251.
36. Menzies D, Ellis H: The role of plasminogen activator in adhesion prevention. Surg Gynecol Obstet 1991;172:362.
37. Dunn RC, Mohler M: Effect of varying days of tissue plasminogen activator therapy on the prevention of postsurgical adhesions in a rabbit model. J Surg Res 1993;54:242.
38. Montz FJ, Fowler JMJ, Wolff AJ, et al: The ability of recombinant tissue plasminogen activator to inhibit post-radical pelvic surgery adhesions in the dog model. Am J Obstet Gynecol 1991;165:1539.
39. Evans DM, McAree K, Guyton DP, et al: Dose dependency and wound healing aspects of the use of tissue plasminogen activator in the prevention of intra-abdominal adhesions. Am J Surg 1993; 165:229.
40. Thompson JN, Whawell SA: Pathogenesis and prevention of adhesion formation. Br J Surg 1995;82:3.
41. Fukasawa M, Girgis W, diZerega GS: Inhibition of postsurgical adhesions in a standardized rabbit model: II. Intraperitoneal treatment with heparin. Int J Fertil 1991;36:296.
42. Andrade-Gordon P, Strickland S: Interaction of heparin with plasminogen activators and plasminogen: Effects on the activation of plasminogen. Biochemistry 1986;25:4033.
43. Jansen RPS: Failure of peritoneal irrigation with heparin during pelvic operations upon young women to reduce adhesions. Surg Gynecol Obstet 1988;166:154.
44. Reid RL, Lie K, Spence JE, et al: Clinical evaluation of the efficacy of heparin-saturated Interceed for the prevention of adhesion reformation in the pelvic sidewall of the human. Prog Clin Biol Res 1993;381:261.
45. Maurer JH, Bonaventura LM: The effect of aqueous progesterone on operative adhesion formation. Fertil Steril 39:485,1983.
46. Montanino-Oviva M, Metzger DA, Luciano AA: Use of medroxyprogesterone acetate in the prevention of postoperative adhesions. Fertil Steril 1996; 65:650.
47. Gehlbach DL, O'Hair KC, Parks AL, Rosa C: Combined effects of tissue plasminogen activator and carboxymethylcellulose on adhesion formation in rabbits. Int J Fertil 1994;39:172.
48. Wiseman DM, Gottlick LE, Diamond MP: Effects of thrombin-induced hemostasis on the efficacy of an absorbable adhesion barrier. J Reprod Med 1992;37:766.
49. diZerega GS: Contemporary adhesion prevention. Fertil Steril 1994;61:219.
50. Haney AF, Doty E: Murine peritoneal injury and *de novo* adhesion formation caused by oxidized-regenerated cellulose (Interceed [TC7]) but not expanded polytetrafluoroethylene (Gore-Tex Surgical Membrane). Fertil Steril 1992;57:202.
51. Bowman MC, Cooke I: The efficacy of synthetic adhesion barriers in infertility surgery. Br J Obstet Gynecol 1994;101:3.
52. Malinak RL: Interceed (TC7) as an adjuvant for adhesion reduction: Clinical studies. In diZerega GS, Malinak LR, Diamond MP, Linsky CB (eds): Treatment of Postoperative Surgical Adhesions. New York, John Wiley & Sons, 1990, pp 193–206.
53. Nordic Adhesion Prevention Study Group: The efficacy of Interceed (TC7) for prevention of reformation of postoperative adhesions on ovaries, fallopian tubes, and fimbriae in microsurgical operations for fertility: A multicenter study. Fertil Steril 1995;63:709.
54. Li TC, Cooke ID: The value of an absorbable adhesion barrier, Interceed, in the prevention of adhesion reformation following microsurgical adhesiolysis. Br J Obstet Gynecol 1994;101:335.
55. Azziz R: Microsurgery alone or with Interceed absorbable adhesion barrier for pelvic sidewall adhesion re-formation. The Interceed (TC7) Adhesion Barrier Study Group II. Surg Gynecol Obstet 1993;177:135.
56. Sekiba K: Obstetrics and Gynecology Adhesion Prevention Committee: Use of Interceed (TC7) absorbable adhesion barrier to reduce postoperative adhesion reformation in infertility and endometriosis surgery. Obstet Gynecol 1992;79:518.
57. Greenblatt EM, Casper RF: Adhesion formation after laparoscopic ovarian cautery for polycystic ovarian syndrome: Lack of correlation with pregnancy rate. Fertil Steril 1993;60:766.
58. Fowler JM, Lacy SM, Montz FJ: The inability of Gore-Tex surgical membrane to inhibit post-radical pelvic surgery adhesions in the dog model. Gynecol Oncol 1991;43:141.
59. Montz FJ, Monk BJ, Lacy SM: The Gore-Tex surgical membrane: Effectiveness as a barrier to inhibit postradical pelvic surgery adhesions in a porcine model. Gynec Oncol 1992;45:290.
60. Montz FJ, Monk BJ, Lacy SM: Effectiveness of two barriers at inhibiting post-radical pelvic surgery adhesions. Gynecol Oncol 1993;48:247.
61. Haney AF, Doty E: Expanded-polytetrafluoroethylene but not oxidized regenerated cellulose prevents adhesion formation and reformation in a mouse uterine horn model of surgical injury. Fertil Steril 1993;60:550.
62. The Surgical Membrane Study Group: Prophylaxis of pelvic sidewall adhesions with Gore-Tex Surgical Membrane: A multicenter clinical investigation. Fertil Steril 1992;57:921.
63. Myomectomy Adhesion Multicenter Study Group: An expanded polytetrafluoroethylene barrier (Gore-Tex Surgical Membrane) reduces post-myomectomy adhesion formation. Fertil Steril 1995;63:491.
64. Haney AF, Murphy AA, Hesla J, et al: Expanded polytetrafluoroethylene (Gore-Tex Surgical Membrane) is superior to oxidized regenerated cellulose (Interceed TC7) in preventing adhesions. Fertil Steril 1995;63:1021.
65. Pagidas K, Tulandi T: Effects of Ringer's lactate, Interceed (TC7) and Gore-Tex Surgical Membrane on postsurgical adhesion formation. Fertil Steril 1992;57:199.
66. Tulandi T, Murray C, Guralnick M: Adhesion formation and reproductive outcome after myomectomy and second-look laparoscopy. Obstet Gynecol 1993;82:213.
67. Hill-West JL, Chowdhury SM, Sawhney AS, et al: Prevention of postoperative adhesions in the rat by *in situ* photopolymerization of bioresorbable hydrogel barriers. Obstet Gynecol 1994;83:59.
68. Urman B, Gomel V, Jetha N: Effect of hyaluronic acid on postoperative intraperitoneal adhesion formation in the rat model. Fertil Steril 1991;56:563.
69. Yaacobi Y, Israel AA, Goldberg EP: Prevention of postoperative abdominal adhesions by tissue precoating with polymer solutions. J Surg Res 1993;55:422.

70. De Iaco P, Pasquinelli G, Costa A, et al: Fibrin sealant in laparoscopic adhesion prevention in the rabbit uterine horn model. Fertil Steril 1994; 62:400.
71. Ar'Rajab AJ, Dawidson I, Sentementes J, et al: Enhancement of peritoneal macrophages reduces postoperative peritoneal adhesion formation. J Surg Res 1993;58:307.
72. Raj SG, Hulka JF: Second-look laparoscopy in infertility surgery: Therapeutic and prognostic value. Fertil Steril 1982;38:325.
73. Trimbos-Kemper TCM, Trimbos JB, van Hall EV: Adhesion formation after tubal surgery: Results of the eighth-day laparoscopy in 188 patients. Fertil Steril 1985;43:395.

14

An Integrated Approach to the Management of Endometriosis

Deborah A. Metzger, PhD, MD

Endometriosis is a painful chronic disease characterized by the growth of endometrial tissue outside the uterus. It most often affects the ovaries, fallopian tubes, ureter, peritoneum, bowel, bladder, and in rare cases the lungs, cesarean section scars, appendectomy scars, and episiotomies. The disease was first described in the 1920s[1, 2] and today is believed to affect 5% to 15% of women of reproductive age. Women diagnosed with endometriosis report more health distress, pain during or after intercourse, and interference with activities than women with other reasons for chronic pelvic pain.[3]

It is important that we acknowledge the chronic recurring nature of this disease and accept the fact that we are unable to prevent recurrences with any one treatment approach, be it surgery, hormones, or pregnancy. Affected women require and deserve long-term integrated care aimed at preserving fertility, improving function, and preventing recurrences. We are limited in providing adequate treatment for these women because universal regimens for integrated medical-surgical treatment of endometriosis are lacking.

Endometriosis is one of the most investigated gynecologic disorders, yet despite this intense academic interest, basic holes in our understanding of this enigmatic disease remain. Of the 4500 articles published on the subject during the past 25 years, descriptive and anecdotal reports have provided varied and incomplete information about endometriosis and its basic treatment. Even the more scientifically rigorous studies are difficult to interpret and apply clinically because the context into which these results are placed is often incomplete or absent. The purpose of this chapter is to attempt to overcome some of these difficulties by providing a basic yet integrated approach to the overall treatment of women with endometriosis.

Pathophysiology of Endometriosis

Endometriosis is a progressive disease involving peritoneal implants, fibrosis, adhesions, and formation of endometriomas. Although many theories have been proposed to explain the development of endometriosis, such as retrograde menstruation, metaplasia, or embryonic rests of müllerian tissue, the most popular and widely accepted theory is that of Sampson, who proposed that during menstruation, viable endometrial cells reflux through the fallopian tubes and implant on the surrounding pelvic structures.[1, 2] By a similar mechanism, viable endometrial cells may implant in open wounds or be transported to distant sites within vascular or lymphatic channels.

Although these theories may explain how endometriosis implants arise, none offers insight into why some women are predisposed but others are protected. Practically all menstruating women have retrograde menstruation and the appropriate hormonal milieu, yet the disease develops in only a few. Clinical and epidemiologic studies have suggested a familial predisposition. Another association has been postulated between the amount of retrograde menstruation and the functional status of the immune system.[4] Several studies have demonstrated that women with a greater amount of retrograde menstruation, such as those with short cycle lengths, menorrhagia, or outflow obstruction, have a much greater chance of developing endometriosis.[4, 5] Intrauterine devices, which increase menstrual flow, are three times as likely to be associated with endometriosis, whereas oral contraceptives, which tend to decrease menstrual flow, are associated with a 50% reduction in the prevalence of endometriosis.[5]

Regardless of how endometrial cells arrive in the abdomen, dysfunction of the immune system results in the inability to remove endometrial cells in a timely way, thus increasing the possibility of endometriosis development. Abnormalities of T-lymphocyte cytotoxicity,[6] B-lymphocyte function, natural killer activity,[7] and complement deposition have been observed in women with endometriosis. Clinical evidence of alterations in immune system function are twice as likely in women with endometriosis, such as chronic yeast infections and environmental allergies,[8] which are often associated with fatigue.

Once the endometrial cells have implanted on peritoneal surfaces, steroid hormones and growth factors provide support for growth and development of the lesions. Thus, the propensity to develop endometriosis is a balance between cell invasiveness, the immune system, the endocrine environment, and the number of endometrial cells that reach the peritoneal cavity.

Once implants of endometriosis develop, a multistep evolution of the disease takes place, involving cyclic menstrual bleeding, an inflammatory reaction, scarring, fibrosis, and sequestration of implants.[9, 10] Hormonal factors are of central importance in the pathogenesis of endometriosis. Like endometrium found in the uterine cavity, endometriosis implants respond to the fluctuating blood levels of ovarian hormones during the menstrual cycle. At the end of each menstrual cycle, endometriosis implants break down and bleed, causing pain or eliciting an inflammatory reaction with subsequent scarring, fibrosis, and adhesions of the affected tissues.[11]

Diagnosis

Endometriosis should be suspected in any patient with the triad of dysmenorrhea, dyspareunia, and infertility. However, it should be kept in mind that the symptoms of endometriosis may be quite variable and are for the most part determined by the areas of involvement. Although it occurs most frequently in the pelvis, endometriosis has been found in most areas of the body. After the pelvic organs, the next most commonly affected locations include the appendix, terminal ileum, cervix, perineum, abdominal scars, umbilicus, inguinal region, and ureter. Only rarely is endometriosis encountered on the diaphragm, extremities, pleura, lungs, gallbladder, spleen, stomach, or kidney.

Symptoms of pain tend to be most severe at the time of menstruation, although some women experience the most intense pain around the time of ovulation. Severity of symptoms does not always correlate with the extent of the disease; not infrequently, patients with extensive disease exhibit minimal symptoms whereas some with minimal disease may have marked symptoms. Patients with infertility may not exhibit any pain or significant dysmenorrhea.

Numerous studies have attempted to identify patient reported symptoms or physical findings that predict the presence of endometriosis. Older reviews a report a poor correlation between preoperative examinations and operative findings.[12, 13] Fedele and colleagues[14] found a relative risk of 3.1 for women reporting two or more of symptoms, which included dysmenorhea, pelvic pain, or deep dyspareunia. Others have found focal tenderness on pelvic examination to be associated with the location of implants.[15, 16] However, these symptoms cannot be consistently identified in all women with endometriosis.

The most common physical findings of pelvic endometriosis are generalized pelvic tenderness, nodular induration of the uterosacral ligaments, ovarian enlargement, and a fixed, retroverted uterus. Just as the symptoms of endometriosis can be quite variable depending on the tissues and organs involved, the pelvic findings may also be confused with other gynecologic disorders such as pelvic inflammatory disease, pelvic masses, and ectopic pregnancy.

A definitive diagnosis of endometriosis can be made only by direct visualization of the pelvis. Laparoscopy is the procedure of choice because it provides a panoramic view of the entire abdomen (see Chapter 12). Several classifications of extent of disease involvement have been developed to determine the effects of therapy and the prognosis for fertility.[17] A significant limitation of all of the classification systems has been the poor correlation between extent of disease and pain symptoms.[16] This apparent lack of correlation may be related to the morphologic and functional heterogeneity of implants, which change over time.[18] Initial implants, which are petechial or clear vesicles, showed the highest level of *in vitro* prostaglandin $F_{2\alpha}$ production, whereas more typical implants (blue, brown or black) were the least active physiologically.[19]

It has been suggested that a relationship exists between the characteristics of a patient's symptoms and the type of endometrial implant present. Characteristics such as color, degree of fibrosis, depth, size, and location may determine the type of symptoms experienced.[18, 20] Moreover, a natural progression may occur in an individual implant with age, from superficial clear and red lesions to powder-burn, diffusely fibrotic peritoneal implants.[21] Adolescents are more likely to have nonpigmented and subtle lesions.[22] Prostaglandin production is increased twofold in these "early" forms, possibly correlating with dysmenorrhea.[19] Together, these findings describe a general progression from dysmenorrhea in younger women to pelvic pain/dysparunia with the development of black, fibrotic lesions in older women. Thus, a staging system that considers the variations of lesion type, location, depth, and size is needed.

Treatment

The goals of treatment of endometriosis are to decrease pain, increase function, limit recurrence of disease, and maintain or enhance fertility. In planning therapy, many variables must be considered, such as age of the patient, extent of disease, degree of symptoms, and desire for immediate or deferred fertility. Hormonal therapy, surgery, and expectant management have been used alone or in combination to treat endometriosis. When treatment is initiated only after patients become symptomatic, both the physician and patient often feel a sense of failure and disappointment. For this reason, it is important to acknowledge that endometriosis is a chronic condition requiring long-term solutions and a multidisciplinary approach. The optimal approach to treatment requires integration of the mind and the body of the patient, medical and surgical treatments, and attention to other medical and health-related issues the patient may face.

The rationale behind treatment is based on the factors thought to be involved in the pathogenesis of endometriosis-related symptoms: retrograde menstruation, implants, estrogen, and the immune system. Optimal treatment of patients can be achieved by a three-pronged approach that includes (1) initial surgery to remove visible implants and (2) a 3- to 6-month course of hypoestrogenemia followed by (3) extended amenorrhea to inhibit retrograde menstruation. Nonspecific enhancement of immune function can be achieved by attention to diet, exercise, and stress management. More specific immunotherapy can be offered to women who have chronic yeast infections or environmental allergies and who may have significant fatigue. If this integrated approach is used, the vast majority of patients experience long-term pain relief with minimal chance of recurrence.

For patients with dysmenorrhea or mild pelvic pain as their presenting symptoms, initial treatment may consist of a 2- to 3-month trial of oral contraceptives (OCPs) and non-steroidal antiinflammatory agents. Patients who fail to obtain adequate relief, who develop recurrence of symptoms while being treated conservatively, or who have more severe pain require definitive diagnosis and aggressive treatment.

Surgical Management

Not surprisingly, many gynecologists have approached endometriosis as a surgical disease under the assumption that if all disease can be excised and proper anatomic relationships restored, a patient could be cured. However, it is now apparent that the initial pain relief experienced by a patient is often short lived: Symptoms may recur in 12% to 54% of all women within a year.[23] Rather than serving as an indicator of a lack of efficacy, these data should focus our attention on what aspects of surgery may be important in achieving pain relief, particularly in the context of a multifaceted approach that includes postoperative hormonal suppression.

Localization of tenderness on physical examination generally corresponds to the location of the anatomic sources of pain, and for this reason, it is important to perform a careful pelvic examination to map the areas of maximal tenderness (see Chapters 7 and 12).

Preoperative hormonal therapy has been advocated by some to lessen the need for extensive tissue dissection and to decrease the risk of postoperative formation of adhesions. On the other hand, preoperative hormonal therapy makes the endometriosis less visible, with the risk of leaving behind disease that may be reactivated with resumption of menstruation.[24] Although no controlled studies have been carried out to determine the best approach, whether or not a surgeon uses preoperative hormonal treatment should have no bearing on the overall approach to the treatment of endometriosis that is described in this chapter.

Conservative resection of endometriosis was tradinationally performed by laparotomy, but laparoscopic surgery is being increasingly used for all stages of disease.[25] In addition to establishing a diagnosis of endometriosis, laparoscopy permits concurrent treatment. However, laparotomy still has a role in the treatment of endometriosis. Regardless of the route of surgery, general principles of surgical management of endometriosis improve success.

Although it may appear obvious, endometriosis cannot be treated unless it is recognized. Thorough intraoperative examination of the pelvis is essential, with particular attention directed to the ovaries, anterior cul-de-sac, broad ligament under the ovaries, uterosacral ligaments, and posterior cul-de-sac (see Chapter 12).

For superficial implants, ablation of the implants is sufficient. However, for implants that demonstrate scarring, retraction, immobility of the peritoneum, or nodularity, wide local excision is necessary to remove the entire implant.[10] Failure to excise deep-seated implants in the cul-de-sac, particularly where there is complete or partial obliteration of the cul-de-sac, may be responsible for rapid recurrence of symptoms after surgery. Moreover, these fibrotic implants do not respond particularly well to hormonal suppression. Bowel resection may be necessary in some cases. Endometriomas also respond poorly to hormonal suppression, and recurrence is common after surgical drainage. The endometrioma capsule must be removed in order to minimize recurrence.

Adhesion formation is common after surgery, and attention to minimizing adhesions helps maintain fertility and prevent subsequent pain due to adhesions (see Chapter 13). Although laparoscopic surgery appears to decrease the risk of adhesion reformation when compared with laparotomy,[26] techniques to decrease adhesion formation should be a part of any surgical procedure. These include strict hemostasis, careful handling of the tissues, minimal use of suture, and use of high-power settings on electrocautery instruments and laser to minimize thermal damage and tissue necrosis. Various adhesion barriers are currently available Interceed, Preclude, and Seprafilm, and many others are under development.

Finally, selected patients may benefit from adjunctive pain-relieving measures such as presacral neurectomy, uterosacral nerve transection, or uterine suspension (see Chapters 18 and 19).

Medical Management

The three commonly used classes of hormonal suppressive agents for endometriosis are progestins, danazol, and gonadotropin-releasing hormone (GnRH) agonists. Although the mechanism of their actions differs, all of these medications produce a hypoestrogenic environment that induces amenorrhea and atrophy of intrauterine endometrium as well as endometriosis implants. All are equally effective; however, cost and patient tolerance of side effects may be the most important determinants in the selection of a specific agent.

Attention is being focused on the GnRH agonists as a versatile method of ovarian suppression because of the ability to ameliorate many of the hypoestrogenic side effects of these medications with hormonal add-back.[27] Many different agents have been added to GnRH agonists to treat symptoms such as loss of bone density, hot flashes, and breakthrough bleeding (Table 14–1). I prefer to use norethindrone acetate 2.5 mg qd during the entire duration of GnRH agonist treatment because it also suppresses ovarian function, prevents hot flashes, and minimizes loss of bone density without adding estrogen.[28]

Some problems that have been observed in approximately 10% of women on GnRH agonists include breakthrough bleeding, breakthrough pain, and inadequate pain relief. Breakthrough bleeding is often accompanied by dysmenorrhea or recurrent pain and when present around the time of monthly injections signifies the need to (1) decrease the interval between injections, (2) increase the amount of GnRH agonist administered at 28-day intervals, or (3) switch to a different GnRH agonist. Women who have inadequate pain relief in the absence of bleeding may have sources of pain in addition to endometriosis. The commonly found problems coexisting with endometriosis include abdominal wall trigger points (see Chapters 25 and 26), hernias (see Chapter 32), interstitial cystitis (see Chapter 22), pelvic congestion (see Chapter 17), irritable bowel syndrome (see Chapter 23), or any of the other syndromes described in this book.

Table 14–1. **MEDICATIONS USED IN CONJUNCTION WITH GnRH AGONISTS**

Norethindrone
Etidronate
Norethindrone + etidronate
Estrogen (oral and transdermal)
Estrogen + progestin (continuous)
Estrogen + progestin (cyclic)
Calcitonin
Calcium
Medroxyprogesterone acetate

Controlled studies show a high degree of efficacy of hormonal therapy when relief of pain and dysmenorrhea are used as endpoints.[29] Although most women continue to experience significant relief of general pelvic pain and dyspareunia once the medications are discontinued, dysmenorrhea invariably returns with the resumption of cyclic menses. Approximately 25% to 30% report recurrence of pelvic pain symptoms within 6 months of treatment.[30–35] It is not clear whether recurrence is due to reactivation of residual disease[36] or acquisition of new implants. Women who are more likely to have recurrences include those with severe disease[37] or large endometriomas.

Continuous Oral Contraceptives

Because pain and dysmenorrhea often recur within a few months of cessation of hormonal therapy, the continuation of amenorrhea with less expensive, more easily tolerated medications is desirable. Because the symptom that returns first is dysmenorrhea and because retrograde menstruation appears to be a factor in the development and recurrence of endometriosis, it seems rational to prevent menstruation. This can be achieved by several methods. First, suppression can be continued with GnRH agonists with hormonal add-back. This is an expensive approach and should be reserved for those patients resistant to other treatments. A second method is the use of depot medroxyprogesterone acetate or high-dose oral medroxyprogesterone acetate (30 to 50 mg qd). Although inexpensive, side effects and breakthrough bleeding may make it unacceptable to many patients. Finally, OCPs may be used to continue the hormonal suppression and symptom improvement initially achieved with GnRH agonists or other hormonal therapy.[38] When given continuously (i.e., only active pills are taken without a break for menses), OCPs are quite versatile, and current formulations minimize breakthrough bleeding and side effects. Treatment is continued until conception is desired or the patient reaches menopause.

Attention to some pitfalls increases the proportion of patients who benefit from continuous OCPs. The goals of treatment are to prevent menses and breakthrough bleeding, which are often associated with an increase in pain. In the past, high-dose OCPs were used and the dose was increased successively to treat breakthrough bleeding. Not surprisingly, this type of treatment has fallen out of favor. Women taking long-term OCPs for the treatment of endometriosis should feel better, not worse because of side effects. Minimize side effects, such as increased appetite, depression, and premenstrual symptoms, by starting with 35-μg estrogen, low-progestin pills containing norethindrone (0.4 to 0.5 mg) or desogestrel. Although triphasic pills are popular, the variation in the estrogen or progestin dose makes it difficult to avoid breakthrough bleeding and dysmenorrhea. Therefore, only monophasic pills, taken at the same time each day, should be used.

The ability to suppress ovulation and menstruation with continuous OCPs is directly related to the age of the patient and the progestin content of the pill. Younger women may require additional progestin to maintain ovarian suppression, and this can be accomplished by switching to a pill with a higher norethindrone content or by adding norethindrone to the current OCP (0.35 to 2.5 mg qd). Women who develop headaches on 35-μg estrogen-containing OCPs can be switched to 20-μg pills. This regimen can be modified for smokers (while they are on a smoking cessation program) by using norethindrone acetate (0.35 to 2.5 mg qd) and oral (0.5 to 1.0 mg bid) or transdermal estradiol (0.375 to 0.1 mg once or twice weekly) to prevent headaches and breakthrough bleeding.

If breakthrough bleeding and side effects of OCPs can be prevented or treated, the vast majority of patients with endometriosis achieve long-term pain relief. The exception are women who continue to experience breakthrough bleeding despite altering the estrogen-to-progestin ratio. With intermittent and prolonged bleeding, pain often recurs. For this reason, women with unresponsive breakthrough bleeding may benefit from a 3-month course of GnRH agonist, after which continuous OCPs can be tried again. Sources of dysfunctional bleeding such as polyps, submucous fibroids, and bleeding disorders should also be sought. A few women have recurrence of pain in the absence of breakthrough bleeding and may be treated by increasing the progestin dose or by eliminating the estrogen. If no improvement occurs, other sources of pain should be sought.

Although not yet approved in the United States, OCPs containing the antiprogestogen gestrinone have gained in popularity in Europe for their efficacy in treating endometriosis without the cholesterol-raising effects of some of the oral contraceptives currently used. Mifepristone (antiprogesterone) and pure anti-estrogens may soon be available as additional long-term treatments.

Additional Treatment Approaches

Treatment of patients with pain associated with endometriosis continues to be a challenge despite the availability of diverse medical and surgical treatments for this condition. Part of the difficulty in managing these patients lies in our limited understanding of the pathophysiology of pain associated with this disease, the subjective nature of pain, and the chronic recurring nature of this disease.

Women with endometriosis want to know about their disease, and health care providers can encourage their patients by answering questions and supplying resources. Information is also available from the Endometriosis Association (8585 North 76th Place, Milwaukee, WI 53223, telephone [414]355-2200). Many women also need help with emotional issues such as disability due to constant or unpredictable pain, repeated unsuccessful attempts at treatment, unpleasant drug side effects, and relationship issues related to dysparunia or inability to have sex. At some point, nearly all women with endometriosis express concern about their future fertility. They are often encouraged to become pregnant right away because it may be impossible later. However, with a well-planned approach, women with endometriosis have an excellent chance of conceiving when they are ready.

Women with endometriosis often describe a feeling of not being in control of their lives. Physicians and health care personnel can go a long way in restoring some of their loss of control by encouraging the patient to be a partner with the physician in determining the best course of treatment. Women with endometriosis should be encouraged to explore diet and nutritional alternatives, chiropractic, acupuncture, psychotherapy (see Chapters 27 and 28), physical therapy (see Chapters 24 and 28), pain clinics (see Chapter 30), and stress management[39] to enhance their quality of life and allow them to regain a sense of control.

Recurrence of Symptoms or Inadequate Pain Relief

Recurrence of symptoms is discouraging for both patient and physician. Table 14–2 lists some of the points to consider when treatment appears inadequate.

Treatment Options for Women with Pain Wanting to Conceive

Women with pain and infertility associated with endometriosis face several dilemmas: (1) The very treatments that provide other women with long-standing pain relief are contraindicated in women trying to conceive, (2) common fertility treatments, such as superovulation or *in vitro* fertilization, may hasten the return of endometriosis symptoms, (3) women attempting to conceive are reluctant to take medication in the luteal phase of the cycle, (4) dysmenorrhea and pelvic pain may progressively worsen as they have regular menses, and (5) these patients may require periodic surgical treatment that may further compromise fertility. Thus, they feel an urgency to become pregnant before the pain symptoms become disabling.

Several approaches may augment fertility and minimize pain. First, a plan for fertility treatment should be mapped out in advance, including a time allottment of 12 to 18 months, depending on the emotional, financial, and social needs of the couple. The proposed treatments should have an appropriate risk-benefit ratio. Aggressive treatment with superovulation and intrauterine insemination or *in vitro* fertilization should be considered for all women but particularly for those older than 35 years.

Some options for management of dysmenorrhea are compatible with conception. Primrose oil (ω3 fatty acids), when taken daily, has been successfully used to decrease dysmenorrhea significantly.[40] In addition, oral progesterone (200 mg tid) or progesterone suppositories may be started 2 days after the luteinizing hormone surge to decrease dysmenorrhea.[41]

Table 14–2. **DEALING WITH LESS THAN SUCCESSFUL TREATMENT OF ENDOMETRIOSIS**

1. The diagnosis may be wrong, or endometriosis may be present in addition to other pain-producing pathology.
2. The focus of treatment is on crisis management rather than long-term continuous suppression of symptoms (i.e., prevention).
3. The patient has an unrecognized chronic pain syndrome (see Chapter 2) or preexisting depression (see Chapter 27).
4. The patient may have endometriosis that is particularly sensitive to estrogen, even in the presence of progestins.
5. You or your patient have unrealistic goals.
6. You do not like taking care of patients with endometriosis/chronic pelvic pain.
7. The patient has endometriosis that is resistant to treatment, or treatment options are limited by side effects or intolerances.
8. Surgical excision was not performed or was incomplete (i.e., fibrotic nodules were not excised).

Hysterectomy

For patients with recurrent or intractable pain associated with endometriosis, hysterectomy remains the definitive treatment. For women who have been treated for infertility, removal of the uterus, tubes, and ovaries is a sensitive issue, and premature recommendation of hysterectomy as the only treatment option may be met with resistance, emotional reaction to impending loss, and bereavement. It is important that the decision to proceed with a hysterectomy be made primarily by the patient, who, with support from her physician, needs to weigh her hope of bearing children despite continued pain against having control over her life. By coming to this important realization herself, she may willingly relinquish her uterus as opposed to feeling she is having it taken from her. This difference in a patient's perception makes the postoperative recovery easier, although a mourning period is not unusual and should be acknowledged by the caregivers.

In young women, remote from menopause, whether bilateral oophorectomy is mandatory to achieve a permanent cure remains controversial. The incidence of symptom recurrence after hysterectomy with ovarian conservation has been reported to be as low as 1% and as high as 85%. Namnoum and colleagues[42] showed that women who had ovarian conservation at the time of hysterectomy for endometriosis were 6.1 times more likely to develop recurrent pain and 8.1 times more likely to require reoperation than women who initially had oophorectomy and were placed on postoperative hormone replacement therapy. Moreover, the women with ovarian conservation had milder disease than those who underwent oophorectomy, and thus conservation of the ovaries was considered valid because of the apparent low risk of recurrence. Thus, ovarian conservation may not fulfill the goals of definitive therapy.

All visible endometriosis should be removed at the time of hysterectomy to prevent recurrence of symptoms due to fibrotic or deep nodules. Postoperative hormonal replacement can be commenced immediately after surgery and should include both estrogen and a progestin. Progestin attenuates the growth-promoting effects of estrogen and decreases the possibility of recurrent pain due to endometriosis. Alternatively, patients can be treated with progestins alone for hypoestrogenic symptoms for 3 to 6 months, followed by either estrogen alone or combined continuous estrogen and progestin.

Recurrence of pain after hysterectomy is not frequent but when it does occur is discouraging to both patient and physician. Table 14–2 lists some of the factors that may be responsible for recurrent pain; others are discussed in Chapter 15.

Summary

1. Pain management of endometriosis requires an integrated therapeutic approach that includes appropriate medical care, education, attention to diet, exercise, and psychologic support.
2. Women with endometriosis often have additional health problems such as environmental allergies and chronic yeast infections that need to be addressed.
3. Optimal management of the pain associated with endometriosis requires an integrated approach to surgical and medical therapy, which includes (1) thorough surgical excision, (2) a period of hypoestrogenemia, and (3) continuous OCPs until conception is desired or menopause occurs.
4. Women with pain and infertility require modifications in treatment to enhance fertility and treat pain.
5. Women who have had complete resection of endometriosis and continue to have pain or develop pain while on hormonal suppression are very likely to have other reasons for pain in addition to endometriosis.
6. Not all of a patient's complaints should be automatically attributed to the effects of endometriosis, and conversely, when a patient has nonspecific gastrointestinal, genitourinary, or pelvic pain symptoms, endometriosis should be suspected.
7. If a patient has pain severe enough to warrant a hysterectomy, both ovaries should be removed. In addition, all visible endometriosis should be removed.
8. Patients who have undergone hysterectomy and bilateral salpingo-oophorectomy should be treated with both estrogen and *progestin* to reduce the risk of recurrence.

References

1. Sampson JA: Perforating hemorrhagic (chocolate) cysts of the ovary. Arch Surg 1921;3:245.
2. Sampson JA: Ovarian hematomas of endometrial type (perforating hemorrhagic cysts of the ovary) and implantation adenomas of endometrial type. Boston Med Surg J 1922;186:445.
3. Mathias SD, Kuppermann M, Liberman RFM, et al: Chronic pelvic pain: Prevalence, health-related

quality of life, and economic correlates. Obstet Gynecol 1996;87:321.
4. Olive DL, Henderson DY: Endometriosis and müllerian anomalies. Obstet Gynecol 1987;69:412.
5. Sangi-Haghpeykar H, Poindexter AN: Epidemiology of endometriosis among parous women. Obstet Gynecol 1995;85:983.
6. Steele RW, Dmowski WP, Marmer DJ: Immunologic aspects of human endometriosis. Am J Reprod Immunol 1984;6:33.
7. Oosterlynck D, Cornillie FJ, Waer M, et al: Women with endometriosis show a defect in natural killer activity resulting in a decreased cytotoxicity to autologous endometrium. Fertil Steril 1991;56:45.
8. Nichols TR, Lamb K, Arkins JA: The association of atopic disease with endometriosis. Ann Allergy 1987;59:360.
9. Koninckx PR, Martin D: Treatment of deeply infiltrating endometriosis. Curr Opin Obstet Gynecol 1994;6:231.
10. Koninckx PR, Meuleman C, Demeyere S, et al: Suggestive evidence that pelvic endometriosis is a progressive disease, whereas deeply infiltrating endometriosis is associated with pelvic pain. Fertil Steril 1991;55:759.
11. Metzger DA: Hormonal responsiveness of ectopic endometrium. Infertil Reprod Med Clin North Am 1992;3:597.
12. Cunanan RG, Courey NG, Lippes J: Laparoscopic findings in patients with pelvic pain. Am J Obstet Gynecol 1983;146:587.
13. Lundberg WI, Wall JE, Mathers JE: Laparoscopy in evaluation of pelvic pain. Obstet Gynecol 1973;42:872.
14. Fedele L, Stefano B, Bocciolone L, et al: Pain symptoms associated with endometriosis. Obstet Gynecol 1992;79:767.
15. Ripps BA, Martin DC: Correlation of focal pelvic tenderness with implant dimension and stage of endometriosis. J Reprod Med 1992;37:620.
16. Fedele L, Parazini F, Bianchi S, et al: Stage and localization of pelvic endometriosis and pain. Fertil Steril 1990;53:155.
17. Buttram VC: Evolution of the revised American Fertility Society classification of endometriosis. Fertil Steril 1985;43:347.
18. Venturini PL, Semino A, DeCecco L: The biological basis of medical treatment of endometriosis. Gynecol Endocrinol 1995;9:259.
19. Vernon MW, Beard JS, Graves K, Wilson EA: Classification of endometriosis implants by morphological appearance and capacity to synthesize prostaglandin F. Fertil Steril 1986;46:801.
20. Metzger DA, Szpak CA, Haney AF: Histologic features associated with hormonal responsiveness of ectopic endometrium. Fertil Steril 1993;59:83.
21. Redwine DB: Age-related evolution on color appearance of endometriosis. Fertil Steril 1987; 48:1062.
22. Vercellini P, Fedele L, Arcaini L, et al: Laparoscopy in the diagnosis of chronic pelvic pain in adolescent women. J Reprod Med 1989;34:827.
23. Candiani GB, Fedele L, Vercellini P, et al: Repetitive conservative surgery for recurrence of endometriosis. Obstet Gynecol 1991;77:421.
24. Evers JLH: The second-look laparoscopy for evaluation of the result of medical treatment of endometriosis should not be performed during ovarian suppression. Fertil Steril 1987;47:502.
25. Crosignani PG, Vercellini P, Biffignandi F, et al: Laparoscopy versus laparotomy in conservative surgical treatment for severe endometriosis. Fertil Steril 1996;66:706.
26. Operative Laparoscopy Study Group: Postoperative adhesions development after operative laparoscopy: Evaluation at early second-look procedures. Fertil Steril 1991;55:700.
27. Lemay A, Surrey ES, Friedman AJ: Extending the use of gonadotropin-releasing hormone agonists: The emerging role of steroidal and nonsteroidal agents. Fertil Steril 1994;61:21.
28. Surrey ES: Steroidal and nonsteroidal "add-back" therapy: Extending safety and efficacy of gonadotropin-releasing hormone agonists in the gynecologic patient. Fertil Steril 1995;64:673.
29. Rock JA, Truglia JA, Caplan RJ: Zoladex (goserelin acetate implant) in the treatment of endometriosis: A randomized comparison with danazol. Obstet Gynecol 1993;82:198.
30. Waller KG, Shaw RW: Gonadotropin-releasing hormone analogue for endometriosis: Recurrence after treatment. Br J Obstet Gynaecol 1993;100:777.
31. Barbieri RL, Evans S, Kistner R: Danazol in the treatment of endometriosis: Analysis of 100 cases with a 4-year follow-up. Fertil Steril 1982;37:737.
32. Biberoglu KO, Behrman SJ: Dosage aspects of danazol therapy in endometriosis: Short-term and long-term effectiveness. Am J Obstet Gynecol 1981; 139:645.
33. Fedele L, Bianchi S, Bocciolone L, et al: Buserelin acetate in the treatment of pelvic pain associated with minimal and mild endometriosis: A controlled study. Fertil Steril 1993;59:516.
34. Dlugi AM, Miller JD, Knittle J: Lupron Depot (leuprolide acetate for depot suspension) in the treatment of endometriosis: A randomized, placebo-controlled, double-blind study. Fertil Steril 1990;54:419.
35. Bergqvist A, Bergh T, Hogstrom L, et al: The effects of the gonadotropin releasing hromone agonist triptorelin versus placebo on symptoms of endometriosis including 12 months follow-up. Fertil Steril (in press).
36. Nisolle-Pochet M, Casanas-Roux F, Donnez J: Histologic study of ovarian endometriosis after hormonal therapy. Fertil Steril 1988;49:423.
37. Waller KG, Shaw RW: Gonadotropin-releasing hormone analogues for the treatment of endometriosis: Long-term follow-up. Fertil Steril 1993;59:511.
38. Vercellini P, Trespidi L, Colombo A, et al: A gonadotropin-releasing hormone agonist versus a low-dose oral contraceptive for pelvic pain associated with endometriosis. Fertil Steril 1993;60:75.
39. Caudill MA: Managing Pain Before It Manages You. New York, The Guilford Press, 1995.
40. Harel Z, Biro FM, Kottenhahn RK, Rosenthal SL: Supplementation with omega-3 polyunsaturated fatty acids in the management of dysmenorrhea in adolescents. Am J Obstet Gynecol 1996;174:1335.
41. Overton CE, Lindsay PC, Johal B, et al: A randomized, double-blind, placebo-controlled study of luteal phase dydrogesterone (Duphaston) in women with minimal to mild endometriosis. Fertil Steril 1994;62:701.
42. Namnoum AB, Hickman TN, Goodman SB, et al: Incidence of symptom recurrence after hysterectomy for endometriosis. Fertil Steril 1995;64:898.

15

Pain After Hysterectomy

John F. Steege, MD

Surveys of patient satisfaction after hysterectomy performed for the purpose of treating painful gynecologic conditions have reported surprisingly high percentages of women remaining pain free for a year after operation. Of 99 women who underwent hysterectomy for pelvic pain of presumed uterine origin, 76% reported relief, but no correlation was found between the presence or absence of uterine pathology and the surgical outcome.[1] In the Maine Women's Health Study,[2] more than 90% of those who underwent surgical treatment for chronic pain had a successful outcome. A relatively small percentage developed new symptoms in other organ systems during the first year after their surgery. Finally, a prospective cohort study of 308 women who had hysterectomy for chronic pelvic pain reported cure in 74%, improvement in 21%, and no change or worsened pain in only 5% at 1 year of follow-up.[3]

Despite these reassuring overall statistics, every gynecologist has seen women with persistent pain after hysterectomy. Indeed, perhaps the most important questions a gynecologist asks before performing hysterectomy to treat pain are, Is there enough pathology present to justify surgery? and Is this person at risk for having continued pain after surgery? The first question might better be rephrased (Table 15–1): Is hysterectomy the most appropriate choice of surgical treatment for the pathology that is present? The lack of a quantitative relationship between the amount of pathology and the intensity of chronic pain is discussed at length in Chapter 2. Regarding the second question, when a person demonstrates the psychologic and behavioral characteristics of a chronic pain syndrome, the surgeon should carefully consider hysterectomy as only one part of an overall treatment plan. When other components, such as functional bowel disease, musculoskeletal problems, and urinary tract symptoms are present, the preoperative discussion must carefully list the physician's impressions about the contribution that each may make to a person's total discomfort and must discuss treatments to be rendered for these components. In my experience, in most situations in which pain persists after hysterectomy, either a chronic pain syndrome or contributions by other organ systems or both of these were present and diagnosable before the surgery.

Table 15–1. **QUESTIONS TO ASK ONESELF BEFORE PERFORMING HYSTERECTOMY**

Is hysterectomy the most appropriate surgical treatment?
Is this person at risk for having continued pain after surgery?
What other measures should be part of the treatment plan, in addition to surgery?

The Postoperative Interview

Another very important interaction in the relationship with the patient's family can take place immediately after completing surgery. At this moment, the family has been apprehensively waiting, often for hours, concerned about both the surgical findings and the recovery of their loved one. They are feeling vulnerable and may be more emotionally open at this time. Find a sufficiently private place in which to discuss the operative findings in detail and with appropriate drawings or photographs. Especially in the case of patients with a chronic pain problem, one might ask in a very simple and open-ended way what the family has felt might be the factors contributing to the patient's pain. Family members are often very insightful about the interactions between life stresses, marital relationship problems, depression problems, and physical factors. When discussing such issues with a surgeon, they are often pleased to know that you understand that there is more to the pain problem than simply the adhesions or the endometriosis you may have found. A sense of teamwork can develop and can be extremely helpful. A favorable outcome of this postoperative discussion depends on the success of your preoperative efforts at patient and family education.

Reappearance of Symptoms After Surgery

In more than an occasional situation, your postoperative patient may greet you on the first day after surgery saying, "I am sore from the surgery, but that pain that I had is gone." In my experience, this kind of reaction almost always bodes well for ultimate recovery from the preoperative pain.

More commonly, the patient is too uncomfortable to tell whether or not the surgery was truly effective until at least 2 to 4 weeks has passed. Unfortunately, even when the pain improves during the first 6 weeks after surgery, one cannot necessarily be reassured that the ultimate outcome will be positive, especially for patients with chronic pain. The dynamics surrounding the surgical process serve to confuse the interpretation of the results. Despite perhaps the best of efforts in treating chronic pain as a disease in its own right, once surgery is suggested, the physician, the patient, and the family often revert to the acute pain model. Medications are again prescribed differently, and the family appropriately rallies around the patient to offer emotional and logistical support. Meals are brought over to her house to help during the first couple of weeks after surgery. Help is offered with household tasks and childcare. In brief, any secondary gain made in response to the chronic pain problem is significantly amplified by the acute events around the time of surgery.

The contributions of other organ systems to the pain problem may also diminish in the postoperative period. Bed rest and longer periods of sleep may diminish musculoskeletal components. A more careful diet may diminish the impact of irritable bowel syndrome, and feelings of depression may be mitigated by the increased level of support and attention supplied by the family. As the recovery continues and the patient becomes more active and resumes more of her usual responsibilities, the other elements of a chronic pain syndrome may gradually begin to reappear. By the 6-week checkup, the pain may be back full force or may have partially returned, ultimately returning completely by 2 to 3 months after surgery.

This entire picture is made more difficult to interpret by the possibility of the profound placebo effect that surgery can provide.[4] This is usually considered to last at least 2 to 3 months after the implementation of a strong therapeutic measure (such as surgery), although it can certainly last longer. When pain returns in this setting, the surgeon is faced with the task of distinguishing between the recurrence of preoperative disease (e.g., pelvic adhesions) and the reemergence of functional disorders.

Such an unhappy outcome is impossible to avoid completely. Nevertheless, the more complicated the chronic pain pattern, the more useful it is preoperatively to educate a patient and her family about the factors affecting how she will feel postoperatively. Emphasize that surgery does not restore the anatomy to a "brand new" condition; some somatic and visceral nociception may very well persist. The degree to which persistent nociceptive signals lead to pain may depend on their filtering at the spinal cord level and their central processing.

Aside from these general concerns, particular categories of posthysterectomy pelvic pain are worth discussing: intrinsic vaginal apex pain, residual ovary, ovarian remnant, postoperative adhesions, and recurrent endometriosis (Table 15–2).

Intrinsic Vaginal Apex Pain

Pain localized to the vaginal apex itself may appear after hysterectomy, sometimes

Table 15–2. **POSTHYSTERECTOMY PAIN: QUALITY AND PATTERNS**

	Timing of Appearance After Surgery	Quality	Relation to Activities
Vaginal apex	Months to years	Sharp; stinging	Deep dyspareunia
Residual ovary	First year	Pressure, aching, sharp	Cyclic
Ovarian remnant	1–3 years	Pressure, aching, sharp	Cyclic increases
Adhesions	3–6 months	Variable, pulling, aching, tearing	Position, exercise, bowel function
Endometriosis	1–5 years	Aching, sharp	Deep dyspareunia, continuous

months or even years after surgery. Deep dyspareunia typically is the chief complaint. Over time it may progress to become a more constant type of pain in some cases. The character of the pain can vary but is generally described as sharp. Occasional patients describe the pain in terms suggesting dysesthesia (i.e., stinging, burning, or tingling sensations).

Attention to the chronology allows the clinician to distinguish this late-appearing group of problems from the more common disorder of deep dyspareunia that appears immediately after the surgery. Lingering induration of the vaginal cuff or, if healing indeed appears to be complete, lack of vaginal expansion due to insufficient sexual arousal can cause this problem. A carefully taken sexual history (see Chapter 9) can clarify the role of sexual dysfunction in the disorder. Supplemental vaginal lubrication, together with sexual counseling suggestions involving coital position changes (see Chapter 28), may be helpful. A preoperative level of sexual adjustment that is less than satisfactory makes postoperative dyspareunia more likely.

For patients with intrinsic vaginal apex tenderness that occurs some time after a hysterectomy, a number of pathologic entities must be considered. These include inclusion cysts, chronic stitch abscess, recurrent endometriosis in the vaginal cuff, residual ovary adherent to the vaginal cuff, and vaginal apex trigger points.

The diagnosis of focal vaginal apex pain can be made relatively easily during pelvic examination. After performing a careful digital examination of the pelvic floor musculature (see Chapter 7), place a vaginal speculum that is sufficiently large to provide a good view of the suture line across the vaginal apex. Then gently and systematically palpate the vaginal sidewalls and the vaginal apex with a cotton-tipped applicator. Unless the patient also has intrinsic vaginal sidewall pain by history, the sidewalls almost invariably are totally comfortable during this palpation. The vaginal apex normally also is entirely comfortable as the applicator is moved across the apex. If focal pathology is present, the patient reliably reports abnormal sensations emanating from a very localized area. In some instances, pathology is also visible, such as the bulging of an epithelial inclusion cyst or a stitch abscess. Perhaps more commonly, the pathology is buried within the vaginal apex tissue itself and is not readily noted by the applicator examination or by subsequent manual palpation.

The findings of the applicator examination are essentially replicated during bimanual palpation if the vaginal examining fingers are carefully moved across the vaginal apex step by step. In a very thin patient, intrinsic vaginal apex pathology may be palpable during the bimanual examination. More commonly, documentation of such pathology awaits surgical exploration.

Inclusion cysts seem to occur when the vaginal cuff is closed somewhat inaccurately, with the cut edges of the vaginal mucosa rolled under and buried in the cuff tissue itself. The reason for the delay in their appearance is unknown, as is their basic pathophysiology. Pathologically, they seem to consist of confused whorls of epithelial cells, sometimes containing chronic inflammatory fluid, but many times they are entirely solid. A stitch abscess may develop years after the original surgery, even when absorbable suture has been used.

Small implants of recurrent endometriosis

can present in a very similar fashion. These extremely focal areas of sensitivity are almost invariably not diagnosable by transvaginal ultrasound examination.

When the initial examination reveals no focal pathology but very localized pain, an intrinsic trigger point may be present. As discussed elsewhere (see Chapters 25 and 30) trigger points may develop virtually anywhere in the body but more commonly occur in areas of previous tissue injury. Their pathophysiology is incompletely understood, but the clinical phenomenon is well documented. Injection with 3 to 5 ml of a local anesthetic is diagnostic, because the block eliminates the pain entirely. More prolonged relief is sometimes obtained by adding a steroid, usually triamcinolone 6 mg (1 ml) per 10 ml of anesthetic. In some cases, relief lasts for weeks or months. When this is not the case, vaginal apex discomfort can sometimes be treated successfully with a topical anesthetic gel. Before intercourse, 2% or 5% lidocaine can be applied to the top of the vagina with a vaginal medication applicator. The dose needs to be carefully adjusted on a trial-and-error basis to avoid excessive anesthesia for the patient and her partner.

If medical therapy is not successful, the vaginal apex can be surgically revised. The transvaginal approach to vaginal apex pathology is traditional and is still a viable option. However, when the margins of the lesion are not obvious on vaginal examination, it is useful to perform laparoscopy and examine the vaginal apex to localize the pathology precisely before excising it. First, perform a rectovaginal examination with one hand while manipulating a smooth-tipped 5-mm laparoscopic probe with the other in order to perform a bimanual palpation of the pelvic floor and vaginal apex (Fig. 15–1). This is a very reliable method for discovering hidden cul-de-sac endometriosis, intrinsic vaginal apex endometriosis, retroperitonealized ovarian remnant tissue, vaginal apex inclusion cysts, and stitch abscesses. Alternatively, one can place a cool light source in the vagina itself and transilluminate the vaginal apex, revealing the pathology in silhouette. The light source can be removed and a 2- or 3-cm diameter smooth-tipped vaginal stent placed to stretch out the vaginal apex and allow easier laparoscopically directed surgical revision of the vaginal apex (Fig. 15–2).

The laparoscopic approach also allows removal of any intestinal adhesions to the vaginal cuff and permits precise identification of the edge of the bladder by filling the bladder via the Foley catheter. It is usually necessary to incise the peritoneum and retract the bladder inferiorly. With the pathology identified and the vaginal apex thus defined, the lesion can then be excised with electrocautery scissors, laser, or any other laparoscopic energy source. With the vaginal stent in place, the pneumoperitoneum is not compromised. At that point, laparoscopic suturing techniques can be used to close the cuff. Alternatively, the laparoscopy can be terminated and the colpotomy closed transvaginally.

In some cases, it is difficult to distinguish the role of possible intrinsic vaginal apex pathology from the potential role of a closely adherent ovary. In this setting, conscious pain mapping (see Chapter 33) may be a useful procedure to perform first. When the offending pathology is then identified, the patient can be placed under general anesthesia and the appropriate procedure performed.

Residual Ovary

Pain in a residual ovary is often intermittent and may be attributed to functional cyst formation. Hormonal suppression (oral contraceptives, continuous medroxyprogesterone, or gonadotropin-releasing hormone [GnRH] agonists), analgesics, and watchful waiting are often sufficient treatment. If the ovary is encased in postoperative pelvic adhesions, then it is more likely to cause pain repeatedly during the course of its normal physiologic functioning. A cyclic pattern of such pain, documented by prospective calendar recording, is helpful in making this diagnosis. Serial pelvic examination may be useful, perhaps coupled with transvaginal ultrasound examination.

Vaginal cuff closure during vaginal hysterectomy sometimes draws the ovary down

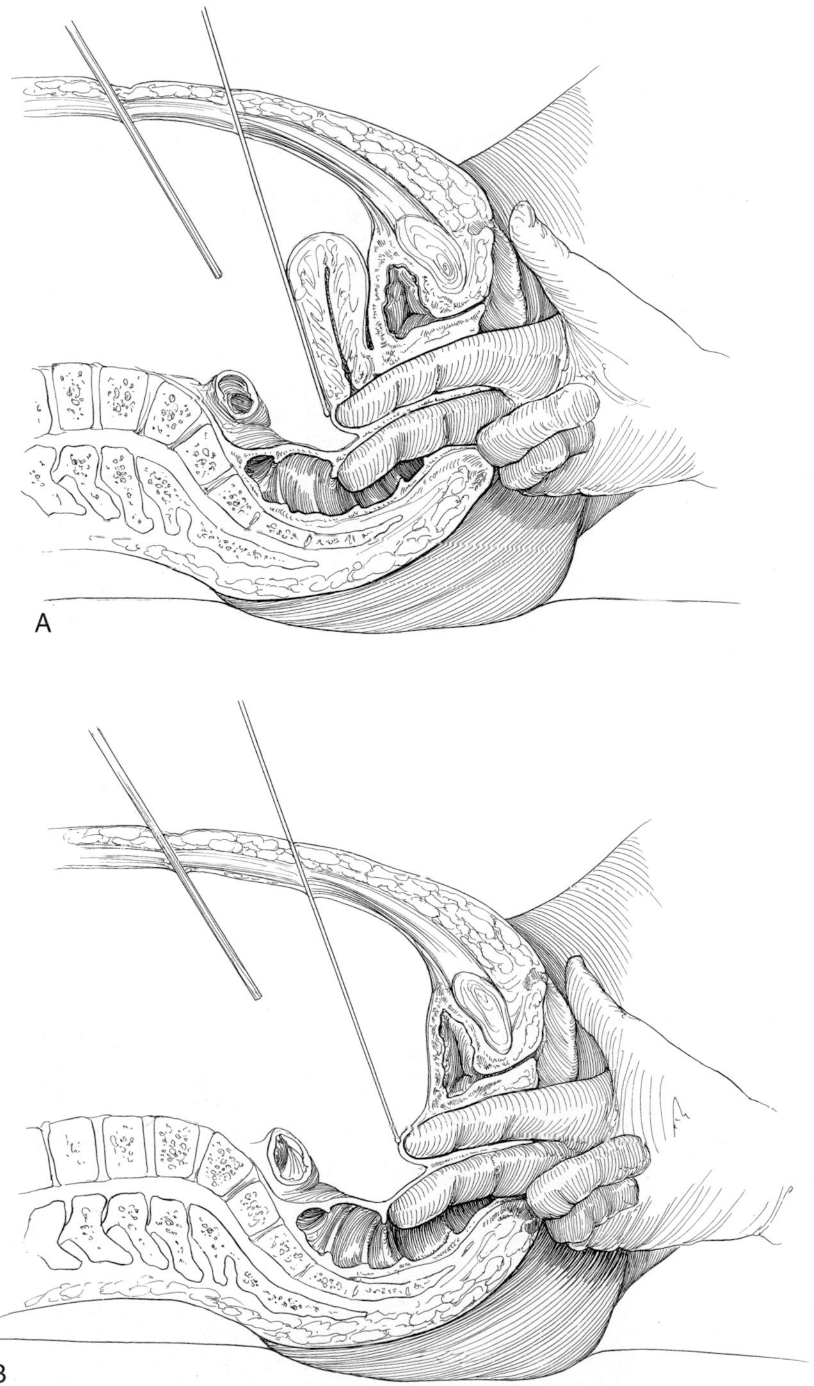

Figure 15–1. Laparoscopic bimanual examination of the pelvic floor and vaginal apex. *A*: The intact pelvis. *B*: After hysterectomy.

toward the vaginal apex. This was a more common problem in decades past, when gynecologists were trained to suture the utero-ovarian ligament intentionally into the vaginal cuff to augment pelvic support. Now that this is less often done, the painful vaginal apex ovary is a less common, although not rare, occurrence. In thinner patients, a bimanual examination usually outlines the anatomy sufficiently to make the diagnosis. In heavier patients, transvaginal ultrasound examination can document that an ovary is

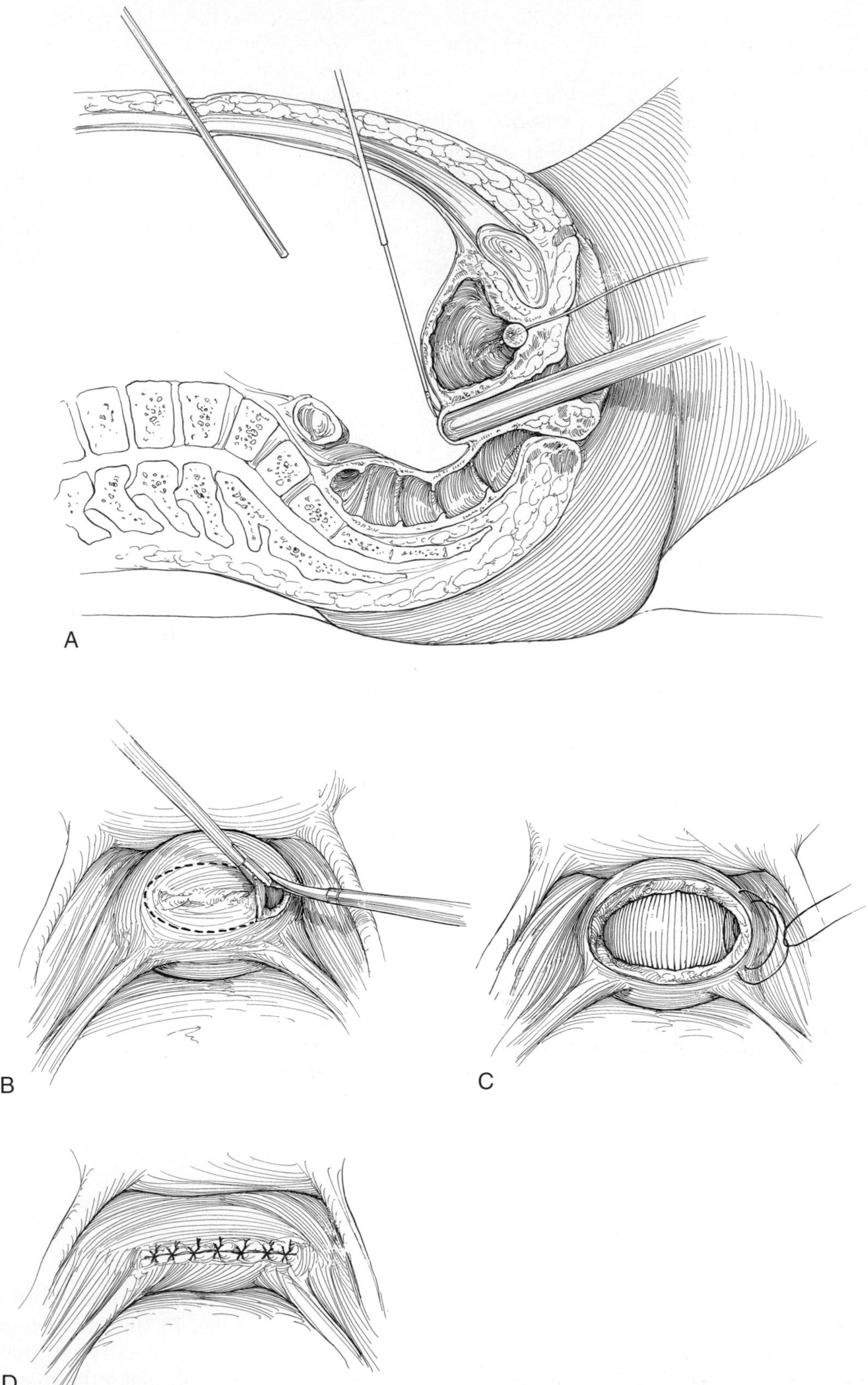

Figure 15–2. Laparoscopic vaginal apex revision. *A*: Vaginal stent in place, taking down the bladder. *B*: Circumferential incision over stent. *C*: Suturing the apex. *D*: Completed apex revision.

adherent to the vaginal cuff, but the study has to be performed carefully to have this degree of accuracy.

When posthysterectomy ovarian pain is refractory to medical therapy, surgical removal may be indicated. In the majority of cases, this can be accomplished by an experienced operative laparoscopist. Care should be taken to visualize the ureter carefully, because it more often closely underlies the ovary after hysterectomy than in an undisturbed pelvis. Cystoscopically placed ureteral stents can facilitate locating the ureters, especially if the pelvic sidewall peritoneum is scarred or the ovary is scarred to the sidewall. Retroperitoneal dissection should be used when necessary to dissect the ureter away from the ovary.

In my experience, the procedure is substantially simplified by isolating and transecting the infundibulopelvic ligament first, rather than trying to free up the ovary entirely before transecting its vascular pedicle. Such an approach follows the technique traditionally taught for performing oophorectomy via laparotomy.

When the causal role of the residual ovary in the pain is unclear, conscious pain mapping (see Chapter 33) should be considered before oophorectomy.

Ovarian Remnant Syndrome

Ovarian remnant syndrome is defined as the persistence of functional or nonfunctional ovarian tissue despite ostensible prior removal of both ovaries. Thought for many years to be quite rare, the syndrome has been increasingly reported in the past decade.[5–8] When unilateral pain is present in a patient who has had prior bilateral salpingo-oophorectomy, ovarian remnant should be considered in the differential diagnosis.

Laboratory study of rats suggests that fragments of ovarian tissue may be capable of attaching to the peritoneal surface and surviving, developing their own independent vascular supply.[9] Far more commonly, however, ovarian remnants appear to develop along the course of the vascular supply of the ovary, anywhere from the origins of the infundibulopelvic ligament, where they cross the common iliac vessels, down to the vaginal cuff itself. One must presume that in such instances, an unrecognized tiny fragment of ovary was left behind in a bed of scar tissue at the time of previous surgery. Such cases most often arise after surgery for extensive pelvic adhesive disease or endometriosis.

Low-cost clinical diagnosis can be made by asking the patient to discontinue hormonal replacement, if she is using it, and observing for the appearance of vasomotor symptoms within the subsequent several weeks. The clinical suspicion can be confirmed by measuring follicle-stimulating hormone and estradiol levels about 3 to 4 weeks after stopping hormonal replacement. Menopausal levels of these hormones should be found if no functioning ovarian tissue is present. However, in three cases I have found remnants that were physically present but hormonally nonfunctional, with preoperative follicle-stimulating hormone levels in the 80 mIU/ml range.

Ultrasonography can be used to confirm the presence of a unilateral pelvic mass; however, caution must be used in interpreting ultrasound examination findings in a patient who has had many previous operations. Computed tomography and magnetic resonance imaging scans are less useful for this diagnosis and are equally prone to artifact.

The presence of a symptomatic ovarian remnant does not necessarily dictate its surgical removal. Hormonal suppression can often be accomplished, with reasonable resolution of symptoms. Oral contraceptives may be a first-line measure, with oral or intramuscular medroxyprogesterone being a reasonable low-cost alternative. If these should fail, suppression of the remnant with GnRH agonists may be very effective. Add-back therapy with estrogen can be used as well. This combination is quite expensive but may be a viable alternative to surgical therapy when the patient is reasonably close to the expected age of menopause. In some patients, the remnant can be suppressed with injections given less frequently than the usual monthly regimen.

Many women who have an ovarian remnant also have postoperative adhesive disease. This makes it difficult to determine which of the two pathologies is more important. Ovarian suppression, particularly with GnRH agonists, can effectively eliminate the ovarian tissue component, thereby allowing estimation of the importance of the pelvic adhesions and other factors. Two caveats to this approach must be mentioned. First, GnRH agonists may have a nonspecific effect on other organ systems, especially possibly improving irritable bowel syndrome. Second, when an ovarian remnant is present and is suppressed by GnRH agonists, it can become so small that it is difficult to find at the time of surgery. When possible, GnRH agonist should be discontinued and surgery delayed until the mass is again detectable or pain recurs.

If the remnant is not detectable by examination or ultrasonography, it can sometimes be stimulated to appear by the use of clomiphene citrate. The impact of the clomiphene test on the patient's pain may also further emphasize the importance of the remnant in the etiology of the pain.

Surgical technique for the removal of the ovarian remnant deserves comment. The majority can successfully be approached laparoscopically.[10] I have treated 15 remnants in this manner and have noted recurrence in only one case. Again, the surgery is facilitated by preoperative placement of a ureteral stent to provide easy identification of the ureter and safe dissection of it away from any remnant ovarian tissue. If the dissection becomes too difficult or too prolonged, the procedure should be converted to laparotomy.[11] The literature reports a recurrence rate of 10% to 20% after removal of an ovarian remnant.

Postoperative Adhesions

The treatment of pelvic adhesive disease is discussed at greater length in Chapter 13. The present discussion focuses on the prevalence of adhesions and techniques that might be useful to prevent their formation after hysterectomy.

Autopsy studies have revealed that between 50% and 80% of women develop pelvic adhesive disease after pelvic surgery. It is readily apparent, then, that not all adhesions are associated with pain. Adhesions are more prevalent in those who have pain than in those without, but the role of the adhesions in the pain problem must be individually assessed (see Chapter 33).

Consideration must be given to the type of person in whom postoperative pain is likely to occur. If the psychologic and behavioral stigmata of a chronic pain syndrome are present preoperatively (see Chapter 2), pain is more likely to recur or persist after surgery. No surgical procedure results in healing that is so complete that tissue is normal. All healing involves scarring, and it is reasonable to suspect that in many, such scarring may create some nociceptive signals. In the vast majority, these signals either can be successfully blocked or can be interpreted centrally as a normal phenomenon. For a person who has become extremely sensitive to pain, the same signals may develop into a pain syndrome.

In this scenario, surgical approaches to pelvic adhesive disease are inherently a trap: The more they are performed, the more they reinforce the expectation that everything can be made normal and that adhesive disease is solely and entirely responsible for the person's pain.

The development of conscious pain mapping (see Chapter 33) has been very helpful in evaluating this problem. In many cases involving adhesions, traction on those adhesions during laparoscopy performed under local anesthesia did not reproduce the pain. Many of these women had undergone one or more laparoscopic lyses of adhesions with transitory relief of the pain. This transitory relief can be the sum of various factors unrelated to the adhesions: the placebo effect, bed rest, transitory alterations in bowel function, increased postoperative pain medication, and so on. In selected instances, reinterpreting the adhesions, followed by careful and systematic treatment of other components of the pelvic pain problem, has resulted in substantial degrees of pain relief despite leaving the adhesions intact.

Reorienting a patient and her family to a more comprehensive approach obviously requires a persistent and substantial educational effort (see Chapter 28). For patients unwilling to accept the notion that anything but the adhesions can be causing a pain problem, it may be useful to undertake a careful preoperative educational session, perform a pain-mapping procedure, and then lyse the adhesions as part of an overall treatment program.

Endometriosis

Hysterectomy with removal of both ovaries is widely accepted as the most successful and aggressive surgical approach to endometriosis. Nevertheless, approximately 10% of women undergoing such a procedure may have recurrence of symptoms, with about 1% to 4% requiring further surgery.[12]

Two clinical points are perhaps the most important in this topic: First, of all women having pelvic pain after hysterectomy for endometriosis, only a small fraction have the pain due to recurrent disease. In my experience, about 90% of women who have such pain have postoperative adhesions with no evidence of recurrent endometriosis. Such a conclusion can of course be reached only after careful laparoscopic examination. (For reasons cited earlier, response to GnRH agonists does not specifically prove that the recurrent pain is due to the recurrent endometriosis.) Second, when recurrent endometriosis is shown to be present, its location should correspond to the location of the pain for it to be held responsible for the discomfort.[13]

The typical person with recurrent endometriosis following hysterectomy feels well for a year or more after the original surgery, only to have pelvic pain return in a very gradual fashion. Here again, the chronology of the return of pain is of key importance: A person whose pain returns within 2 to 3 months after surgery is far more likely to suffer from postoperative adhesions or other components rather than the regrowth of endometriosis itself.

The pain of recurrent endometriosis often starts out as deep dyspareunia but is soon joined by a noncyclic, more general central pelvic pain. The diagnostic evaluation should of course include a careful pelvic examination, perhaps with careful cotton-tipped applicator mapping of the vaginal apex as described in this chapter, as well as with transvaginal ultrasound examination. However, the vast majority of the current endometriosis implants are small and not specifically palpable or able to be visualized by ultrasound techniques. Laparoscopy therefore remains an essential ingredient in diagnosis.

When performing laparoscopy for endometriosis in any case, but perhaps especially after hysterectomy, it is most helpful to perform a bimanual examination (see Fig. 15–1). Retroperitoneal disease can be readily appreciated in this manner. In a similar way, a lighted bougie can be placed in the vagina and the vaginal apex and cul-de-sac transilluminated to isolate any hidden endometriosis lesions.

Further hormonal therapy after such surgery may or may not be necessary, depending on how much of the recurrent disease could be excised.

Postoperative Care: What to Do When You Have Performed Another Operation to Cure Postoperative Pain

As suggested earlier, discussion with the patient and her family before and after a repeat operation is of critical importance. Great care must be taken to place the importance of that surgery in proper perspective vis-à-vis treatment of other components such as affective disorder, musculoskeletal complaints, and bowel complaints. For a person requiring the extreme measure of a repeat operation, it is important to emphasize that rehabilitation may be slow and gradual. This is contrary to the usual surgeon's style and is also contrary to the patient's and patient's family's belief that surgery is the most effective form of treatment.

A further useful generalization is that any person who has had the unhappy experience of three or more operations within the space of a year should be considered to be depressed until proven otherwise. This observation can be viewed from two angles:

Either depression developed early and the recurrence of the pain may be aggravated by the presence of the depression but was missed in the preoperative assessment, or many normal emotionally healthy individuals when subjected to the stress of three operations have good reason to develop depression.

Finally, an important part of the rehabilitation process may be the need to establish supportive care to help patients develop cognitive approaches for dealing with continued postoperative discomforts. In many cases, the fear of further surgery, the fear of the return of pain, and the chronic disability previously experienced all may contribute to a negative interpretation of any nociceptive signals that may occur after surgery. Patients need to be encouraged to manage discomforts on a day-to-day basis, focusing on the present rather than fearing the future. This is by no means an easy task and often cannot be accomplished over the telephone or in the context of a busy gynecology office. This is the time when supportive mental health care can be extremely helpful; it is better accepted by a patient and her family when the possibility of such help is introduced early in the evaluation of chronic pelvic pain (see Chapter 28).

References

1. Stovall TG, Ling FW, Crawford DA: Hysterectomy for chronic pelvic pain of presumed uterine etiology. Obstet Gynecol 1990;75:676.
2. Carlson KJ, Miller BA, Fowler FJ Jr: The Maine Women's Health Study: II. Outcomes of nonsurgical management of leiomyomas, abnormal bleeding, and chronic pelvic pain. Obstet Gynecol 1994;83:566.
3. Hillis SD, Marchbanks PA, Peterson HB: The effectiveness of hysterectomy for chronic pelvic pain. Obstet Gynecol 1995;86:941.
4. Turner JA, Deyo RA, Loeser JD, et al: The importance of placebo effects in pain treatment and research. JAMA 1994;271:1609.
5. Steege JF: Ovarian remnant syndrome. Obstet Gynecol 1987;70:64.
6. Pettit PD, Lee RA: Ovarian remnant syndrome: Diagnostic dilemma and surgical challenge. Obstet Gynecol 1988;71:580.
7. Webb MJ: Ovarian remnant syndrome. Aust N Z J Obstet Gynecol 1989;29:433.
8. Price FV, Edwards R, Buchsbaum HJ: Ovarian remnant syndrome: Difficulties in diagnosis and treatment. Obstet Gynecol Surv 1990;45:151.
9. Minke T, DePond W, Winkelmann, Blythe J: Ovarian remnant syndrome: Study in laboratory rats. Am J Obstet Gynecol 1994;171:1440.
10. Nezhat F, Nezhat C: Operative laparoscopy for the treatment of ovarian remnant syndrome. Fertil Steril 1992;57:1003.
11. Elkins TE, Stocker RJ, Key D, et al: Surgery for ovarian remnant syndrome: Lessons learned from difficult cases. J Reprod Med 1994;39:446.
12. Namnoum AB, Gehlbach DL, Hickman TN, et al: Incidence of symptom recurrence after hysterectomy for endometriosis. Fertil Steril 1995;64:898.
13. Stout AL, Steege JF, Dodson WC, et al: Relationship of laparoscopic findings to self-report of pelvic pain. Am J Obstet Gynecol 1991;164:73.

16

Miscellaneous Causes of Pelvic Pain

Barbara S. Levy, MD

The approach to diagnosis of chronic pelvic pain (CPP) and its treatment poses a unique problem distinctly different from the evaluation of recent-onset acute pelvic pain. In our eagerness to analyze and diagnose the cause of CPP and to find a cure for the underlying disease, we frequently overlook the complex and insidious predisposing factors that lead to chronic pain syndromes. As physicians and scientists, we believe that our task lies in finding the physical lesion or disease that we can excise or treat, and we expect that this management will cut out the pain. In fact, it is rare for any single disease entity or physical problem to be the isolated cause of chronic pain. Treatment certainly must include proper diagnosis and treatment of underlying disease; however, an integrated approach that includes attention to the psychologic and social predisposing factors is required for ultimate improvement in a patient's quality of life and the outlook for long-term cure. If we do not address these issues, we may be successful in managing one source of pain, but another area of disability will soon surface.

This chapter addresses several entities that have been associated with pelvic pain. Readers must keep in mind that although these physical findings may be present in patients with chronic pain, they may have little relevance to the actual cause of the pain. These anatomic abnormalities may have initiated a series of events that predisposed a patient to chronic pain. Acute pain in a particular region may cause splinting, muscle spasm, decreased circulation, change in habit patterns, and ultimately chronic pain. Treating the original source without addressing the consequences of the pain (e.g., chronic muscle tension, fatigue, depression) is unsuccessful because perpetuation of the pain had more to do with the body's response to the initial pain than to the inciting event itself. Care must be taken, therefore, in assigning causation to these anatomic factors that we find in our diagnostic evaluation for pathology in patients with CPP. Treatment of CPP requires appropriate medical and surgical management of *relevant* pathology coupled with interventions by experts in other disciplines who can address the psychologic, social, and emotional components of a patient's problem. Several miscellaneous problems associated with pelvic pain are addressed in that context in this chapter. Table 16–1 tabulates several other entities that have been associated with CPP.

Fibroids

Leiomyomas are the most common tumors found in the female genital tract. Almost one of four women has palpable fibroids by

Table 16–1. **OTHER CAUSES OF CHRONIC PELVIC PAIN**

Claudication
Arteriovenous malformations
Antecedent tubal sterilization
Uterine anomalies with hematometra
Levator ani myalgia
Endosalpingiosis
Postabortal pelvic inflammatory disease
Interstitial cystitis
Irritable bowel syndrome
Antecedent pelvic fracture

the time she reaches the fourth decade of life. The incidence of small, nonpalpable tumors discovered by endovaginal ultrasound examination or laparoscopy is even higher. In general, myomas cause no symptoms. They are benign tumors made up predominantly of smooth muscle fibers and some connective fibrous tissue, and they grow under the influence of cyclic estrogen and progesterone. Rapid growth of these tumors is common in pregnancy with the increase in estrogen and progesterone. Degeneration of the fibroids results from alteration in the blood supply to the tumor. This may occur with rapid growth, torsion or atrophy resulting from menopause, or the use of gonadotropin-releasing hormone agonists. Pain can result from degeneration. It is usually gradual in onset and intermittent in nature, with the exception of the pain due to torsion, which is acute as the blood supply to the tumor is suddenly and completely occluded. Signs of peritoneal irritation accompany acute torsion of a pedunculated myoma, along with leukocytosis and fever. More commonly, fibroids are associated with a sensation of pressure in the pelvis because their bulk rests on adjacent organs. Urinary frequency may be a presenting complaint. Cramping pain may result as the uterus attempts to deliver a large pedunculated submucous myoma. Physical examination reveals a dilated cervix with a smooth fibrous mass protruding through the os.

We may expect to find leiomyomas frequently as we assess patients with CPP. Determining their contribution to a patient's symptoms requires a bit more evaluation. Pain mapping, beginning with the patient's demonstrating the area of maximal discomfort on a line drawing of the pelvis and proceeding to careful physical examination, must isolate the region of the myoma as the only source of discomfort if we are to conclude that it is the cause of the patient's problem. Laparoscopy under local anesthesia has been described as a method for determining how various pathologic conditions contribute to a patient's pain. This may offer a significant advance in the study of CPP because it offers a means of distinguishing between causative versus associated pathology. Nezhat and colleagues,[3] in a series of 121 women who had myomectomies, investigated the associated symptoms and pathology. They found that 42% of the women had preoperative complaints of pelvic pain. In this group, endometriosis or adenomyosis was found in association with the fibroids in 79%. In contrast, only 29% of patients with fibroids but no pelvic pain had associated endometriosis or adenomyosis. Based on these data, we must question the true relationship between fibroids and pelvic pain. Surgery for removal of large fibroids certainly is successful in decreasing uterine bulk and diminishing pressure on adjacent organs, but the long-term results in managing chronic pain must be determined and the risks versus potential benefits of major surgery discussed in detail with patients.

Chronic Appendicitis

Acute appendicitis is the result of obstruction of the appendiceal lumen by a fecalith or proliferative lymphoid tissue. The closed loop obstruction results in increasing intraluminal pressure as the mucosal secretions accumulate, and necrosis ensues when the intraluminal pressure limits adequate circulation. The pain is initially diffuse, dull, and vague. Continued distention further stimulates local nerve endings and leads to nausea, vomiting, increased peristalsis with cramping abdominal pain, and eventually localized peritoneal irritation as bacterial invasion reaches the serosa. This process, once initiated, generally progresses and requires immediate surgical intervention. On rare occasions, however, episodes of acute appendicitis resolve spontaneously. Some patients report intermittent attacks of right lower quadrant pain that remits gradually over a short period. Pathologic evaluation of their appendices when removed demonstrates thickening and scarring, presumably from previous inflammatory reaction. Endometriosis may also obstruct the appendiceal lumen and cause acute appendicitis. In addition, endometriosis may invade the appendix, causing more chronic right lower quadrant symptoms. The incidence of these problems is unknown. Localized right lower quadrant chronic pain unresponsive to conservative measures deserves careful evaluation at laparoscopy, with the capability for appendectomy should pathology be identified.

Adenomyosis

Adenomyosis is a condition in which endometrial glands and stroma grow within the myometrium, usually without direct connection to the endometrium. In the past, the diagnosis was made only at hysterectomy; however, modern imaging modalities such as transvaginal ultrasonography and magnetic resonance imaging techniques are becoming sensitive enough to distinguish this entity without requiring hysterectomy or myometrial biopsy. The symptoms of adenomyosis include increasing menorrhagia and pelvic pain that occurs before, during, and after menses. In addition, women may suffer from aching discomfort after orgasm and vigorous exercise. On physical examination, the uterus is enlarged in a globular configuration, and marked tenderness is elicited on bimanual palpation of the uterine contour. When adenomyosis is suspected on examination and conservative testing, medical management is appropriate to confirm that suppression of ovulation and menses will reduce or eliminate pain. This can be accomplished with use of continuous oral contraceptives, progestins, danazol, or gonadotropin-releasing hormone agonists. Failure of medical management should lead to a search for alternate diagnoses before proceeding with extirpative surgery. Hysterectomy remains the only definitive treatment for adenomyosis and should be reserved for those patients in whom conservative measures have failed and childbearing is no longer a consideration. Advocates of endometrial ablation for management of menorrhagia and dysmenorrhea have found that adenomyosis is the chief culprit in failure of ablation to control symptoms in the long term.

Recurrent Ovarian Cysts

Adnexal masses are rarely a cause of pelvic pain. The ovary normally produces a functional cyst during each menstrual cycle. The late onset of symptoms in patients with ovarian cancer is testimony to the fact that enlargement of the ovary is generally asymptomatic. Frequently, however, patients with CPP have been led to believe that their normal ovarian cysts are causing episodes of acute exacerbation of pain. In the absence of torsion, rupture with significant peritoneal irritation, or enlargement significant enough to create a mass effect, functional ovarian cysts do not cause pain. Our desire to find and treat pathology in patients presenting with recurrent pelvic pain and our fear of undiagnosed ovarian malignancy often lead us to intervene in these cases. We must resist this temptation because it only serves to reinforce a sense of physical illness in these patients and delays the appropriate multidisciplinary approach to management of chronic pain. Patients with chronic pain have frequently tolerated many surgical procedures for functional ovarian cysts. Reoperation must be avoided because it increases the probability of ovarian dysfunction, adhesions, and further pathology.

Large cystic pelvic masses cause pelvic pressure, urinary frequency, and often dyspareunia. It is not unreasonable to monitor such a patient with examinations through one or two menstrual cycles, if the patient can tolerate the delay. If the cyst is persistent, it most often may be approached laparoscopically when the risk of malignancy is small. Even when suspicion is high, laparoscopy may help avoid laparotomy in some cases in which endometriomas or dermoid cysts have mimicked the characteristics of malignant ovarian tumors.

Painful Normal Ovary

The ovaries, like their counterpart, the testes, are tender when palpated. Under normal circumstances, these freely mobile structures do not cause discomfort. However, when they are bound in adhesions and tethered in place, pain may occur with movement, sexual activity, or normal ovulation. Endometriosis, pelvic inflammatory disease, and adhesions from prior surgical intervention all may contribute to fixation of the ovary and consequent pain when the ovary is touched. Ovarian suppression may be successful in ameliorating these symptoms by shrinking the ovaries and preventing the distention of the ovarian capsule or the stretching of surrounding adhesions that occurs during normal ovulation. At times, however, surgical intervention may be required. Once again, it is important to rule out other causes, especially for patients suffering from chronic pain syndromes. When the pain pattern and the physical findings are consistent, surgical mobilization may be quite successful in alleviating these symptoms. The addition of barrier substances, once adequate mobilization has been achieved, may help to prevent subsequent adhesion formation.

Uterine Malposition

Retroversion of the uterus has been implicated as a cause of chronic back pain and dyspareunia. Retrodisplacement of the uterus is a normal anatomic variant and is rarely, by itself, associated with pelvic symptoms. Many conditions, however, lead to pathologic fixation of the uterus in a retroverted position, causing dyspareunia and possibly low back pain. Once these underlying conditions have been adequately treated, the pain is likely to improve despite continued retroversion of the uterus. Pelvic relaxation with prolapse of the uterus may lead to chronic low back pain and dyspareunia. Because low back pain is such a common complaint, it is imperative to document improvement in pain with restoration of normal anatomy before recommending surgery for pain alone. The uterus may be repositioned with the use of a mechanical device, (pessary) to restore its normal location within the pelvic cavity. Pessaries of various shapes and sizes are available, and although they may not be acceptable to a patient as a long-term solution for her problem, they are excellent devices for documenting the contribution of uterine position to the patient's complaints. If her back pain is not resolved when her uterus is supported, surgery is unlikely to be successful in improving her symptoms.

Cervicitis/Endometritis

Chronic infection of the cervix or endometrium may contribute to CPP and dyspareunia. Cervicitis is manifested by purulent cervical mucus and tenderness to motion and palpation of the cervix. Cultures are frequently negative for the usual pathogens, including *Chlamydia;* nevertheless, treatment with antibiotics for 2 to 4 weeks may be successful in improving the symptoms. Tetracyclines or erythromycins are the drugs of choice for this situation. There is no reason to use expensive and exotic antimicrobials. Ureoplasmas and mycoplasmas may be the etiologic agents. When signs and symptoms of cervicitis are not present, no other pathology has been identified, and the uterus remains significantly tender, endometritis may be present. Endometrial biopsy demonstrating plasma cells in the endometrial stroma is required for the definitive diagnosis. A short course of antibiotics should be successful in relieving the symptoms. If that is not the case, other causes of pelvic pain must be considered.

Conclusion

Many pathologic conditions may be present in the pelvis. Clinicians must be skeptical about the cause-and-effect relationship between these conditions and CPP in most patients. Diligent clinical evaluation is quite likely to uncover *some* aberrant anatomy in almost everyone. We must be critical in our thinking and our approach to our patients. Only when pathology can be demonstrated to contribute substantially to a patient's presenting problem are we justified in medically or surgically treating it.

References

1. Danforth DN (ed): Obstetrics and Gynecology, 3rd ed. New York, Harper & Row, 1977, pp 943–953.
2. Schwartz SI, Lillehei RC, Shires GT, et al: Principles of Surgery. New York, McGraw-Hill, 1964, pp 1167–1175.
3. Nezhat CH, Bess O, Nezhat C: Pelvic pain and dysmenorrhea in the presence of myomas are largely due to associated adenomyosis and endometriosis. J Am Assoc Gynecol Laparosc 1995;3:1.

17

Pelvic Congestion

Deborah A. Metzger, PhD, MD

A well-described but frequently overlooked cause of chronic pelvic pain (CPP) is pelvic congestion. This is a syndrome of many names that has been described in the gynecologic, surgical, and general medical literature. It is associated with pelvic varicosities and pelvic pain and is often found in women in whom no obvious pathologic cause of their pelvic pain can be found.

Gynecologists have divided opinions about the legitimacy of pelvic congestion as a physical diagnosis. Many factors contribute to this dispute, including the lack of specific diagnostic criteria, the significant proportion of these women with emotional distress, and the tradition of classifying pain as "real" or "all in the head." As we have discussed throughout this book, it is impossible to separate the physical and emotional components of pain. The purpose of this chapter is to review the literature on pelvic congestion with the goal of providing readers with alternative approaches to treating these women.

Historical Perspective

The pelvic congestion syndrome is a condition of CPP occurring in the setting of pelvic varicosities. Since Richet's first description in 1857[1] of a case of tubo-ovarian varicocele, many clinical reports have implicated varicosities in the infundibulopelvic and broad ligaments as having a causative relationship to CPP.[2–8] This condition in women is analogous to scrotal varicocele in men.[9]

Others have rejected this association and have argued that pelvic congestion is purely a psychosomatic complaint,[10] based on the high prevalence of emotional disturbance in women with CPP.[10–12] Based on in-depth interviews with 36 women with pelvic congestion, Duncan and Taylor[10] found that with few exceptions, these women were "psychologically ill individuals, exhibiting conversion hysteria, anxiety hysteria, obsessive-compulsive neuroses, reactive depression and schizoid personality structure manifested by emotional immaturity and strong dependency needs." Furthermore, they observed a correlation between emotional responses during the interview and variations in the blood flow of the vaginal wall. Increased blood flow occurred during periods of tension. On the basis of these findings, it was postulated that "along with the emotional disturbance incident to the precipitating stresses, the patients also reacted with sustained pelvic hyperemia leading ultimately to congestion, edema and pain." Thus, the implication was that stress causes this type of pelvic pain. However, a later publication, which included a control group, concluded that these vascular changes in response to stress occur in *all* women.[13]

Taylor's publications[10, 14–18] had a profound influence on attitudes toward women with pelvic pain in general and pelvic congestion in particular, despite the lack of controls and the small sample size. With additional reports of nervous symptoms such as depression, headache, and insomnia among these patients,[14, 19] it is not surprising that a significant number of gynecologists continue to regard pelvic congestion as a psychosomatic disease. Taylor's work was done at a time when investigative tools such as laparoscopy, pelvic venography, and ultrasonography were not available. Given the evolving attitudes in our approach to CPP, it seems rational to investigate the etiology of this type of pelvic pain from a more objective perspective and to promote an integrated approach to management.

With the advent of laparoscopy, pelvic venography, and ultrasonography, the pathophysiology of the condition has become clearer. The vast majority of our understanding of pelvic congestion comes from the careful and systematic studies performed by Beard's group of gynecologists working at St. Mary's Hospital in London.[12, 20–38] In addition, Hobbs, a general surgeon working at a special vein clinic, has also written extensively about his observations of vulvar varices, varicose veins of the leg, and pelvic pain associated with dilated ovarian veins.[39–41]

Pathophysiology

The observation of rich anastomotic plexuses among the different visceral components of the pelvis and the relative scarcity of valves in the pelvic venous system have contributed to the understanding of the pathophysiology of pelvic congestion. The female pelvis has a complex network of venous structures. The visceral system is composed of various extensive venous plexuses that surround the rectum, bladder, vagina, uterus, and ovaries. All these are interconnected by anastomoses, are essentially valveless, and normally have their major drainage into the internal iliac system. The large uterine and vaginal plexuses drain mainly through two or three veins at the uterine pedicle into the internal iliac veins. The ovarian plexus drains superiorly via the ovarian veins: The left ovarian vein almost always drains into the left renal vein, and the right usually directly into the vena cava.[42]

The internal iliac vein and its numerous visceral and parietal tributaries serve as an important collateral pathway in case of obstruction of the iliocaval segment. The relative scarcity of valves encountered in the pelvic plexuses is thus beneficial and contributes to the development of collateral circulation, because blood can flow in either direction.[43]

The importance of valves in the hemodynamics of the venous circulation and in the pathophysiology of varicose veins has been long recognized. Anatomic studies have shown that 13% to 15% of women lack valves in the left ovarian vein; the corresponding figure for the right vein is 6%.[44, 45] When present, 43% of the valves on the left and 35% to 41% on the right are incompetent.[44, 45] Mean values of ovarian venous diameter at this level are 3.8 mm in the presence of competent valves and 7.5 mm when the valves are incompetent. The upper limit of normal diameter for ovarian veins is 5 mm.[46]

Special anatomic characteristics of the pelvic veins make them particularly likely to dilate in the nonpregnant state, given the appropriate stimulus.[24] The complex venous drainage system in the pelvis comprises many thin-walled unsupported veins that are devoid of valves and that have weak attachments between the adventitia and supporting connective tissue[47]—quite different from veins elsewhere in the body. The histology of the vessel walls of pelvic varicosities is similar to that of varicose veins elsewhere, including fibrosis of the tunica intima and media, muscle hypertrophy, and proliferation of capillary endothelium.[48]

Varicose veins may develop not only as a result of valvular incompetence but also as a result of genetic anomalies and disturbances in the collagen structure of the venous wall.[43] Aside from the genetic, hormonal, and valvular disorders, important anatomic and physiologic factors during pregnancy contribute to the development of hypertension in the pelvic veins. As the veins dilate during pregnancy, the valve cusps separate and become incompetent.[49] The larger number of cases in women with children indicates that pregnancy is a risk factor for the development of a varicocele.[50] During pregnancy, the vascular capacity of the ovarian veins may increase 60 times over the nonpregnant state[51] thus contributing to both valvular incompetence and venous dilatation.

It has been shown by pelvic venography that more than 80% of women without an obvious cause of their pain at laparoscopy have marked venous congestion in the major pelvic veins, which are frequently dilated up to three times their normal diameter.[21] Using transuterine venography, 91% of patients with CPP had evidence of varicocele, compared with 11% of control patients.[21] Further studies using the specific venoconstrictor dihydroergotamine, administered intravenously to women during an acute attack of pain, have shown that this drug causes narrowing of the veins with improvement of the congestion and a significant reduction in pain.[32] These findings suggest that venous congestion in the pelvis is a common cause of pain in women and that it can be temporarily diminished by venoconstriction.

Evidence also suggests widespread physical changes in the pelvic organs of women with pelvic congestion. Adams and colleagues[20] found that in a group of 55 women with chronic pain due to pelvic congestion, ultrasound measurement revealed that they had a larger uterus and thicker endometrium than did a group of normal women matched for age and parity. In patients with evidence of ovarian vein varicocele, disorders of the menstrual cycle, such as menorrhagia and polymenorrhea, were more frequently reported than in patients without varicocele ($P < .05$).[50] Morever, 56% of the women with pelvic congestion were found to have cystic changes in their ovaries that ranged from a classic polycystic pattern to the appearance of clusters of four to six cysts in bilaterally enlarged ovaries.[18, 20]

Symptoms

Owing to the variability in the veins that are dilated and congested, it follows that a patient's symptoms vary depending on the organ systems affected. In general, pain in women with pelvic congestion is brought on or exacerbated by any stimulus that increases intraabdominal pressure and congestion, such as prolonged standing, walking, or lifting, whereas lying down provides relief.[24, 35] The pain is commonly present only on one side, but direct questioning usually reveals that in most women it occasionally occurs on the other side. Patients typically are in their late 20s or early 30s and are more likely to have had children than not. The pain is described as a dull aching pain in the pelvis that is worsened by walking and other postural changes. Cyclic changes in intensity of the pain have also been noted. Dysfunctional bleeding and dysmenorrhea of the congestive type are common.[50] Dyspareunia may be a symptom, but patients more commonly report a postcoital ache that may last for hours or days. Acute episodes of severe pain may have provoked hospital admission or emergency room visits, often with the discharge diagnosis of pelvic inflammatory disease (PID).[24]

Although patients may have bowel symptoms, a consistent change in bowel habits is not reported, in contrast to patients diagnosed as having irritable bowel syndrome.[26] Bladder irritability was found in 24% to 45% of patients with pelvic congestion,[15, 39] with no pathology evident on cultures or cystoscopy. In some of these patients, the late films of the vulval venogram series showed filling defects at the bladder base due to dilated veins of the vesical plexus.[39] Others have noted congestion and edema of the trigone in some of the women at cystoscopy.[15] Virtually all researchers have pointed out that in addition to pelvic symptoms, a substantially high proportion of the patients have various symptoms in other organ systems, including functional gastrointestinal symptoms,[26, 52] chronic headache, fibromyalgia, backache, excessive vaginal discharge, deep dyspareunia, and emotional disorders. Some of these symptoms may be related to alterations in pelvic organ structure and function that result from generalized venous congestion.[20]

Clinicians faced with these diverse symptoms must decide if a patient has multiple causes of her symptoms unrelated to pelvic congestion, whether all of the symptoms are related to pelvic congestion, or whether a condition such as endometriosis coexists with pelvic congestion. In one series, only 10 of 21 women with symptoms of pelvic congestion had pelvic varicosities as the sole finding.[53, 54] The differential diagnosis includes virtually any diagnosis that affects the abdominopelvic organs.

Physical Examination

Beard and colleagues[25] compared the clinical features of 35 women with pelvic pain

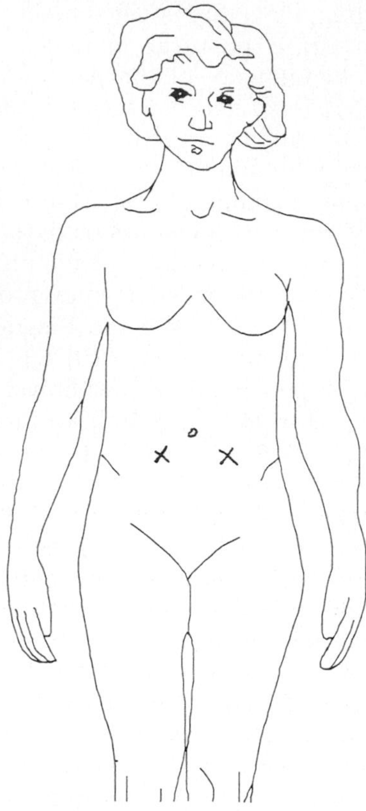

Figure 17–1. Localization of tenderness on abdominal examination. The ovarian point is located at the junction of the upper and middle thirds of a line drawn from the anterior superior iliac spine to the umbilicus.

and demonstrable congestion on pelvic venography versus those of 22 women with pelvic pain due to classic pathology. On abdominal examination, pressure over the ovarian point (Fig. 17–1) produced pain in the pelvis identical to that of which the patient complained. Pressure at this point results in compression of the ovarian vein over the transverse processes of the lumbar vertebrae, which results in back-pressure on the plexus of veins at the hilum of the ovary.[23]

The cervix is often blue as a result of engorgement.[23] On bimanual examination, cervical motion tenderness is common. The position of the uterus, its size, and tenderness of the uterosacral ligaments did not prove to be useful distinguishing features. The most useful distinguishing physical sign is marked ovarian tenderness elicited by gentle compression on bimanual vaginal examination, which reproduced the pain being complained of.[25] The similarities of these signs to those of PID explain why almost half of the women in Beard's study had a previous diagnosis of recurrent PID. The combination of tenderness on abdominal palpation over the ovarian point and a history of postcoital ache was 94% sensitive and 77% specific for discriminating pelvic congestion from other causes of pelvic pain.

It should be noted, however, that not all researchers are in agreement with the findings of Beard's group. In contrast, both Renaer (1980)[55] and Taylor (1949)[15] emphasize that tenderness of the posterior parametrium and uterosacral ligaments is the most useful diagnostic sign, present in more than 80% of their patients. Frequently reported symptoms and signs are summarized in Table 17–1.

Diagnostic Testing

Because of the nonspecific nature of the symptoms of pelvic congestion, the diagnosis is difficult to establish on the basis of

Table 17–1. **SIGNS AND SYMPTOMS SUGGESTIVE OF PELVIC CONGESTION**

Symptoms
- Dull, aching pelvic pain, worse with standing, activity, or Valsalva's maneuver
- Urinary urgency/frequency with negative urine culture and cystoscopy
- Gastrointestinal symptoms that do not fit diagnostic criteria for irritable bowel syndrome
- Postcoital ache lasting hours or days*
- Pain that moves between the right lower quadrant and left lower quadrant (one may predominate)
- Low back pain
- Secondary dysmenorrhea
- Dysfunctional uterine bleeding
- Migraine headaches
- Family history of varicosities

Signs
- Ovarian point tenderness on abdominal examination
- Cervical motion tenderness
- Adnexal tenderness*

Diagnostic studies
- Polycystic ovaries on ultrasound examination
- Normal findings on pelvic examination at laparoscopy

*These two symptoms/signs, when both present, are 94% sensitive and 77% specific for pelvic congestion.

From Beard RW, Reginald PW, Wadsworth J: Clinical features of women with chronic lower abdominal pain and pelvic congestion. Br J Obstet Gynaecol 1998;95:153.

history and physical examination alone. An integrated approach to these patients includes attention to physical assessment as well as psychosocial functioning. Thorough evaluation of a patient's gastrointestinal and urologic systems is important, when symptoms are present. Treatment with antidepressants, bladder and bowel antispasmodics, fiber, exercise, diet, and therapy aimed at improving coping skills all should be instituted as indicated. In addition, patients should be reevaluated during this treatment phase, because the nature of the primary problem may become more apparent. Additional testing, aimed at assessment of the pelvic vasculature, is needed to establish the diagnosis before performing surgical procedures such as laparoscopy.

Giacchetto and colleagues[50] estimated, based on a study of 35 women with CPP, that valvular incompetence of the genital venous system occurs rather frequently, affecting half of the women studied. Despite the fact that it is a common problem,[54, 56] it has been difficult to diagnose except by invasive techniques. Whereas the diagnosis of a varicocele in the males is made first clinically and then confirmed by Doppler studies, until recently, the same diagnosis in females has been possible only with invasive techniques such as venography.[21, 57–59] With the introduction of transvaginal ultrasound examination, laparoscopy, and other techniques, we now have the ability to diagnose pelvic congestion specifically.

Laparoscopy

Virtually all women with CPP undergo laparoscopy, which is quite useful in diagnosing many but not all of the causes of CPP (see Chapter 12). However, dilated veins often cannot be seen because of their retroperitoneal position, increased intraabdominal pressure, and increased venous drainage with Trendelenburg positioning. It should be noted that a nondiagnostic laparoscopy in a woman with CPP is highly suspicious of pelvic congestion. Beard and associates[21] showed that 91% of women seeking relief of CPP, with no other pelvic pathology on laparoscopic examination, had dilated veins and vascular congestion in the broad ligaments and ovarian plexus demonstrated on venography. Although this high proportion of affected women can be attributed to referral bias, others have also reported high rates of pelvic congestion in laparoscopy-negative women.[50]

Venography

Various venographic techniques for imaging the dilated pelvic venous plexus have been described, including injection of radiopaque medium into the pelvic vessels,[57, 58, 60] transfemoral selective venography,[61] and transuterine injection of water-soluble contrast. This latter technique was first described in 1925 by Heinen and Siegel[62] and has since been reported by several European and American researchers.[63] The technique is straightforward, particularly for those familiar with hysterosalpingography and transcervical tubal cannulation (Fig. 17–2).

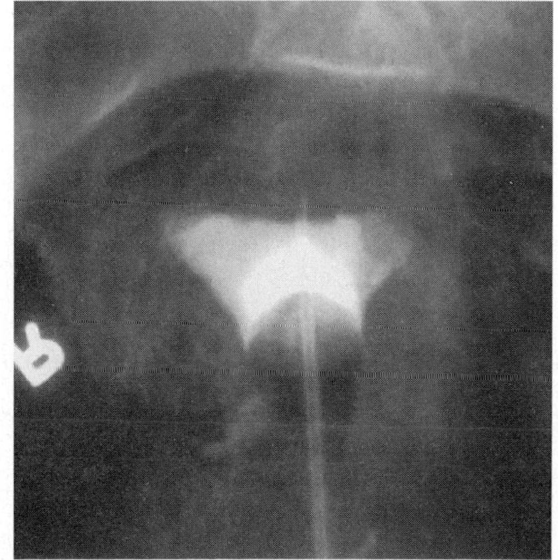

Figure 17–2. Transcervical venogram. The patient is positioned on the examination table in a frog-legged position. An intrauterine access balloon catheter (Cook) is passed transcervically, and the balloon is inflated with saline. Water-soluble contrast is injected into the uterine cavity, and the position of the balloon is confirmed fluoroscopically. A 17-gauge single-lumen oocyte retrieval needle (Rocket USA) is passed through the intrauterine access catheter, and using fluoroscopic guidance, the needle is advanced into the muscle of the uterine fundus. While maintaining the position of the needle, 10 ml of hyaluronidase is injected, immediately followed by 30 ml of water-soluble contrast. Pictures are taken in rapid sequence over a period of 30 to 60 seconds.

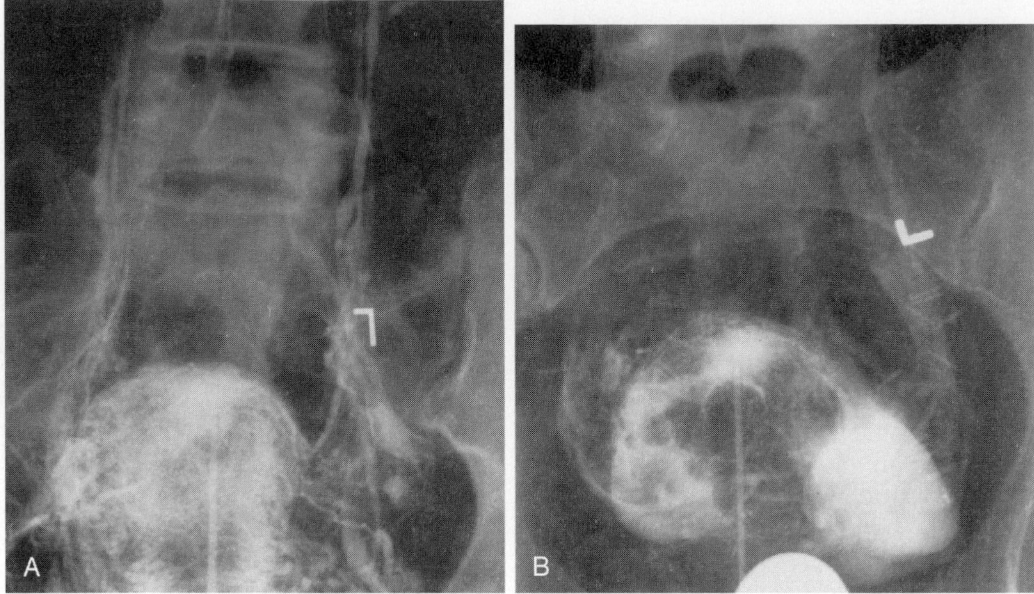

Figure 17–3. Normal (*A*) and abnormal (*B*) transcervical venograms. Note the dilated and tortuous ovarian vein in *B*. This patient subsequently underwent left ovarian vein ligation, which provided partial relief.

In addition to visualizing the veins of the broad ligaments, transuterine venography also gives information about the volume, structure, and vascularity of the uterus (Fig. 17–3). Specific criteria of the venogram that are assessed in order to make the diagnosis are summarized in Table 17–2.

Transuterine venography has a few drawbacks. Although large varices may be seen in the broad ligament, the ovarian veins are not always filled, even with unilateral pressure on the iliac fossa. In some patients, the ovarian veins were subsequently found to be grossly dilated by selective ovarian venography.[40] The cervix occasionally cannot be penetrated and may require dilatation. Patients may experience discomfort when the contrast medium is injected, and because of the need to maintain positioning of the needle, we have heavily sedated the majority of our patients with midazolam and propofol. Perforation of the uterus has been reported but has not caused major sequelae.[64] In our series of 12 patients, we have not encountered any of the foregoing difficulties (Metzger DA, Epstein FB: Unpublished data).

Other attempts at venography have included cannulation of the dorsal vein of the clitoris after surgical exposure, injection of vulvar varices, and direct ovarian venography. Selective transfemoral ovarian venography is performed by passing a catheter into the femoral vein and guiding it under fluoroscopy into the left ovarian vein. The right ovarian vein is more difficult to access because it drains directly into the inferior vena cava. Any of the following is suggestive of pelvic congestion syndrome: an ovarian ve-

Table 17–2. **SCORING SYSTEM FOR TRANSUTERINE VENOGRAMS**

	Points		
Parameter	1	2	3
Maximum diameter of ovarian vein (mm)	1–4	5–8	>8
Time of disappearance of contrast from end of injection (seconds)	0	20	40
Congestion of ovarian plexus*	Normal	Moderate	Extensive

*Congestion of the ovarian venous plexus is defined according to the classification of Kaupilla.[48] Veins that are small, straight, similar in caliber, and easily visualized are classified as normal. Veins that are variable in caliber, tortuous, and difficult to see separately are classed as moderately congested. Veins that are very wide with great variation in caliber and marked tortuosity are considered severely congested.

Total venogram scores of >5 (sum of the scores for the three parameters) have been shown to have a sensitivity of 91% and a specificity of 89% when compared with the clinical physical diagnosis. Moreover, the venogram score is not influenced by the stage of the menstrual cycle or parity.[21]

nous diameter 10 mm at its widest point, uterine venous engorgement, moderate or severe congestion of the ovarian plexus, filling of veins across the midline, or filling of vulval or thigh varicosities.[65] The presence of more than one of the foregoing factors is considered strong supportive evidence for the diagnosis. Selective ovarian venography has the significant advantage that the pelvic, ovarian, and iliac venous anatomy can be demonstrated together with any communicating ovarian, vulvar, or leg varicosities. The venous caliber in pelvic congestion is generally greater than that in male varicoceles.

Ultrasonography

Ultrasonography with or without color Doppler capabilities has been used to document pelvic venous congestion and to describe both diminished flow and increased diameter of pelvic veins.[42, 66] Pelvic ultrasound examination is a valuable noninvasive screening procedure that may prove useful in selecting patients for venography. Moreover, ultrasonography allows an assessment of individual venous plexuses such as the bladder, paracervical, and ovarian. It must be noted, however, that a nondiagnostic ultrasound examination does not preclude the condition, and if the clinical history is strongly suggestive, further investigation is merited.

Giacchetto and colleagues[60] compared ultrasonography findings in 35 women with pelvic pain with the appearance on ovarian vein venography. They found that the presence of linear or circular anechogenic structures lateral to the uterus and cervix with a diameter greater than 5 mm was indicative of pelvic varices. The vascular nature of these structures was confirmed with Valsalva's maneuver and, better yet, in the upright position. These findings on vaginal ultrasound examination were confirmed by retrograde phlebography. In contrast, in those patients seen to have an intact pelvic vein valvular system, ultrasonography demonstrated the presence of vascular structures lateral to the uterus with a diameter less than 5 mm. No changes in the diameter occurred with Valsalva's maneuver or in a standing position. Another advantage of transvaginal ultrasound examination is that it is possible to observe the veins continuously and to measure responses to medications.[34]

Miscellaneous Methods

Xenon 133 clearance has been studied as a noninvasive means of diagnosing pelvic congestion.[67] Seventy-six patients ages 20 to 56 years scheduled for gynecologic surgery were questioned preoperatively about pelvic pain symptoms. Clearance curves for ^{133}Xe were determined in all women after injection of the isotope into the anterior lip of the cervix. At laparotomy, signs of pelvic congestion were present in 40 patients and absent in 36. Blood flow was significantly slower in women with pelvic congestion than in nonaffected women. However, the predictive value of xenon clearance was altered by pathology such as fibroids and ovarian cysts, with sufficient overlap of findings that doubtful results were obtained in 16 patients.

Treatment

Despite abundant literature that has been generated on the subject for at least 150 years, few effective treatments have been developed (Table 17–3). Part of the difficulty in identifying effective treatments has been

Table 17–3. **TREATMENTS FOR PELVIC CONGESTION**

Not effective
Uterine suspension[8, 40]
Gonadotropin-releasing hormone agonists[29]
Oral contraceptives
Antidepressants
Tranquilizers
Possibly effective
Psychotherapy
Ergots
Effective
Hysterectomy/bilateral salpingo-oophorectomy
Oophorectomy
Ovarian vein ligation
Medroxyprogesterone acetate
Ovarian vein embolization

the problems encountered in diagnosing pelvic congestion. Another obstacle is that the symptoms of pelvic congestion may encompass other organ systems, to which ineffectual treatment is directed. Our challenge as physicians is to diagnose and treat these patients as specifically as possible.

Patients with pelvic congestion present many diagnostic and management challenges, as detailed earlier. Some of these patients are reassured by an evaluation that demonstrates a lack of pathology (see Chapter 12). Others may derive significant benefit from symptomatically directed treatment. It is unclear what proportion of patients with pelvic congestion ultimately require surgery, but this should be reserved until more conservative measures have failed and the diagnosis has been confirmed by either venography or ultrasonography.

Medical Therapy

Treatment with medroxyprogesterone acetate (MPA) in women with demonstrable pelvic congestion leads to narrowing of the veins with a reduction in pelvic congestion and an associated reduction in pelvic pain in 18 of 22 patients treated.[31] Reported side effects of the use of a relatively high dose of MPA (30 to 50 mg) include weight gain, increased appetite,[31] and bloating.[28] Breakthrough bleeding is troublesome in a significant proportion of women (18%).[31] Pelvic pain frequently returns when treatment is stopped. However, the improvement that these women experience while on treatment is reassuring that a correct diagnosis has been made.

More importantly, MPA has been compared with other treatments in controlled trials. When compared with psychotherapy alone or in combination with MPA, MPA showed a significant benefit in pain reduction compared with controls (73% versus 33% reporting at least a 50% improvement). Nine months after the end of therapy, no overall significant effect of MPA or psychotherapy was noted, but an interaction between MPA and psychotherapy was found, with 71% of the women in this group showing a greater than 50% reduction in pain score. The explanation for these findings is likely to be complex because of the known interaction between psychologic and somatic factors in pain. On the somatic side, the data support the hypothesis that pelvic congestion is in some way dependent on the effects of ovarian hormones. Treatment with MPA may provide a means of temporary relief from a pain that has often been crippling for many years and allows a woman to gain a sense of control over the pain. She may then find it easier to practice the coping strategies taught during psychotherapy once MPA is discontinued and the pain returns.[28] Alternatively, MPA and psychotherapy may allow a woman to modify the way in which she interprets nociceptive signals.

Ovarian suppression alone does not appear to have a beneficial effect on the symptoms of pelvic congestion. Use of oral contraceptives to treat patients with pelvic congestion does not appear to have significant benefit. In fact, some patients have an increase in symptoms while taking oral contraceptives.[68] Gangar and associates[29] studied 21 women with pelvic congestion treated with gonadotropin-releasing hormone (GnRH) agonists with continuous estradiol valerate 1 mg daily and MPA 5 mg daily. They had no significant relief of pain. Unfortunately, no control group treated with GnRH agonists alone was included.

One conclusion that can be drawn from these studies is that treatment directed toward constricting the dilated pelvic veins is effective in relieving pain, as demonstrated in studies with MPA[31] and dihydroergotamine,[32] both of which have demonstrated venoconstrictor activity. Unfortunately, the beneficial effect of the treatment lasts only as long as the medication is taken, and this observation has prompted a search for more long-lasting approaches.

Surgical Therapy

Although Taylor decried the use of major surgery for pelvic congestion, only one in his whole series of patients was classified as completely cured, and that was by hysterectomy.[17] Others have described the impact that hysterectomy has on the symptoms of pelvic congestion quite eloquently: "... where the patient has her family, vaginal hysterectomy ... is likely to convert an ill, anemic and fatigued wife into a happy, congenial companion."[69] Beard and colleagues[22] prospectively monitored 36 women with pelvic congestion; 33 had failed to obtain long-term relief of pain on medical therapy. All underwent total abdominal hysterectomy and bilateral salpingo-oophorectomy. Median pain score on visual analogue scale fell from a preoperative value of 10 to 0 at 1 year. Twelve of the 36 women had some residual pain 1 year postoperatively, but in only one woman was the pain affecting her daily life. The median frequency of sexual intercourse increased from once per month preoperatively to eight times per month 1 year postoperatively.

The results of this study help to resolve the cause-and-effect controversy about whether the emotional disturbance to daily life displayed by so many women is caused by or results in their long-standing pelvic pain.[55, 70] As a group, the women in Beard's study[22] had the most disturbed marital and social lives of all the women attending the pelvic pain clinic. The fact that 35 of 36 women reported that their lives returned to normal with the disappearance of pelvic pain suggests that much of the preoperative overt disturbance of behavior in their daily lives was the product of the pain rather than the cause of it.

The severity of disruption of the life of a woman is an important factor influencing the decision to perform radical surgery. Other factors include duration of pain, age, parity of the patient, and response to prior therapy. Less radical approaches, which preserve reproductive function, have been gaining favor and include venous ligation and venous embolization.

Treatment of ovarian vein varicosities originally consisted of ligation and resection of the ovarian vein via the transperitoneal route.[2, 7, 53, 54] Analogous with extraperitoneal resection of the spermatic vein above the inguinal ligament for treatment of varicocele of the testis[71] is a method developed by Rundqvist and colleagues.[56] This method consists of extraperitoneal resection of the left ovarian vein in women with pelvic varicosities. Overall results of venous ligation for pelvic pain due to pelvic congestion are presented in Table 17–4. Based on these small series of patients, consistent evidence seems to show that ovarian vein ligation is an effective treatment for symptomatic ovarian vein varicosities.

Several observations that have been made may improve the outcome of ligation procedures. First, the venous caliber in pelvic congestion is generally greater than that in male varicoceles, and distal venous blockade alone may lead to significant amounts of thrombus in the proximal vein.[72] The potential complication of pulmonary embo-

Table 17–4. **HISTORICAL RESULTS WITH DIFFERENT TREATMENTS**

Reference		No. of Patients	Follow-up	Cured	Improved	No Change
Ligation						
Edlundh[53]		6	"Short"		6	
Mattson[6]		25	1–3 years	25		
Metzger (unpublished)		20	0.5–1.5 years	14	3	3
Miller and Kanavel[7]		4	?	4		
Rundqvist et al[56]		15	0.5–8 years	8	3	4
Sharp and Sharp (unpublished)		1	7 years	1		
	Total	71		52 (73%)	12 (17%)	7 (10%)
Embolization						
Edwards et al[72]		1	0.5 year	1		
Giacchetto et al[50]		3	1 year	3		
Machan et al (unpublished)		22	2 years	16		6
Sichlau et al[38]		3	1 year	2	1	
	Total	29		22 (79%)	1 (4%)	6 (22%)
Total Abdominal Hysterectomy/Bilateral Salpingo-Oophorectomy						
Beard et al[22]		36	1 year	24 (67%)	12 (33%)	0

lism should be avoided by ligation of the proximal vessel also. Second, Lechter[73] ligated only the ovarian vein on the side involved when he began his study but then became convinced that both sides needed to be treated because the rich cross-communications in the pelvis may lead to recurrence on the contralateral side. Third, patients must be carefully selected because this procedure is effective only for the symptoms of pelvic congestion mediated by the ovarian veins. Central pelvic and other general congestive symptoms would not be expected to respond. Finally, advances in laparoscopic surgery now make day surgery for this condition a reality, and my colleagues and I have successfully used this approach in a series of patients (see Table 17–4).

Interventional radiologic techniques were previously used successfully to treat only testicular varicoceles in men. Reports now (see Table 17–4) attest to the success of the analogous embolization procedure in women with CPP and pelvic congestion. The treatment is comparable to surgical ligation of the ovarian veins but is less invasive and is performed as an outpatient procedure. Unfortunately, the right ovarian vein may be difficult to access via the transfemoral route, and the radiation exposure for this fluoroscopic procedure can be considerable. Although certain features resemble the male varicocele, for which transcatheter embolization is an established treatment,[74] several differences in ovarian anatomy necessitate a modified embolization technique. Communications may exist between the left ovarian vein and the inferior mesenteric veins, splenic vein, and ureteric veins.[40] For this reason, the use of liquid sclerosants may be hazardous and should be avoided.

The effect of venous ligation or embolization on ovarian function is unknown, but ovarian venous drainage is unlikely to be impaired, owing to communications with the uterine plexus and hence the internal iliac vein. In fact, several investigators have observed improvement in menstrual symptoms and regulation of cycles.[72] One of my first patients to undergo laparoscopic bilateral ovarian vein ligation conceived within 6 months. However, because of the lack of long-term studies, ovarian vein ligation/embolization should be reserved for patients in whom the benefits clearly outweigh the risks and for patients who are willing to accept possible ovarian failure as a consequence.

Summary

Pelvic varicosities are associated with vascular stasis, congestion of the pelvic organs, and pain in the same way as varicose veins in the legs may produce pain. That intravenous injection of the selective vasoconstrictor dihydroergotamine causes constriction of the pelvic varicosities and improvement in symptoms suggests a direct link. Varicosities have been reported in 91% of women in one clinic with otherwise unexplained CPP but only rarely in symptom-free controls. Valvular incompetence of the ovarian veins has been suggested by some as a cause. Others have concentrated on ovarian hormones because the condition affects only women in the reproductive age group. Endocrine studies have not been carried out, but ultrasonography has been used to investigate the physical dimensions of target organs for accurate measurement of uterine size, endometrial thickness, and ovarian volume. Adams and colleagues[20] suggested that either an excess of estrogen or an excessive response to it might not only be responsible for pelvic congestion but might also cause uterine and endometrial hypertrophy: These features were indeed observed in women with pelvic varicosities. Another common finding was the presence of polycystic ovaries. Further studies have used transvaginal ultrasound examination, which gives high-quality images of pelvic organs and can show pelvic varicosities without the need for venography.

As with other sources of CPP, an integrated approach is essential, given the significant proportion of women who have pelvic congestion and pain as well as emotional difficulties and multisystem symptoms. Treatment options directed toward the pelvic congestion include high-dose MPA, venous ligation, venous embolization, and hysterectomy.

It remains for clinicians and radiologists alike to become more aware of the pelvic congestion syndrome and the symptoms, signs, and ultrasonographic findings that characterize this disabling and often overlooked but readily treatable condition.

References

1. Richet MA: Traité Pratique d'Anatomie Medico-Chirurgicale. Paris, E. Chamerot Libraire Editeur, 1857.
2. Castano CA: Pelvic varicocele. Surg Gynecol Obstet 1925;40:237.
3. Dudley AP: Varicocele in the female: What is its influence upon the ovary? N Y Med J 1888;48:147.
4. Emge LA: Varicose veins of the female pelvis. A preliminary report. Acta Obstet Gynecol Scand 1921;32:133.
5. Fothergill WE: Varicocele in the female. BMJ 1921;2:925.
6. Mattson CH: Varicose veins of the broad ligament. Minn Med 1936;19:376.
7. Miller SM, Kanavel AB: Uncomplicated varicose veins of the female pelvis. Am J Obstet Gynecol 1905;51:480.
8. Lefevre H: Broad ligament varicocele. Acta Obstet Gynecol Scand 1964;43(Suppl 7):122.
9. Chidekel N: Female pelvic veins demonstrated by selective renal phlebography with particular reference to pelvic variocosities. Acta Radiol 1968;193:1.
10. Duncan CH, Taylor HC: A psychosomatic study of pelvic congestion. Am J Obstet Gynecol 1952;64:1.
11. Benson R, Hanson K, Matarazzo J: Atypical pelvic pain in women: Gynecologic psychiatric considerations. Am J Obstet Gynecol 1959;77:806.
12. Beard RW, Belsey EM, Lieverman MV, Wilkinson JCM: Pelvic pain in women. Am J Obstet Gynecol 1977;128:566.
13. Osofshy HJ, Fisher S: Pelvic congestion: Some further considerations. Obstet Gynecol 1968;31:406.
14. Taylor HC: Vascular congestion and hyperemia, their effect on structure and function in the female reproductive system. Part I. Physiologic basis and history of the concept. Am J Obstet Gynecol 1949;57:211.
15. Taylor HC: Vascular congestion and hyperemia, their effect on structure and function in the female reproductive organs. Part II. The clinical aspects of the congestion-fibrosis syndrome. Am J Obstet Gynecol 1949;57:637.
16. Taylor HC: Vascular congestion and hyperemia, their effect on structure in the female reproductive organs. Part III. Etiology and therapy. Am J Obstet Gynecol 1949;57:654.
17. Taylor HC: Pelvic pain based on a vascular and autonomic nervous disorder. Am J Obstet Gynecol 1954;67:1177.
18. Taylor HC: The problem of pelvic pain. In Meigs JV, Somers HS (eds): Progress in Gynecology, vol 3. New York, Grune & Stratton, 1957, pp 191–207.
19. Benson R, Hanson K, Matarazzo J: Atypical pelvic pain in women: Gynecologic psychiatric considerations. Am J Obstet Gynecol 1959;77:806.
20. Adams J, Reginald PW, Granks S, et al: Uterine size and endometrial thickness and the significance of cystic ovaries in women with pelvic pain due to congestion. Br J Obstet Gynecol 1990;97:583.
21. Beard RW, Highman JH, Pearce S, Reginald PW: Diagnosis of pelvic varicosities in women with chronic pelvic pain. Lancet 1984;2:946.
22. Beard RW, Kennedy RG, Gangar KF, et al: Bilateral oophorectomy and hysterectomy in the treatment of intractable pelvic pain associated with pelvic congestion. Br J Obstet Gynaecol 1991;98:988.
23. Beard RW, Reginald PW, Pearce S: Pelvic pain in women. BMJ 1986;293:1160.
24. Beard RW, Reginald PW, Pearce S: Psychological and somatic factors in women with pain due to pelvic congestion. Adv Exp Biol Med 1988; 245:413.
25. Beard RW, Reginald PW, Wadsworth J: Clinical features of women with chronic lower abdominal pain and pelvic congestion. Br J Obstet Gynaecol 1988;95:153.
26. Farquhar CM, Hoghton GBS, Beard RW: Pelvic pain–pelvic congestion or the irritable bowel syndrome? Eur J Obstet Gynecol Reprod Biol 1990;37:71.
27. Farquhar CM, Rae T, Thomas DC, et al: Doppler ultrasound in the nonpregnant pelvis. J Ultrasound Med 1989;8:451.
28. Farquhar CM, Rogers V, Franks S, et al: A randomized controlled trial of medroxyprogesterone acetate and psychotherapy for the treatment of pelvic congestion. Br J Obstet Gynecol 1989;96:1153.
29. Gangar KF, Stones RW, Saunders C, et al: An alternative to hysterectomy? GnRH analogue combined with hormone replacement therapy. Br J Obstet Gynaecol 1993;100:360.
30. Pearce S, Knight C, Beard RW: Pelvic pain—a common gynecological problem. J Psychosom Obstet Gynecol 1982;1:12.
31. Reginald PW, Adams J, Franks S, et al: Medroxyprogesterone acetate in the treatment of pelvic pain due to venous congestion. Br J Obstet Gynaecol 1989;96:1148.
32. Reginald PW, Kooner JS, Samarage SU, et al: Intravenous dihydroergotamine to relieve pelvic congestion with pain in young women. Lancet 1987;8:351.
33. Saxon DW, Garquhar CM, Rae T, et al: Accuracy sound measurement of female pelvic organs. Br J Obstet Gynaecol 1990;97:695.
34. Stones RW, Rae T, Rogers V, et al: Pelvic congestion in women: Evaluation with transvaginal ultrasound and observation of venous pharmacology. Br J Radiol 1990;63:710.
35. Thomas DC, McArdle FJ, Rogers VE, et al: Local blood volume changes in women with pelvic congestion measured by applied potential tomography. Clin Sci 1991;81:401.
36. Thomas DC, Stones RW, Farquhar CM, Beard RW: Measurement of pelvic blood flow changes in response to posture in normal subjects and in women with pelvic pain owing to congestion by using a thermal technique. Clin Sci 1992;83:55.
37. Stones RW, Thomas DC, Beard RW: Suprasensitivity to calcitonin gene-related peptide but not vasoactive intestinal peptide in women with chronic pelvic pain. Clin Auton Res 1992;2:343.
38. Stones RW, Loesch A, Beard RW, Burnstock G: Substance P: Endothelial localization and pharmacology in the human ovarian vein. Obstet Gynecol 1995;85:273.
39. Craig O, Hobbs JT: Vulval phlebography in the pelvic congestion syndrome. Clin Radiol 1974;25:517.
40. Hobbs JT: The pelvic congestion syndrome. Practitioner 1976;216:529.

41. Hobbs JT: The pelvic congestion syndrome. Br J Hosp Med 1990;43:200.
42. Frede TE: Ultrasonic visualization of varisocities in the female genital tract. J Ultrasound Med 1984;3:365.
43. LePage PA, Villavicencio JL, Gomez ER, et al: The valvular anatomy of the iliac venous system and its clinical implications. J Vasc Surg 1991;14:678.
44. Ahlberg NE, Bartley O, Chidekel N: Circumference of the left gonadal vein. An anatomical and statistical study. Acta Radiol 1965;3:503.
45. Ahlberg NE, Bartley O, Chidekel N: Right and left gonadal veins. An anatomical and statistical study. Acta Radiol 1966;4:593.
46. Kennedy A, Hemingway A: Radiology of ovarian varices. Br J Hosp Med 1990;44:38.
47. Von Peham H, Amreich J: Operative Gynecology, Vol. 1, Philadelphia, Lippincott Co, 1934, p 156.
48. Kaupilla A: Uterine phlebography with venous compression. A clinical and roentgenological study. Acta Obstet Gynecol Scand 1970;49:33.
49. Tamvakopoulos SK: Non-invasive estimation of lower limb venous dynamics in pregnant women. Proceedings of the VI European American Symposium on Venous Diseases. Abstract No. 02.3, Washington DC, 1987.
50. Giacchetto C, Cotroneo GB, Marincolo F, et al: Ovarian varicocele: Ultrasonic and phlebographic evaluation. J Clin Ultrasound 1990;18:551.
51. Hodgkinson CP: Physiology of the ovarian veins during pregnancy. Obstet Gynecol 1953;1:26.
52. Manning P, Thompson WG, Heaton KW, Morris AF: Towards positive diagnosis of the irritable bowel syndrome. BMJ 1978;2:653.
53. Edlundh KO: Pelvic varicosities in women: A preliminary report. Acta Obstet Gynecol Scand 1964;43:399.
54. Edlundh KO: Pelvic varisocities in women. Acta Obstet Gynecol Scand 1964;43:399.
55. Renaer M: Chronic pelvic pain without obvious pathology in women. Eur J Obstet Gynecol Reprod Biol 1980;10:415.
56. Rundqvist E, Sondholm LE, Larsson G: Treatment of pelvic varicosities causing lower abdominal pain with extraperitoneal resection of the left ovarian vein. Lancet 1984;i:339.
57. Topolanski-Sierra R: Pelvic phlebography. Am J Obstet Gynecol 1958;76:44.
58. Hughes RR, Curtis DD: Uterine phlebography: Correlation of clinical diagnoses with dye retention. Am J Obstet Gynecol 1962;83:156.
59. Bellina JH, Dougherty CM, Mickal JA: Transmyometrial pelvic venography. Obstet Gynecol 1969; 34:194.
60. Helander CG, Lindbaum A: Varicocele of the broad ligament. A venographic study. Acta Radiol 1960;53:97.
61. Ahlberg NE, Bartley O, Chidekel N: Retrograde contrast filling of the left gonadal vein. Acta Radiol 1965;3:385.
62. Heinen G, Siegel T: Zur Grage des lokalen Kontrast Mittel Schadkgung bei der Uterus Phlebography. A Cl Gynak 1925;87:829.
63. Hammen R: The technique of pelvic phlebography. Acta Obstet Gynecol Scand 1965;44:370.
64. Murray E, Comparato M: Uterine phlebography. Am J Obstet Gynecol 1968;102:1088.
65. Lechter A, Alvarez A: Pelvic varices and gonadal veins. Phlebology 1986;85:225.
66. Hodgson TJ, Reed MWR, Peck RJ, Hemingway AP: Case report: The ultrasound and Doppler appearances of pelvic varices. Clin Radiol 1991;44:208.
67. Pellegri PP, Montanari GD: The preoperative diagnosis of pelvic congestion by means of 133 Xenon injected into the cervical myometrium. Acta Obstet Gynecol Scand 1981;60:447.
68. Allen WM: Chronic pelvic congestion and pelvic pain. Am J Obstet Gynecol 1971;109:198.
69. Stearns HC, Sneeden VD: Observations on the clinical and pathologic aspects of the pelvic congestion syndrome. Am J Obstet Gynecol 1966;94:718.
70. Reiter RC, Gambone JC: Demographic and historic variables in women with idopathic chronic pelvic pain. Obstet Gynecol 1990;75:428.
71. Fritjofsson A, Sandholm LE: Extraperitoneal resecton of the left ovarian vein in women with pelvic varicosities. J R Coll Surg 1974;2:1299.
72. Edwards RD, Robertson IR, MacLean AB, Hemingway AP: Case report: Pelvic pain syndrome—successful treatment of a case by ovarian vein embolization. Clin Radiol 1993;47:429.
73. Lechter A: Pelvic varices: Treatment. J Cardiovasc Surg 1985;26:111.
74. White RI, Kaufman SL, Barth KH, et al: Occlusion of varicoceles with detachable balloons. Radiol 1981;139:327.

18

Nerve Cutting Procedures for Pelvic Pain

Deborah A. Metzger, PhD, MD

Dysmenorrhea severe enough to limit social activities affects more than 18 million women in the United States.[1] In addition, the majority of women with endometriosis report dysmenorrhea that is not correlated with the extent of disease. Nonsteroidal antiinflammatory drugs (NSAIDs), oral contraceptives, progestins, danazol, and gonadotropin-releasing hormone analogues have provided much needed relief to the majority of women with dysmenorrhea, but 20% to 25% fail to obtain relief or experience side effects that limit the usefulness of these medications. For this latter group of women, nerve-cutting procedures that interrupt transmission of pain signals from the uterus and cervix provide an alternative.

For women with lateral chronic pelvic pain unresponsive to more traditional modes of treatment, other types of nerve-cutting procedures have been proposed (Table 18–1). Although the benefits and risks have not yet been tested in the appropriate settings, these procedures are included for completeness.

Indications and Patient Selection

It should be noted that uterosacral transection and presacral neurectomy benefit only those women with midline pain. Those with predominantly lateral pain fail to obtain relief from these procedures and may be candidates for ovarian sympathectomy (discussed later). Lateral and midline pain differs both anatomically and physiologically, as reflected in the difference in innervation (see Chapter 5): Lateral structures receive their innervation mostly via nerve fibers traversing the infundibulopelvic ligaments, which are not transected with either uterosacral transection or presacral neurectomy.

Preoperative evaluation and counseling of patients is imperative to determine if a patient is an appropriate candidate for one of the procedures and to make sure that her expectations about pain relief are realistic. Appropriate candidates are women with intractable dysmenorrhea that limits their activities each month and fails to respond to NSAIDs, oral contraceptives, or luteal phase progesterone. For women with primary or secondary dysmenorrhea as the only identified pathology, a hysterosalpingogram should be performed to rule out uterine septa or submucous fibroids. Some clinicians have also advocated administration of a paracervical block during menstrual pain to verify that interruption of nerve transmission will alleviate the pain. However, except for unpublished anecdotal reports, no study has been undertaken to demonstrate a correlation between response to paracervical block and response to interruption of these nerve fibers.

Patients should be fully informed about the potential risks and potential for emergency laparotomy should vascular or ureteral injury occur. They also need to be aware that pain relief after surgery may be incomplete and that pain recurrence is a possibility. Other risks include bowel injury and postoperative bladder or bowel dysfunction in the case of presacral neurectomy. For procedures that are not established in medical practice, it is important to

Table 18–1. **NERVE-CUTTING PROCEDURES**

Procedure	Indications	Complications
Uterosacral transection	Severe dysmenorrhea	Ureteral injury Uterine prolapse Temporary pain relief
Presacral neurectomy	Severe dysmenorrhea	Intraoperative hemorrhage Bowel/bladder dysfunction
Uterovaginal ganglion excision	Unilateral or bilateral lower pelvic pain	Ureteral injury Urinary retention
Ovarian sympathectomy	Ovarian pain	Cystic enlargement of ovary

convey to patients the experimental nature of the surgery.

Two methods of surgical interruption of midline nerve pathways have been described: uterosacral transection (laser uterine nerve ablation—LUNA; laser neurectomy; uterosacral ligation; paracervical uterine denervation; uterosacral nerve resection), in which the nerve fibers are cut in close proximity to the uterus, and presacral neurectomy, which results in transection of the superior hypogastric plexus at the level of the sacrum. The optimal choice of procedure remains controversial and is further complicated by the fact that uterosacral transection is technically easier to perform than presacral neurectomy.

Uterosacral Transection

Pain impulses from the uterus, cervix, and proximal fallopian tubes pass through nerve fibers that merge into the paracervical Frankenhäuser's plexus at the base of the uterosacral ligaments and exit through the uterosacral ligaments to the inferior and superior hypogastric plexuses. Because of this sensory pathway, transection of the uterosacral ligaments has been suggested as a method of managing some types of pelvic pain. Before the advent of oral contraceptives and NSAIDs, Doyle[2] designed a vaginal approach to interrupt the uterosacral ligaments as an alternative to presacral neurectomy, which required a laparotomy and long convalescence. His results were similar to those obtained with presacral neurectomy. He described his technique of paracervical uterine denervation as a transection of the area at the back of the cervix deep enough to interrupt the lowest portions of the uterosacral ligaments at their point of insertion into the cervix and vaginal apex. The techniques that are popular today are laparoscopic variations of the same procedure.

Efficacy and Complications

Lichten and Bombard[3] reported relief of incapacitating primary dysmenorrhea in 9 of 11 (81%) patients subjected to uterosacral nerve transection. None of the patients allocated to the control arm of the study reported alleviation of menstrual pain. By the 12th month after surgery, however, only 5 of 11 (45%) continued to have significant pain relief.[3] Gurgan and colleagues[4] reported that 19 of 23 women showed improved dysmenorrhea, with an average pain reduction of only 33%. Similarly, Sutton[5] reported a 63% mean reduction in pain scores. Thus, uterosacral transection should not be regarded as a cure but as a secondary procedure that may provide partial amelioration of pain, particularly in conjunction with NSAIDs.

If uterosacral transection is unsuccessful, it is presumed that either interruption of the nerve fibers was incomplete or that the nerves regenerated. Lichten[6] reported that repeating the procedure did not relieve dysmenorrhea, implying that the course of the nerve fibers in these individuals may represent an anatomic variation. In cadaver dissections, it has been found that 30% of women have significant deviations of nerve pathways from normal,[7] thus explaining the high rate of failure with this procedure. Several patients with failed uterosacral transection did obtain relief from subsequent presacral neurectomy.[8]

When compared with the results obtainable with presacral neurectomy (discussed later), uterosacral transection is indicated for dysmenorrhea only because of its poorer results. It is less useful for control of central pelvic pain. Intraoperative complications include ureteral injury[9] as well as long-term complications such as uterine prolapse.[10, 11]

Laparoscopic Procedure

Uterosacral transection is a relatively easy procedure to perform laparoscopically. A standard three-puncture technique is used (10- to 12-mm umbilical trocar, two 5-mm lateral suprapubic accessory trocars). The uterosacral ligaments are put on tension by anteverting the uterus using a uterine manipulator (Cohen cannula, Zumi, Hulka, or Pelosi). With a carbon dioxide or contact laser, cautery, or scissors, the ligaments are interrupted at their insertion into the cervix, using an axial motion from medial to lateral (Fig. 18–1*A*). Transection at this location is advocated as a means of maximizing the number of nerve fibers transected because of dispersion of the fibers as they pass farther along the length of the uterosacral ligaments. Unfortunately, this segment of the uterosacral ligament is also the portion that is closest to the uterine vessels and to the ureter. The suction-irrigator can be used as a backstop, as a way of making the uterosacral ligament more prominent, and as protection for the ureter (see Fig. 18–1*A*). At frequent intervals, the depth of the incision should be examined to assess the degree of ligament transection, because the goal is to transect the uterosacral ligament *completely*. However, attention must also be given to an artery that extends along the lateral aspect of the uterosacral ligament. Bleeding from this vessel is a particular concern because of the proximity of the ureter, uterine vessels, and rectum when electrocautery is used to achieve hemostasis. Some surgeons also vaporize a path across the base of the cervix between the uterosacral ligaments (Fig. 18–1*B*), although no controlled studies indicate whether this is necessary to provide optimal pain relief. If the uterosacral ligaments are not easily identifiable, the procedure may entail significant risks of injury to adjacent tissues, and the procedure is not recommended under these circumstances.

Because ureteral injury is a serious complication associated with this procedure, the location of the ureter should be identified from the pelvic brim to the paracervical tissue. The distance between the ureter and the uterosacral ligaments usually is 2 to 3 cm. If the ureter lies closer to the uterosacral ligament, a relaxing peritoneal incision is made along the lateral side of the uterosacral ligament to allow lateral retraction of the ureter before the ligament is transected (Fig. 18–1*C*).

Presacral Neurectomy

Presacral neurectomy offers an alternative for the amelioration of intractable dysmenorrhea, deep dyspareunia, sacral backache, and chronic recurrent pain in the center of the pelvis. Since its introduction in 1899 by Jaboulay,[12] presacral neurectomy for relief of pelvic pain and dysmenorrhea has encountered periods of fluctuating enthusiasm. Cotte[13] was the first surgeon to perform the procedure in the United States and reported some 1500 cases in 1937,[14] with a 98% success rate. For the next two decades, presacral neurectomy was performed frequently for both primary and secondary dysmenorrhea. Black, who compiled almost 10,000 cases from the literature, physician questionnaires, and personal experience, reported an overall success rate ranging from 75% to 80%.[15] Just as presacral neurectomy became accepted as the surgical treatment for dysmenorrhea, various medical therapies, such as oral contraceptives and NSAIDs, became widely available and presacral neurectomy became much less frequent. With the ability to perform presacral neurectomy endoscopically rather than by laparotomy, however, there has been a resurgence in interest for the women who fail to obtain adequate relief with medical therapy.

Efficacy and Indications

Presacral neurectomy is most commonly performed for severe, intractable dysmenor-

have been reported frequently. Urinary complaints include long-term urinary urgency[28, 29] and short-term postoperative urinary retention in 50%.[15, 30] Constipation has been reported in as many as 90% of patients.[15, 19, 21, 22, 28] Although some investigators have reported that the constipation was mild and responded to dietary changes,[21] others reported moderate or severe constipation that developed or worsened in one third of patients who underwent a presacral neurectomy, but no such changes were observed in controls.[19] One had recurrent subocclusive crises due to the formation of fecal masses in the rectal ampulla. Not every study has reported bowel and bladder dysfunction. Metzger and colleagues[20] did not find any significant bowel and bladder dysfunction in patients undergoing presacral neurectomy compared with controls, and this conclusion was based on the individual practices of three different surgeons and on preoperative and postoperative questionnaires that specifically addressed these issues. Anecdotal reports from others regularly performing presacral neurectomies also attest to the relative rarity of bowel and bladder complications. Thus, the question that must be answered is this: Does a difference in technique account for the variability in the incidence of bowel and bladder dysfunction?

Other significant complications associated with presacral neurectomy include painless labor[15, 19]; vaginal dryness in as many as 15%, resolving within 6 months[31]; adhesions resulting in intermittent ileal obstruction[15]; and additional surgery for pain.[22] No reports relating postoperative sexual dysfunction to presacral neurectomy could be found. It should be noted that the majority of reports involving presacral neurectomy state that either no complications occurred or that they were transient and resolved without sequelae. Recurrence rates of 0% to 18%[15, 22] have been reported, although some of the recurrences were related to lateral pain.

Given these complications, it is essential that patients be carefully evaluated, screened, and counseled before surgical treatment. Only patients who have failed to respond to medical therapy should be considered. Moreover, because presacral neurectomy is not effective for adnexal pain, those patients with predominantly adnexal pain are not appropriate candidates.

Operative Procedure

Presacral neurectomy, unlike uterosacral transection, requires a significant degree of surgical skill. It should be undertaken by only those surgeons familiar with the retroperitoneal anatomy of the presacral space.

At the level of the bifurcation of the aorta, the intermesenteric nerves join to form the superior hypogastric plexus, interiliac plexus, or presacral nerve, which is the chief sympathetic nerve supply of the bladder, the rectum, and the internal genitalia except for the ovary and the distal part of the fallopian tube (Fig. 18–2). The hypogastric plexus is moderately wide and is formed from two or three incompletely fused trunks of the intermesenteric nerves. Perhaps 20% of patients have complete fusion with the formation of a single nerve. Considerable variability exists in the course of these nerve fibers (Fig. 18–3), which spread out behind the peritoneum in a bed of loosely meshed areolar tissue that lies on the bodies of the fourth and fifth lumbar vertebrae. In the midline, the middle sacral artery is situated between the nerves and the anterior surface of the vertebral bodies.

The superior hypogastric plexus may or may not form a middle hypogastric plexus, a flat expanse of neurofibrous tissue overlying the sacral promontory and extending just below it. This plexus divides to form the bilateral inferior hypogastric plexuses, which pass downward and follow the course of the uterosacral ligaments from the sacrum to the lateral surface of the rectal ampulla to join the pelvic plexus (uterovaginal plexus, cervical ganglion, or Frankenhäuser's plexus) lateral to the cervix, where they join fibers from the nervi erigentes.[32]

Meticulous dissection and hemostasis are required during presacral neurectomy. Adequate exposure of the sacral promontory, aortic bifurcation, and ureters is essential. The boundaries for resection are as follows:

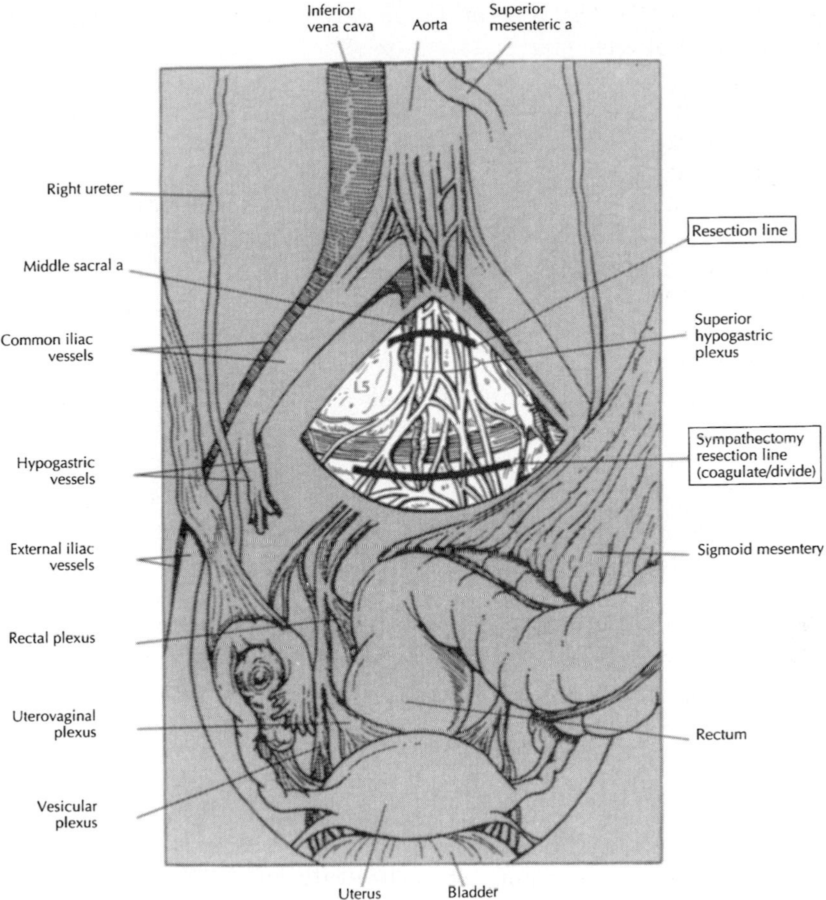

Figure 18–2. Anatomy of the superior and inferior hypogastric plexus and level of transection for presacral neurectomy and sympathectomy. (From Mann WJ, Stovall TG: Gynecologic Surgery. New York, Churchill Livingstone, Inc, 1996, Figure 41–2.)

superior—the bifurcation of the aorta; on the right—the right internal iliac artery and right ureter; on the left—inferior mesenteric and superior hemorrhoidal arteries; and deep—the periosteum of the vertebral bodies (Fig. 18–4).

Standard laparoscopic instruments and techniques are used. In addition to immediately available bipolar cautery, the surgeon requires graspers and instruments for cutting, such as scissors, monopolar cautery, or laser. The patient is positioned supine in leg supports. Steep Trendelenburg's positioning with left lateral tilt is required to keep the bowel out of the operative field. Preoperative bowel preparation may also be indicated to improve visualization. After a pneumoperitoneum is established, the laparoscope is inserted through a 10-mm trocar placed in an umbilical incision. Two 5-mm trocars are inserted approximately 4 cm above the pubic symphysis and lateral to

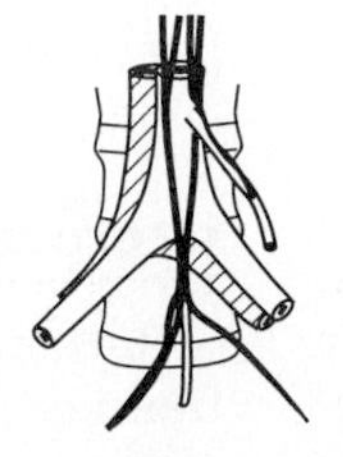

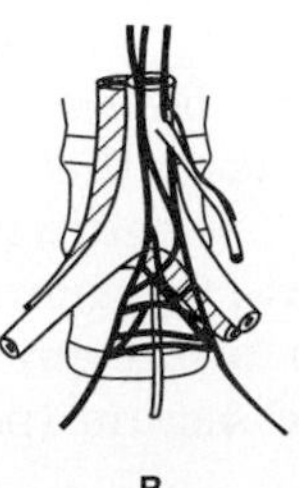

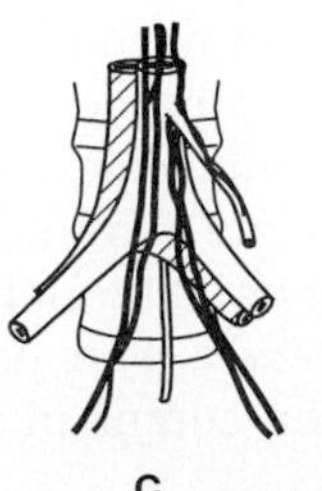

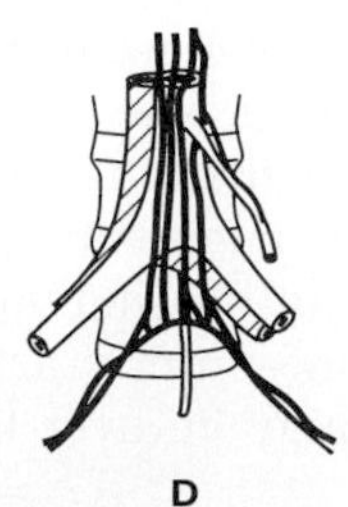

Figure 18–3. Different patterns of nerve fibers in the superior hypogastric plexus. *A*: Single nerve type, 24%. *B*: Plexus type, 58%. *C*: Parallel type, 16%. *D*: Arch-shaped type, 2%. (From Fliegner JRH, Umstad MP: Presacral neurectomy—a reappraisal. Aust N Z J Obstet Gynaecol 1991;31:76.)

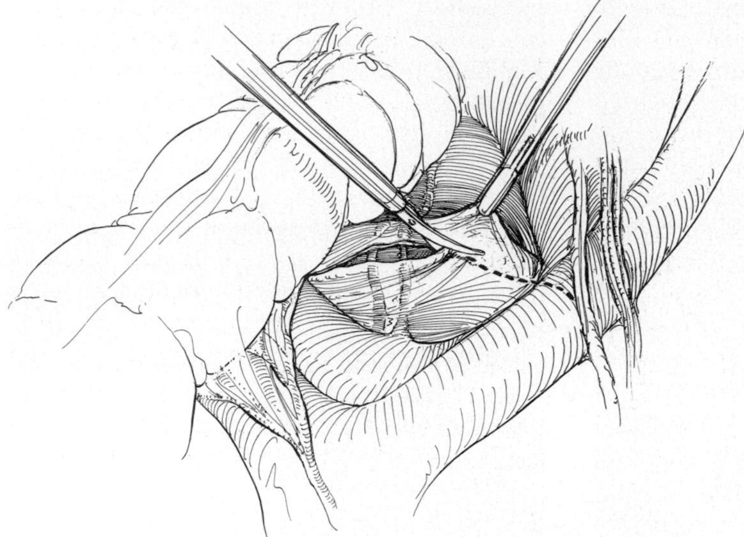

Figure 18–4. Landmarks for performing a presacral neurectomy as viewed from the laparoscope inserted into the umbilical trocar.

the rectus muscles. A third 5-mm trocar may be placed in the midline, if necessary. An alternative approach is to place the laparoscope in a midline suprapubic port to view the sacrum from a caudal direction.

The sacral promontory, ureters, and iliac vessels are identified, and the peritoneum overlying the sacral promontory is elevated and incised transversely. Bleeding points are controlled with either bipolar cautery or mono/bipolar scissors. The common iliac arteries, ureter, inferior mesenteric artery, and superior hemorrhoidal artery are identified under the peritoneum. The fatty presacral tissue anterior to the fascia that covers the sacrum contains the sympathetic nerves that supply the uterus. This loose areolar tissue is carefully incised down to the level of the vertebral periosteum between the right ureter and the inferior mesenteric artery/hemorrhoidal artery. This incision gapes open and separates the proximal and distal portions of the nerve plexus. The retroperitoneal space is copiously irrigated, and bleeding points are controlled with a defocused laser or cautery. The edges of the peritoneum are left open without suturing.

Deviations from normal anatomy are common. The pelvic mesocolon may be inserted in front of the interiliac trigone so that the hypogastric plexus cannot be reached without ligating the chief branches of the inferior mesenteric artery.[29] The path of the ureter may be over the center of the sacrum (personal observations). Finally, the convergence of the common iliac veins may be over the sacral promontory (personal observations).

The success rate in relieving pelvic pain by presacral neurectomy is directly related to two factors. Proper patient selection identifies those who are most likely to benefit from the procedure. Those who have failed medical therapy and who have primarily central pain are the patients who have been reported to have the highest rates of success. Some evidence suggests that women with primary dysmenorrhea have a higher cure rate than those with secondary dysmenorrhea (65% to 89% compared with 37% to 53%).[22] The second factor that contributes to success is the thoroughness of the operative dissection of the nerve plexus and the extent to which the afferent pain fibers of the presacral plexus are completely resected. Some surgeons, fearful of bleeding as a result of injury to the middle sacral artery, perform an incomplete procedure, leaving the nerves intact. An additional and often unrecognized problem is that fibers from the preaortic plexus may pass behind the common iliac vessels and enter the inferior hypogastric plexus, bypassing the interiliac trigone.[29]

Uterovaginal Ganglion Excision

Presacral neurectomy and uterosacral transection interrupt only a portion of the nerve fibers from the uterus and cervix. In addition to the sympathetic nerves that pass from the hypogastric plexus via the uterosacral ligament to the uterovaginal plexus lateral to the cervix, fine sympathetic and parasympathetic fibers (nervi erigentes) arise from the anterior roots of the sacral nerves (S2–S4) and enter the uterovaginal plexus via the vaginal artery, ureter, and pelvic sidewall. Perry proposed that continued transmission of sensory information through these latter nerves limits the efficacy of both uterosacral transection and presacral neurectomy.

In 1990, Gillespie performed the first procedure to ablate selectively a portion of the uterovaginal ganglia.[33] In her series of 175 patients who underwent bilateral plexus ablation, 64% reported significant relief, 33% had moderate improvement, and 3% failed to benefit. However, the pudendal nerve latency test she used has never been validated and most likely represents motor effects rather than sensory. Moreover, success was highly correlated with return of this test result to normal, which is very unusual in nerve conduction studies. More than 60% of the subjects also had other procedures performed at the same time, making it difficult to assess the true outcome. Finally, no postoperative urodynamic studies, voiding diaries, or other attempts were made to look for complications. Despite these concerns, destruction of the vesicoureteric plexus has been used since then in the treatment of pain due to hypersensitive bladder disorders such as interstitial cystitis.

Other preliminary results are based on Perry's experience with seven patients with unilateral and three patients with bilateral laparoscopic uterovaginal ganglion excision (LUVE) procedures. Patients complaining of persistent unilateral or bilateral lower pelvic pain were considered for LUVE. Pain scores were compared before and 1 hour after a paracervical block. Those patients who noted a decrease in their pain score and who had failed other surgical attempts at amelioration of pelvic pain were considered candidates for LUVE. Four patients reported excellent relief and four good relief, with two failures. Although not reported by Perry, Gillespie reported a high incidence of urinary retention and bladder insensitivity postoperatively, requiring permanent self-catherization.[33]

The uterovaginal ganglion is located on each side of the cervix, superficial and deep to the ureter as it traverses the uterine artery tunnel. It spreads into the base of the broad ligament and parallels the pelvic sidewall, ureter, and vaginal artery. Ureteric catheters are placed to facilitate dissection of the ganglion and to safeguard the ureter. The peritoneum is incised over the ureter, and blunt dissection isolates the loose connective tissue and retroperitoneal fat containing the ganglion. Hemostatic clips are preferred over bipolar coagulation to diminish periureteral fibrosis. A segment of tissue that is bordered by the ureter above, uterosacral ligament below, ureteric tunnel caudally, and the miduterosacral ligament level cephalad is removed. This is submitted for pathologic study to confirm ganglion and peripheral nerves. The peritoneum remains open.

No recommendations can yet be made about patient selection or long-term benefit. At this point, however, it can be advised that this procedure *not* be undertaken except in a research program with institutional review board approval.

Ovarian Sympathectomy

A discussion of the role of pelvic neurectomy would be incomplete without mentioning ovarian sympathectomy. The ovary derives its nerve supply mainly from the ovarian plexus, a meshwork of nerve fiber bundles that arise from the aortic and renal plexuses and accompany the ovarian artery and vein throughout their course.

Adnexal pain is common but may be difficult to differentiate from uterine pain, particularly just before and during menstruation. The ovarian nerves have a separate anatomic distribution along the psoas muscle to the region of the kidneys and the inferior mesenteric plexus. However, because these nerves intercommunicate with the presacral nerves, clinical symptoms for a specific ovarian pain syndrome may be confusing. It is obvious, therefore, that if one is selecting an operation for the relief of pelvic pain, the distribution of the pain fibers as identified by the site of origin of the symptoms is most important. This can be accomplished by selective nerve blocks or careful pelvic mapping of the areas of tenderness by pelvic examination (see Chapter 7) or by conscious pain mapping (see Chapter 33).

To perform an ovarian sympathectomy, the infundibulopelvic ligaments are divided and ligated. It is not possible to strip the sympathetic nerves from the ovarian vessels so that the ovarian vessels have, of necessity, to be divided.[29] Ovarian sympathectomy has been reported to improve ovarian pain or ovarian dysmenorrhea significantly.[34] Browne's technique consisted of division of both infundibulopelvic ligaments, their nerves, and their blood vessels. Of 21 ovarian denervations, he reported 80.9% complete success, 4.7% partial success, and 14.2% failure. Fliegner and Umstad[29] reported that two of the three patients who had a presacral neurectomy plus ovarian sympathectomy responded completely and that the other had recurrence of central pain but not adnexal pain.

Ovarian sympathectomy is infrequently used, and its value in routine application is therefore difficult to assess. Moreover, the major reason that has been offered for its infrequent use is the complication of cystic ovarian enlargement due to a compromised blood supply, which often requires subsequent oophorectomy.[35] However, ovarian sympathectomy occurs as a result of interruption of the infundibulopelvic ligament for management of symptomatic ovarian vein varicosities, and this complication has not been reported (see Chapter 17). A solution to this problem would be to undertake a meticulous dissection of the ovarian nerves from around the ovarian artery and vein with preservation of the blood supply to the ovary, a procedure with high risk of trauma to the fragile vessels and retroperitoneal hematoma formation.[35]

References

1. Henzl MR: Dysmenorrhea: Achievements and challenge. Sex Med Today 1985;9:8.
2. Doyle EB: Paracervical uterine denervation by transection of the cervical plexus for the relief of dysmenorrhea. Am J Obstet Gynecol 1955;70:11.
3. Lichten EM, Bombard J: Surgical treatment of primary dysmenorrhea with laparoscopic uterine nerve ablation. J Reprod Med 1987;32:37.
4. Gurgan T, Urman B, Aksu T, et al: Laparoscopic CO_2 laser uterine nerve ablation for treatment of drug resistant primary dysmenorrhea. Fertil Steril 1992;58:422.
5. Sutton C: Laser uterine nerve ablation. In Donnez J (ed): Laser Operative Laparoscopy and Hysteroscopy. Leuven, Belgium, Nauwelaerts Publishing, 1989, p 43.
6. Lichten E: Three years experience with L.U.N.A. Am J Gynecol Health 1989;3:9.
7. Elant L: Surgical anatomy of the so called presacral nerve. Surg Gynecol Obstet 1933;57:51.
8. Perez JJ: Laparoscopic presacral neurectomy. J Reprod Med 1990;35:625.
9. Gomel V, James C: Intraoperative management of ureteral injury during operative laparoscopy. Fertil Steril 1991;55:416.
10. Good MC, Copas PR, Doody MC: Uterine prolapse after laparoscopic uterosacral transection. J Reprod Med 1993;72:995.
11. Davis GD: Uterine prolapse after laparoscopic uterosacral transection in nulliparous airborne trainees: A report of three cases. J Reprod Med 1996;41:279.
12. Jaboulay M: Le traitement de la devralgie pelvienne par la paralysie due sympathetique sacre. Lyon Med 1899;90:102.
13. Cotte MG: Sur le traitment des dysmenorrhees rebelles par la sympathectomie hypogastrique perarterielle ou la section de nerf presacre. Lyon Med 1925;135:153.
14. Cotte MG: Resection of the presacral nerve in the treatment of obstinate dysmenorrhea. Am J Obstet Gynecol 1937;33:1030.
15. Black WT: Use of presacral sympathectomy in the treatment of dysmenorrhea. Am J Obstet Gynecol 1964;89:16.
16. Polan M, DeCherney A: Presacral neurectomy for pelvic pain in infertility. Fertil Steril 1980;34:557.
17. Tjaden B, Schlaff WD, Kimball A, Rock JA: The efficacy of presacral neurectomy for the relief of midline dysmenorrhea. Obstet Gynecol 1990;76:89.
18. Nezhat C, Metzger DA, Nezhat F: A simplified approach to laparoscopic presacral neurectomy. Br J Obstet Gynecol 1992;99:659.
19. Candiani G, Fedele L, Vercellini P, et al: Presacral neurectomy for the treatment of pelvic pain associated with endometriosis: A controlled study. Am J Obstet Gynecol 1992;167:100.
20. Metzger DA, Montanino-Oliva M, Davis GD, Redwine D: Efficacy of presacral neurectomy for the relief of midline pelvic pain. Paper presented at the annual meeting of the American Association of Gynecologic Laparoscopists, New York, October 19–23, 1994.
21. Chen FP, Chang SD, Chu KK, Soong YK: Comparison of laparoscopic presacral neurectomy and laparoscopic uterine nerve ablation for primary dysmorrhea. J Reprod Med 1996;41:463.
22. Lee RB, Stone K, Magelssen D, et al: Presacral neurectomy for chronic pelvic pain. Obstet Gynecol 1986;69:517.
23. Patsner B, Ozz WJ: Intractable venous sacral hemorrhage: Use of stainless steel thumbtacks to obtain hemostasis. Am J Obstet Gynecol 1990;162:452.

24. Davis AA: The technique of resection of the presacral nerve (Cotte's operation). Br J Surg 1933; 20:516.
25. Cotte MG: Technique of presacral neurectomy. Am J Surg 1949;78:50.
26. Fontaine R, Herrmann LG: Clinical and experimental basis for surgery of pelvic sympathetic nerves in gynecology. Surg Gynecol Obstet 1932;54:133.
27. Buttram VC, Reiter RC: Endometriosis. In Buttram VC, Reiter RC (eds): Surgical Treatment of the Infertile Female. Baltimore, Williams & Wilkins, 1985, pp 89–147.
28. Meigs JV: Excision of the superior hypogastric (presacral nerve) for primary dysmenorrhea. Surg Gynecol Obstet 1939;68:723.
29. Fliegner JRH, Umstad MP: Presacral neurectomy—a reappraisal. Aust N Z J Obstet Gynecol 1991;31:76.
30. Black WT: Presacral sympathectomy for dysmenorrhea and pelvic pain. Am Surg 1936;103:903.
31. Rock J, Jones H: Reparative and reconstructive surgery of the female generative tract. Baltimore, Williams & Wilkins, 1983, pp 136–138.
32. Curtis AH, Anson BM, Ashley FL, Jones T: The anatomy of the pelvic autonomic nerves in relation to gynecology. Surg Gynecol Obstet 1942;75:743.
33. Gillespie L: Destruction of vesicoureteric plexus for the treatment of hypersensitive bladder disorders. Br J Urol 1994;74:40.
34. Browne OD: Survey of 113 cases of primary dysmenorrhea treated by neurectomy. Am J Obstet Gynecol 1949;57:1053.

19

Uterine Suspension

Deborah A. Metzger, PhD, MD

By the middle of the 18th century, uterine retrodisplacement was firmly established as a pathologic entity producing general constitutional disturbances and local functional disorders.[1] After Alexander and Adams described the first operation for suspending the uterus in 1882,[1] many variations of the procedure were introduced,[2] and it became a frequent gynecologic procedure for dysmenorrhea, pelvic pain, infertility, backache, and cystic degeneration of the ovaries.[3] Most of the older indications for suspension of a retroverted uterus have not stood the test of time.[4, 5]

Uterine suspension has become a relatively infrequent procedure, but a few clinical conditions remain as indications for this type of conservative surgery. The main indication for uterine suspension is dyspareunia secondary to uterine retroversion. Laparoscopy in this situation facilitates diagnosis and treatment of previously undetected causes of dyspareunia and, when no other pathology is present, allows uterine suspension to be performed without laparotomy. The only other indication for uterine suspension is selected cases of severe endometriosis involving the cul-de-sac and rectum when re-formation of adhesions is a significant concern.[6]

Evaluation of a patient with dyspareunia includes conducting a thorough history and physical examination. Particular attention should be paid to the position of the uterus and to clinical signs of cul-de-sac pathology. Women with dyspareunia secondary to uterine position have a retroverted, retroflexed uterus, and palpation of the uterine-cervical junction or fundus on vaginal examination reproduces the pain (Fig. 19–1). Although some investigators have advocated a trial of a pessary before surgical correction of the retroversion,[7] others have noted that with a Smith-Hodge pessary in place, dyspareunia is eliminated in the patient and experienced by the male partner instead.[8]

The efficacy of laparoscopic uterine suspension has been demonstrated in a number of studies,[9–12] with approximately 90% of patients reporting complete or partial relief of dyspareunia.[10] The two reports that failed to show improvement after ventrosuspension[4, 5] were performed for various indications such as chronic pelvic pain, backache, infertility, and dysmenorrhea—the conditions for which uterine suspension has no demonstrated value. However, when only women with deep dyspareunia and no other pathology were analyzed, 80% reported alleviation of symptoms at the 6-month follow-up.[4] Thus, there appears to be universal agreement that uterine suspension for deep dyspareunia is worthwhile and effective.

Several studies have noted that uterine suspension appears to be a long-term solution for women with dyspareunia secondary to uterine retroversion.[7, 11] However, I have seen a patient with a recurrence of dyspareunia and retroversion after a full-term pregnancy during which the round ligaments were stretched. This particular patient required a repeat uterine suspension, which has continued to be effective 2 years after the repeat procedure.

Uterine suspension may be accomplished at laparotomy or laparoscopy with the goal of securing the uterus in an anterior position and bringing the ovaries and fallopian tubes forward and out of the posterior pelvis. The round ligaments can be folded, plaited, ligated, transplanted, banded, or shirred[1, 12] to reposition the uterus in an anterior or midplane position. Alternatively, the uterine fundus itself can be attached to the ante-

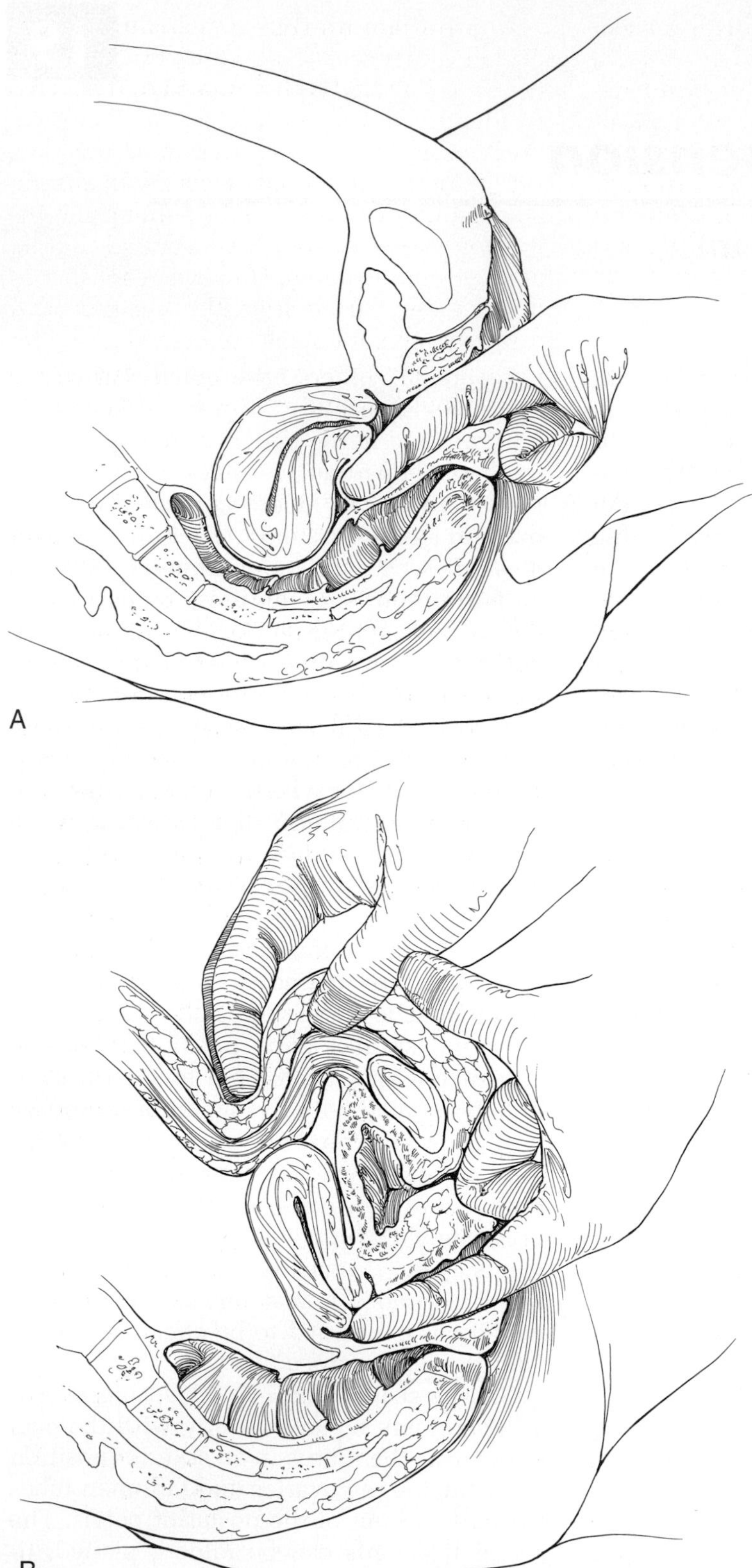

Figure 19–1. Physical examination for dyspareunia secondary to uterine position. *A*, Dyspareunia reproduced by palpation of the retroverted uterus. *B*, Bimanual palpation of the anteverted uterus.

rior abdominal wall, although this has anecdotally been reported to lead to chronic pelvic pain in some women. Steptoe[13] described the modern technique of laparoscopic ventrosuspension, which has been modified by various clinicians. Although numerous methods of uterine suspension have been described, three currently are worth presenting.

Ventrosuspension of the Round Ligament

This procedure involves umbilical location of the laparoscope and insertion of two 5-mm suprapubic accessory trocars, which are placed in an avascular area 4 cm above the pubic symphysis and lateral to the rectus muscles (Fig. 19–2). Grasping forceps are introduced through the trocars,[7, 8, 10, 13] or long Kelly clamps can be introduced through the suprapubic stab incisions. Both round ligaments are grasped near their midpoint, and the pneumoperitoneum is allowed to escape partially. The knuckle of round ligament is gently and firmly pulled through the incision in the fascia.

Appropriate uterine suspension is confirmed by laparoscopic visualization, and the bowel and fallopian tubes are inspected to identify bowel entrapment or abnormal positioning. The round ligaments are then sutured to the abdominal fascia with absorbable suture material. It is important that the fixation suture include a substantial portion of the round ligament. However, care should be taken not to encircle the ligament and cause strangulation. The skin is closed after evacuation of the remainder of the pneumoperitoneum and removal of the laparoscope.

The most serious problem encountered with this procedure is avulsion of the round ligament because of an inadequate fascial incision, undue force on the round ligament, or positioning the round ligaments with a full pneumoperitoneum. The inferior epigastric arteries may be lacerated during placement of the suprapubic trocars. Although transillumination of the abdomen may be of some benefit in avoiding this complication, it may not be effective in obese patients. Although the use of nonabsorbable suture has been reported, I have encountered a patient who developed chronic pain

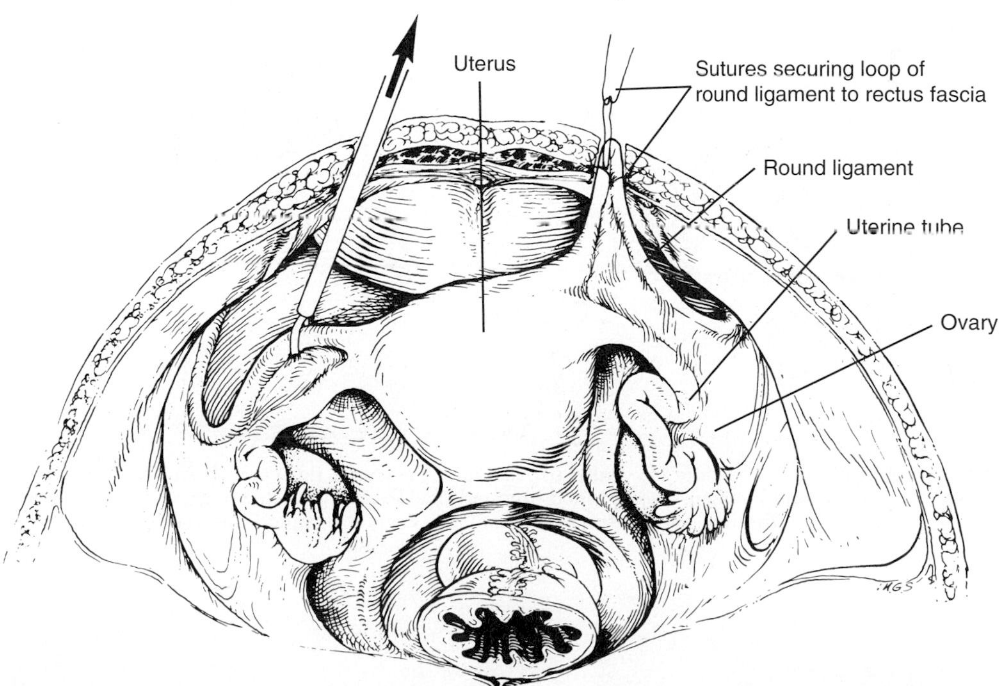

Figure 19–2. Ventrosuspension of the round ligament. (From Mann WJ, Stenger VG: Uterine suspension through the laparoscope. Obstet Gynecol 1978;51:564.)

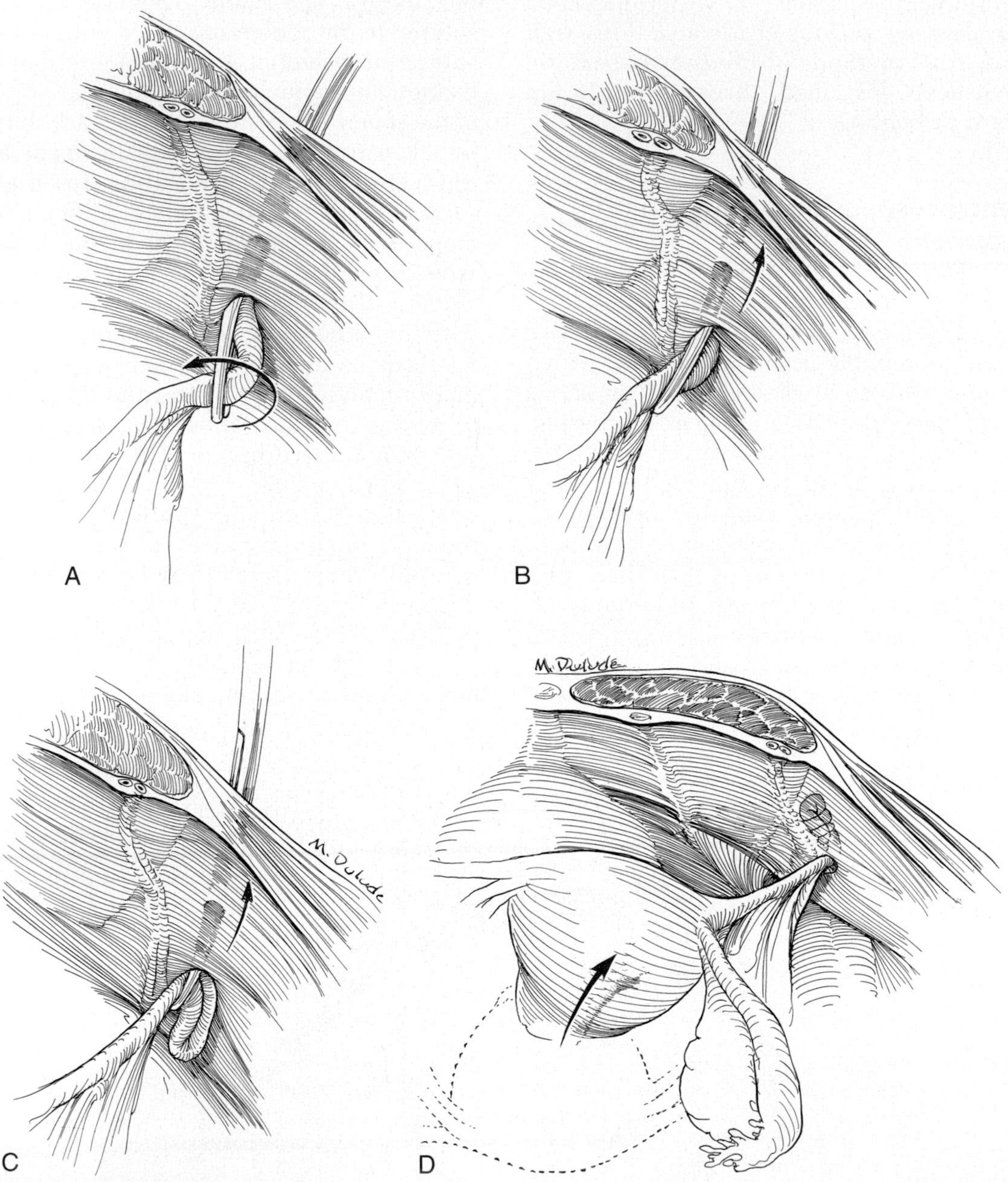

Figure 19–3. Modification of procedure for ventrosuspension of the round ligament. *A*, Atraumatic clamp inserted retroperitoneally along round ligament, then pushed intraperitoneally and pronated to grasp round ligament. *B* and *C*, Round ligament pulled through retroperitoneal tunnel. *D*, Round ligament sutured to posterior aspect of rectus sheath.

in an incision site; this was relieved when the suture was removed. For this reason, delayed absorbable suture (polydioxanone, Vicryl, Dexon) may be a better alternative. Most patients have some degree of incisional pain, which is readily managed with mild analgesics and a heating pad. A patient may on occasion have more significant postoperative discomfort due to spasms of the rectus muscles. This can be managed with local heat, muscle relaxants, and analgesics.

Lose and Lindholm[14] reported a case of intermittent urinary retention in a young woman who had a retroverted, retroflexed uterus and who had undergone a uterine suspension for dyspareunia. At the time of corrective surgery, it appeared that the rearranged uterus caused a type of obstruction that may have been exacerbated by the patient's low voiding pressures. Another type of serious complication occurs when the bowel becomes incarcerated in the space between the round ligament and the anterior abdominal wall, resulting in bowel obstruction. Incarcerated bowel can occur at any time after this type of uterine suspension.

A modification of this procedure, which minimizes the risk of bowel incarceration, is to make incisions bilaterally over the internal inguinal rings (Fig. 19–3). A long Kelly clamp is then passed through the fascia retroperitoneally and directed toward the internal inguinal canal. The peritoneum is entered, and the midpoint of the round ligament is grasped and brought through the previously made tunnel to the fascial incision, where it is sutured in place.

Falope Rings

Falope rings have been used for many years for laparoscopic tubal sterilization. A special instrument is fitted through a 5-mm accessory trocar sleeve and simultaneously grasps the tube, retracts it into the instrument, and places a very small, tight silicone band around the knuckle of the tube. A similar type of procedure can be used to shorten the round ligaments.[12] Placement of several Falope rings may be necessary to achieve the proper degree of tension on the round ligaments (Fig. 19–4).

Falope ring placement on the round ligaments is associated with the same complications as the procedure performed on the fallopian tubes. The most common is laceration of the broad ligament, followed by laceration of the round ligament. The resultant bleeding can be managed using bipolar cautery.

Modified Olshausen's Uterine Suspension

Uterine suspension can also be accomplished by using a modification of Olshausen's[15] round ligament plication (Fig. 19–5). Either delayed absorbable or permanent suture is passed transabdominally via the lower quadrant trocar sites using a swaged needle. While the round ligament is placed on stretch, several bites are taken from the point where the round ligament enters the inguinal canal along the length of the round ligament toward the uterus. Approximately 2 cm from the uterus, the direction of the needle is reversed, and again several bites are taken along the length of the round ligament going toward the inguinal canal. The needle is again passed transabdominally. Once both sides are completed, some of the pneumoperitoneum is allowed to escape and the suture is tied above the fascia.

This procedure should be viewed as an alternative to ventrosuspension of the uterus described earlier. It is associated with the same risk of complications, although the risk of round ligament avulsion may be less. In addition, the risk of bowel incarceration is less. This procedure requires more surgical skill than the other procedures because it uses intracorporeal suturing techniques.

Recommendations

Although the uterine suspension procedures described earlier are the most frequently used methods, no long-term studies have attested to the lasting benefits. Nor have any studies systematically assessed the risks associated with these procedures. Until such information is available, the most prudent approach is carefully to select pa-

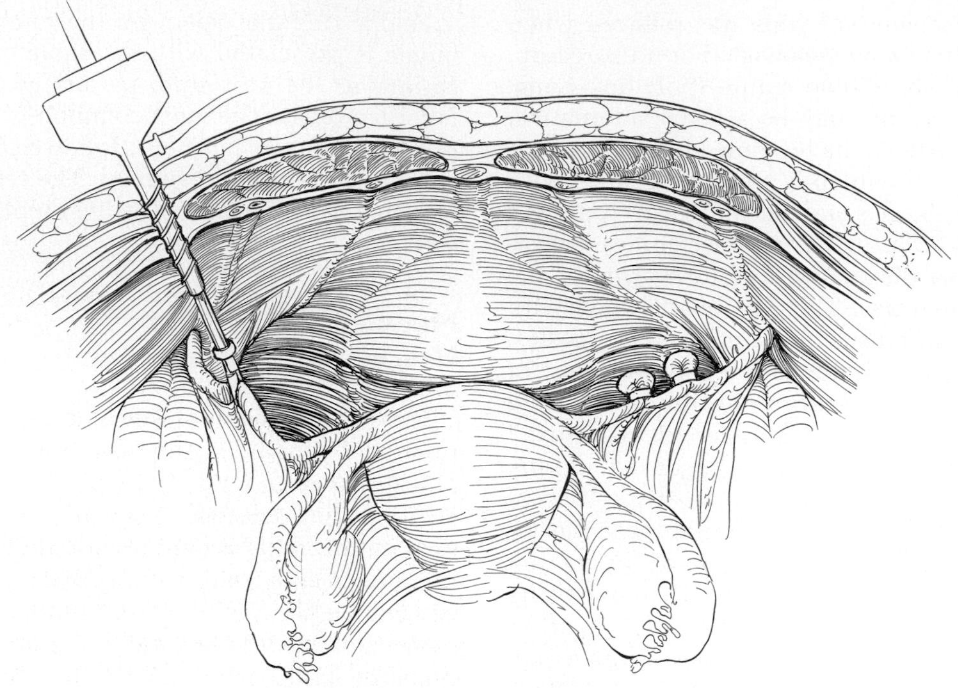

Figure 19–4. Placement of Falope rings.

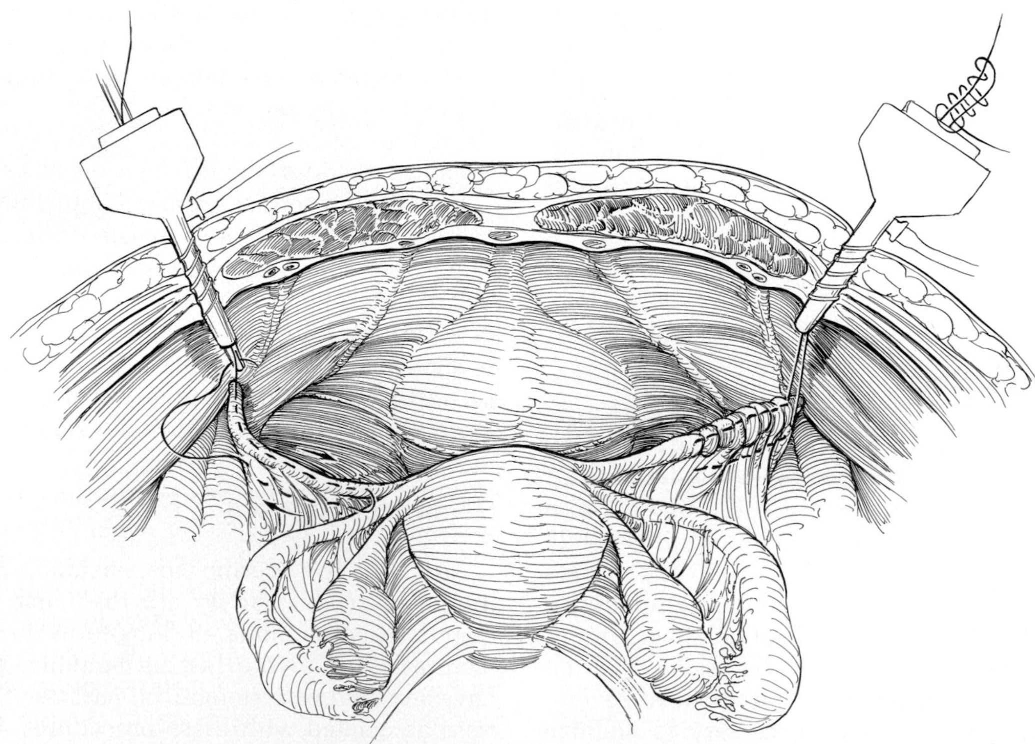

Figure 19–5. Modified Olshausen's uterine suspension.

tients who have an excellent chance of success based on the presence of uterine retroversion and dyspareunia and to use the procedure that is most appropriate for one's level of skill.

References

1. Fluhmann CF: The rise and fall of suspension operations for uterine retrodisplacement. Bull Johns Hopkins Hosp 1955;96:59.
2. Kelly HA: The history of retrodisplacements of the uterus. Surg Gynecol Obstet 1915;20:598.
3. Donaldson JK, Sanderlin JH, Harrell WB: A method of suspending the uterus without open abdominal incision. Am J Surg 1942;15:537.
4. Gleeson NC, Gaffney GM: Ventrosuspension—five years of practice at the Rotunda Hospital reviewed. J Obstet Gynecol 1990;10:415.
5. Yoong AFE: Laparoscopic ventrosuspensions: A review of 72 cases. Am J Obstet Gynecol 1990;163:1151.
6. Jones HW, Rock JA: Endometriosis externa. In Jones HW, Rock JA (eds): Reparative and Constructive Surgery of the Female Generative Tract. Baltimore, Williams & Wilkins, 1983, pp 121–144.
7. Smith DB, Kelsey JF, Sherman RL, et al: Laparoscopic uterine suspension. J Reprod Med 1977;18:98.
8. Candy JW: Modified Gilliam uterine suspension using laparoscopic visualization. Obstet Gynecol 1976;47:242.
9. Paterson MEL, Jordan JA, Logan-Edwards R: A survey of 100 patients who had laparoscopic ventrosuspensions. Br J Obstet Gynecol 1978;85:468.
10. Mann WJ, Stenger VG: Uterine suspension through the laparoscope. Obstet Gynecol 1978;51:563.
11. Servy EJ, Aksu MF, Tzingounis VA: Laparoscopic hysteropexy and the position of the fallopian tubes. In Phillips JM (ed): Endoscopy in Gynecology. Santa Fe Springs, CA, American Association of Gynecologic Laparoscopists Department of Publications, 1978, p 87.
12. Massouda D, Ling FW, Muram D, Stovall TG: Laparoscopic uterine suspension with Falope rings. J Reprod Med 1987;32:859.
13. Steptoe PC: Laparoscopy in Gynecology. London, Livingstone, 1967, p 78.
14. Lose G, Lindholm P: Impaired voiding efficiency and urinary retention after laparoscopic ventrosuspension ad modum Steptoe. Acta Obstet Gynecol Scand 1984;63:371.
15. Olshausen R: Uber ventrale operation bei prolapsus und retroversio uteri. Zentralbl Gynakol 1886; 10:698.

20

Vulvar Vestibulitis

John M. Gibbons, Jr., MD

In 1987, Friedrich suggested the term *vulvar vestibulitis* to describe a chronic syndrome defined by three criteria: severe pain on vestibular touch or attempted vaginal entry, tenderness to light pressure localized within the vulvar vestibule, and gross physical findings limited to vestibular erythema of various degrees.[1] Although the true incidence is unknown, most authorities agree that this condition affects an increasing fraction of their patients with vulvar disorders. Readers should refer to the next chapter to learn the place of this syndrome in the broader context of vulvodynia.

History

Historical descriptions of this symptom-sign complex date back more than 100 years. Skene, in his *Treatise on the Diseases of Women,*[2] referred to "hyperaesthesia of the vulva," which he characterized as supersensitiveness of those tissues. He described his findings as follows: "Pruritus is absent, and on examination of the parts affected no redness or other external manifestation of the disease is visible. When, however, the examining finger comes in contact with the hyperaesthetic part, the patient complains of pain, which is sometimes so great as to cause her to cry out. . . . Sexual intercourse is equally painful, and becomes in aggravated cases impossible." Discussing treatment, he noted that "The sensitive tissue has been dissected off and relief obtained for a time, the hyperaesthesia returning, however, as before the operation." He advised that the best treatment for these patients was to "build them up with tonics and nutritious food, and, if possible, to send them away so that they can have the benefit of a change of air and of scene, and at the same time be removed from the irritation of sexual intercourse. . . ." Kelly, in his 1928 textbook on gynecology, described "exquisitely sensitive deep-red spots in the mucosa of the hymeneal ring as a fruitful source of dyspareunia."[3] For almost 50 years thereafter, the gynecologic literature provided no further references to the syndrome.

In 1976, Pelisse and Hewitt described a similar entity, which they referred to as "erythematous vulvitis en plaques."[4] Articles that appeared in rapid succession discussed an increasing population of patients with "focal vulvitis," "vestibular adenitis," and "infection of the minor vestibular glands." The 1987 article by Friedrich presented the definitive description of the syndrome.

Vestibule

The outer margin of the vulvar vestibule was defined by Hart in 1882.[5] He described "a line of demarcation between the skin and mucous membrane . . . running along the base of the inner aspect of each labium minus and passing into the fossa navicularis separating its skin boundary, the fourchette, from the mucous membrane of the hymen." The vestibule itself extends from this perimeter inward to the hymen, which marks its boundary with the vagina. This ring of tissue is covered with nonpigmented, nonkeratinized, or thinly keratinized squamous epithelium. There are no hair follicles or other skin appendages. The area contains the external urethral meatus as well as the ostia of Skene's paraurethral glands and the Bartholin's gland ducts. Simple tubular mucus-secreting glands, the minor vestibular glands, are noted in some specimens.

The embryologic development of the vestibule is from the anterior segment of the primitive cloaca, the urogenital sinus. This structure divides into the urethra and bladder and the distal vagina, the portion directly connected to the genital skin. The vestibule, therefore, is derived principally from endoderm and shares the anlage of the penile urethra in males. This narrow ring of tissue is sandwiched between the vaginal epithelium and the skin of the fourchette, both of which are derived from ectoderm. The association of vestibulitis with interstitial cystitis in some women is interesting in this regard.

Etiologic Theories

The cause of vulvar vestibulitis is unknown but thought to be multifactorial. A number of plausible theories have been advanced, but none has succeeded in explaining the syndrome in every case. Quite early, investigators noted the association of koilocytotic atypia in biopsy and surgical specimens and proposed human papillomavirus (HPV) as the etiologic agent. In Friedrich's 1987 study,[1] 18% of questionnaire respondents indicated a prior history of condylomata acuminata. In 1982, Pyka and colleagues reported a 27% incidence of koilocytosis in 41 operative specimens from patients with vulvar vestibulitis.[6] Turner and Marinoff in 1988 found HPV DNA by Southern blot in all specimens obtained from a group of seven women with clinical vulvar vestibulitis.[7] Convincing evidence now shows that the occurrence of HPV DNA in surgical specimens from these patients is no more frequent than that in unaffected women, even if clinical papillomatosis is observed.[8, 9]

Another popular theory involved vestibular hypersensitivity to *Candida* organisms. In Friedrich's original group, 63% related a past history of repeated and severe vulvovaginal candidiasis,[1] but Marinoff and Turner in their series published in 1987 had noted in their patients no evidence of active candidiasis or hypersensitivity to the organisms on the basis of intradermal testing.[10] These same researchers, incidentally, failed to find active infection with *Neisseria gonorrhoeae, Gardnerella, Trichomonas,* or herpes simplex.

In 1991, Solomons and colleagues proposed a possible etiologic role for the urinary excretion of large amounts of oxalate crystals.[11] The investigators noted that sharp oxalate crystals, particularly of plant origin, were known to cause burning and itching when in contact with epithelial surfaces. They presented a patient who had recalcitrant vestibular pain and in whom urinary oxalate excretion, although normal over 24 hours, exhibited sharp peaks of transient hyperoxaluria. Her vestibular symptoms responded significantly over 3 months to modification of her diet and to administration of calcium citrate. When this agent was withdrawn, her symptoms recurred. No further detailed reports have described such patients and their response to dietary modification and calcium citrate.

Diagnosis

A woman suffering from vulvar vestibulitis most commonly presents with longstanding dyspareunia. The onset is often strikingly abrupt. The coital pain is experienced first on penetration and may increase if sexual activity is continued. The episode is often followed by a variable period of discomfort described as aching pain or burning. The association of discomfort with coitus is invariable. As time goes on, patients have no days of remission. A truly cyclic relationship to the menstrual cycle is not characteristic, although sanitary pads can be irritating. The repetitive and predictable pain most often leads to total abstinence from vaginal intercourse. In many women, tight clothing and bicycling or horseback riding provoke the symptoms. Some experience pain during ordinary daily activities including sitting. Most patients have abandoned tampon use.

In taking the history, the physician should inquire about allergies, local irritants, oral contraceptive use, and previous treatment including psychotherapy. Gentle questioning may uncover episodes of childhood sexual abuse, rape, or other dramatic genital trauma. (Sexual trauma is not more common in women with vestibulitis but may make treatment more difficult.) A careful review of urinary symptoms, especially noting significant nocturia, may point to relevant bladder problems. Some authorities have suggested an association with the irritable bowel syndrome. Careful inspection of the vulva and vestibule as part of a complete pelvic evaluation is essential. Vulvar dermatoses should be carefully noted and described. Vaginal examination should include determination of pH and the usual wet mount preparations. In women with classic vestibulitis, the vestibular epithelium exhibits no more than patchy erythema. A distinct red halo is often obvious at the ostia of the ducts of Bartholin's glands. Papillae of the inner labia minora are often observed in normal women and are not necessarily indicative of HPV infection. The examiner should also pay careful attention to the periurethral area and the tissue beneath the frenulum of the clitoral prepuce.

The cardinal, striking finding in patients with vestibulitis is exquisite tenderness to light pressure when the vestibular epithelium is touched with a cotton-tipped applicator. The woman is asked to characterize her discomfort on a scale of 0 to 10, and her answers are plotted on a diagram of the vestibule. Once again, the examiner must pay close attention to the periurethral area. The pain is generally most marked when Bartholin's duct orifices are touched and only a bit less so when light pressure is applied in the hymeneal sulcus. Tenderness, although often present, is usually less dramatic more distally toward the fourchette and superiorly in the periurethral area. Severe pain in this latter area presents a therapeutic problem and is thought by some to be a poor prognostic indicator. The prevalence of sensitivity to light touch in various areas of the vestibule is indicated in Figure 20–1.

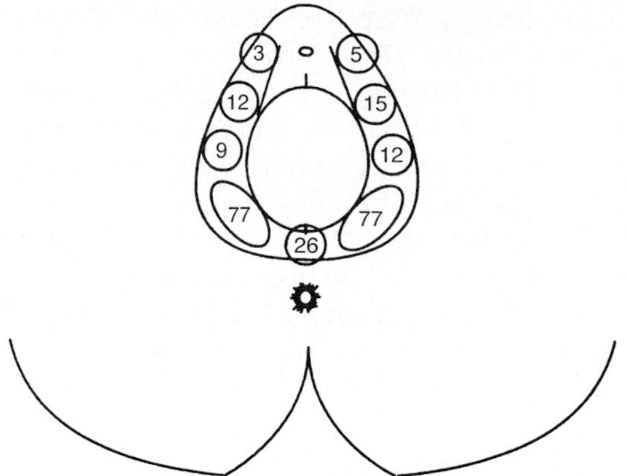

Figure 20–1. The vulvar distribution of 236 lesions of focal vulvitis in 67 patients after 4 and 5 o'clock and 6 and 7 o'clock positions are combined. Numbers inside circles represent total number of lesions encountered at that location. (From Peckham BM, Maki DG, Patterson JJ, Hafez CH: Focal vulvitis: A characteristic syndrome and cause of dyspareunia. Am J Obstet Gynecol 1986;154:855.)

Colposcopic evaluation of the vulvar vestibule (vulvoscopy) adds little to the diagnosis. As mentioned, papillary epithelial projections are noted on the inner surfaces of the labia minora in approximately half of women. These papillations generally exhibit a normal staining reaction to Lugol's solution but may demonstrate acetowhite changes when exposed to 3% acetic acid, which itself may cause intense burning in women with vestibulitis. Even these latter patterns, however, do not correlate with HPV infection when sophisticated diagnostic techniques are applied to biopsy specimens. In fact, colposcopy in some hands may lead to inappropriate treatment with caustic chemicals or the carbon dioxide laser.

The histopathologic findings of vestibular biopsies performed on women meeting Friedrich's clinical criteria are consistent with chronic nonspecific inflammation. According to Prayson and colleagues,[12] who studied specimens from 36 women, the infiltrate consisted primarily of T-lymphocytes and plasma cells with smaller numbers of B-lymphocytes. The infiltrate was seen most commonly in the lamina propria and, to a lesser extent, in the periglandular/periductal connective tissue of the minor vestibular glands. Foci of squamous metaplasia were frequently seen in patients exhibiting vestibular ducts or glands, forming so-called vestibular clefts. Silver stains in the cited study, performed on seven patients, failed to identify fungi, and in this series, morphologic findings of HPV infection were not present in any case. DNA studies of surgical specimens were referred to earlier and serve to impeach the HPV virus as a causative agent.[8, 9] In the clinical setting, therefore, the diagnosis is based on the signs and symptoms of the syndrome and need not be supported by biopsy evidence.

In closing the discussion of diagnosis, note should be made of the growing association of this syndrome with interstitial cystitis (see Chapter 22). Interstitial cystitis is a debilitating bladder disorder characterized by pain, often relieved by bladder emptying, accompanied by urinary frequency and nocturia. The cause is unknown. Urine cultures are negative. The absence of nocturia virtually precludes interstitial cystitis; the diagnosis is usually made during cystoscopy under anesthesia. McCormack cites a Finnish estimate of the incidence of this disorder in women as 0.018% in a study describing the coexistence of this syndrome in 11 of 36 women with "focal vulvitis."[13] Fitzpatrick and colleagues describe three patients with both vulvar vestibulitis and interstitial cystitis and suggest that the coincidence reflects a common disorder of urogenital sinus–derived epithelium.[14] If a gynecologist encounters a patient with vulvar vestibulitis and suspects the coexistence of interstitial cystitis, prompt referral to a urologist is indicated. Treatment for the vestibulitis alone does nothing to ameliorate the urologic condition, and the patient will still be (unhappily) in pain. Conversely, a perceptive urologist may refer to a gynecologic practice those women who have interstitial cystitis and who have satisfied the criteria for vestibulitis and benefited from treatment. To sound a cautionary note, however, patients with interstitial cystitis have long been known to complain of dyspareunia, presumably because of bladder and urethral tenderness.

Treatment

Experience suggests that spontaneous remissions of vulvar vestibulitis do occur, particularly in women with symptoms of less than 6 months' duration. Response to nonspecific medical therapy also seems to happen occasionally in early cases. For this reason, the initial treatment of patients with mild symptoms or those whose complaints are of less than 6 months' duration should be conservative. Clinicians should identify and manage any vulvar dermatitis or vaginitis. Local irritants and potential allergens should be eliminated. A mild hydrocortisone cream or ointment has proved helpful in some patients and may be safely used almost indefinitely. The application of lidocaine as an ointment or as a 4% solution just before intercourse may make coitus possible without serious discomfort. Some authorities have advised their patients to discontinue use of oral contraceptives, although others have recommended their use in therapy. If an element of vaginismus is present, appropriate counseling and treatment should be offered.

More severe cases of vestibulitis of long duration, especially more than 18 months, are unlikely to benefit from conservative measures. Several treatment options can be proposed to these women. To begin with, carbon dioxide laser has no place in the therapy of this disorder. As a matter of fact, some of the early patients seen with this syndrome dated its onset to their recovery from vulvar laser surgery performed for other reasons. At least one investigator has presented encouraging early results using flashlamp-excited dye laser therapy in single or serial treatments, but the criteria for selection of suitable patients remain unclear.[15]

The initial conviction that HPV infection played a major causative part in vestibulitis led to its management with various modalities. Carbon dioxide laser, mentioned earlier, was disappointing, but the use of trichloracetic acid applied to vestibular papillations may offer some relief in milder cases. Recombinant α-interferon, however, was reported to be effective in women demonstrating histologic evidence of HPV infection in biopsy specimens.

Interferon may be administered in two ways: intralesional (intravestibular) injections or intramuscular injections. In 1989, Horowitz described the use of intravestibular interferon to treat a group of women with "condylomatous vulvitis."[16] Fifteen of 17 patients had favorable responses. The technique involved the injection of 1 million units of α-26-interferon into the vestibular tissue circumferentially three times weekly during a 4-week period for a total dose of 12 million units. Side effects included local discomfort and the occurrence of flulike symptoms in some patients after the early injections. Marinoff and colleagues used intralesional α-interferon as the initial treatment for 55 women with or without histologic features suggesting HPV.[17] Although the response rate did not match the earlier study, 49% experienced substantial or partial improvement. The researchers suggested the use of this protocol as an initial step in treatment, reserving surgery for nonresponders, and presented evidence of its cost-effectiveness compared with immediate operation. Bornstein and associates reported treating seven women with vestibulitis using intramuscular β-interferon.[18] All the patients had biopsy histologic features of HPV. Of the two regimens tried, the more successful involved administration of human β-interferon, 3 million IU daily for 5 days followed by 3 million units on alternate days for 20 days (10 injections) to a total of 45 million IU. Follow-up was reported after 6 to 18 months. All three of the patients receiving this dose reported complete remissions, as did two of the four given a total dose of 30 million units.

The most consistent and reproducible results in the treatment of severe vulvar vestibulitis have been reported after surgery. In our unit as in others, the operation is termed *U-shaped vestibulectomy with perineoplasty.* The procedure is based on the surgical approach described in 1981 by Woodruff and coworkers for the treatment of dyspareunia.[19] Axe and colleagues applied a modification of this operation to treat "infection of the minor vestibular gland," and during the next 3 years, 64 patients underwent the procedure, with good response in 80% of the cases.[20] In its latest version, the operation involves, as described by Marinoff and Turner, an incision extending from below the periurethral area on one side (about 9 o'clock), along Hart's line, down into and including a portion of the fourchette, and back along Hart's line to just below the periurethral area on the other side (about 3 o'clock). The inner incision line is behind (cephalad to) the hymeneal ring.[21] The depth of dissection need be only about 2 mm. After the specimen is excised and hemostasis secured, the posterior vaginal epithelium is undermined, mobilized, and brought forward to cover the defect. Closure is accomplished by the placement of two layers of relatively fine synthetic absorbable sutures. The first consists of interrupted simple or horizontal mattress sutures to approximate the deep layers, and the second consists of a running locked suture that brings vaginal epithelium to the skin of the perineum. The single most common error in novice surgical approaches to vestibulitis is the performance of a less-inclusive resection. Injection of marcaine into the operative area at the end of surgery ameliorates immediate postoperative pain. Aftercare involves rest, analgesics, and sitz baths.

Early complications include wound hematoma and dehiscence. Patients may later complain of nodular excrescences along the suture line due to uneven healing. These, if troublesome, are easily handled by office revision under local anesthesia. Much more rarely—remarkably, when one considers the geography of the surgery—the Bartholin's duct becomes blocked and results in cyst formation. This problem is ordinarily managed in the office with a Word's catheter. Very unusually, a patient presents with intermittent pain and swelling in the tissues just overlying the presumed duct orifice. This may be due to the secretions of Bartholin's gland that occur during sexual arousal. Examination discloses a small tender vesicular structure. The Word's catheter is much too large and the "cyst" much too superficial to allow conventional marsupialization. Drainage provides relief, but the problem recurs every 2 to 3 weeks. At the very helpful suggestion of Marinoff, a patient with this problem was treated by the insertion of a polyethylene venous catheter into the duct under colposcopic magnification. A small amount of indigo carmine solution was injected to dilate the duct, which was then fishmouthed and the enlarged orifice sutured in place. The operation was completely successful.

Good results are achieved by surgery in

60% to 90% of patients.[21] Unreported data from our series indicate that 70% of our patients experience complete resolution of the problem, whereas another 15% achieve enough improvement to return to generally comfortable coital activity. Fifteen percent report no improvement, although, unlike results with the carbon dioxide laser, these women are not made worse by the therapy. An occasional patient who has complete relief from the operation may return in 12 to 18 months with a unifocal area of discomfort in the vestibule. Simple local excision in the office invariably restores the good result.

Surgical aftercare requires a physician's time and close attention. Patients are asked to return in 6 weeks. Remnants of suture material may still be evident, and healing may not be quite complete. Nevertheless, many women report less tenderness and discomfort in the vestibular area. This is an excellent opportunity to advise a patient that her next visit in 2 to 3 weeks will begin the process of return to normal sexual activity and to outline the steps she will take. Women who have suffered severe vulvar vestibulitis for more than 6 months have long since abandoned intercourse and almost certainly have acquired some degree of vaginismus. Their return to normal activity, therefore, must be preceded by advice on relaxation techniques, the appropriate use of dilators, and exercises designed to regain trust in their sexual partners. Physicians must be prepared to spend several visits instructing patients in these steps. Early involvement of the partner in the process often accelerates the patient's progress.

Summary

Vulvar vestibulitis is a chronic clinical syndrome of unknown cause defined (by Friedrich) by the constellation of severe pain on vestibular touch or attempted vaginal entry, tenderness to pressure localized within the vulvar vestibule, and physical findings confined to vestibular erythema of various degrees. Conservative treatment is often of benefit to women with mild symptoms of short duration, but severe cases require immunologic or, more commonly, surgical therapy. Pursued to the conclusion of a treatment protocol, good to satisfactory results are obtained in approximately 85% of patients. A physician's understanding of differential diagnoses, associated conditions, and the psychosexual issues of the syndrome is essential to achieving optimal results.

References

1. Friedrich EG Jr: Vulvar vestibulitis syndrome. Gen Reprod Med 1987;32:110.
2. Skene AJC: Treatise on the Diseases of Women. New York, D Appleton & Co, 1889.
3. Kelly HA: Gynecology. New York, D Appleton & Co, 1928.
4. Pelisse M, Hewitt J: Erythematous vulvitis en-plaques. In Proceedings of the Third Congress of the International Society for the Study of Vulvar Disease, Cocoyoc, Mexico. Milwaukee, International Society for the Study of Vulvar Disease, 1976.
5. Hart DB: Selected Papers in Gynaecology and Obstetrics. Edinburgh, W & AK Johnston, 1893.
6. Pyka RE, Wilkinson EJ, Friederich EG, et al: The histopathology of vulvar vestibulitis syndrome. Int J Gynecol Pathol 1982;7:249.
7. Turner MLC, Marinoff SC: Association of human papillomavirus with vulvodynia and the vulvar vestibulitis syndrome. J Reprod Med 1988;33: 533.
8. De Deus JM, Focchi J, Stavale JN, et al: Histologic and biomolecular aspects of papillomatosis of the vulvar vestibule in relation to human papillomavirus. Obstet Gynecol 1995;86:758.
9. Wilkinson EJ, Guerrero E, Daniel R, et al: Vulvar vestibulitis is rarely associated with human papillomavirus infection types 6, 11, 16, or 18. Int J Gynecol Pathol 1993;12:344.
10. Marinoff SC, Turner MLC: Hypersensitivity to vaginal candidiasis or treatment vehicles in the pathogenesis of minor vestibular gland syndrome. J Reprod Med 1987;31:796.
11. Solomons CC, Melmed MH, Heitler SM: Calcium citrate for vulvar vestibulitis. J Reprod Med 1991;36:879.
12. Prayson RA, Stoler MH, Hart WR: Vulvar vestibulitis: A histopathologic study of 36 cases, including human papillomavirus in situ hybridization analysis. Am J Surg Pathol 1995;19:154.
13. McCormack WM: Two urogenital sinus syndromes: Interstitial cystitis and focal vulvitis. J Reprod Med 1990;35:873.
14. Fitzpatrick CC, DeLancey JOL, Elkins TE, et al: Vulvar vestibulitis and interstitial cystitis: A disorder of urogenital sinus-derived epithelium? Obstet Gynecol 1993;81:860.
15. Reid R, Omoto KH, Precop SL, et al: Flashlamp-excited dye laser therapy of idiopathic vulvodynia is safe and efficacious. Am J Obstet Gynecol 1995;172:1684.
16. Horowitz BJ: Interferon therapy for condylomatous vulvitis. Obstet Gynecol 1989;73:446.

17. Marinoff SC, Turner ML, Hirsch RP, et al: Intralesional alpha interferon: Cost-effective therapy for vulvar vestibulitis syndrome. J Reprod Med 1993;38:19.
18. Bornstein J, Pascal B, Abramovici H: Intramuscular β-interferon treatment for severe vulvar vestibulitis. J Reprod Med 1993;38:117.
19. Woodruff JD, Genadry R, Poliakoff S: Treatment of dyspareunia and vaginal outlet distortions by perineoplasty. Obstet Gynecol 1981;57:750.
20. Axe S, Parmley T, Woodruff JD, et al: Adenomas in minor vestibular glands. Obstet Gynecol 1986;68:16.
21. Marinoff SC, Turner MLC: Vulvar vestibulitis syndrome: An overview. Am J Obstet Gynecol 1991;165:1228.

21

Vulvodynia

Marilynne McKay, MD

The international Society for the Study of Vulvar Disease (ISSVD) defines vulvodynia (from the Greek *odynia,* "pain") as chronic vulvar discomfort, especially that characterized by the patient's complaint of burning, stinging, irritation, or rawness.[1] Pruritus vulvae (chronic itching) is different, but patients with *Candida* or a vulvar dermatosis may complain of both.[2] Vulvodynia accompanied by dyspareunia is usually a multifactorial problem, from both an etiologic as well as a psychologic standpoint.

The *chronicity* of vulvodynia is its most important feature. Vulvodynia that has persisted for more than 6 months has more in common with chronic pain syndromes than it does with other gynecologic disorders. Inability to cure a genital problem causes patients significant psychologic stress, especially when discomfort leads to dyspareunia.[3] Vulvodynia is only a symptom; it is not a disease. Lack of knowledge is what leads to the diagnosis of idiopathic or essential vulvodynia. A careful work-up to preclude the most common factors contributing to the problem is required. To choose an effective treatment program, the therapist must recognize the sign and symptom patterns of vulvar burning. Vulvar biopsy is typically of little benefit in the diagnosis of vulvodynia unless skin changes are visible.

Ongoing investigations of the nature and etiology of vulvodynia have resulted in an ever-changing terminology. Some terms introduced early in the study of chronic vulvar pain disorders are no longer valid; persistent use of these words or phrases for conditions they no longer describe further confuses the caregiver seeking current knowledge. This chapter uses 1996 ISSVD-approved terminology.

Symptom Patterns and Demographics

My experience with more than 3000 patients with vulvodynia has revealed several distinct clinical variants. These categories have changed somewhat since they were first described,[4–6] and revisions will undoubtedly continue. This overview of clinical presentations of vulvar pain syndromes divides vulvodynia into three broad categories: (1) vulvar burning and/or dyspareunia *with* skin changes, (2) dyspareunia without skin changes, and (3) vulvar burning without skin changes (Table 21–1). Some treatment regimens are clearly more effective than others for certain conditions.[7]

Vulvodynia is a chronic rather than an acute problem; symptoms present for less than 3 months are likely to resolve spontaneously or with conservative treatment measures. Cases of persistent vulvodynia for a year or more are more difficult, and many of these patients have been told that their problem is primarily psychologic, especially when dyspareunia is the major complaint.[8–10] These women are often resentful and angry at the medical profession when a diagnosis cannot be made. Dyspareunia is a dramatic problem to women, and they may have unrealistic therapeutic expectations, demanding that the physician "do something—anything—to take away the pain." Older patients with neuropathic pain may undergo many work-ups for nonexistent "vaginitis." The inability to communicate symptoms accurately to family and physicians may delay recognition of the problem and initiation of appropriate therapy.

Patients with vulvodynia may experiment

Table 21–1. **DIFFERENTIAL DIAGNOSIS OF VULVODYNIA: PATTERNS OF PAIN**

Symptom Pattern	Dyspareunia	Physical Findings	Typical Patient	Diagnostic Test	Diagnosis	Treatment
Vulvar Burning and/or Dyspareunia with Skin Changes						
Itching and burning, cyclic (often related to menses); responds to anticandidal agents but recurs (topical drugs may irritate, however)	Postcoital irritation, sometimes edema; severe with flares	Variable erythema and edema, minimal vaginal discharge; fissures may occur with intercourse; episodic scaling and pustules	Premenopausal (or estrogen replacement), history of frequent *Candida* infection; frequent use of antibiotics (sinusitis, acne, urinary tract infection); better on anticandidals but often recurs	Vaginal smear and culture for *Candida* and *Gardnerella;* biopsy not helpful	*Cyclic vulvovaginitis* seems related to *Candida* infection or colonization, but exact mechanism unknown (see steroid rebound dermatitis, below)	4–6 months of low-dose systemic fluconazole (150 mg/wk) or vaginal anticandidal agents (terconazole, clotrimazole less irritating)
"Irritated" mucosa; poor tolerance of topical medications; corticosteroids may help, then flare symptoms	Often irritated after coitus, sometimes with swelling	Variable erythema; telangiectasias, hyperplasia of sebaceous glands on inner minora and/or papular rash on labia majora	History of frequent or chronic use of fluorinated or full-strength topical steroid: often culture-positive *Candida*	Vaginal smear and culture for *Candida;* history of allergies	*Steroid rebound dermatitis* due to topical steroids or *irritant reaction; Candida* infection common	Taper steroids, treat with anticandidal drugs every other day while patient on steroids; avoid irritating topical agents
Itching and burning, variable	No	Visible skin changes with loss of vulvar architecture; skin may be thickened or thinned	Any age	Skin biopsy of thickest area or lesion edge	*Lichen sclerosus* (if vagina involved, *lichen planus*)	Topical clobetasol proprionate 0.05% bid for 1 month, daily for 1 month, then as needed for symptoms
Dyspareunia Without Skin Changes						
Pain mainly with intercourse	Specific pain at entry; may prevent intercourse	Point tenderness to cotton-tipped swab palpation of vestibular gland orifices	Usually sexually active until onset of pain; previous inflammatory episodes likely (including laser surgery)	Cotton-tipped palpation of vestibule; not biopsy	*Vulvar vestibulitis* (may be acute and self-limited or chronic)	Excisional surgery reported most consistently effective; intralesional interferon helps <50%
Pain mainly with intercourse	Pain and guarding prevent intercourse	Intercourse virtually impossible	Variable age, reports some pain with all sexual activity; difficult to examine; guarded and fearful; possibly abused	None; physical examination	*Vaginismus*	Psychologic counseling; sex therapy; physical therapy with biofeedback; surgery rarely advisable
Vulvar Burning Without Skin Changes						
Constant burning, not related to touch or pressure	Not necessarily	Variable or no erythema, normal skin; often other perineal symptoms or sciatica	Usually postmenopausal, often not receiving estrogen replacement	Neurologic examination of pudendal branches	*Dysesthetic vulvodynia* or pudendal neuralgia	Low-dose amitriptyline (30–50 mg/d) for control of symptoms

with nontraditional folk remedies or nutritional alterations (such as special diets), but they are also likely to seek surgical intervention for dubious indications. Patient support groups can be helpful but vary in focus: They may emphasize specific patient populations,[11] a spectrum of treatment options,[12] or favorite therapeutic regimens.[13] Computer-literate patients may become extremely knowledgeable about vulvodynia through literature searches, the World Wide Web, and Internet support groups. Vulvodynia is a real challenge to the patient-physician relationship.

Differential Diagnosis

Infections

Patients may complain of vaginitis, but long-standing vulvodynia rarely improves after treatment for *Trichomonas,* bacterial vaginosis (*Gardnerella*), or *Streptococcus.* I hasten to add, however, that secondary infection of chronic vaginitis due to a mucosal disease (desquamative vaginitis, erosive lichen planus) can and does occur. In these cases, mucosal healing depends on elimination of the invading organism(s) and treatment of the underlying disorder. Patients may mistakenly insist on treatment for a physiologic discharge; the care provider should not be misled into prescribing a long course of antibiotics that will enhance the likelihood of *Candida* colonization.

Bacterial infection is an uncommon cause of vulvar discomfort. Streptococcal cellulitis can cause localized erythema and pain, particularly in the perianal area; it occurs more often in children.[14, 15] The presence of follicular pustules (at the base of hairs) with inflammation and peeling of the skin suggests the diagnosis of staphylococcal furunculosis. Fungal infection (tinea cruris) is relatively rare in women; although tinea may cause itching, it is not associated with vulvodynia.

Herpes simplex virus (HSV) is the only sexually transmitted disease that can sometimes be associated with chronic episodic vulvar pain; in individuals who are not immunosuppressed, cycles of recurrence typically last 5 to 7 days and almost never recur more frequently than monthly. A patient with chronic symptoms suggestive of HSV deserves a culture (preferably of an early, intact lesion) to confirm the diagnosis; it is unfair to put her through the psychic trauma of telling her she has herpes on the basis of history alone. A positive serum test does not confirm the diagnosis of HSV (previous cold sores or fever blisters cause permanent seroconversion, and titers are useless); the serum test is helpful only if it is negative. Systemic therapy with acyclovir or valacyclovir is helpful; topical acyclovir is not efficacious for recurrences. Herpes zoster (varicella-zoster virus) is a dermatomal recurrence of childhood chickenpox; lesions may involve the inner thigh or leg as well as one side of the vulva. Recurrences are unlikely, but postzoster neuralgia can be persistent; it responds to the same treatment regimen as dysesthetic vulvodynia (discussed later).

Candida and Cyclic Vulvitis

By far the most ubiquitous infectious organism for genital mucosa is *Candida* (*Monilia,* candidosis, yeast infection).[16] In contrast to the white discharge and itchy rash of acute candidiasis, *cyclic vulvitis* is characterized by cyclic symptomatic flares (or, conversely, days at a time without symptoms). Patients describe episodic vulvar redness, burning, and even edema and fissuring, especially after coitus. Topical medications of any kind may sting the irritated mucosa, causing the patient and care provider to think that she is "allergic to everything." Reports of an accompanying itch or discharge are variable.

Patients with cyclic vulvitis usually improve with topical or systemic anticandidal agents[5] but complain of recurrent symptoms within a month after stopping them. Previous bouts of vulvovaginitis with administration of antibiotics suggest that the patient is colonized with *Candida* (about one of every eight women). Long-term systemic therapy with intermittent or daily ketoconazole[17, 18] or weekly fluconazole[19] can be subsequently tapered to low-dose cyclic therapy at the time when symptoms tend to recur.

The mechanism of cyclic vulvitis is unknown. Symptomatic response to systemic or topical anticandidal agents suggests a cause-and-effect relation to *Candida,* but it is not known whether this is infection, reinfection, allergy, colonization in *Candida*-sensitive patients, or a combination of *Candida* and other factors yet to be identified. Reports of localized vaginal hypersensitivity to candidiasis[20] suggest the possibility of a vaginal allergic response leading to persistent vulvodynia in some patients. Elimination of *Candida* with long-term low-dose antifungals may allow the inflamed vaginal mucosa to regain its normal barrier function. My current preferred *Candida* suppression regimen is oral fluconazole (Diflucan) 100 to 150 mg weekly for 2 to 3 months, tapering to every 10 to 14 days for 2 to 3 months, then monthly. For itching or irritation, I also prescribe pramoxine-hydrocortisone (Pramasone) 1% ointment, a nonsensitizing topical preparation that contains a mild topical anesthetic to apply two to three times daily as needed for irritation. Topical antifungal creams can be used in a similar tapering treatment program: for example, terconazole vaginal cream daily for 2 weeks, then half an applicator Monday-Wednesday-Friday (M-W-F) for 6 weeks, tapering to a weekly dose.

Besides making patients more comfortable, control of chronic cyclic vulvitis may prevent some cases of vulvar vestibulitis. Although the cause of this complication is not known with certainty, most investigators believe that it may be preventable.[21] Acute *Candida*-induced vestibular tenderness generally resolves with or soon after treatment of infection, but chronic vestibulitis may persist for months or years. A commonly accepted theory is that the vestibular glands are altered by local inflammation of some type; if the inflammation resolves, the vestibular glands should gradually recover. Long-standing vestibular inflammation, however, may permanently damage the glands and make the nerves in the area hyperesthetic. Vestibular pain that has been present for more than a year generally has a poorer prognosis, but recovery can be very slow; treatment trials should continue for at least 2 to 3 months. Local inflammation can be reduced by eliminating provoking factors, such as *Candida,* and applying a mid-potency topical steroid cream to the vulvar vestibule for 4 to 6 weeks. If some improvement has been noted after 2 months, then conservative treatment should be continued for another 4 to 6 months. If pain-free intercourse has been possible even once or twice in the 2-month interval between visits, the prognosis is favorable.

Vulvar Dermatoses (Formerly Dystrophies)

The expression *vulvar dystrophy* was coined in the 1960s by gynecologists with limited understanding of dermatologic disease, and the term was then used to distinguish benign from malignant skin disease.[22] In 1987, the term *dystrophy* was replaced by a new ISSVD classification[23] that recognizes dermatologic diagnoses by their traditional medical names, much to the relief of dermatologists and pathologists, who were perplexed by the need to rename well-known skin disorders simply because they affected the vulva. The major vulvar dermatoses, lichen sclerosus (LS), lichen planus (LP), and lichen simplex chronicus (LSC), are histologically distinct; each has a typical clinical presentation and responds to different treatments.

Lichen Sclerosus

This classic genital dermatosis usually presents as a symmetric whitened keyhole pattern on the vulva. The thickened (sclerotic) dermis is white, and the thin atrophic epidermis may be finely wrinkled or scaly. The skin is easily traumatized; bruises and purpura are common. Lesion extent does not seem to correlate with discomfort. LS has no known relationship to hormones or age; it can occur at any time in infants or the elderly, in males as well as females, and virtually anywhere on the body (although disease limited to the genitalia is most common).

It was long accepted that topical steroids are effective in thickened pruritic lesions of LS, but it has now been shown that a several-week course of a superpotent topical corticosteroid (such as clobetasol) also heals erosive or fissured LS.[24] Superpotent corticosteroids may also reverse the disease process.[25] There is no longer any rationale for using testosterone ointment; new studies have shown it to be no better than petrolatum.[26] Fortunately for patients with LS limited to the vulva, this area is more responsive to treatment than other parts of the body.

Clobetasol is not the only topical steroid that can be used to treat LS; slightly lower-potency ointment-based steroids are better tolerated by some patients and have the same effect, although they may need to be used more frequently. If a patient feels that she needs to apply a cream or ointment on a daily basis, then I recommend hydrocortisone 1% ointment two to three times daily as needed to control itching for an indefinite time.

Erosive Vaginitis

Also called desquamative vaginitis, this chronic vaginal disease often proves histologically to be erosive LP, a mucosal form of a relatively common skin disorder. Mucosal LP often affects the gingiva and oral mucosa as well as the vagina.[27] LP tends to flare and remit, often for no apparent reason. A biopsy of the inflamed but healed edge of a lesion is preferred; dermatopathology consultation should be considered for interpretation if the diagnosis is unclear. No single treatment is satisfactory, but some measures have proved better than others. Decreasing bacterial and candidal colonization of the inflamed vaginal mucosa may hasten healing; clindamycin 2% vaginal cream may be inserted daily for 1 week, then M-W-F.[28] A weekly dose of oral fluconazole (100 to 150 mg) prevents *Candida* superinfection. After the first week, I recommend alternating the clindamycin 2% vaginal cream with insertion of a midpotency water-based corticosteroid (i.e., 2% clindamycin vaginal cream on M-W-F and intravaginal corticosteroid using the clindamycin applicator on Tu-Th-Sat) at bedtime. This regimen reduces inflammation and helps the mucosa to regain its normal barrier function. When the condition is inactive, it is not necessary to use any topical agents; with flares, topical steroid and antibiotic should be alternated until the discharge is controlled. Alternatives include topical cyclosporine, an expensive and not very satisfactory vaginal therapy that has been more beneficial for oral lesions.[29] Surgical release of adhesions with follow-up steroid therapy can restore vulvovaginal architecture. These adhesions are often limited to superficial epithelium, and blunt dissection under anesthesia is all that is necessary.

Lichen Simplex Chronicus (Squamous Cell Hyperplasia)

With chronic rubbing or scratching, the skin on any part of the body thickens and develops an intrinsic itch that persists even when the original stimulus resolves. The preferred treatment is a high-potency topical steroid applied twice daily to begin, then tapering to daily over 1 to 2 months. As symptoms improve, application should be decreased to an as-needed basis. On the vulva, *Candida* is often the initiating factor that provokes the itching, and prophylaxis with weekly anticandidal therapy can help to prevent flares while topical steroids are applied. Intralesional corticosteroids (triamcinolone acetonide suspension 10 mg/ml) may also be used for localized areas; this is far more effective than subcutaneous injection of absolute alcohol, an outmoded treatment.

Steroid Rebound Dermatitis

As the use of superpotent topical steroids becomes more widespread (and when they are inappropriately used for disorders other than LS and LSC), it comes as no surprise that side effects are encountered with greater frequency. Complications include striae formation on the inner thighs and inflammatory changes on the labia majora and minora and vulvar vestibule. The normal sebaceous glands on the outer portion of the inner minora appear more prominent; in some cases there is petechial staining of the periurethral area. Steroid rebound dermatitis occurs when high-potency (or even midpotency) topical steroids are applied for longer than 3 to 4 weeks at a time on skin that is not significantly thickened or architecturally altered.[7] The erythema is a result of rebound vasodilation following steroid-induced vasoconstriction; patients typically complain of burning and apply more medication, maintaining the condition. Dermatologists have described this phenomenon on the face (perioral dermatitis), where it develops for the same reason. Apparently the vulva and the face both are thin-skinned steroid-sensitive areas with high concentrations of sebaceous glands.

Symptomatic burning subsides gradually over several weeks when the steroids are discontinued or tapered. In general, topical steroids more potent than hydrocortisone 1% should not be applied to the vulva unless a patient has visible or biopsy evidence of a dermatosis such as LS or lichen simplex.

Dysesthetic Vulvodynia (Formerly Essential Vulvodynia)

The term *essential vulvodynia* was originally used to describe end-stage vulvodynia for which no cause could be determined. When it was subsequently found that treatment for cutaneous neuralgia was effective in most of these patients, *essential* was replaced by the more appropriate *dysesthetic vulvodynia*.[31] Included in this category are pudendal neuralgia and possibly reflex sympathetic dystrophy (see Chapter 25).

The diagnosis is based on a history of unremitting or constant vulvar burning or tingling that may also involve the urethra, the perianal area, or both. Symptoms may vary from morning to night (usually worsening as the day goes on), but the discomfort is remarkably consistent and in some patients may be more intense on one side than the other. The pain is often described as "under the skin" and is rarely worsened with tight clothing or touch. Many patients complain of chronic low back pain or sciatica. This pattern of discomfort is more common in postmenopausal women and young women with a history of low back injury. In my experience, women with dysesthetic vulvodynia may also be more likely to have been diagnosed with interstitial cystitis, urethral syndrome, irritable bowel syndrome, fibromyalgia, or migraines. It is not known whether this might indicate a type of hypersensitivity to somatic pain, but low-dose tricyclic antidepressants such as amitriptyline or nortriptyline appear to be very beneficial.

During the physical examination, a cotton-tipped applicator should be used to compare the sensation of a light stroke on the right side of the vulva and the right inner thigh. The sensations on the left side are compared, and then each side of the vulva is compared with the other. It is not unusual for affected patients to note increased sensation to light touch in the saddle distribution of the pudendal nerve, and a difference from one side to the other is sometimes found. If the patient says that discomfort increases when she sits on the toilet, this may indicate an element of pelvic floor relaxation or dysfunction. Patients who have constant vulvar burning and who also complain of urethral discomfort with urination may have a common pain pathway (urogenital sinus syndrome[32]).

Antidepressants are effective in the management of certain types of pain with or without clinical depression. Because patients often resent the implication that they need a "psychiatric drug," they should be reassured that the medication has been prescribed for its effect on cutaneous nerves and not because of depression.[33] I start amitriptyline at a dose of 10 mg at bedtime, increasing by one tablet weekly as tolerated to a dose of 30 to 50 mg. This dose range has been most helpful in controlling these symptoms. If a patient is able to tolerate 40 to 50 mg per day (divided dose or all at bedtime) without difficulty, then the prescription can be changed to 25-mg tablets for convenience and the dose can be increased to 75 to 100 mg if necessary. Alternatives to amitriptyline for pain relief include the other tricyclics (nortriptyline, imipramine, and desipramine), trazodone, and the benzodiazepine clonazepam. Unfortunately, fluoxetine, a popular drug for treatment of depression with fewer side effects than the tricyclics, has not proved helpful for pain management.

Examination Techniques

Smears and Cultures

A vaginal smear and culture for *Candida* and *Gardnerella* should be part of the workup of vulvodynia, although patients with a chronic low-grade inflammatory response to *Candida* (cyclic vulvitis) may have nondiagnostic fungal cultures at the time of a symptom flare. If possible, the species of *Candida* should be determined, because some are resistant to fluconazole, the oral anticandidal of choice. *Candida krusei* is resistant to oral fluconazole but sensitive to oral ketoconazole and topical terconazole. About a third of the strains of *Candida* (*Torulopsis*) *glabrata* are resistant to terconazole and fluconazole.[34] Antibiotic treatment of culture-proven *Gardnerella* should be initiated while a patient is on an anticandidal suppression regimen to avoid secondary candidiasis.

Colposcopy

As a dermatologist, I have not been impressed with vulvar colposcopy as a diagnostic tool. Unless a woman has a previous history of biopsy-proven vulvar intraepithelial neoplasia, magnification adds little to the recognition of a dermatologic disease on the vulva. It is far more important to develop familiarity with related findings on other parts of the body that may give important diagnostic clues to the diagnosis. Search and treatment for subclinical human papillomavirus (HPV) as the presumed cause of most symptomatic vulvar conditions is fortunately becoming a thing of the past. Without a history of vulvar intraepithelial neoplasia, there is little justification for aggressive treatment of biopsy reports that are merely suggestive of HPV. Vestibular papillae (small, nonkeratinized, symmetric, fingerlike projections at the introitus) rarely have DNA evidence of HPV; papillae are now considered a normal variant. In my experience, it is far more common for symptomatic vulvodynia to respond to anticandidals than to treatment for HPV.

Biopsy

If a vulvar lesion is present, a biopsy specimen should be taken at the thickest portion(s). If the lesions are eroded or ulcerated, the best location to sample is the lesion periphery, so that the pattern of inflammation can be appreciated in intact skin. Erosive vaginitis may be due to an autoimmune blistering disease, and thus a biopsy for immunofluorescence should also be performed. A special fixative other than formalin is required. The histopathologic finding of nonspecific inflammation can be attributed to various problems, including dermatitis due to irritants, cell-mediated allergic reactions, overuse of topical steroids, and *Candida* hypersensitivity; the advice of a dermatopathologist is encouraged.

Treatment

Steroids

Systemic steroids are rarely indicated in the treatment of vulvar dermatoses. High–potency topical steroids such as clobetasol should be prescribed only for thick, scaly dermatoses (LS, LSC) or for erosive vaginitis (LP). I generally start with a twice-daily dose for 3 to 4 weeks, then taper to once daily for 3 to 4 weeks, then to M-W-F or only when symptoms recur. If a patient likes the soothing effect of more frequent application of a cream or ointment, then I recommend a lower-potency preparation, which can be applied more often. When a patient has no evidence of thick, scaly plaques or erosive disease, I do not prescribe a superpotent steroid.[35]

Estrogens, Androgens, Progesterone

The complaint of mild postcoital introital irritation with or without urethral discomfort is consistent with lack of estrogen. This pattern of vulvar symptoms responds well to topical estrogen creams, and if a patient is perimenopausal or postmenopausal, topical estrogen could be tried on an empirical basis for a month or two. The use of topical androgens or topical progesterone has been superseded by topical steroids (discussed earlier). Hormones do not toughen vulvar skin and should not be used for this purpose.

Antipruritics

In general, antipruritics are not effective in the treatment of vulvodynia. *Candida* is the most common cause of vulvar itching, and a treatment trial of a topical or oral anticandidal agent for a few months is certainly warranted for a patient who has itched for months or years. If the skin is thickened (lichenified) as a result of scratching, then a topical steroid is necessary to restore the normal thickness (discussed earlier). Doxepin hydrochloride 5% (Zonalon) cream has been shown to be effective for eczema, but trials have not been conducted on pruritus vulvae. A mixture of betamethasone valerate and crutamiton cream is sometimes helpful for mild itching but causes irritation when used for vulvar burning. Unfortunately, there is no good "antiitch pill." Patients who awaken frequently because they itch may be helped by antihistamines that shorten the time needed to fall asleep.

Antidepressants and Anxiolytics

As a rule, dermatologists do not prescribe anxiolytics for skin diseases that are chronic in nature and tend to recur. Dysesthetic vulvodynia generally responds well to low-dose tricyclic antidepressants such as amitriptyline or nortriptyline. Psychologic counseling should be encouraged for patients with marital or family problems as a result of their chronic symptoms. These sometimes take the form of obsessive-compulsive behavior or fear of having or contracting a sexually transmitted disease.

Alcohol Neurolysis

Injection of absolute alcohol into the vulva is not recommended for the treatment of symptomatic vulvar burning; in fact, intralesional corticosteroids (e.g., triamcinolone acetonide suspension) are more effective for vulvar itching. Vulvar skin slough is a complication of alcohol injection, and this procedure is strongly discouraged.

Vulvectomy

Although vestibulectomy may be helpful for vulvar vestibulitis, vulvectomy is rarely appropriate for a benign vulvar disease. Vestibuloplasty may be performed when the introitus has been compromised by progressive scarring (LS, LP, desquamative vaginitis, bullous dermatoses), but procedures should be delayed until the condition is controlled by topical steroids. The vaginal adhesions are the result of erosive surfaces healing together; they are not deep and can be bluntly dissected apart without much difficulty when a patient is under anesthesia.

Summary

A patient's fears often center on cancer or contagion; she may demand tests to "find out exactly what I have." Reassurance that infection and cancer have been ruled out can give substantial comfort, but a patient should be advised of the laboratory's limitations. Negative results do not mean that the problem is all in her head. Doctor-patient communication to avoid misunderstanding should be a major therapeutic goal, because vulvodynia is more of a condition than a disease. Physicians should understand that the different types of vulvodynia can be recognized by different symptom patterns. Therapy should take into account the typically slow improvement in symptoms; documentation of initial impairment and progressive increments of improvement is recommended.

References

1. Burning vulva syndrome: Report of the ISSVD task force. J Reprod Med 1984;29:457.
2. McKay M: Vulvodynia versus pruritus vulvae. Clin Obstet Gynecol 1985;28:123.
3. McKay M, Farrington J: Vulvodynia: Chronic vul-

var pain syndromes. In Stoudemire A, Fogel B (eds): Medical Psychiatric Practice, vol 3. Washington, DC, American Psychiatric Press, 1995.

4. McKay M: Subsets of vulvodynia. J Reprod Med 1988;33:695.
5. McKay M: Vulvodynia: A multifactorial problem. Arch Dermatol 1989;125:256.
6. McKay M: Vulvodynia: Diagnostic patterns. Dermatol Clin 1992;10:423.
7. McKay M: Vulvodynia and pruritus vulvae. In Black MM, McKay M, Braude P, (eds): Color Atlas and Text of Obstetric and Gynecologic Dermatology. London, Mosby-Wolfe, 1995, pp 101–108.
8. Dodson MG, Friedrich EG Jr: Psychosomatic vulvovaginitis. Obstet Gynecol 1978;51:23s.
9. Lynch PJ: Vulvodynia: A syndrome of unexplained vulvar pain, psychologic disability and sexual dysfunction. J Reprod Med 1986;31:773.
10. Friedrich EG Jr: The vulvar vestibule. J Reprod Med 1983;28:773.
11. Interstitial Cystitis Association, PO Box 1553, Madison Square Station, New York, NY 10159.
12. National Vulvodynia Association, PO Box 4491, Silver Springs, MD 20914-4491.
13. Vulvar Pain Foundation, 433 Ward Street, Graham, NC 27253.
14. Kokx NP, Comstock JA, Facklam RR: Streptococcal perianal disease in children. Pediatrics 1987; 30:659.
15. Rehder PA, Eliezer ET, Lane AT: Perianal cellulitis: Cutaneous group A streptococcal disease. Arch Dermatol 1988;124:702.
16. McKay M: Cutaneous manifestations of candidiasis. Am J Obstet Gynecol 1988;158:991.
17. Sobel JD: Management of recurrent vulvovaginal candidiasis with intermittent ketoconazole prophylaxis. Obstet Gynecol 1985;65:435.
18. Sobel JD: Recurrent vulvovaginal candidiasis. A prospective study of the efficacy of maintenance ketoconazole therapy. N Engl J Med 1986;315:1455.
19. Sobel JD: Fluconazole maintenance therapy in recurrent vulvovaginal candidiasis. Int J Gynecol Obstet 1992;37(Suppl):17.
20. Witkin SS, Jeremias J, Ledger WJ: A localized vaginal allergic response in women with recurrent vaginitis. J Allergy Clin Immunol 1988;81:412.
21. McKay M, Frankman O, Horowitz BJ, et al: Vulvar vestibulitis and vestibular papillomatosis: Report of the ISSVD committee on vulvodynia. J Reprod Med 1991;36:413.
22. International Society for the Study of Vulvar Disease: New nomenclature for vulvar disease. Obstet Gynecol 1976;47:122.
23. Wilkinson E, Ridley CM, McKay M, et al: The ISSVD classification of vulvar nonneoplastic epithelial disorders and intraepithelial neoplasia. Am J Dermatopathol 1991;13:428.
24. Dalziel KL, Millard PR, Wojnarowska F: The treatment of vulvar lichen sclerosus with a very potent topical corticosteroid (clobetasol propionate 0.05%) cream. Br J Dermatol 1991;124:461.
25. Dalziel KL, Wojnarowska F: Long-term control of vulval lichen sclerosus after treatment with a potent topical steroid cream. J Reprod Med 1993;38:25.
26. Sideri M, Origoni M, Spinaci L, Ferrari A: Topical testosterone in the treatment of vulvar lichen sclerosus. Int J Gynecol Obstet 1994;46:53.
27. Pelisse M: The vulvo-vaginal-gingival syndrome. A new form of erosive lichen planus. Int J Dermatol 1989;28:381.
28. Sobel JD: Desquamative inflammatory vaginitis: A new subgroup of purulent vaginitis responsive to topical 2% clindamycin therapy. Am J Obstet Gynecol 1994;171:1215.
29. Becherel PA, Chosidow O, Boisnic S, et al: Topical cyclosporine in the treatment of oral and vulvar erosive lichen planus: A blood level monitoring study. Arch Dermatol 1995;131:495.
30. McKay M: Dysesthetic ("essential") vulvodynia: Treatment with amitriptyline. J Reprod Med 1993;38:9.
31. McCormack WM: Two urogenital sinus syndromes. J Reprod Med 1990;35:873.
32. France RD: The future for antidepressants: Treatment of pain. Psychopathology 1987;20(Suppl 1):99.
33. Sobel JD: Controversial aspects in the management of vulvovaginal candidiasis. J Am Acad Dermatol 1994;31:S10.
34. McKay M: Topical steroids in the therapy of vulvar diseases (appendix B). In Black MM, McKay M, Braude P (eds): Color Atlas and Text of Obstetric and Gynecologic Dermatology. London, Mosby-Wolfe, 1995, p 173–179.

22

Bladder and Urethral Syndromes

Jill M. Peters-Gee, MD

Urinary frequency, urgency, dysuria, and suprapubic pressure are common complaints expressed to physicians and other health care providers. These complaints sometimes are transient but often are chronic. The differential diagnosis of these irritative voiding complaints includes many easily treated problems as well as some more elusive diseases.

Evaluation

The first step in evaluating a woman with voiding complaints is taking a very thorough history, followed by performing an equally thorough physical examination. Key points in the history include time of onset of symptoms, relationship of symptoms to the menstrual cycle, frequency of urination, nocturia, dysuria, dyspareunia, aggravating factors, alleviating factors, exposure to irritating substances, and relationship to intercourse. Equally helpful is a voiding log that outlines the dated time of void, voided volume, and any related symptoms such as pain, incontinence, urgency, and so on. Irritative symptoms that are worse premenstrually may be due to endometriosis involving the urinary tract or fibroids causing extrinsic compression. Some women can experience obstructive voiding symptoms or even retention related to fibroids that increase in size premenstrually. The presence of associated problems may provide clues to the underlying disease process in selected patients. Patients should be questioned about incontinence, difficulty emptying, and related problems such as the presence of fibromyalgia, migraines, irritable bowel disease, and recurrent urinary tract infections (UTIs). Patients with interstitial cystitis have an increased incidence of fibromyalgia, migraines, vulvodynia, and irritable bowel disease, whereas recurrent UTI should lead one to consider the possibility of an anatomic abnormality such as urethral diverticulum or a foreign body within the urinary tract (i.e., suture, stone). The incidence of bladder carcinoma is increased in patients with a history of smoking, exposure to aniline dyes, and exposure to cyclophosphamide. Long-term indwelling catheters and other causes of chronic inflammation have been associated with squamous cell carcinoma of the bladder. If a patient has a history of recurrent UTIs, it is important to see positive cultures as documentation. Many women with "recurrent cystitis" really do not have true bacterial cystitis. They may be treated as such, but they often have urethritis, interstitial cystitis, or other problems.

While taking a history, it is helpful to have the patient describe exactly where and when she feels pain. Also note whether anything aggravates or alleviates the symptoms. Pain localized to the urethra may indicate urethritis, urethral diverticulum, or vaginitis. Pain felt deeper in the bladder may be related to cystitis, interstitial cystitis, bladder spasms, and so on. The timing of the pain and when it occurs during voiding are also noteworthy. The classic pain of interstitial cystitis, for example, is typically described as a suprapubic pressure that is relieved by voiding.

A thorough physical examination includes an abdominal examination, pelvic examination, and assessment for urethral or anterior vaginal wall tenderness. If urethral discharge is seen when the anterior vaginal wall is milked, one should think of urethral diverticulum. Patients should be assessed for uterine or cervical motion tenderness, a pelvic mass, or pelvic pain. A postvoid residual assessment by catheterization or bladder ultrasound examination is occasionally necessary.

Finally, a urinalysis is mandatory and is really an extension of the physical examination. Both microscopic analysis and dipstick testing can be used. The dipstick is a rapid office detection test that may assess for leukocytes, nitrite, glucose, hemoglobin, protein, and even specific gravity. The nitrite test depends on the conversion of urinary nitrate to nitrite by bacterial action. The test is often integrated with an esterase test that suggests the presence of leukocytes by a color change caused by esterase present in the leukocytes. Microscopic analysis can be performed on either spun or unspun urine. The presence of red blood cells, white blood cells, or bacteria may be significant. Almost all women with acute cystitis have pyuria, and about one half have microhematuria. Pyuria can also be found in women with urethritis, but it is not usually encountered in vaginitis. Persistent pyuria with negative cultures can occur in genitourinary tuberculosis. In these cases, urine testing for acid-fast bacilli may be needed.

Irritative symptoms such as frequency, nocturia, and urgency can be caused by physical irritants inside the lumen of the bladder, extrinsic irritants outside the bladder, or muscular/neurologic factors. Urinalysis and culture are a good beginning, followed by cytologic study to assess for carcinoma *in situ* (CIS) in heavy smokers and older women. Cystoscopy may be indicated for evaluation of irritative symptoms, especially if associated with hematuria. Radiographic studies such as intravenous pyelography, renal ultrasonography, and voiding cystourethrography may be needed to rule out anatomic problems. Urodynamics may be required to assess bladder function in cases of incontinence or voiding disorders.

Cystometry can be performed very simply in the office using a urethral catheter and a water manometry setup. After the patient voids, a 16 French catheter is inserted and the postvoid residual urine volume is measured. The urethral catheter is then connected to the water manometric cystometer, and water is instilled into the bladder at a rate of 1 ml/sec. The patient is asked to report when she first feels the desire to urinate and when a strong urge to void is present. The cystometric pressures are recorded every 50 ml and plotted on a cystometrographic sheet. Electronic urodynamic equipment can record multiple channels such as urethral pressure, abdominal pressure, vesical pressure, and electromyography of the sphincter. Urodynamic study is performed when one suspects a neurogenic bladder or detrusor instability and the patient fails an empirical trial of anticholinergic medication such as hyoscyamine, oxybutynin, propantheline bromide, or flavoxate.

Differential Diagnosis

The differential diagnosis for irritative symptoms consists of many different entities (Table 22–1). The diagnostic evaluation is really a process of elimination. History alone can rule out some entities, but others require a methodic evaluation.

Urinary Tract Infections

One of the most common causes of irritative voiding symptoms in women is recur-

Table 22–1. **DIFFERENTIAL DIAGNOSIS OF IRRITATIVE VOIDING SYMPTOMS**

Cystitis: acute and chronic
Urethritis: acute and chronic
Urethral diverticulum
Urethral syndrome
Interstitial cystitis
Unstable bladder, detrusor instability, neurogenic bladder
Bladder or urethral carcinoma, carcinoma *in situ*
Urinary stones
Radiation cystitis
Cyclophosphamide cystitis
Endometriosis
Atrophic urethritis
Other inflammatory process outside bladder (e.g., diverticulitis, mass)

rent UTIs. Prevalence rates of bacteriuria are estimated to be 2% in females 15 to 24 years old and 10% in women 55 to 64 years old.[1] *Cystitis* is the term typically used to describe infection localized to the bladder and sometimes associated with urethritis. Symptoms include frequency, urgency, dysuria, nocturia, urge incontinence, suprapubic discomfort, and occasionally hematuria.

Sexual activity is positively correlated with the incidence of UTIs in women. One study of women seen at a sexually transmitted disease clinic noted a higher prevalence of bacteriuria within 24 hours of coitus.[2] Both the frequency and recency of sexual intercourse are related to the risk of cystitis. As much as a 60-fold increased risk of bacteriuria is noted in women who have engaged in intercourse within the previous 48 hours, when compared with women who have not.[3] This increase appears to be related to inoculation of the bladder with periurethral bacteria. Those women who do have not have colonization of their periurethral or vaginal areas with coliforms introduce normal vaginal flora that are rapidly cleared with voiding and thus do not produce infection. In women who are colonized with pathogenic coliform bacteria, such as *Escherichia coli,* infection may result. UTIs in nonpregnant symptomatic women are usually caused by enteric strains of gram-negative aerobic organisms. *E. coli* is the predominant organism in 80% to 85% of patients. The remaining causative bacteria are *Klebsiella, Enterobacter, Proteus* sp., *Enterococcus,* group D *Streptococcus,* and *Staphylococcus saprophyticus.*[4]

Elderly women have low levels of estrogen and increased susceptibility to UTIs. Reid and associates have shown that uropathogens attach in larger numbers to uroepithelial cells from women older than 65 years when compared with cells from premenopausal women.[5] In addition, postmenopausal estrogen-deficient women have higher vaginal pH, increased vaginal colonization with *E. coli,* and higher rates of recurrent UTIs than premenopausal women. Estrogen replacement therapy has been shown to lower vaginal pH, decrease vaginal colonization with *E. coli,* and decrease the frequency of UTIs.[6]

Postcoital Urinary Tract Infections

Postcoital UTIs can be prevented in part by encouraging patients to void after intercourse and with the use of prophylactic antibiotics before or after intercourse. Vosti first demonstrated that nitrofurantoin given after intercourse prevented UTI.[7] Other antibiotics such as trimethoprim-sulfamethoxazole, nalidixic acid, and sulfonamides have been shown to be effective as well.[8] When compared with continuous low-dose prophylaxis, postcoital antibiotic use may reduce medication costs and side effects as well as decrease the emergence of resistant bacterial strains.

As many as 25% of women presenting to a primary care practitioner because of irritative symptoms are found not to have a UTI.[9] Four important conditions may also present with irritative voiding symptoms: urethral syndrome, interstitial cystitis, CIS of the bladder, and detrusor instability.

Urethral Syndrome

Urethral syndrome consists of a symptom complex that can include dysuria, frequency, urgency, suprapubic discomfort, and voiding dysfunction such as stranguria. Stranguria is the slow and painful discharge of urine, often due to spasm of the bladder or urethra. Urethral syndrome is a diagnosis of exclusion often used to label a condition for which no other explanation can be found for the symptoms. Urethral syndrome is estimated to account for as many as 5 million office visits a year in the United States. The etiology remains controversial; popular hypotheses include infection, urethral spasm, urethral obstruction, hypoestrogenism, and neurologic, traumatic, allergic, and psychogenic causes.[10]

The diagnosis of urethral syndrome is made by first ruling out the possibility of infection. A symptomatic patient with a urine culture in which the bacteria count exceeds 100/ml should be considered and treated as having cystitis. A close look at urethral anatomy and any discharge, tenderness, or mass is necessary. The Skene's glands are located superiolateral to the urethral meatus. An infection or obstruction in one of these glands may present as exquisite point tenderness or as a cystic lesion lateral to the meatus.

Treatment for urethral syndrome consists of empirical antibiotic therapy. If symptoms appear to arise after a recent documented UTI, long-term use of suppressive antibiotics for 8 to 12 weeks has proved helpful. If sterile pyuria is found in association with acute symptoms consistent with urethral syndrome, *Chlamydia trachomatis* should be suspected, especially in young, sexually active women. Urethral culture for *Chlamydia* can be performed by using an intraurethral swab. These women can be treated empirically with a 10-day course of tetracycline or doxycycline. Stamm and colleagues demonstrated convincing evidence for an infectious cause in acute urethral syndrome, with 11 of 59 women demonstrating *C. trachomatis.*[11] Other possible infectious agents include *Lactobacillus, S. saprophyticus, Corynebacterium,* and fastidious organisms such as *Ureaplasma urealytica.* If symptoms persist and pyuria is still present after treatment with doxycycline, erythromycin should be used as the second-line drug. If symptoms and pyuria still persist, further urologic work-up should be considered to rule out stones, tumors, or other causes of pyuria.

Urethral stenosis or obstruction has long been believed to cause symptoms consistent with urethral syndrome. Many urologists have routinely treated symptomatic women with urethral dilation, assuming organic stenosis was present. Part of the problem has been failure to recognize the variation in normal urethral caliber. In addition, the criteria for diagnosis of stenosis have been inconsistent. The mean caliber of the urethra has been shown to be approximately 22 French, with a range of 18 to 28 French.[12] Bergman and colleagues randomized 60 patients with urethral syndrome into three groups: placebo, 10-day course of doxycycline, or three successive urethral dilations. The subjective improvement rate was 75% in the urethral dilation group. This was significantly higher than in either of the other groups.[13] If a woman has symptoms of decreased urinary stream, hesitancy, and interrupted stream, urethral dilation certainly should be considered if she has no evidence of infection.

Urethral spasm may have a role in causing symptoms associated with urethral syndrome.[14] Encouraging results have been obtained with biofeedback, diazepam administration, behavior modification, and electric stimulation. Hypoestrogenism can be an etiologic factor in postmenopausal women. The urethra is embryologically derived from the urogenital sinus, with the lower two thirds covered with stratified squamous epithelium. Estrogen supplementation administered either orally or topically in postmenopausal women can decrease symptoms of frequency, urgency, and dysuria.

In summary, urethral syndrome can be treated in a number of ways. Empirical therapy with antibiotics is indicated when pyuria is identified and bacterial cystitis has been ruled out. Estrogen supplementation in postmenopausal patients should be considered, especially when atrophic changes are present. Some physicians use urethral dilation when antibiotics fail or as a first-line therapy. Other treatments including dimethyl sulfoxide (DMSO), silver nitrate, antiinflammatory agents, skeletal muscle relaxants such as clidinium bromide–chlordiazepoxide, or α-antagonists such as terazosin or doxazosin have been used with some success. If a patient describes symptoms of irregular voiding patterns with hesitancy, stranguria, or intermittency, pelvic floor spasticity or dysfunction may be contributing to the symptoms. In these cases, biofeedback techniques, perhaps in conjunction with electric stimulation, may be helpful. It is important to remember that the best results (85% to 100%) often occur with observation alone.[15, 16]

Urethral Diverticulum

Women with persistent lower urinary tract symptoms that have been unresponsive to traditional treatment should be suspected of having a urethral diverticulum. The incidence of urethral diverticulum is thought to be between 1% and 6%. The majority of cases are diagnosed in women between 20 and 60 years of age and are more commonly found in the black population.[17] The number of urethral diverticula diagnosed is in part related to the effort that a practitioner puts forth in looking for them. The classic triad of symptoms consists of dysuria, dyspareunia, and postvoid dribbling or incontinence.[18] The most frequent complaints are those associated with lower urinary tract irritation, such as frequency, dysuria, and urgency. It is believed that urethral diverticula may arise from the periurethral glands, subsequent to infection or obstruction; however, the true etiology remains a subject of debate.

Diagnosis of a urethral diverticulum may be based on physical examination, in which milking the anterior vaginal wall demonstrates loss of a small amount of urine or purulent discharge. A cystic mass on the anterior vaginal wall may indicate a diverticulum. If the diverticulum is small or empty, it is difficult to palpate. Radiographic tests such as intravenous pyelography, voiding cystourethrography, or double balloon urethrography may demonstrate filling of the diverticulum. The orifice of the diverticulum can occasionally be seen on endoscopy.

The optimal treatment for most symptomatic urethral diverticula is surgical excision or obliteration. Distal diverticula may be marsupialized, as described by Spence and Duckett.[19] A small number of diverticula can develop stones or even carcinoma within them, presumably secondary to chronic stasis and infection.

Interstitial Cystitis

It is possible that urethral syndrome represents a milder or earlier form of interstitial cystitis. Interstitial cystitis is a symptom complex typically presenting as frequency, nocturia, urgency, and suprapubic pain often relieved by voiding. As many as 60% of patients may have dyspareunia. It is a chronic and often disabling disease of unknown cause and variable management. Since it was first described by Skene in 1887, its cause has been sought.

Interstitial cystitis is best considered a syndrome. Wide variations in type and severity of symptoms are characteristic. The milder earlier presentations of interstitial cystitis may be called *urethral syndrome, urethrotrigonitis, urgency-frequency syndrome,* or *pseudomembranous trigonitis.* Many patients are not diagnosed with interstitial cystitis until symptoms have become chronic and are more classic. In fact, in an epidemiologic study performed in 1987, it was found that it takes an average of 4.5 years and five doctors to make the diagnosis of interstitial cystitis. In the United States, it is believed that for every patient diagnosed with interstitial cystitis, at least five remain undiagnosed.[20]

Because of the complexities of syndrome definition, it is difficult to estimate the true incidence of interstitial cystitis. Oravisto, in a Finnish study of 103 people with interstitial cystitis, estimated an annual incidence of 1.2 cases per 100,000 and a prevalence of about 10 to 11 per 100,000.[26] It has been estimated that as many as 450,000 individuals in the United States may have interstitial cystitis, and 90% of these are women. The median age of diagnosis is between 40 and 46 years in most series.[20, 21] As many as 30% of patients were found to be younger than 30 years at onset of symptoms in one study of 565 patients with interstitial cystitis.[22] The disease appears mostly in whites but is also reported in blacks.[22] Also reported is an increase as great as 400% in Jewish persons.[23] This disease has a profound effect on patients. According to Koziol, in an epidemiologic study of 565 patients with interstitial cystitis, 30% of patients are unable to work and an additional 32% are unable to work at a position for which they are qualified.[22] When quality of life indicators were assessed, patients with interstitial cystitis scored lower than patients on renal dialysis.[20] Overall, substantial numbers of patients report psychologic difficulties such as anxiety, depression, and strained emotional ties with loved ones.[22]

Although interstitial cystitis was first described more than 100 years ago, its etiology still remains elusive. A number of theories have been set forth, but none has been proved conclusively. Indeed, the pathogenesis most likely is multifactorial. Some of the hypothesized causes of interstitial cystitis include infections, autoimmune disorders, neurogenic factors, inflammatory (especially increased mast cells) conditions, lymphatic obstruction, endocrinologic factors, psychosomatic dysfunction, allergy, and impaired permeability or alteration of the glycosaminoglycan layer.[24]

The diagnosis of interstitial cystitis is in part a diagnosis of exclusion. The diagnosis is linked to its definition, which has been as elusive as the disease itself. To help develop a concise definition of the disease, the National Institute of Arthritis, Diabetes, Digestive and Kidney Diseases (NIDDK) held workshops in August 1987 and November 1988.[25, 26] Consensus criteria (Table 22–2) were established for the diagnosis of interstitial cystitis to help provide uniform criteria for researchers. Many patients who do not fulfill these criteria still can have the disease but should not be considered for research studies.

Office cystoscopy does not reveal the classic findings of interstitial cystitis. Accurate diagnosis can be made only by cystoscopy and hydrodistention under general or regional anesthesia. In this procedure, the bladder is distended to 80 to 100 cm H_2O using gravity filling for 1 to 2 minutes. The bladder may be filled and emptied twice before evaluation. After distention, the typical cystoscopic findings include glomerulations that look like small petechiae or submucosal hemorrhages, fissures, and ulcers. Glomerulations must be diffuse (present in at least three quadrants of the bladder), and there must be at least 10 glomerulations per quadrant. Hemorrhages on the trigone or posterior bladder wall do not constitute a positive finding because these can be caused by scope trauma. It is important to document bladder capacity under anesthesia because this can be a useful prognostic indicator. The bladder of a normal woman holds more than 1000 ml under anesthesia, whereas less than 850 ml capacity is typical for a patient with interstitial cystitis.[27] The average bladder capacity for patients with interstitial cystitis is between 550 and 650 ml.[28]

Bladder biopsy is helpful to preclude other causes of symptoms, such as eosinophilic cystitis, endometriosis, chronic cystitis, and CIS. One should always obtain a biopsy specimen of the bladder after hydrodistention, never before, because bladder rupture or perforation may occur. Interstitial cystitis is not a pathologic diagnosis. Many nonspecific findings may be seen on biopsy, including inflammation, increased numbers of mast cells, mucosal hemorrhage, and mucosal rupture.[29]

Therapy for interstitial cystitis is not usually curative; rather, it is aimed at alleviating the symptoms of the disease. Many treatments are available including pharmacologic, intravesical, nonsurgical, and surgical (Table 22–3). Patients with interstitial cystitis often complain more of pain or pressure symptoms and are less bothered by their underlying urinary frequency. For these patients, amitriptyline has been very helpful. As much as 90% subjective improvement has been noted using 25 to 75 mg of amitriptyline at bedtime.[30] Patients with primary complaints of urinary frequency but fewer complaints of pain or pressure seem to fare well with DMSO or DMSO combination therapy. DMSO has many properties includ-

Table 22–2. **DIAGNOSTIC CRITERIA FOR INTERSTITIAL CYSTITIS**

Automatic Exclusions
Younger than 18 years
Benign or malignant bladder tumors
Radiation cystitis
Tuberculous cystitis
Bacterial cystitis
Vaginitis
Cyclophosphamide cystitis
Symptomatic urethral diverticulum
Uterine, cervical, vaginal, or urethral cancers
Active herpes
Bladder or lower urethral calculi
Waking frequency less than 5 times in 12 hours
Nocturia less than twice nightly
Symptoms relieved by antibiotics, urinary antiseptics, urinary analgesics
Duration less than 12 months
Involuntary bladder contractions (urodynamics)
Capacity greater than 400 ml, absence of sensory urgency

Automatic Inclusions
Hunner's ulcer

Positive Factors
Pain on bladder filling relieved by emptying
Pain (suprapubic, pelvic, urethral, vaginal, or perineal)
Glomerulations after hydrodistention on cystoscopy

Table 22–3. **TREATMENT MODALITIES IN INTERSTITIAL CYSTITIS**

Nonsurgical

Pharmacologic
Antihistamines
Antiinflammatories
Sodium pentosan polysulfate (Elmiron)
Anticholinergics

Intravesical
Dimethyl sulfoxide (DMSO)
$DMSO_2$ (investigational)
DMSO cocktails
Silver nitrate
Sodium oxychlorosene (Chlorpactin)
Cystostat (investigational)
Cromolyn (a mast cell inhibitor) (investigational)

Other
Electric stimulation
Biofeedback
Transcutaneous electric nerve stimulation (TENS)
Epidural block
Bladder pillar block

Surgical
Endoscopic procedures
  Hydrodistention
  Transurethral resection and fulguration
  Neodymium : yttrium-aluminum garnet (Nd : YAG) laser
Open surgical procedures
  Denervation procedures
  Bladder augmentation procedures
  Urinary diversion

ing antiinflammatory, analgesic, muscle relaxant, mast cell inhibition, and collagen dissolution.[31] Overall response rate varies from 50% to 90%, with a relapse rate of 35% to 40%.[32] DMSO is the intravesical treatment used most often, primarily because of its affordability, safety, and ease of office administration. DMSO is administered via a small 8 to 10 French urethral catheter after first anesthetizing the urethra with lidocaine (Xylocaine) 2% jelly. The bladder is drained, and 50 ml of DMSO is instilled by gravity. The patient is instructed to hold the solution for 15 to 20 minutes. DMSO should not be given in the presence of a UTI or immediately after bladder biopsy. It is teratogenic in animals and therefore should not be used in pregnancy. DMSO is sometimes used in combination with additives such as heparin, steroids, sodium bicarbonate, and bupivacaine. Patients may experience a garliclike breath odor or taste in their mouths from the DMSO.

Sodium oxychlorosene (Chlorpactin) has a germicidal activity within the bladder, as well as a detergent effect on the bladder mucosa. A 0.04% solution is typically instilled under general anesthesia. Messing and Stamey reported a 79% success rate after six instillations.[33] Single-lavage therapy has demonstrated improvement in 50% to 60% of patients.[32] Many other intravesical agents have also been used (see Table 22–3).

Hydrodistention of the bladder for diagnosis of interstitial cystitis can also have therapeutic effects in 30% to 60% of patients with interstitial cystitis.[20] Hydrodistention of the bladder may cause ischemia or mechanical damage to the submucosal nerve plexus and stretch receptors in the bladder, and this in turn may lead to reduced pain and frequency and increased bladder capacity.[34]

Conservative measures are especially helpful in patients with milder symptoms. The role of diet, bladder training, stress reduction, and so forth cannot be underestimated. Noninvasive treatments such as biofeedback and electric stimulation can provide relief for some patients. It is important when dealing with patients with interstitial cystitis to have a treatment plan, not only for the current therapy but also for the next step if initial therapy fails. This approach always offers hope to patients trying to cope with this aggravating disease. A tremendous research effort is under way to help determine the cause of interstitial cystitis and improve treatment for this disease.

References

1. Kass EH, Savage W, Santamaria BAG: The significance of bacteriuria in preventive medicine. In Kass ED (ed): Progress in Pyelonephritis. Philadelphia, FA Davis, 1979, pp 3–100.
2. Kelsey MC, Mead MG, Gruneberg RN, et al: Relationship between sexual intercourse and urinary tract infection in women attending a clinic for sexually transmitted disease. J Med Microbiol 1979;12:511.
3. Karram MM: Lower urinary tract infection. In Walters MD, Karram MM (eds): Clinical Urogynecology. St. Louis, CV Mosby, 1993, pp 314–316.
4. Teichman JMH, Parsons CL: Urinary tract infections. In Buchsbaum HJ, Schmidt JD (eds): Gynecologic and Obstetric Urology, 3rd ed. Philadelphia, WB Saunders, 1993, pp 429–440.
5. Reid G, Zorzitto ML, Bruce AW, et al: Pathogenesis of urinary tract infection in the elderly: The role

of bacterial adherence to uroepithelial cells. Curr Microbiol 1984;11:67.
6. Raz R, Stamm WE: A controlled trial on intravaginal estriol in postmenopausal women with recurrent urinary tract infections. N Engl J Med 1993;329:753.
7. Vosti KL: Recurrent urinary tract infection: Prevention by prophylactic antibiotics after sexual intercourse. JAMA 1975;231:934.
8. Pfau A, Sacks T, Englestein D: Recurrant urinary tract infections in premenopausal women. Prophylaxis based on an understanding of the pathogenesis. J Urol 1983;129:1152.
9. Berg AO, Hiedrich FE, Fihn SD, et al: Establishing the cause of genitourinary symptoms in women in a family practice: Comparison of clinical examination and comprehensive microbiology. JAMA 1984;251:620.
10. Karram MM: Frequency, urgency, and painful bladder syndromes. In Walters MD, Karram MM (eds): Clinical Urology and Gynecology. St. Louis, CV Mosby, 1993, pp 285–287.
11. Stamm WE, Wagner KC, Amset R, et al: Causes of the acute urethral syndrome in women. N Engl J Med 1980;303:409.
12. Uehling DT: The normal caliber of the adult female urethra. J Urol 1978;120:176.
13. Bergman A, Karram MM, Bhata NN: Urethral syndrome. A comparison of different treatment modalities. J Reprod Med 1989;34:157.
14. Kaplan WE, Firlit CF, Schoenberg HW: The Female urethral syndrome: External sphincter spasm as etiology. J Urol 1980;124:48.
15. Zufill R: Ineffectiveness of treatment of urethral syndrome in women. Urology 1978;12:337.
16. Carson CC, Segura JW, Osborne DM: Evaluation and treatment of the female urethral syndrome. J Urol 1980;124:609.
17. Davis BL, Robinson DG: Diverticula of the female urethra; assay of 120 cases. J Urol 1970;104:850.
18. Boyd DB, Raz S: Female urethral diverticula. In Raz S (ed): Female Urology. Philadelphia, WB Saunders, 1983, pp 378–393.
19. Spence HM, Duckett JW: Diverticulum of the female urethra: Clinical aspects and presentation of a simple operative technique for cure. J Urol 1970;104:432.
20. Held PJ, Hanno PM, Pauly MV, et al: Epidemiology of interstitial cystitis: 2. In Hanno PM, Staskin DR, Krane RJ, et al: Interstitial Cystitis. New York, Springer-Verlag, 1990, pp 29–48.
21. Ratliff TL, Klutke, CG, McDougall EM: The etiology of interstitial cystitis. Urol Clin North Am 1994;21:21.
22. Koziol JA: Epidemiology of interstitial cystitis. Urol Clin North Am 1994;21:7.
23. Wein AJ, Hanno PM, Gillenwater JY: Interstitial cystitis: An introduction to the problem. In Hanno PM, Staskin DR, Krane RJ, Wein AJ (eds): Interstitial Cystitis. New York, Springer-Verlag, 1990.
24. Johansson SL, Fall M: Pathology of interstitial cystitis. Urol Clin North Am 1994;21:55.
25. Gillenwater JY, Wein AJ: Summary of the National Institute of Arthritis, Diabetes, Digestive and Kidney Diseases workshop on interstitial cystitis. J Urol 1988;140:204.
26. Oravisto KJ: Epidemiology of interstitial cystitis: I. In Hanno PM, Staskin DR, Krane RJ, et al (eds): Interstitial Cystitis. New York, Springer-Verlag, 1990, pp 25–28.
27. Koziol JA: Epidemiology of interstitial cystitis. Urol Clin North Am 1994;21:7.
28. Parsons CL: Interstitial cystitis. In Kursch ED, McGuire EJ (eds): Female Urology. Philadelphia, JB Lippincott, 1994, pp 421–438.
29. Pool TL: Interstitial cystitis: Clinical considerations and treatment. Clin Obstet Gynecol 1967;10:185.
30. Kirkemo AK, Miles BJ, Peters JM: Use of amitriptyline in the treatment of interstitial cystitis. J Urol 1990;143:279A.
31. Sant GR: Intravesical 50% dimethyl sulfoxide (RIMSO 50) in treatment of interstitial cystitis. Urology 1987;29 (Suppl):17.
32. Sant GR, LaRock DR: Standard intravesical therapies for interstitial cystitis. Urol Clin North Am 1994;21:73.
33. Messing EM, Stamey TA: Interstitial cystitis: Early diagnosis, pathology and treatment. Urology 1978;13:389.
34. Hanno PM, Wein AJ: Conservative therapy of interstitial cystitis. Semin Urol 1991;9:143.

23

Gastrointestinal Disorders

William E. Whitehead, PhD

The first section of this chapter briefly describes gastrointestinal (GI) disorders that are associated with pelvic pain and presents information for differential diagnosis. Subsequent sections focus on the irritable bowel syndrome (IBS) because it is the most common GI abdominal pain syndrome and the one most likely to occur in association with (or to be confused with) gynecologic disorders. The chapter describes the overlap between IBS and dysmenorrhea and provides a description of the etiology and management of IBS.

Gastrointestinal Causes of Pelvic Pain: Differential Diagnosis

Irritable Bowel Syndrome. An international committee of experts[1] reported concensus criteria for the diagnosis of IBS. These include abdominal pain that is relieved by defecation or associated with a change in the frequency or consistency or stools, plus two or more of a list of five additional symptoms: altered stool frequency, altered stool form, dyschezia or urgency, passage of mucus, and bloating. Alternative explanations for these symptoms should be sought through a limited set of investigations that include flexible sigmoidoscopy, stool guaiac testing, simple blood chemistry tests to detect any immune reaction (e.g., sedimentation rate or white blood cell count), and thyroid function tests.[2] Figure 23–1 shows the recommended diagnostic algorithm.

Lactose Intolerance. Lactase enzyme deficiency can produce symptoms of abdominal pain, bloating, and diarrhea that may be difficult to distinguish from IBS. However, the occurrence of the symptoms 2 to 3 hours after eating and their relationship to ingestion of milk or milk products distinguish lactase deficiency from other pelvic pain syndromes. Lactose intolerance can be objectively diagnosed by the noninvasive breath hydrogen technique, in which the concentration of hydrogen in expired air is tested at 30-minute intervals for 3 hours after the patient ingests 50 g of lactose. A positive test result is a rise in hydrogen concentration exceeding 20 ppm between 1 and 3 hours after ingestion. Lactose intolerance should be suspected in African Americans (in whom the prevalence is 70%) and in other racial or ethnic groups whose ancestors were indigenous to tropical climates.

Small Bowel Bacterial Overgrowth. Abdominal pain that is associated with bloating and diarrhea and occurs immediately after eating (within 1 hour) and is unrelated to the type of food eaten may be due to proliferation of bacteria in the proximal small intestine. This should be suspected in patients with prior gastric surgery (especially Roux-en-Y) or vagotomy, but it may also occur in patients with idiopathic GI motility disorders (discussed later). Small bowel bacterial overgrowth can be diagnosed by the noninvasive hydrogen breath test. Breath samples should be taken at 15-minute intervals, and a positive response is a rise in hydrogen concentration exceeding 20 ppm within 2 hours after ingesting 80 g of sucrose or other readily absorbed sugar.

Chronic Intestinal Pseudo-Obstruction (CIP). CIP comprises a spectrum of motility abnormalities of the small intestine that give rise to intermittent symptoms that mimic bowel obstruction—that is, rapid abdominal distention unrelated to meals and abdominal pain that is usually severe. These functional bowel obstructions are frequently ac-

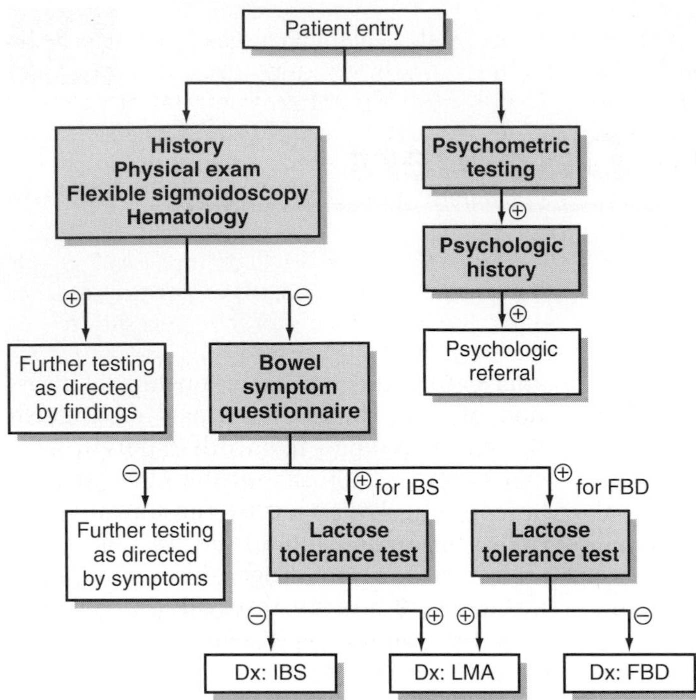

Figure 23–1. Diagnostic algorithm for patients with abdominal pain and altered bowel habits that are refractory to the usual initial treatments. The parallel pathways at the top of the diagram indicate that all patients should receive psychometric testing as well as a history and physical examination on their initial visit. IBS refers to patients who meet Rome diagnostic criteria for irritable bowel syndrome. FBD refers to patients who have abdominal pain or altered bowel habits but who do not meet Rome diagnostic criteria for IBS. LMA refers to lactose malabsorbers. (From Whitehead WE, Schuster MM: Irritable bowel syndrome. In Winawer SJ (ed): Management of Gastrointestinal Diseases. New York, Gower Medical, 1992, p. 32.15.)

companied by nausea, vomiting, and diarrhea. The symptoms typically are unrelated to eating and may be infrequent, with periods of days to weeks between episodes. However, the motility abnormalities that are responsible for these symptoms predispose patients to small bowel bacterial overgrowth, and when this occurs, symptoms may follow most meals.

The diagnosis of CIP is often made on clinical grounds but should be confirmed by a small bowel motility study. This requires that a catheter containing several pressure transducers or perfusion ports be passed transnasally and migrated beyond the pylorus so that pressures can be recorded from at least three points in the small intestine and at least one point in the gastric antrum for a prolonged period (18 to 24 hours is optimal). Fasting small bowel motility is normally characterized by bursts of contractions at 10 to 12 cycles per minute that sweep down the bowel. This is referred to as phase III of the migrating motor complex. The small bowel motility study should also include measurement of gastric and small bowel motility in response to a meal.

Two types of CIP are distinguished on the basis of small bowel motility testing: a myogenic and a neurogenic variety. The myogenic form of CIP is characterized by decreased numbers and decreased amplitudes of contractions and decreased or absent stimulation of contractions after eating a meal. However, when phase III motility patterns occur, these are peristaltic. Myogenic CIP frequently occurs secondary to other disorders such as scleroderma, in which segments of the bowel are atonic and dilated.

The neurogenic variety of CIP is characterized by normal amplitudes and numbers of contractions, but these contractions are disorganized or nonperistaltic. Phase III motility patterns can usually be seen on motility recordings, but they are fragmented and nonperistaltic. The response to eating may include a failure to inhibit the fasting motility pattern (i.e., the cycling of phase III motility patterns) or a normal increase in numbers of contractions following the meal.

Inflammatory Bowel Disease (IBD). Both Crohn's disease and ulcerative colitis may give rise to symptoms of abdominal pain, but the distinguishing sign is bloody diarrhea. Also associated may be signs of fever, an elevated white blood cell count, and swollen joints. The symptoms are unrelated to the phase of the menstrual cycle and are therefore rarely confused with dysmenorrhea. However, in the early stages of the disease before bloody diarrhea has become a prominent symptom, IBD may be confused with IBS or endometriosis affecting the bowel. The differential diagnosis of colonic IBD depends on colonoscopy, and the diagnosis of small bowel IBD depends on upper GI imaging studies (barium follow-through or computed tomography scan).

Diverticular Disease. In diverticular disease, pockets develop adjacent to blood vessels and penetrate into the muscle wall of the bowel. Most diverticula occur in the sigmoid colon. Diverticular disease is usually asymptomatic unless an infection develops in these pockets, after which patients experience abdominal pain, fever, and tenderness on palpation of the abdomen. Diverticulitis is not usually confused with IBS or IBD because of its acute presentation. Differential diagnosis may require a barium enema, which is preferred to sigmoidoscopy because of the risk of perforation. Diverticulitis requires aggressive treatment with antibiotics or surgery or both.

Levator Ani Syndrome and Proctalgia Fugax. Levator ani syndrome[3] is diagnosed when a patient has chronic or recurrent rectal pain or aching in the absence of evidence of an alternative disease process to explain the symptoms. The pain should be described as aching, tenderness, or a feeling of stool in the rectum; it should not be described as burning or stinging, which is characteristic of hemorrhoid disease or anal fissure. The symptoms of levator ani syndrome are usually described as being worse with sitting (as compared with standing or lying down), and the discomfort may be relieved or lessened by hot baths or other applications of heat. The physiologic mechanism for levator ani syndrome is believed to be tonically overcontracted (spastic) striated pelvic floor muscles, and confidence in the diagnosis is increased if the pain is reproduced by traction on the pelvic floor during rectal examination.

Proctalgia fugax is diagnosed on the basis of a fleeting sharp pain in the anal canal or rectum that lasts for seconds or minutes (< 20 minutes) and is followed by long intervals without pain. More than 50% of patients with proctalgia fugax report that the pain occurs fewer than five times per year. Differential diagnosis requires ruling out other anorectal pathology, but the brief and infrequent nature of the symptoms is not consistent with any other common disease entity.

Endometriosis Affecting the Bowel. A relatively common occurrence is implantation of endometrial tissue on the serosal side of the bowel. This tissue is sensitive to reproductive hormone cycling.[4] It may give rise to symptoms of bowel obstruction, including abdominal pain and bloating. This disorder may be difficult to distinguish from other GI disorders such as CIP, IBS, and IBD on the basis of symptoms alone because the symptoms do not reliably vary with the phase of the menstrual cycle. When suspected, the diagnosis requires confirmation by laparoscopy.

Overlap Between Irritable Bowel Syndrome and Dysmenorrhea

A well-documented association is noted between dysmenorrhea and IBS. In a study of 383 women ages 20 to 40 years who were recruited through Planned Parenthood clinics in Maryland, functional bowel disorders were identified in 61% of women with dysmenorrhea but in only 20% of women without dysmenorrhea.[5] A similar high prevalence was observed by Prior and colleagues,[6] who found an overall prevalence of IBS in 37% of patients referred to a gynecology clinic as compared with 28% in dermatology and otorhinolaryngology clinics. These researchers reported that 50% of gynecology patients referred because of abdominal pain, dyspareunia, or dysmenorrhea had IBS.

Gynecologists' failure to identify patients who have IBS and to target treatment at the bowel disorder may lead to unsatisfactory health outcomes. Prior and Whorwell[7] found that women with IBS who consulted gynecologists were less likely to receive a firm diagnosis (8% versus 44%) and were more likely to remain symptomatic at the end of 1 year (65% versus 32%). Whitehead and colleagues[8] found that the prevalence of hysterectomy in women with IBS was three times the national average. Two other research teams[6, 9] also reported that women with IBS were significantly more likely to receive a hysterectomy and less likely to report an improvement in symptoms after this operation.

It is unclear whether the strong association between IBS and dysmenorrhea represents diagnostic confusion or whether dysmenorrhea and IBS have a common physiologic basis. Crowell and coworkers[5] could find no bowel symptoms that reliably distinguished patients with IBS from those with dysmenorrhea, although they did find scales on the Moos[10] Menstrual Distress Questionnaire (scales for water retention, pain, negative affect, and behavior change) that distinguished between IBS and dysmenorrhea.

Whitehead and colleagues[11] found that patients with IBS were significantly more likely than healthy controls or women with a nonspecific functional bowel disorder to report an exacerbation of their bowel symptoms during menses, suggesting a possible physiologic basis for the overlap in diagnoses. The principal bowel symptoms that were worse during menses were bloating and diarrhea. This worsening of bowel symptoms during menses was independent of psychologic symptoms of neuroticism, which were common in these women. Heitkemper and colleagues[12] made similar observations of an exacerbation of bowel symptoms during menses in patients with IBS.

Observations such as these suggested the hypothesis that this exacerbation of bowel symptoms during menses might be related to prostaglandins. Crowell and colleagues[5] tested this hypothesis but found no association between IBS and prostaglandins; levels of prostaglandins E_2 and $F_{2\alpha}$ were higher in women with dysmenorrhea than in women without dysmenorrhea, independently of whether the women had IBS. Thus, it is possible that prostaglandin levels or response to prostaglandin inhibitors may help clinicians to distinguish IBS from dysmenorrhea.

Physiologic Mechanisms for Irritable Bowel Syndrome

Visceral Hyperalgesia. The key symptom in IBS is abdominal pain that is recognized to be GI in origin because it is relieved by defecation or associated with a change in the frequency or consistency of stools.[1, 8] The physiologic basis for this symptom is believed to be increased pain sensitivity, because as a group patients with IBS report pain at a lower threshold when a balloon is distended in the sigmoid colon[13, 14] or rectum.[15, 16] However, some have questioned whether hypersensitivity to rectal distention can account for all IBS cases or only for a subgroup, because only 40% to 60% of patients with IBS report pain at levels of distention below the range of normal values.[17] Others[16] have argued, however, that pain sensitivity is a biologic marker for IBS and that the specificity of this marker is high (i.e., 94%) if multiple pain indicators are combined (i.e., intensity of the reported pain sensation and the pattern of somatic referral of pain elicited by balloon distention of the bowel, in addition to the threshold volume of the balloon at which pain is reported).

A decreased threshold to report pain could reflect a psychologic tendency to label as painful those sensations that others would label as nonpainful, rather than a difference in the sensitivity of peripheral stretch receptors or afferent pathways. This hypothesis is suggested by the frequent observation that patients with IBS tend to report multiple non-GI symptoms and to score high on scales for somatization and hypochondriasis.[18] Data that favor a physiologic explanation over a psychologic explanation for increased pain sensitivity are (1) reports of lower thresholds for nonpainful intensities of sensation such as gas and urgency to defecate[19] and (2) the absence of a significant correlation between pain thresholds and general psychologic measures such as the global symptom index of the SCL-90R scale.[14, 16] However, contrary data on both points have been cited. Some investigators have been unable to show a difference in the threshold for nonpainful sensations resulting from rectal distention,[16] and other investigators do find a correlation between pain thresholds and measures of psychologic distress. No conclusions on the role of psychologic factors in visceral hyperalgesia can be reached at this time.

Colon Motility. Although no distinct pattern of motility is noted only in patients with IBS, these patients show an exaggerated motility response to provocative stimuli including balloon distention of the colon[14] or rectum,[15] psychologic stress,[20] and eating. However, an overlap is observed between patients with IBS and controls, rendering this pattern of hyperreactivity of limited usefulness as a diagnostic marker.

Small Bowel Motility. Patients with IBS also exhibit discrete clustered contractions (i.e., bursts of two to three contractions occurring at intervals of 60 to 120 seconds). Such discrete clustered contractions also occur in healthy subjects, but they are more frequent in patients with IBS and they are more likely to be associated with abdominal pain[21] in IBS. These patients are also more likely to report pain in association with ileal giant propagated contractions, but the frequency of such contractions is no greater than in healthy controls.[22] A third pattern of small bowel motility in IBS is interruption or fragmentation of the phase III motor patterns that characterize fasting small bowel motility.[23, 24] This fragmentation of the normal fasting motility pattern is observed only during waking.

None of the physiologic markers described earlier is specific enough to be used as a diagnostic sign of IBS. This may mean that IBS is a heterogeneous group of disorders, in which case these physiologic events could be markers for subgroups who might respond to specific treatments. This hypothesis is currently being investigated.

Psychologic Mechanisms for Irritable Bowel Syndrome

A majority of patients with IBS who are identified through their attendance at medical clinics have psychiatric disorders or personality disorders.[18] This observation has led some to infer that IBS is a psychiatric disorder without any physiologic basis.[25] However, this is probably not the case because (1) no specific pattern of psychologic traits or symptoms is specific to IBS and (2) people with IBS who have not consulted physicians appear to have no more symptoms of psychologic distress than the rest of the population.[27, 27] This has been interpreted to mean that psychologic symptoms do not cause IBS but do influence which patients seek treatment. Although psychologic symptoms are not useful diagnostic markers for IBS, they affect the management of the disorder and may become the focus of treatment.

Fifty to 85% of patients with IBS report that psychologic stress triggers exacerbations of their bowel symptoms.[28] The effects of stress are independent of the psychologic trait of neuroticism.[29] This strong association between stress and the symptoms of IBS has led to the use of stress management training in the form of progressive muscle relaxation training and biofeedback as a treatment for IBS, as outlined later.

Studies suggest that a history of sexual or physical abuse may contribute to the development of IBS. Drossman and colleagues[30] reported that 53% of gastroenterology clinic patients who had functional GI disorders acknowledged a history of sexual abuse, as compared with 37% of patients with organic diagnoses. This observation of an increased incidence of sexual abuse in women with IBS has been replicated by other investigators.[31, 32] However, the majority of patients with IBS do not report a history of abuse, and the majority of women who report abuse do not have IBS. The mechanisms by which abuse contributes to the development of IBS have not been elucidated.[33]

As the previous review suggests, many physiologic and psychologic factors show a significant association with IBS, but none is specific to IBS. This suggests that IBS is best thought of as a multifactorial disorder in which physiologic, psychologic, and sociocultural factors interact to influence the expression of IBS and the extent of disability and health care use.[34] This model provides a rationale for the usefulness of many different approaches to treatment, either singly or in combination.

Medical Management of Irritable Bowel Syndrome

Medical management of IBS is directed toward management of symptoms rather than treatment of the underlying disorder. Treatment is individualized on the basis of the predominant symptom (Table 23–1).

Diarrhea. Diarrhea in patients with IBS rarely consists of the passage of large-volume watery stools. Rather, it involves the frequent passage of loose stools or defecation accompanied by a strong urge or fecal incontinence. Loperamide (Imodium) has been shown to be effective for reducing stool frequency and urgency,[35] but overdosing and precipitating a slow-transit type of constipation pose a significant risk. This is especially a problem when patients self-medicate with this over-the-counter medication without a physician's supervision. Diphenoxylate, which is combined with atropine in the combination drug Lomotil, may also be effective in diarrhea-predominant IBS, but diphenoxylate crosses the blood-brain barrier and may cause euphoria and addiction (the primary reason it is combined with atropine).

Anticholinergics and smooth muscle relaxing drugs may also be helpful to patients with diarrhea-predominant IBS. A meta-analysis[36] found the anticholinergic cimetropium bromide, the calcium channel blockers pinaverium bromide and octylonium bromide, the opiate antagonist trimebutine, and mebeverine (a β-phenylethylamine with anticholinergic properties) to be superior to placebo. None of these compounds is approved for marketing in the United States, but the older anticholinergics hyoscyamine sulfate (Levsin, Donnatal) and dicyclomine hydrochloride (Bentyl), although not endorsed by this meta-analysis because they have not been adequately tested by controlled studies, appear to be effective in clinical practice. Anticholinergic side effects (e.g., dry mouth, blurred vision) often limit the use of these medications.

The tricyclic antidepressants desipramine (Norpramin)[37] and trimipramine (Surmontil)[38] have also been found to be effective for diarrhea-predominant IBS. Other tricyclic antidepressants may be equally effective, but data on their use in patients with IBS are inadequate to evaluate their efficacy. It is not known whether the beneficial effects of the tricyclics are due to peripheral anticholinergic activity, visceral hyperalgesia, or central nervous system effects on depres-

Table 23–1. **PHARMACOLOGIC TREATMENT OF IRRITABLE BOWEL SYNDROME**

Symptom	Drug	Daily Dose	Major Side Effects
Diarrhea	Loperamide (Imodium)	Titrate: 4 mg average	Constipation
	Diphenoxylate HCl	20 mg	Euphoria, sedation, dry mouth, constipation
	Hyoscyamine sulfate (Levsin, Donnatal)	<1.5 mg	Dry mouth, blurred vision, dizziness
	Dicyclomine HCl (Bentyl)	80–160 mg	Dry mouth, blurred vision, dizziness
	Desipramine HCl (Norpramin)	150 mg	Dry mouth, sedation, confusional states, hypertension, hypotension, constipation
	Trimipramine maleate (Surmontil)	50 mg	Dry mouth, sedation, confusional states, hypertension, hypotension, constipation
Constipation	Fiber from any source	≥30 grams	Bloating, abdominal pain
	Lactulose (Chronulac, Duphalac)	10–30 grams	Bloating
	Sorbitol	10–30 grams	Bloating
	Cisapride (Propulsid)	40–80 mg	Dizziness, headaches
Abdominal pain	Desipramine HCl (Norpramin)	150 mg	Dry mouth, sedation, confusional states, hypertension, hypotension, constipation
	Trimipramine maleate (Surmontil)	50 mg	Dry mouth, sedation, confusional states, hypertension, hypotension, constipation
	Hyoscyamine sulfate (Levsin, Donnatal)	<1.5 mg	Dry mouth, blurred vision, dizziness
	Dicyclomine HCl (Bentyl)	80–160 mg	Dry mouth, blurred vision, dizziness

sion. However, the fact that IBS patients enrolled in treatment studies to date were not selected on the basis of the presence of depression suggests that the central nervous system antidepressant action of these compounds is not what makes them effective.

Constipation. Constipation in patients with IBS is associated with transit times within the normal range but with symptoms of infrequent stools and straining with defecation. Symptoms attributable to pelvic floor dyssynergia (i.e., paradoxic contraction of the pelvic floor muscles rather than relaxing these muscle when straining to defecate) should be precluded. The paradoxic contraction that defines pelvic floor dyssynergia can be detected by digital examination: The anal sphincter should relax around the examining finger rather than contract when the patient strains to defecate.

Conservative management of constipation-predominant IBS is a high-fiber diet or fiber supplementation from artificial sources to achieve an average of at least 30 grams of dietary fiber dialy. This regimen is generally effective if the patient is compliant.[39, 40] However, a diet containing 30 grams of fiber per day is unpalatable to many patients, and adherence frequently falls to 50% or less within 3 months of initiating treatment.[41] This has severely limited the usefulness of fiber supplementation. An osmotic laxative such as lactulose (Chronulac, Duphalac) or sorbitol may be used daily for chronic constipation. Cisapride (Propulsid) has also been reported by some researchers to be effective for constipation-predominant IBS,[42] but not all trials have been positive; therapeutic benefits are modest and the drug is costly.

Pain. Pain in patients with IBS is reported to be improved by use of tricyclic antidepressants.[37, 38] The mechanism by which this is achieved is not known. Some believe the effect is via direct effects on central or peripheral serotonin pathways mediating pain perception,[43] but an indirect effect via central nervous system modulation of depression or other psychologic symptoms, which in turn influences pain perception, has not been precluded. The serotonin reuptake inhibitors have not been investigated in patients with IBS. However, studies show that selective 5-HT3 receptor antagonists lower pain sensitivity in IBS.[44] These compounds may be available for the management of abdominal pain in the future. Two of these agents, ondansetron (Zofran) and granisetron (Kytril), are currently marketed but are licensed only for the short-term treatment of nausea and vomiting associated with chemotherapy. The anticholinergics dicyclomine hydrochloride and hyoscyamine sulfate are also reported anecdotally to decrease the frequency and severity of abdominal pain in IBS.

Psychologic Treatments for Irritable Bowel Syndrome

Relaxation Training. The simplest behavioral treatment for IBS is progressive muscle relaxation training. This is a form of stress or anxiety management that involves teaching patients to tense and relax groups of skeletal muscles systematically while attending to the sensations in the muscles. Two studies have reported that progressive muscle relaxation training was effective at reducing the symptoms of pain and diarrhea.[45, 46] In addition, progressive muscle relaxation has been combined with other psychologic treatment approaches in several successful treatment studies.[47, 48]

Cognitive-Behavioral Therapy. Cognitive-behavioral therapy refers to techniques for teaching patients to recognize self-defeating thoughts that contribute to depression or anxiety and to substitute more positive thoughts for them. An example would be teaching patients to recognize that they react to any sensation from the GI tract with the thought that they will inevitably develop pain and diarrhea, which will make it impossible for them to do their work or to socialize. They might be taught to try to catch themselves thinking along these lines and to substitute thoughts that they can now control these bowel symptoms by relaxation or biofeedback. Blanchard and colleagues[47] conducted a series of studies in which such an approach was successfully used to reduce the frequency and severity of IBS.

Hypnosis. How hypnosis works has not been established, but it involves a hypersuggestible state that can be induced by (1) narrowing the subject's focus of attention and (2) reinforcing the subject's natural tendency to follow the therapist's suggestions by "suggesting" experiences that will occur naturally. For example, hypnotic induction frequently begins by having subjects stare at a fixed object without blinking and then suggesting that their eyelids are becomming heavy. This reinforces the sensations associated with fatigue of the extraocular muscles and makes the subject more inclined to follow further suggestions. This may be followed by suggesting that the subject use imagery to help him or her achieve skeletal muscle relaxation. Weekly or biweekly training sessions of this kind may be combined with home practice of autohypnosis using an audiotape. Whorwell and colleagues[49] reported that hypnosis of this type was associated with significantly greater decreases in abdominal pain and diarrhea than was achieved by a placebo pill and discussions of the role of emotions in IBS. These benefits were well maintained at follow-up a year later if patients continued to use autohypnosis.[50] However, subjects older than 55 years and subjects with significant amounts of anxiety and depression were less likely to benefit. Other research groups have also found that hypnosis is beneficial for IBS.[51]

Psychotherapy. Brief interpersonal psychotherapy was reported in two studies to be superior to continuation of medical therapy for the treatment of IBS.[48, 52] In the more recent of these two very similar studies, Guthrie and colleagues[48] provided psychotherapy that consisted of discussions of interpersonal problems that patients were currently experiencing, which the psychotherapist used to demonstrate to patients how they were using maladaptive coping mechanisms. The therapist encouraged more appropriate coping techniques and taught patients progressive muscle relaxation training. The psychotherapist saw patients on six occasions during a 3-month period. This approach to psychotherapy was associated with significant improvements in abdominal pain and diarrhea as well as psychologic distress, and these improvements were still present at 12-months' follow-up. Guthrie and colleagues noted that their treatment was more effective in patients who were aware of a relationship between stress and bowel symptoms and in patients who were anxious. Interpersonal psychotherapy was less effective in patients who reported chronic unremitting abdominal pain.

Overview of Psychologic Treatments for Irritable Bowel Syndrome. No studies have directly compared the effectiveness of these different psychologic interventions, and in fact available data suggest that they may produce similar outcomes. The skill of the therapist as determined by training and experience may have more to do with the outcome than the particular technique used. Limited data suggest that hypnosis may work better than psychotherapy in young patients who report little stress or anxiety. Conversely, interpersonal psychotherapy, relaxation training, or cognitive behavior therapy may work better for more anxious patients.

A disadvantage of all these psychologic techniques is that they require special skills and training not possessed by most internists. This means that patients must be referred to a psychologist or psychiatrist, and many patients will not comply with the recommendation to see a mental health care provider. Thus, for both practical and economic reasons, it is recommended that the first approach to treatment consist of fiber supplementation for constipated patients, anticholinergics for diarrhea-predominant patients, or a tricyclic antidepressant for patients whose main complaint is pain. If these interventions fail or if psychologic distress is significant, referral to a psychologist or a psychiatrist should be considered.

Summary

Many GI conditions may cause abdominal pain, but the GI disorder most likely to be confused with painful gynecologic conditions is IBS. IBS affects 50% to 60% of women who consult gynecologists for pelvic pain, and it is often unrecognized. This may have consequences for management because women with IBS are more likely to receive a hysterectomy and are less likely to benefit from this operation.

The cause of IBS is poorly understood, and a multifactorial model of disease in which physiologic and psychosocial causes interact provides the best approach to understanding and treating this disorder. Medical management of IBS is targeted at the bowel symptoms that are most troublesome for the individual patient: For patients with diarrhea-predominant symptoms, use of loperamide or anticholinergics has been helpful, whereas for patients with constipation-predominant symptoms, increased dietary fiber is the most conservative treatment. Pain-predominant IBS may respond to tricyclic antidepressants or anticholinergics. When medical management alone does not provide adequate relief of IBS symptoms, psychologic treatments should be considered. Psychologic treatments found to be effective for the management of IBS in controlled trials include relaxation training, hypnosis, cognitive-behavioral therapy, and interpersonal psychotherapy.

Acknowledgment

Preparation Supported in Part by Grants KO5 MH00133 and RO1 DK31369

References

1. Thompson WG, Creed F, Drossman DA, et al: Functional bowel disease and functional abdominal pain. Gastroenterol Int 1992;5:75.
2. Whitehead WE, Schuster MM: Irritable bowel syndrome. In Winawer SJ (ed): Management of Gastrointestinal Diseases, vol 2. New York, Gower Medical, 1992, pp 32.1–32.25.
3. Whitehead WE, Devroede G, Habib FI, et al: Report of an international workshop on functional disorders of the anorectum. Gastroenterol Int 1992;5:92.
4. Zwas FR, Lyon DT: Endometriosis: An important condition in clinical gastroenterology. Dig Dis Sci 1991;36:353.
5. Crowell MD, Dubin NH, Robinson JC, et al: Functional bowel disorders in women with dysmenorrhea. Am J Gastroenterol 1994;89:1973.
6. Prior A, Wilson K, Whorwell PJ, Faragher EB: Irritable bowel syndrome in the gynecological clinic. Dig Dis Sci 1989;34:1820.
7. Prior A, Whorwell PJ: Gynaecological consultation in patients with the irritable bowel syndrome. Gut 1989;30:996.
8. Whitehead WE, Crowell MD, Bosmajian L, et al: Existence of irritable bowel syndrome supported by factor analysis of symptoms in two community samples. Gastroenterology 1990;98:336.
9. Longstreth GF, Preskill DB, Youkeles L: Irritable bowel syndrome in women having diagnostic laparoscopy or hysterectomy. Relation to gynecologic features and outcome. Dig Dis Sci 1990;35:1285.
10. Moos RH: Perimenstrual symptoms: A manual and overview of research with the Menstrual Distress Questionnaire. Palo Alto, CA, Department of Psychiatry and Behavioral Sciences, Stanford University School of Medicine, 1985.
11. Whitehead WE, Cheskin LJ, Heller BR, et al: Evidence for exacerbation of irritable bowel syndrome during menses. Gastroenterology 1990;98:1485.
12. Heitkemper MM, Jarrett M, Cain KC, et al: Daily gastrointestinal symptoms in women with and without a diagnosis of IBS. Dig Dis Sci 1995; 40:1511.
13. Ritchie J: Pain from distention of the pelvic colon by inflating a balloon in the irritable colon syndrome. Gut 1973;14:125.
14. Whitehead WE, Holtkotter B, Enck P, et al: Tolerance for rectosigmoid distention in irritable bowel syndrome. Gastroenterology 1990;98:1187.
15. Whitehead WE, Engel BT, Schuster MM: Irritable bowel syndrome: Physiological and psychological differences between diarrhea-predominant and constipation-predominant patients. Dig Dis Sci 1980;25:404.
16. Mertz H, Naliboff B, Munakata J, et al: Altered rectal perception is a biological marker of patients with irritable bowel syndrome. Gastroenterology 1995;109:40.
17. Lembo T, Munakata J, Mertz H, et al: Evidence for the hypersesitivity of lumbar splanchnic afferents in irritable bowel syndrome. Gastroenterology 1994;107:1686.
18. Whitehead WE: The disturbed psyche and the irritable gut. Eur J Gastroenterol Hepatol 1994;6:483.
19. Prior A, Maxton DG, Whorwell PJ: Anorectal manometry in irritable bowel syndrome: Differences between diarrhoea and constipation predominant subjects. Gut 1990;31:458.
20. Fakudo S, Suzuki J: Colonic motility, autonomic function, and gastrointestinal hormones under psychological stress in irritable bowel syndrome. Tohoku J Exp Med 1987;151:373.
21. Kellow JE, Gill RC, Wingate DL: Prolonged ambulant recordings of small bowel motility demonstrate abnormalities in the irritable bowel syndrome. Gastroenterology 1990;98:1208.
22. Kellow JE, Phillips SF, Miller LJ, Zinsmeister AR: Dysmotility of the small intestine in irritable bowel syndrome. Gut 1988;29:1236.
23. Kumar D, Wingate DL: The irritable bowel syndrome: A paroxysmal motor disorder. Lancet 1985;2:973.
24. Kumar D, Thompson PD, Wingate DL, et al: Abnormal REM sleep in the irritable bowel syndrome. Gastroenterology 1992;103:12.
25. Walker EA, Roy-Byrne PP, Katon WJ: Irritable bowel syndrome and psychiatric illness. Am J Psychiatry 1990;147:565.
26. Drossman DA, McKee DC, Sandler RS, et al: Psychological factors in the irritable bowel syndrome. A multivariate study of patients and nonpatients with irritable bowel syndrome. Gastroenterology 1988;95:701.
27. Whitehead WE, Bosmajian L, Zonderman AB, et al: Symptoms of psychologic distress associated with

irritable bowel syndrome: Comparison of community and medical clinic samples. Gastroenterology 1988;95:709.
28. Drossman DA, Sandler RS, McKee DC, Lovitz AJ: Bowel patterns among subjects not seeking health care. Gastroenterology 1982;83:529.
29. Whitehead WE, Crowell MD, Robinson JC, et al: Effects of stressful life events on bowel symptoms: Subjects with irritable bowel syndrome compared with subjects without bowel dysfunction. Gut 1992;33:825.
30. Drossman DA, Leserman J, Nachman G, et al: Sexual and physical abuse in women with functional or organic gastrointestinal disorders. Ann Intern Med 1990;113:828.
31. Longstreth GF, Wolde-Tsadik G: Irritable bowel-type symptoms in HMO examinees: Prevalence, demographics, and clinical correlates. Dig Dis Sci 1993;38:1581.
32. Talley NJ, Fett SL, Zinsmeister AR, Melton LJ III: Gastrointestinal tract symptoms and self-reported abuse: A population-based study. Gastroenterology 1994;107:1040.
33. Drossman DA, Talley NJ, Leserman J, et al: Sexual and physical abuse and gastrointestinal illness: Review and recommendations. Ann Intern Med 1995;123:782.
34. Drossman DA, Creed FH, Fava GA, et al: Psychosocial aspects of the functional gastrointestinal disorders. Gastroenterol Int 1995;8:47.
35. Cann PA, Read NW, Holdsworth CD, Barends D: Role of loperamide and placebo in management of irritable bowel syndrome (IBS). Dig Dis Sci 1984;29:239.
36. Poynard T, Naveau S, Mory B, Chaput JC: Meta-analysis of smooth muscle relaxers in the treatment of irritable bowel syndrome. Aliment Pharmacol Ther 1994;8:499.
37. Greenbaum DS, Mayle JE, Vanegeren LE, et al: Effects of desipramine on irritable bowel syndrome compared with atropine and placebo. Dig Dis Sci 1987;32:257.
38. Myren J, Lovland B, Larssen SE, and the Multicentre Group of Practitioners Conducted by Specialists in Gastroenterology: A double-blind study of the effect of timipramine in patients with the irritable bowel syndrome. Scand J Gastroenterol 1984;19:835.
39. Cann PA, Read NW, Holdsworth CD: What is the benefit of coarse wheat bran in patients with irritable bowel syndrome? Gut 1984;25:168.
40. Kumar A, Kumar N, Vij JC, et al: Optimum dosage of ispaghula husk in patients with irritable bowel syndrome: Correlation of symptom relief with whole gut transit time and stool weight. Gut 1987;28:150.
41. Kruis W, Winszierl M, Schussler P, Holl J: Comparison of the therapeutic effect of wheat bran, mebeverine and placebo in patients with the irritable bowel syndrome. Digestion 1986;34:196.
42. Mueller-Lissner SA: Cisapride in chronic idiopathic constipation: Can the colon be re-educated? Bavarian Constipation Study Group. Eur J Gastroenterol Hepatol 1995;7:69.
43. Mayer EA, Gebhart GF: Basic and clinical aspects of visceral hyperalgesia. Gastroenterology 1994; 107:271.
44. Talley NJ: Review article: 5-Hydroxytryptamine agonists and antagonists in the modulation of gastrointestinal motility and sensation: Clinical implications. Aliment Pharmacol Ther 1992;6:273.
45. Voirol MW, Hipolito J: Anthropo-analytical relaxation in irritable bowel syndrome: Results 40 months later. Schweiz Med Wochenschr 1987; 117:1117.
46. Blanchard EB, Greene B, Scharff L, Schwarz-McMorris SP: Relaxation training as a treatment for irritable bowel syndrome. Biofeedback Self Regul 1993;18:125.
47. Blanchard EB, Schwarz SP, Suls JM, et al: Two controlled evaluations of a multicomponent psychological treatment of irritable bowel syndrome. Behav Res Ther 1992;2:175.
48. Guthrie E, Creed F, Dawson D, Tomenson B: A controlled trial of psychological treatment for the irritable bowel syndrome. Gastroenterology 1991;100:450.
49. Whorwell PJ, Prior A, Faragher EB: Controlled trial of hypnotherapy in the treatment of severe refractory irritable-bowel syndrome. Lancet 1984;2:1232.
50. Whorwell PJ, Prior A, Colgan SM: Hypnotherapy in severe irritable bowel syndrome: Further experience. Gut 1987;28:423.
51. Harvey RF, Hinton RA, Gunary RM, Barry RE: Individual and group hypnotherapy in treatment of refractory irritable bowel syndrome. Lancet 1989;1:424.
52. Svedlund J, Sjodin I, Otosson J-O, Dotevall G: Controlled study of psychotherapy in irritable bowel syndrome. Lancet 1983;2:589.

24

Musculoskeletal Problems

Patricia King Baker, MA, PT

Musculoskeletal dysfunctions have been clearly demonstrated as significant factors, both primary and secondary, in the etiology and clinical manifestation of chronic pelvic pain (CPP).[1–15] Although the relationship between musculoskeletal dysfunctions and CPP is established and reports of successful management are statistically impressive,[6, 9, 10, 13] the information available in the literature on musculoskeletal aspects of this frustrating clinical problem remains somewhat sparse. Detailed attention to screening for musculoskeletal dysfunctions and consultation with practitioners skilled in musculoskeletal examination and treatment contribute importantly to the treatment of this population.

Many musculoskeletal structures of the back and lower extremities share segmental innervation with urogenital structures. Table 24–1 illustrates the segmental innervation and referred pain sites of musculoskeletal structures commonly involved in CPP. Pain referred from these musculoskeletal structures could easily mimic urogenital pelvic pain; this theory is supported by clinical reports.[6, 9, 10, 13–18] Because of overlapping pain patterns as well as the potential comorbidity of musculoskeletal and urogenital dysfunctions, practitioners dealing with CPP on a routine basis need skills in screening the musculoskeletal system or close referral relationships with practitioners skilled in this area.

This chapter addresses the musculoskeletal dysfunctions and diseases commonly associated with CPP in terms of their etiology, clinical signs and symptoms, and treatment recommendations. Presented here is a musculoskeletal screening examination that can help gynecologists, internists, or family practice physicians determine if referral to a musculoskeletal practitioner is warranted. Detailed diagnostic procedures that might be performed by a physical therapist or orthopedic physician are described.

Basic Biomechanics of the Low Back and Pelvis

Bony Structure and Function

The bony pelvis is composed of the innominate, sacrum, and coccyx (Fig. 24–1).[19] The innominate has three components—the ischium, ilium, and pubis—which are fused in an adult. The mobile articulations present in the pelvis include the two sacroiliac joints, the pubic symphysis, and the sacrococcygeal articulation. Additionally, the acetabulum of the innominate articulates with the femoral head (the hip), and the base or superior aspect of the sacrum articulates with the fifth lumbar vertebra (L5–S1).

The primary functions of the bony pelvis are to (1) transfer weight-bearing forces between the trunk and lower extremities, (2) support and protect the pelvic viscera, (3) provide attachments for the muscular and ligamentous structures, and (4) serve as the birth canal and provide support and protection for the fetus in women.

Weight-bearing forces are transferred downward from the lumbar spine through the sacroiliac articulations and out to the hips. This process occurs in reverse as weight-bearing forces are transferred superiorly from the lower extremity to the trunk in the stance phase of the gait cycle. Understanding these normal force transmission relationships can facilitate the interpretation of history and clinical signs of pathologic states. For example, a traumatic force ex-

Table 24–1. **MUSCULOSKELETAL ORIGINS OF CHRONIC PELVIC PAIN**

Structure	Innervation	Referred Pain Site(s)	Common Disorders
Hip	T12–S1	Lower abdomen; anterior medial thigh; knee	DJD; capsular stiffness or inflammation; bursitis
Lumbar ligaments, facets/disks	T12–S1	Low back; posterior thigh and calf; lower abdomen; lateral trunk; buttock	DJD; capsular entrapments; instability; herniation; capsular stiffness and inflammation
Sacroiliac joints	L4–S3	Posterior thigh; buttock; pelvic floor	Acute strain; laxity, displacement
Abdominal muscles	T5–L1	Abdomen; anteromedial thigh; sternum	Weakness; strain; diastasis; trigger points
Iliopsoas	L1–L4	Lateral trunk; lower abdomen; low back; anterior thigh	Adaptive shortening; trigger points; protective guarding
Piriformis	L5–S3	Low back; buttock; pelvic floor	Adaptive shortening; trigger points; protective guarding
Pubococcygeus	S1–S4	Pelvic floor; vagina; rectum; buttock	Adaptive shortening; weakness; lengthening strain; trigger points
Obturator internal/external	L3–S2	Pelvic floor; buttock; anterior thigh	Adaptive shortening; protective guarding; weakness
Quadratus lumborum	T12–L3	Anterior lateral trunk; anterior thigh; lower abdomen	Adaptive shortening weakness

DJD, degenerative joint disease.

From King Baker P: Musculoskeletal origins of chronic pelvic pain. Obstet Gynecol Clin North Am 1993;20:719.

erted through the lower extremity upward into the acetabulum (as might occur when an individual slips off a curb or misses a step) may result in sprain or strain of the sacroiliac joints or pubic symphysis as the innominate is driven posteriorly by the upward force. This is pertinent to this discussion of pelvic pain because sacroiliac trauma, particularly when severe, may be accompanied by some strain or even separation of the pubic symphysis, which produces anterior lower abdominal pain. Osteoporosis of the spine may predispose to thoracic or lumbar spinal compression fracture, with referred pain in the abdomen.

Consistent with the primary supportive and protective functions of the pelvis, the articulations are designed principally for

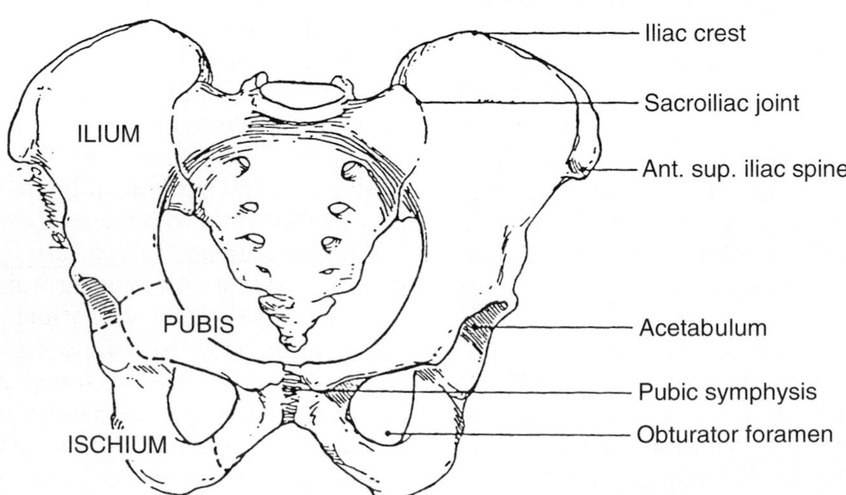

Figure 24–1. Osseous anatomy of the pelvic girdle. (From Gould SF: Anatomy. In Gabbe SG, Neibyl JR, Simpson JL: Obstetrics: Normal and Abnormal Pregnancies, 2nd ed. New York, Churchill Livingstone, 1991.)

stability.[20–24] The sacroiliac articulations are classified as synovial joints but are atypical in that the iliac surface is covered with fibrocartilage rather than hyaline cartilage. The sacral surface is covered by a thick hyaline cartilage. Fibrocartilaginous joint surfaces are covered with hyaline cartilage. The length, width, and shape of the articular surfaces vary significantly between individuals and along gender lines. The smaller surface area of the female sacroiliac makes it potentially more mobile than that of the male. The variations and irregularities in the sacroiliac articulation are thought to contribute to the degenerative changes noted in both sexes. The pubic symphysis is a stable yet mobile cartilaginous joint. Superior and inferior movement of the pubis occurs in normal gait and in response to torsional movements of the ilium in other activities. Its movement in pregnancy and childbirth is well established.[23, 25–27]

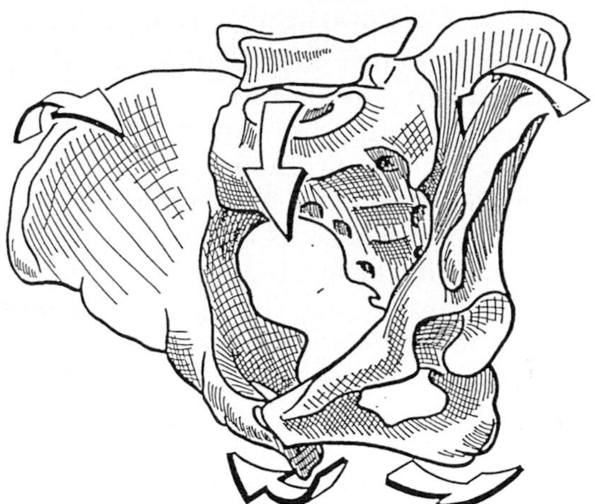

Figure 24–2. Inflare of the ilium and nutation of the sacrum. (From Kapandji IA: The Physiology of the Joints, vol 3. The Trunk and Vertebral Column. New York, Churchill Livingstone, 1994.)

Kinematics

The significance of mobility in the sacroiliac joints and pubic symphysis has been and continues to be debated among practitioners. However, that these articulations are mobile and remain so throughout most of adulthood, particularly in females, is well documented.[20] The mechanical relationships in the pelvic girdle have been studied by osteopaths, physical therapists, and radiologists.[25–31]

The principal movements of the sacrum relative to the ilium are nutation and counternutation (Fig. 24–2). In nutation, the base or superior surface of the sacrum tilts anteriorly and the sacral apex or inferior pole tilts posteriorly. This movement is thought to combine with extension of the sacrococcygeal articulation in childbirth to increase the anteroposterior diameter of the birth canal. Slight sacral nutation is considered normal in standing posture, as is a slight lumbar lordotic curve. Sacral nutation accompanies lumbar flexion or forward bending during active movement. Nutation places a shear force on the sacroiliac articulations and an anteroposterior strain on the posterior sacroiliac ligaments, including the sacrotuberous and sacrospinous, which resist that movement. Counternutation or posterior tilting of the base of the sacrum is usually accompanied by lumbar flexion or forward bending (flat back posture) when present as a postural adaptation. Side bending and rotation movements of the sacrum are thought to occur in combination with nutation and counternutation in normal gait.

The principal movements of the ilium in reference to the sacrum are anterior and posterior torsion (sometimes referred to as *rotations*), inflare and outflare, upslip and downslip (see Fig. 24–2). Anterior and posterior torsional movements occur in the normal gait cycle. A slight anterior tilt of the pelvis with the anterior superior iliac spines (ASIS) being approximately one-fourth inch lower than the posterior superior iliac spines (PSIS) is expected in normal standing posture. Repetitive strains due to faulty postural habits such as standing on one foot, prone sleeping, and pregnancy contribute to exaggerations of pelvic tilt and ilial torsion unilaterally and bilaterally. Traumatic events such as motor vehicle accidents and childbirth may also contribute to dysfunctions and even result in anterior displacement of the articulation. The anterior sacroiliac ligaments are often torn in childbirth, diminishing the likelihood of return of optimal pelvic stability postpartum without specific attention to posture and strengthening exercises to compensate for ligamentous strain and protect from further stretching secondary to faulty posture.

Posterior rotation and outflare of the ilium normally occur in pregnancy as the abdominal cavity is enlarged to accommodate the fetus. These movements are checked by the ligaments and capsule of the pubic symphysis and anterior sacroiliac joints. Outflare and inflare are commonly assessed by comparing the distances between the ASIS and the umbilicus bilaterally. Outflare, the common position in pregnancy, is usually accompanied by external rotation of the hips. Without attention to postpartum stretching, chronic stiffness with loss of internal rotation and extension in the hips may manifest as a chronic condition postpartum. A reduction in internal rotation range of motion of the hip has been identified as a common occurrence in the pelvic pain[9, 10] and low back pain[32] populations and may be associated with sacroiliac dysfunction as either a primary or secondary problem. Joint hypomobility is not likely to cause nociceptive activity until the stiff joint is strained or inflamed, as often happens when sedentary individuals engage in physical activity that is not part of their ordinary routine. Joint hypomobility is thought to be an etiologic factor in the development of a neighboring joint hypermobility, which often presents clinically with signs of acute inflammation. For example, many practitioners report stiff hips accompanying painful, hypermobile sacroiliac joints or lumbosacral joints.[33, 34]

Neighboring articulations outside the pelvis proper have a role in pelvic mechanics and in the etiology of some of the dysfunctions associated with CPP. Both the L5–S1 and hip articulations contribute to altered pelvic mechanics and CPP symptoms. Although the L5–S1 articulation does not directly move the sacroiliac or pubic symphysis, it indirectly affects the mechanics of the pelvic girdle through articular and myofascial kinetic relationships. The base or superior surface of the sacrum articulates with the body and lateral facets of the fifth lumbar (L5) vertebra, and the posterior aspect of the iliac crest gives rise to the iliolumbar ligament, which attaches to the transverse processes of L4 and L5 in females and usually to L4 alone in males. The iliolumbar ligament, for example, whose sensory innervation arises from L1, has been incriminated in anterior iliac crest pain.[35] Spondylolisthesis and other changes in lumbar position and mobility as well as iliosacral torsional strains may contribute to irritation of the iliolumbar ligament and the development of anterior, low abdominal pain.

Muscles: Mechanical Relationships, Function and Dysfunction

Changes in hip posture and mobility alter pelvic mechanics via direct muscle action and myofascial length/tension relationships. Hip flexion, extension, abduction, adduction, and internal and external rotation affect the anteroposterior and lateral tilt of the pelvis by both articular and myofascial kinematic relationships. A mechanism for altered hip rotation range of motion secondary to pregnancy posture was mentioned earlier. The position of hip flexion is usually accompanied by posterior rotation or torsion of the ilium (Fig. 24–3*A* and *B*) and hip extension by an anterior ilial torsion (Fig. 24–3*C*). The relationship between hip external and internal rotation and ilial inflare and outflare was already presented.

Muscles attaching to the bony pelvis and influencing its function include the muscles of the pelvic floor or levator ani and to a lesser degree the muscles of the external genitalia and urogenital diaphragm; the abdominals; the flexors, extensors, adductors, abductors, and rotators of the hip; and the extensors and rotators of the thoracic and lumbar spine. The length and hence resting tone and strength of all these muscles may be altered by changes in the posture and mobility of the bony pelvis as well as by metabolic and neurophysiologic changes.

Pelvic Floor

The pelvic floor muscles or levator ani support the pelvic viscera[36, 38] and in doing so must counteract gravitational as well as intraabdominal forces. The levator ani comprises two distinct muscles, the iliococcygeus and the pubococcygeus. The strength

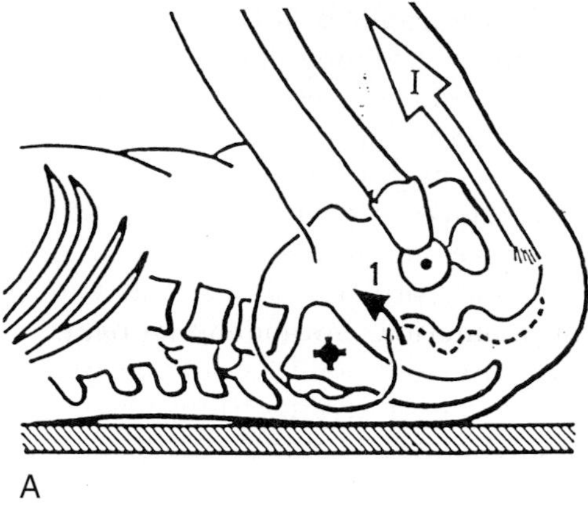

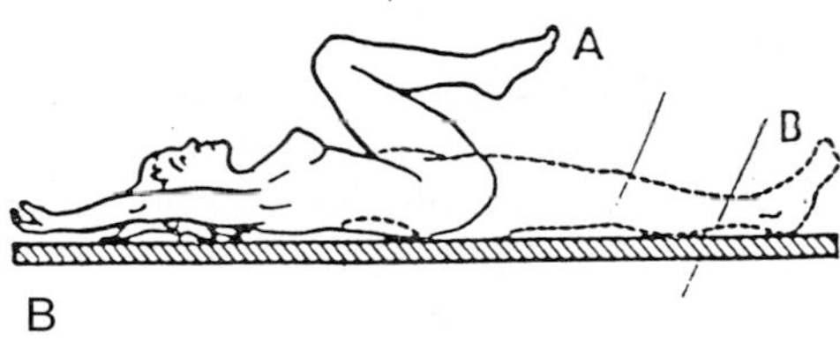

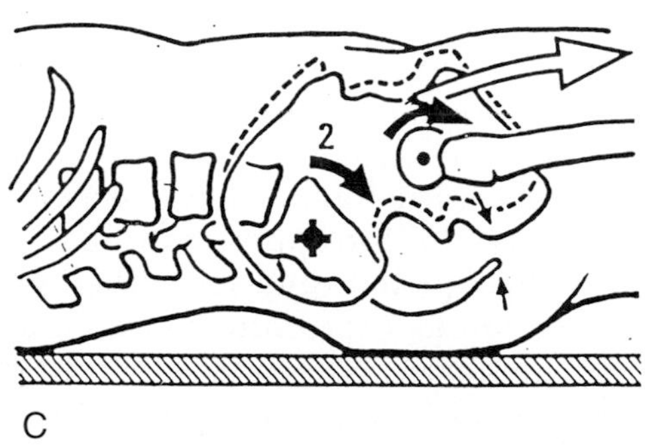

Figure 24–3. *A* and *B*: Posterior ilial rotation occurring with hip flexion; *C*: Anterior ilial rotation and sacral nutation (black arrows) occurring with hip extension (white arrows). (From Kapandji IA: The Physiology of the Joints, vol 3: The Trunk and Vertebral Column. New York, Churchill Livingstone, 1994.)

of the levator ani is considered the primary factor in the maintenance of normal anatomic relationships of the pelvic viscera, with ligamentous tension counteracting downward forces only when pelvic floor muscle support is diminished.[37, 39] Intraabdominal pressure is increased with Valsalva's manuever, which often occurs in lifting, childbirth, and defecation. This musculature also functions during sexual intercourse, has a primary role in continence, and must relax and distend during labor and delivery.

Muscle has a normal physiologic resting tone that is increased with active contraction, fatigue, and stress and diminished by disuse and by metabolic and neurophysiologic compromise. Type I muscles fibers, designed for sustained contraction and endurance, account for a large portion of pelvic floor muscle tissue.[37] Disuse and denervation appear to be major factors in the development of pelvic floor relaxation dysfunctions. Like degenerative joint disease (DJD) of the hip,[40] pelvic floor relaxation has been associated with sedentary Western lifestyles and is known to be rare in societies that use squatting more than sitting posture. Squatting does not stretch the pelvic floor musculature, whereas prolonged sitting does.[40, 41] Patterns of muscle imbalance common in patients with pelvic pain and low back pain[9, 10, 42] may also exert stretching forces on the pelvic floor. Western methods of childbirth, which minimize assistance from gravity and the ability of the birth canal to increase its anteroposterior diameter because the mother is supine on a hard surface, are thought to contribute to pelvic floor strain. Women delivering in this position often resort to Valsalva's pushing, with resultant pelvic floor strain and the now expected phenomenon of postpartum hemorrhoids. This type of strain should also be considered a possible factor in the development of postpartum pelvic pain.

Abdominals

The abdominals principally serve to support the abdominal viscera and have a slight role in maintaining the normal lordotic curve in upright posture. The abdominals contribute to stabilization of the trunk during lifting and work in synergy with the levator ani. Weakening of the abdominals may occur secondary to sustained stretching in the excessive anterior pelvic tilt position, which is pronounced during pregnancy and in the CPP population.

Prime Movers of the Hip

Specific muscles with the principal function of moving the sacroiliac articulations do not exist. Pelvic girdle movement occurs as a result of the action of hip and low back muscles attached to the bony pelvis and of kinetic forces exerted through articular structures (ligaments, capsules, discs) of the lumbar spine to the pelvis. The piriformis, for example, attaches to the anterior aspect of the sacrum and moves the sacral base anteriorly (nutation) when the femur is fixed. Its principal action is hip external rotation. The hip adductors attach to the pubis, and with a fixed femur their contraction exerts a downward force, contributing to anterior rotation of the innominate. The action of the hip flexors (e.g., iliopsoas and rectus femoris) produces an anterior torsional force on the ilium, whereas the hip extensor muscles (gluteus maximus and others) work in a force couple with the abdominals to rotate the ilium posteriorly.

Iliopsoas

The iliopsoas muscle is active in upright, resting posture and attaches to the ilium, femur, lumbar spine, and diaphragm. Its length is frequently compromised in conjunction with faulty posture in persons with pelvic pain and low back pain.[9, 10, 42, 43] Hypertonus in this muscle is also a common finding in those groups. Referred pain from the iliopsoas is usually reported to occur in the lower abdominal area, lateral to the rectus and superior to the inguinal ligament—the exact location of most CPP complaints, in my experience. Its action or adaptive shortening serves to increase hip flexion, anterior pelvic tilt/rotation, and lumbar extension and rotation—all associated with musculoskeletal pelvic pain (see the later discussion on typical pelvic pain [TPP] posture).

Evolution of Musculoskeletal Problems

Musculoskeletal problems identified as primary causative factors in CPP appear to occur most commonly in response to chronic repetitive stress and strain associated with faulty posture, poor body mechanics, and poor physical conditioning. Table 24–2 lists musculoskeletal dysfunctions reported in the CPP population. Direct trauma to musculoskeletal structures is described less frequently but is reported secondary to accidents, surgical procedures, and more "normal" types of trauma such as childbirth. Musculoskeletal problems may also present as secondary problems in patients with pelvic pain, as in the muscular hypertonus that occurs with segmental facilitation from primary urogenital dysfunction, postsurgical disuse, healing complications, or psychogenic disturbance.

Musculoskeletal problems are further categorized as either dysfunctions or diseases. Dysfunctions of the musculoskeletal system have been defined by Paris[34] as "a state of altered mechanics, clinically manifested as either an increase or decrease in expected range of motion or by the presence of an aberrant motion." Musculoskeletal dysfunctions include sprains, strains, abnormal strength and flexibility, and degenerative conditions. Musculoskeletal dysfunctions are identified and managed by physical therapists. Musculoskeletal disease states, however, should be diagnosed and managed by orthopedic or other appropriately prepared physicians. Fractures do not fit the explicit definition of dysfunction or disease but belong in the jurisdiction of physicians, usually orthopedic, for appropriate management. Orthopedic physical therapists routinely conduct screening examinations for the presence of disease and fractures. The examination of the patients with CPP should be conducted with the possibility of such pathologies in mind.

Primary Musculoskeletal Problems

Shared segmental innervation exists between many musculoskeletal structures of the lower quarter and the organs and soft tissues of the urogenital system, allowing the clinical phenomenon of referred pain. The close anatomic proximity of urogenital structures to the site of pain as well as the commonly reported cyclic nature of symptoms leads both patients and practitioners to suspect a urogenital cause. Table 24–1 lists the musculoskeletal structures most

Table 24–2. **MUSCULOSKELETAL DYSFUNCTIONS REPORTED IN CHRONIC PELVIC PAIN CASES**

Report	Dysfunction	Treatment
Hunter and Zihlman[6]	Intrapelvic muscle strain; faulty posture	Posture education; therapeutic exercise
King et al[10]	Trunk, hip, and abdominal muscle imbalance—various dysfunctions; faulty posture	Posture education; therapeutic exercise; passive stretching; heat/cold/ electrotherapy modalities
Paradis and Marganoff[11]	Levator ani spasm; slumped posture	Massage
Sinaki et al[14]	Pelvic floor myalgia; poor posture; deconditioned muscles	Massage; deep heat; exercise
Sicuranza et al[13]	Strain of abdominal, paravertebral, and gluteal muscles secondary to short leg	Heel lift
Slocumb[15]	Abdominal trigger points	Injection

From King Baker P: Musculoskeletal origins of chronic pelvic pain. Obstet Gynecol Clin North Am 1993;20:719.

commonly associated with CPP, their levels of segmental innervation, sites of referred pain, and common disorders. Table 24–3 lists the structures of the female urogenital system, their segmental innervation, and common sites of referred pain. Comparison of these two tables illustrates the difficulty of identifying etiologic factors for CPP by symptom location alone. Cyclic pain worsened with menses would seem to distinguish musculoskeletal from urogenital disturbances; however, it can be hypothesized that capsuloligamentous instability may be increased during the luteal phase and menses as a result of elevated relaxin and progesterone levels. This theory is supported by clinical reports of the behavior of musculoskeletal symptoms.[9, 10, 44]

Typical Pelvic Pain Posture

A typical pattern of faulty posture has been observed in patients with musculoskeletal CPP.[9, 10] This faulty pattern is consistent with the lordosis and kyphosis-lordosis postures described by Kendall and McCreary[45] (Fig. 24–4). This same posture pattern is associated with pregnancy and may in some cases begin during pregnancy and become dysfunctional when postpartum attention to posture and strengthening is inadequate. In my experience, many nulliparous women with CPP also present with this posture. The primary mechanical changes occurring in TPP posture include the following:

- Anterior tilt of the pelvis (usually anterior rotation of the innominate and increased nutation of the sacrum)
- Increased lumbar lordosis (increased lumbosacral angle)
- Hyperextension of the knees
- Line of gravity displaced anteriorly in the lower extremities and pelvis

Musculoskeletal dysfunctions associated with TPP and CPP include the following:

- Adaptive shortening and hypertonus of the iliopsoas muscle

Table 24–3. **REFERRED PAIN: FEMALE UROGENITAL SYSTEM**

Structure	Segmental Innervation	Potential Site for Local Referred Pain
Ovaries	T10–T11	Lower abdomen, low back
Uterus	T10–L1	Lower abdomen, low back
Fallopian tubes	T10–L1	Lower abdomen, low back
Perineum	S2–S4	Sacral apex, suprapubic, rectum
External genitalia	L1–L2, S3–S4	Lower abdomen, medial anterior thigh, sacrum
Kidney	T10–L1	Ipsilateral low back and upper abdominal
Urinary bladder	T11–L2, S2–S4	Thoracolumbar, sacrococcygeal, suprapubic
Ureters	T11–L2, S2–S4	Groin, upper and lower abdomen, suprapubic, anteromedial thigh, thoracolumbar

From King PM, Myers CA, Ling FW, Rosenthal RH: Musculoskeletal factors in chronic pelvic pain. J Psychosom Obstet Gynecol 1991;12:87.

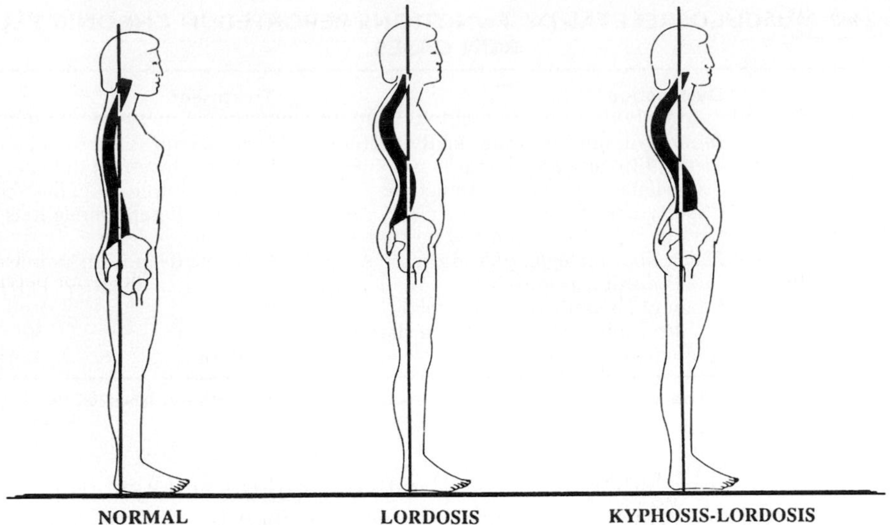

Figure 24–4. Normal and faulty posture. Both lordosis and kyphosis-lordosis occur in typical pelvic pain posture. (From King PM, Meyers CA, Ling FW, et al: Musculoskeletal factors in chronic pelvic pain. J Psychosom Obstet Gynecol 1991;12:87.)

- Adaptive shortening and hypertonus of the hip external rotators (piriformis, obturators)
- Lengthening strain on the iliofemoral ligament (Y ligament of Bigelow) and anterior capsule of the hip
- Loss of capsular extensibility, synovitis, and DJD of the hips; iliopectinius bursitis
- Lengthening strain on abdominals, with resultant weakness or trigger points
- Sacroiliac strain
- Hypermobility and DJD of the thoracolumbar articular facets (see the later discussion on thoracolumbar syndrome)

Interestingly, the principal muscular components of this dysfunctional pattern are also reported by Jull and Janda[42] as common in other patients with musculoskeletal dysfunctions, particularly that associated with low back pain.

Table 24–4 summarizes the musculoskeletal changes associated with lordosis and swayback posture, as described by Kendall and McCreary.[45] Characteristics of both these faulty posture patterns occur in TPP.

Thoracolumbar Syndrome

Thoracolumbar syndrome, described by Paris,[34] includes anterior abdominal and lateral hip pain referred from the thoracolumbar area in patients who have had lumbar fusion. The mechanism for this syndrome is attributed to hypermobility at the thoracolumbar junction, which occurs adaptively when the low and midlumbar segments are fused. Patients' complaints of anterior and lateral hip and abdominal pain often resolve with stabilization exercises and antiinflammatory modalities such as therapeutic cold and electrotherapy. Irritation of the lateral femoral cutaneous nerve is a potential source of symptoms in this syndrome, because patients often adopt a lordotic lumbar posture, which stretches that nerve and increases the opportunity for its compromise at the anterior superior iliac spine. A similar mechanical pattern occurs with TPP posture, in which the mid and low lumbar articulations lose range of motion owing to the prolonged faulty lordotic posture, which closely packs the lumbar facet joints. Hypermobility develops at the thoracolumbar junction, with resultant inflammation and referred anterior abdominal and thigh pain. Kopell and Thompson[46] describe entrapment of the ilioinguinal nerve at the ASIS secondary to loss of hip extension range of motion and increases in anterior pelvic tilt. They further describe the mechanical relationships between those changes and upper lumbar hypermobility, consistent with Paris'

Table 24–4. **FAULTY POSTURE, SIDE VIEW: ANALYSIS AND TREATMENT**

Postural Fault	Anatomic Position of Joints	Muscles in Shortened Position	Muscles in Lengthened Position	Treatment Procedures, if Indicated on the Basis of Tests for Alignment and Muscle Length and Strength Tests
Lordosis posture	Lumbar spine hyperextension Pelvis; anterior tilt	Low back erector spinae	Abdominals, especially external oblique	Stretch low back muscles if tight Strengthen abdominals by posterior pelvic tilt exercises and, if indicated, by trunk curl. Avoid sit-ups because they shorten hip flexors. Stretch hip flexors when short. Strengthen hip extensors, if weak.
	Hip joint flexion	Hip flexors	Hip extensors	Instruct about proper body alignment. Depending on degree of lordosis and extent of muscle weakness and pain, use support (corset) to relieve strain on abdominals and to help correct the lordosis

From Kendall FD, McCreary EK, Provanoc PG: Muscles—Testing and Function. Revised 4th ed, Baltimore, Williams & Wilkins, 1993.

theory of the etiology of thoracolumbar syndrome.

Iliopectineal Bursitis

The iliopectineal bursa is located on the anterior aspect of the hip joint just lateral to the pubis and underneath the iliopsoas muscle (Fig. 24–5). It usually communicates with the hip joint anteriorly between the pubofemoral and iliofemoral ligaments. Inflammation of this relatively large bursa is thought to be a factor in the anterior pain associated with DJD of the hip and may also contribute to symptoms of CPP. The iliopectineal bursa may become irritated, with an increase in friction associated with adaptive shortening of the iliopsoas as well as with hip joint synovitis. When inflamed, this bursa is palpable just lateral to the pubis and distal to the ASIS. As with all bursae, it is not palpable unless inflamed and is even then difficult to palpate. Magnetic resonance imaging or ultrasound examination should confirm this diagnosis.

Degenerative Joint Disease of the Hip

DJD of the hip is endemic in Western societies and appears to be associated with sedentary life and the commonness of sitting.[40] This dysfunction often eventually leads to a total hip replacement. Anterior hip and groin pain often occurs. DJD is thought to begin with alterations in range of motion—either hypermobilities or hypomobilities that disturb normal nutrition and lubrication processes within the joint—and lead to destruction of articular cartilage. Stiff hips (reduced capsular extensibility) are often the precursor to more extensive degeneration. Loss of internal rotation is an early sign of capsular restriction in the hip and is a common finding in patients with both pelvic pain and low back pain.[9, 10, 32] Normal internal rotation range of motion is near 45 degrees. Ranges of 15 to 25 degrees are common in young adult and middle-aged women with CPP that I have examined. Loss of internal rotation range of motion encourages adaptive shortening of the external rotator muscles of the hip, including the piriformis and obturators, which when shortened or hypertonic contribute to pelvic floor tension myalgia. Range of motion values less than the expected should be considered indicative of dysfunction predisposing to DJD, and affected persons should be referred to physical therapy.

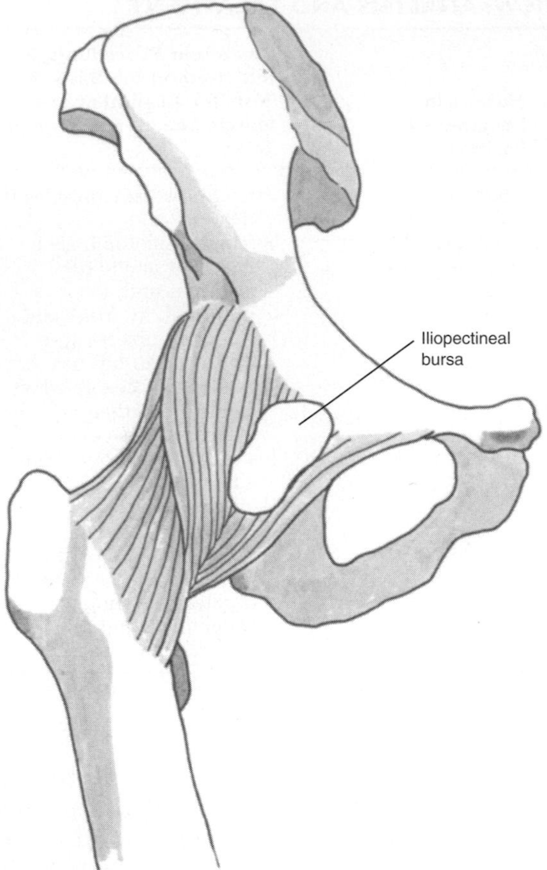

Figure 24–5. Iliopsoas (iliopectineus) bursa. (From Kessler RM, Hertling D: Management of Common Musculoskeletal Disorder: Physical Therapy Principles and Methods, 2nd ed. Philadelphia, JB Lippincott, 1990.)

In the early stages of DJD, significant changes are not visible on radiographs because the degeneration occurs first in the articular cartilage and only later in the subchondral bone. Interestingly, articular cartilage, the first structure to undergo degeneration, is both avascular and aneural. Its avascular status contributes to its early degeneration. Its aneural status explains the significant destruction that can develop before the joint become symptomatic. Palpation of the anterior aspect of the joint for edema and tenderness is also recommended. Joint manipulation and active exercise are appropriate treatments for restoring range of motion in the early stages of degeneration and for maintaining range of motion in the latter stages. Antiinflammatory modalities and medications such as nonsteroidal antiinflammatory drugs (NSAIDs) are used to manage associated pain and edema.

Pubic Separations and Sprains

An increase in separation at the pubic symphysis may occur during labor and delivery and if unresolved in the postpartum period may lead to chronic lower abdominal discomfort and perhaps tension myalgia in the pelvic floor and hips. More severe cases of sympholysis are likely to be accompanied by painful alterations in gait and possibly a posture of hip external rotation and ilial outflare.[28] Strain or adaptive shortening of the hip adductors in either acute trauma or long-term adaptive shortening may produce abnormal superior/inferior separation of the pubis via their action at the pubis. A palpable difference in the comparative superior/inferior heights of the pubis right to left in conjunction with tenderness and edema in the suprapubic area may be indicative of dysfunction in this articulation. Unilateral pelvic floor tension associated with faulty pelvic posture, sacroiliac dysfunction, or gynecologic or psychologic phenomena may produce strain on the pubic symphysis. Table 24–5 presents common dysfunctions of

Table 24–5. **JOINT DYSFUNCTIONS IN THE PELVIS**

Pubic symphysis
Inferior pubic shear
Superior pubic shear
Pubic separation
Sacroiliac
Anterior sacral torsion
Posterior sacral torsion
Bilaterally flexed sacrum
Bilaterally extended sacrum
Unilateral sacral flexion (inferior sacral shear)
Unilateral sacral extension (superior sacral shear)
Iliosacral
Anterior rotation of the ilium
Posterior rotation of the ilium
Ilial upslip (superior innominate shear)
Ilial downslip (inferior innominate shear)
Outflare of the ilium
Inflare of the ilium
Sacrococcygeal
Lateral subluxations
Anteroposterior subluxations

From Bookhout MM, Boissonnault JS: Musculoskeletal dysfunction in the female pelvis. Orthop Phys Ther Clin North Am 1996;5:1.

the pubic symphysis and sacroiliac articulations.

Sacroiliac Sprains/Strains/Displacements

Sacroiliac dysfunction may occur in response to the repetitive strain of faulty postures or a traumatic event such as a fall on the ischium. Asymmetric adaptations of the sacroiliac articulation combined with the trauma of labor and delivery may also sprain or displace these articulations. Sensory innervation to the sacroiliac joints arises from segments L4–S4, and thus the range of referred pain is wide, often including the entire posterior thigh and leg and the ventral surface of the foot, as well as local pain and tenderness. Pain may occasionally be referred from the sacroiliac to the pelvic floor. Sacroiliac dysfunctions may alter pubic symphysis function and in that manner contribute to the development of anterior pelvic pain.

Diastasis Recti

Separation of the rectus abdominis is a common occurrence during the second and third trimesters of pregnancy, as well as in the postpartum period, and may contribute to CPP in pregnancy. It is not clear whether this is a true tear or a relaxation of tissue. The separation is at or near the umbilicus.[41, 47] A diastasis signals abdominal weakness, diminished visceral support, and diminished facilitation for pelvic floor muscle activity, because these groups work in synergy.[48] Exercises to strengthen the abdominals are modified to avoid further strain. Vertical placement of the examiner's fingers at the linea alba identifies this dysfunction. If a separation of greater than two fingers exists, abdominal function likely is significantly impaired. Diastasis recti may contribute to trigger points in the abdominals and requires modified exercise.

Coccydynia

A fall or other direct trauma can cause coccygeal pain. Childbirth-related sprains and fractures may occur when delivery is attempted on a hard surface, limiting the sacrococcygeal extension necessary to increase the anteroposterior diameter of the birth canal during delivery. The coccyx is innervated by S1–S4 and may refer pain throughout the pelvic floor. Tension myalgia may occur as a secondary response to the inflammation of traumatic coccyx injury in both acute and chronic states. Length and tone of the pelvic floor muscles may be altered by coccyx displacements due to sprain or fracture. For example, hypertonus in the pelvic floor muscles may lead to local trigger points and introital dyspareunia. Similarly, the gluteus maximus has tendinous attachments in the sacrococcygeal capsule. Reproduction of pelvic floor pain with resisted hip extension is indicative of coccyx dysfunction due to that relationship. Pelvic pain arising from the coccyx may be reported to be worsened with hip extension activities such as stair climbing.

Pelvic Floor Dysfunction

The muscles of the pelvic floor often become symptomatic owing to decreased strength, hypotonus, or hypertonus. The term *pelvic floor relaxation* is often used to describe hypotonus and strength reduction. Pelvic floor relaxation may be a direct cause of symptoms in some CPP cases; however, this is rare in my experience. Pelvic floor relaxation in early stages, without notable symptoms or signs, may be significant in the rehabilitation of patients with musculoskeletal CPP because even mild to moderate strength and length changes may contribute to other pain-producing muscle imbalances within the pelvis and abdominal wall. Relaxation of the pelvic floor frequently develops in association with birth trauma and inadequate postpartum strengthening.

Much debate centers on the various methods of childbirth and the impact that birthing positions and methods have on the tissues of the pelvic floor. The merits and details of those arguments are beyond the scope of this discussion. It is generally agreed, however, that prolonged or precipitous labor, high-birth-weight infants, and instrument-assisted deliveries place exceptional strain on the pelvic floor musculature in childbirth. Obesity, chronic constipation, and Valsalva's lifting have also been linked to increased strain on the pelvic floor, although DeLancey[37] has questioned the role of obesity. Inadequate relaxation of the pelvic floor during delivery due to maternal tension or lack of training is thought to increase risks of tears or episiotomies, both of which impair recovery of pelvic floor strength and extensibility. Patients with pelvic relaxation commonly complain of a feeling of "falling out" and in later stages often suffer prolapse of the urogenital organs. They often become incontinent. Early attention to training of the pelvic floor muscles should correct the majority of relaxation dysfunctions. If rehabilitation is not instated early, the physiology and length of the muscles may be altered to the point that rehabilitation potential is limited. Many women seem to accept some degree of pelvic floor relaxation or incontinence as normal; for this reason, practitioners may need to question patients very specifically about the history to identify early symptoms of relaxation. (Further discussion on myofascial dysfunction and clinical assessment of pelvic floor function are found in Chapters 7 and 26.)

Peripheral Entrapment Neuropathies

The abdominals are commonly recognized by gynecologic practitioners as potential entrapment sites for the ilioinguinal and iliohypogastric nerves (see Chapter 25). Kopell and Thompson[46] describe several cases of peripheral entrapment neuropathies associated with mechanical impingement of neural tissue by musculoskeletal neighbors. Faulty postures and repetitive activities creating excessive fibrous tissue and muscle length changes are associated with the development of entrapment neuropathy in many of their cases. They describe cases of entrapment of ilioinguinal and obturator nerve near the ASIS and abdominal wall. Faulty posture and muscle imbalances are reported to contribute to the ilioinguinal entrapment. Osteitis pubis and obturator hernia are presented as factors in the obturator entrapment. As the obturator nerve enters and exits the obturator foramen, it is closely related to the abdominal musculature and the obturator internus. Tension or length changes in those muscles can be theorized as potential contributions to entrapment of the obturator nerve, which produces pain in the groin and anterior thigh. Work similar to that of Kopell and Thompson has been presented by Dawson and colleagues.[49]

It seems logical to theorize that adaptive changes in tone and length of pelvic musculature might also result in local entrapments, with diminished muscle tone or pain being potential consequences. The genitofemoral, ilioinguinal, and iliohypogastric nerves all lie in close anatomic proximity to the iliopsoas muscle (Fig. 24–6), which was described earlier as commonly shortened and hypertonic in the CPP population.[9, 10] Entrapment of the sciatic nerve secondary to shortening and tone changes in the piriformis has been reported to create neuropathy.[46, 49] A similar phenomenon has been theorized to occur in our physical therapy clinic when CPP has been relieved by myofasical manipulation techniques at sites of anatomic juxtaposition of peripheral nerves supplying the painful area and shortened myofascial tissues. Based on anatomic relationships, the genitofemoral nerve appears to be at particular risk because it normally bifurcates the iliacus, sometimes above and sometimes below its separation into genital and femoral branches. A similar situation of bifurcation of the piriformis by the sciatic is also thought by some to increase risk of entrapment.

In cases of peripheral entrapment neuropathy, nerve blocks may provide temporary relief; however, if the anatomic compromise remains, the symptoms will likely return once anesthetics have ceased their activity. Transcutaneous neurolysis is sometimes performed when blocks have only short-term effect. In the case of these three peripheral nerves, entrapment in the iliopsoas, commonly shortened in the pelvic pain population, should be considered. If mechanical entrapment is occurring, stretching and myofascial release techniques directed at the involved soft tissues may produce symptomatic change. Lateral femoral cutaneous nerve entrapment was discussed in the section on thoracolumbar syndrome. Pudendal neuropathies are also reported in the gyne-

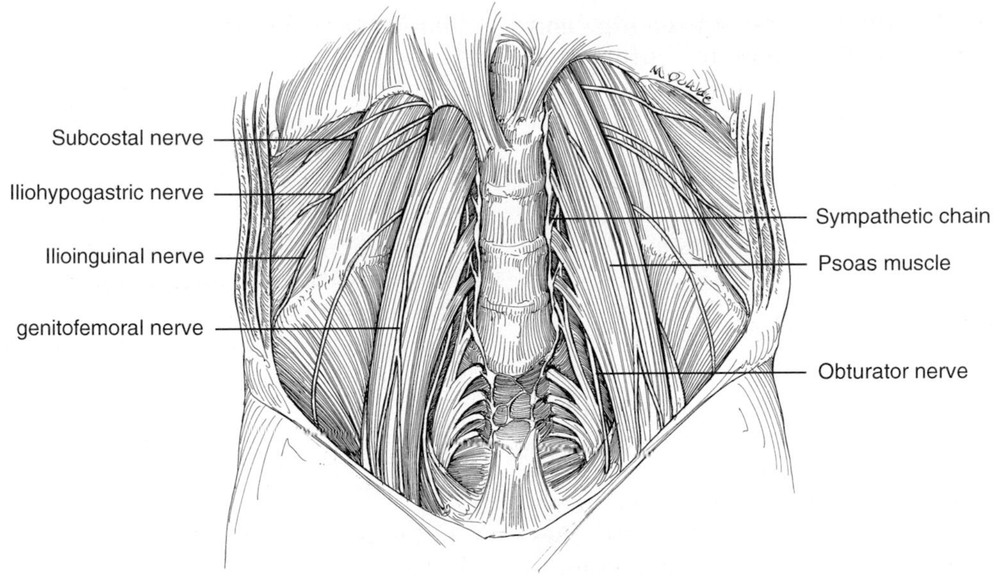

Figure 24–6. Anatomic relationships between the iliopsoas muscle and the iliohypogastric, ilioinguinal, and genitofemoral nerves. (From Williams PL, Warwick R: Gray's Anatomy, 36th ed. New York, Churchill Livingstone, 1980.)

cologic literature and are most commonly associated with stretching injuries during childbirth. The pudendal nerve is in close anatomic proximity to the sacrospinous ligament and piriformis muscle. The high incidence of decreased internal rotation at the hip (which places the piriformis in a shortened position) in the CPP population can lead to a theory of possible pudendal entrapment or irritation secondary to changes in the length or tone of the piriformis.

Lumbar Disk Protrusion/Herniations

Most lumbar disk protrusions and herniations occur in the L4–L5 or L5–S1 interspace, with pain located primarily in the low back, buttock, and posterior leg and calf. The upper lumbar segments are more likely to refer pain to the abdomen and anterior pelvis, and disk pathology is rare at those segments.

Secondary Musculoskeletal Problems

Abdominal Trigger Points

Abdominal trigger points have gained popularity as a focus of treatment in individuals with CPP.[15] Trigger point discomfort may be temporarily relieved with the Fluori-Methane "spray and stretch" techniques advocated by Travell and Simons,[50] as well as by massage, electrotherapy modalities, and myofascial stretching. According to Travell and Simons, trigger points result from muscle spindle dysfunction in muscles held in chronic states of shortening or lengthening. Trigger points may then be caused by the muscle length problem. Chronic shortening of muscle tissue may occur when a state of hypertonus is maintained in response to segmental facilitation or local pathology. Muscle length is commonly altered in response to prolonged faulty postures. Abdominal trigger points may occur secondary to the lengthening strain on the abdominals in the lordosis posture common in CPP. Additional trigger points in CPP patients might occur in response to central summation to dysfunction or disease of urogenital structures that share innervation with the abdominal musculature.[50]

Pelvic Floor Trigger Points

Trigger points often occur in the pelvic floor musculature and produce exquisite pain with radiation on palpation. Length changes secondary to sacroiliac, hip, and sacrococcygeal dysfunctions; protective hypertonus from dysfunction in other structures sharing innervation with the involved muscles; and psychogenic tension all should be considered as etiologic factors. (For more information, see the discussion of myofascial dysfunction in Chapter 26.)

Tension Myalgia Secondary to Psychosocial Disturbances

That psychosocial stress produces physical response is well known. Cortisol levels, blood pressure, and muscle tone, among other physical factors, are elevated in response to stress. Tension myalgia that does not respond to management of related musculoskeletal or urogenital disorders may respond to treatment of generalized anxiety and environmental stressors. A history of sexual abuse is common in this population.[51, 52] Patients with chronic pain often have tension myalgia related to a combination of stress, inflammation, and instability. A structured system of assessment and a multidisciplinary approach including psychologists and physical therapists assist in identifying the relationships among these factors.

Postsurgical Scar Dysfunction

Postsurgical scarring is less common after laparoscopic surgery than after laparotomy, but abdominal incisions may produce chronic pain. Cutaneous nerve entrapments at scar sites may respond to therapeutic heat and myofascial manipulation. In obese patients, special care must be taken to maintain abdominal scar and skin length during postsurgical healing. Gentle muscle contractions beginning with isometrics in the abdominal wall are excellent means to enhance physiologic mechanisms and to improve healing in abdominal and pelvic floor myofascia and skin. Pelvic tilt exercises in supine position, performed simultaneously with a gentle exhale, may be instated immediately after operation. Progression may be facilitated by supervision by a physical therapist to evaluate both healing and strength responses to treatment.

Direct manual cross-friction massage is often used by physical therapists to promote healing and flexibility during scar formation.[31] This technique may be applied by the therapist or self-administered by patients. The massage must be applied with deep enough palpation contact to avoid cutaneous irritations such as blisters but with intensity sensitive to patients' tolerance. Very small-amplitude massage strokes are applied perpendicular to the fiber orientation of the healing tissue.

Cardiovascular Endurance and Functional Limitations

Individuals experiencing chronic pain often have diminished cardiovascular endurance because of inactivity. Shortness of breath that occurs with the activity required in musculoskeletal screening is usually indicative of poor exercise capacity or acute pain. Limited aerobic capacity restricts function and promotes a vicious cycle of inactivity, dysfunction, and pain. Therapeutic goals in the management of chronic pain usually include attention to aerobic capacity.

Musculoskeletal Diseases and Fractures

Although not common, fractures have been reported in patients with CPP and should be considered. Stress fractures of the pubis and the ilium have been associated with pregnancy, labor, and delivery. Osteoporosis is a common problem in postmenopausal women. Fractures of the femoral neck, sacrum, and vertebrae occur in conjunction with osteoporosis. Pain markedly exacerbated by weight-bearing is a key finding indicating possible fracture. Fractures in any of the mentioned sites could produce pain in the usual CPP locations.

Night pain, pain progressively worse at rest, and pain not clearly affected by position changes or specific movements are red flags in the history for a nonmusculoskeletal etiology. Paget's disease, tuberculosis, ankylosing spondylitis, and other inflammatory or infectious diseases may affect the articulations of the pelvic girdle and produce symptoms mimicking sacroiliac pain or CPP. The intracapsular blood supply of the hip puts that joint at particular risk for necrosis when the joint is edematous or degenerative.[32] Tumors of the skeleton should also be considered when pain patterns and physical findings do not fit a musculoskeletal or urogenital pattern. Osteonecrosis of the hip, often associated with diabetes or alcoholism, is another pathologic condition that may produce anterior thigh and groin pain.

Diagnosis

History and Interview

Characteristics of Musculoskeletal Pain

The fact that musculoskeletal and urogenital dysfunctions can mimic each other in terms of location of symptoms has been established. That musculoskeletal dysfunctions may be exacerbated during menses has also been discussed. The difficulty of differenting these two groups of potential pathologies and their comorbidity complicates the diagnostic process. When key elements of history implicate the musculoskeletal system, additional screening procedures or consultation with a musculoskeletal practitioner such as a physical therapist are appropriate.

The characteristic most commonly ascribed to pain of musculoskeletal origin is its pattern of improvement with rest and exacerbation with activity. Musculoskeletal pain should not awaken a patient at night or be exacerbated at rest. The exception to this might be later stages of DJD of the hip aggravated by side sleeping. Patients experiencing this, however, should report the ability to return to sleep after changing positions. The musculoskeletal history usually includes specific activities or positions that are most comfortable, as well as others described as least comfortable or most aggravating. Pain that is constant and unaffected by activity or position is not indicative of musculoskeletal dysfunction except in the most acute stages of the inflammatory process.

Acute inflammatory musculoskeletal conditions should respond quickly to rest and antiinflammatory medications. A specific activity or position can usually be identified as being most aggravating. In lumbar disk pathology, for example, sitting is often the position of greatest discomfort.

Most musculoskeletal problems common in CPP are associated with joint laxity and muscle weakness. Pain that worsens later in the day or with any prolonged, constrained posture is characteristic of hypermobility or instability dysfunctions.[34] Connective tissue creep or lengthening associated with gravitational torque is the mechanism held responsible for this pattern. In later stages of instability, patients have difficulty maintaining static postures for even short periods and may be noted to shift and alter positions constantly during the interview process.

Another important key to identifying musculoskeletal dysfunction is the presence of low back pain or a history of low back or lower extremity injury. Patients may not offer this information because it seems unrelated to the problem they have often defined as gynecologic.

Associated Sexual Dysfunction

Musculoskeletal dysfunctions of the pelvic girdle and low back may be manifested as dyspareunia. Hypertonus of the pelvic floor and pelvic floor trigger points can contribute to entrance dyspareunia. Finally, weakness of the pelvic floor can reduce sexual satisfaction for both partners. Deep thrust dyspareunia may be related to sacroiliac or low back dysfunction. Dyspareunia symptoms reduced in alternate positions may indicate a musculoskeletal component, especially when other signs and symptoms characteristic of musculoskeletal dysfunction are also present.

Associated Menstrual Dysfunction

Dysmenorrhea complaints are often a component of the pelvic pain history. Pain exacerbated during the menstrual cycle may have a primary musculoskeletal origin. Abnormal bleeding such as changes in frequency, duration, or amount do not indicate primary musculoskeletal pathology, although comorbidity should not be ruled out without further screening.

Associated Urologic Dysfunction

Incontinence may be directly associated with musculoskeletal dysfunction of the pelvic floor and complaints of pelvic pain. Assessment of the strength of the pelvic floor is indicated. Other signs of urologic dysfunction such as frequency, urgency, and painful urination are not indicative of musculoskeletal involvement, but again, comorbidity should not be ruled out without further investigation.

Musculoskeletal Screening Examination (Table 24–6)

Posture, Structure, and Ergonomic Assessment

Posture should be observed from anterior, posterior, and lateral views while the patient is standing. First observe the patient's self-selected pattern of standing, which may indicate a tendency to unilateral weight-bearing or other faulty habits. The clinician may wish to inquire about the patient's usual or most comfortable posture, which the patient may or may not be able to articulate. Postures are often subconscious habits that patients cannot accurately describe without conscious appraisal after return to the home or work environment.

Once observation of self-selected standing posture is complete, the patient should be asked to place her feet about shoulder width apart and to stand comfortably. Posterior assessment should focus on palpation of the iliac crests and greater trochanters to identify any lateral obliquity of the pelvis or leg length descrepancies. The PSIS and ASIS are compared from the lateral view to determine the amount of anterior or posterior pelvic tilt. Lateral assessment of the spinal curvatures should be conducted. A bilateral comparison of PSIS heights and ASIS heights provides information about asymmetric ilial torsion. All landmark relationships should be confirmed in non–weight-bearing prone and supine positions. In the supine position, bilateral symmetry of the pubis may be assessed with fingertip palpation on the superior aspect of the pubis, right and left. A finding of right pubis superior to left, right ASIS superior to left, and right PSIS lower than left could be labeled as either a posterior torsion of the right ilium or an anterior torsion of the left. If symptoms are unilateral, the symptomatic side is usually chosen as the reference for labeling the postural asymmetry. Mobility and provocation tests later in the evaluation confirm the involvement of one or both sacroiliac or pubic symphysis articulations.

On posterior assessment, an area or band of segmental muscle hypertrophy/hypertonus may be noted, indicating instability (ligamentous laxity; spondylolisthesis) at a specific vertebral level.[34] Other common components of typical pelvic pain posture such as hyperextended knees (genu recurvatum), unilateral stance, exaggerated lumbar lordosis or thoracic kyphosis, and forward head may be noted as well. Patients presenting with obvious kyphosis and forward head posture (the auditory meatus is located anterior to the acromion on a lateral view of posture) should be questioned about signs and symptoms such as headaches, neck pain, and thoracic outlet and carpal tunnel syndromes.

Ergonomic contributions to faulty posture are primarily investigated by inquiry about sleeping, standing, and sitting postures common at home and at work. Length of time in various positions and the relationships of positions to symptom behavior should be determined. Patients may have to self-assess postural habits and report back at a follow-up visit. Prone and side-lying sleeping postures often contribute to pelvic girdle dysfunction. If individuals rest with one hip in flexion and the other in extension, torsional strains result in the pelvis. Prolonged sitting may contribute to pelvic floor stretching and increased intradiskal pressure. Standing with knees in hyperextension contributes to the anterior pelvic tilt and lumbar lordosis so common in pelvic pain. Unilateral stance contributes to torsional strains on the sacroiliac and pelvic floor.

Range of Motion and Flexibility

Screening for active range of motion of the lumbar spine is recommended because this range is often limited in TPP. From

Table 24–6. **MUSCULOSKELETAL SCREENING EXAMINATION**

Posture
- Habitual standing pattern
  - Anterior/posterior
    - Unilateral
    - One lower extremity externally rotated
    - Scoliosis
    - PSIS and iliac crest horizontal symmetry

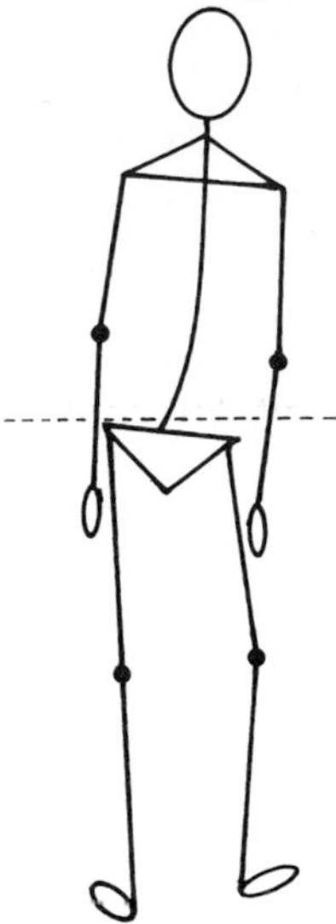

- Lateral
  - Pelvic tilt
  - Spinal curvatures
  - Knee hyperextension
  - Head position

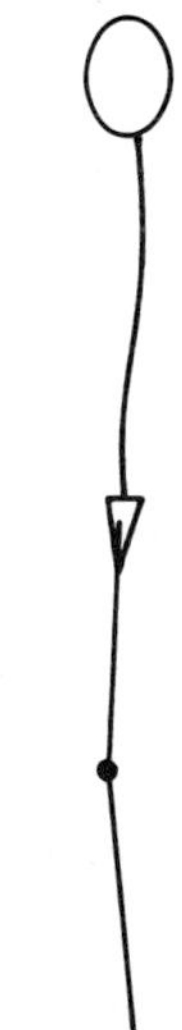

- Supine
  - Pubis symmetry
  - ASIS symmetry

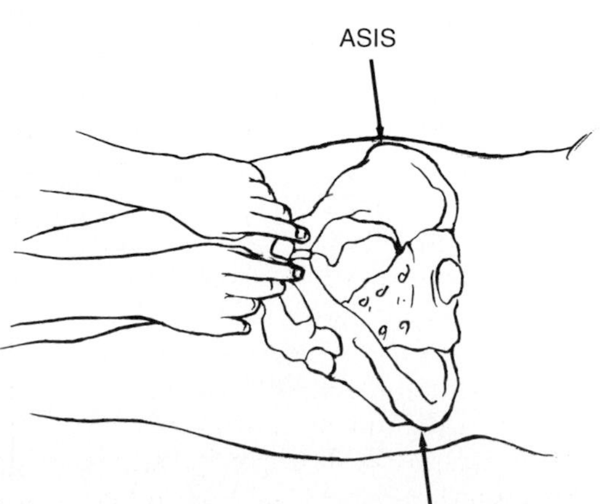

Table continued on following page

Table 24–6. **MUSCULOSKELETAL SCREENING EXAMINATION** *(Continued)*

Range of motion and flexibility
  Active range of motion
    Forward bending
      Reversal of lordosis is normal

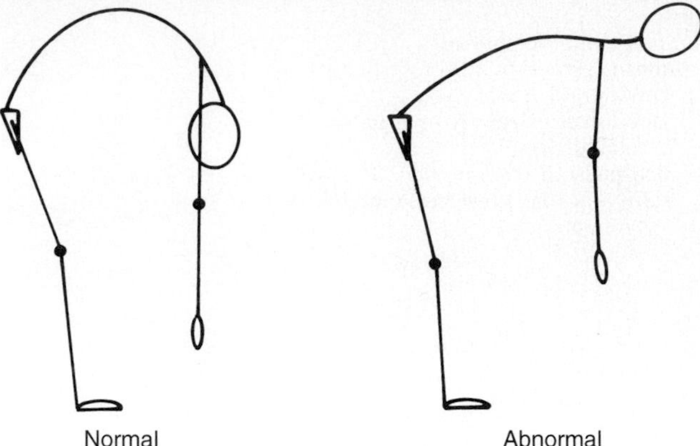

Passive range of motion
  Hip rotation (see Fig. 24–7)
  Straight leg raise (hamstring length)
    Normal length: 80 degrees
    Excessive length: 110 degrees
    Short length: 50 degrees
    Thomas test (see Fig. 24–8)

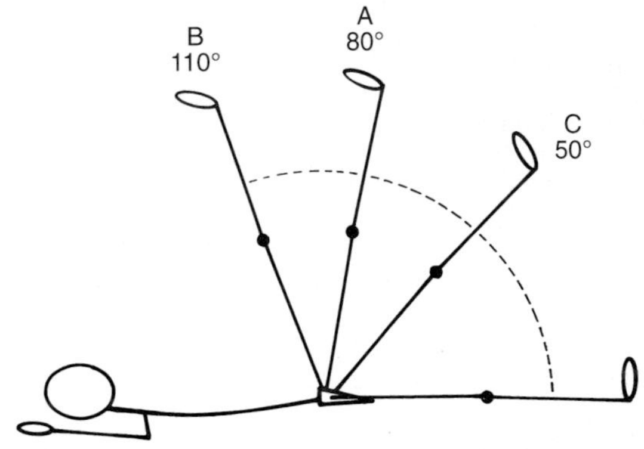

Strength and stability
  Trendelenburg test
    Dropping of non–weight-bearing iliac crest
    Balance and control

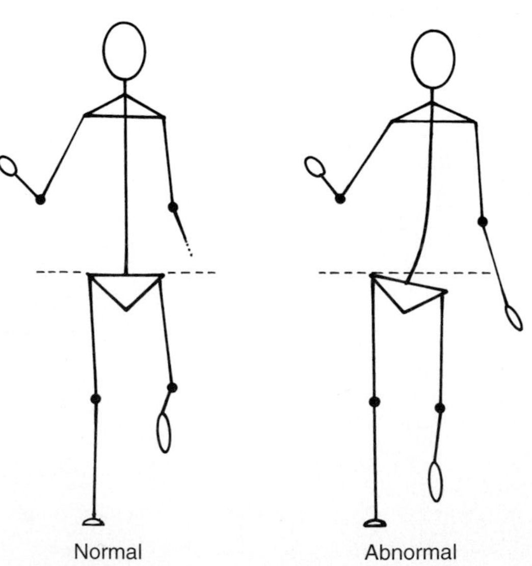

Table 24–6. **MUSCULOSKELETAL SCREENING EXAMINATION** *(Continued)*

Quadruped position, with alternate arm and leg horizontal
- Neutral lumbar position
- Balance and control

Pelvic floor (see Chapter 7)
- Manual examination
- Reported volitional control of urine flow

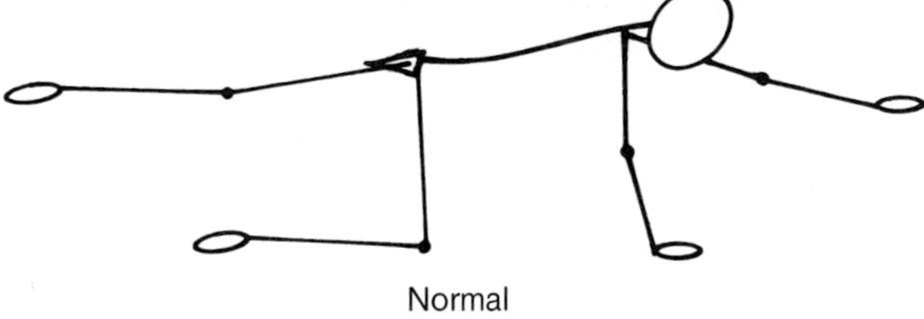

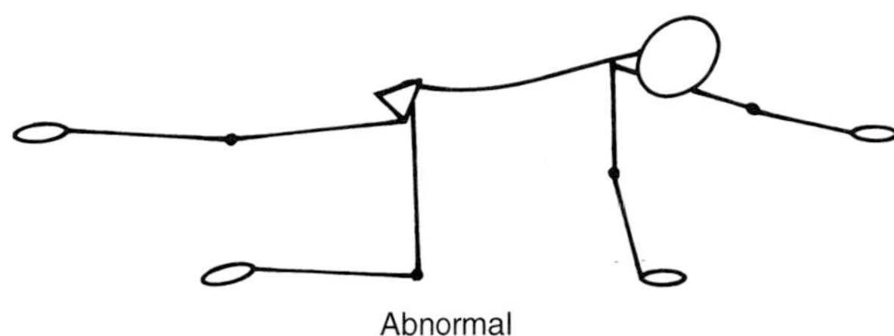

Abdominal
- Sit-up: flex vertebral column:
  - 50% (fair grade): with forearms extended forward
  - 60% (fair plus grade): hold it flexed while coming to a sitting position with forearms extended forward
  - 80% (good grade): hold it flexed while coming to a sitting position with forearms folded across chest
  - 100% (normal grade): hold it flexed while coming to a sitting position with hands clasped behind head

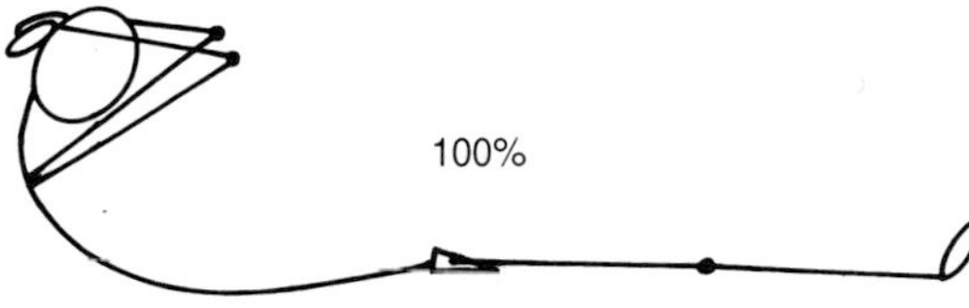

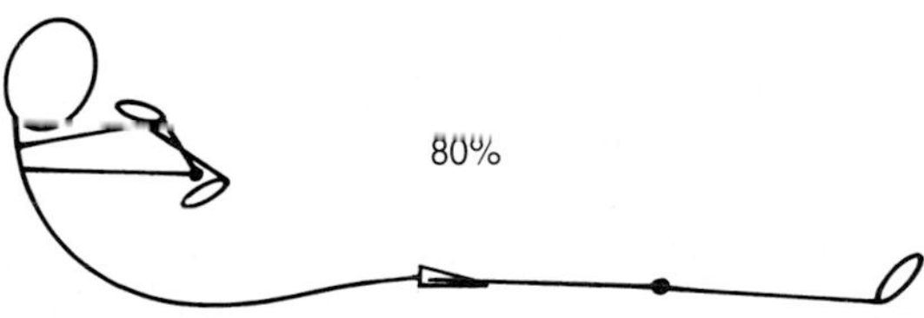

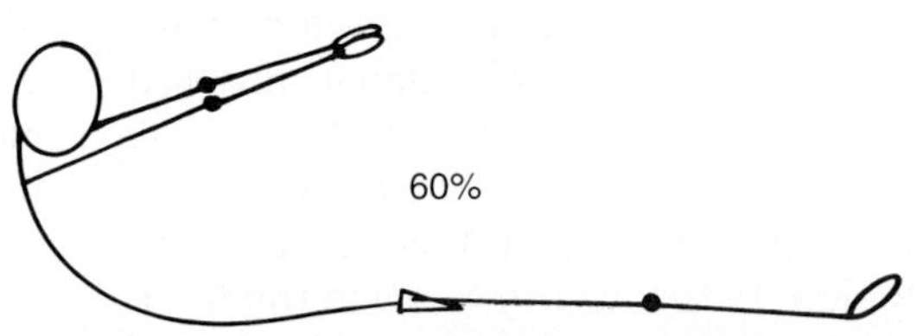

Table continued on following page

Table 24–6. **MUSCULOSKELETAL SCREENING EXAMINATION** *(Continued)*

Leg lowering: hold low back flat on table with legs at given angle 60% (fair plus grade): 60-degree angle 80% (good grade): 30-degree angle 100% (normal grade): horizontal	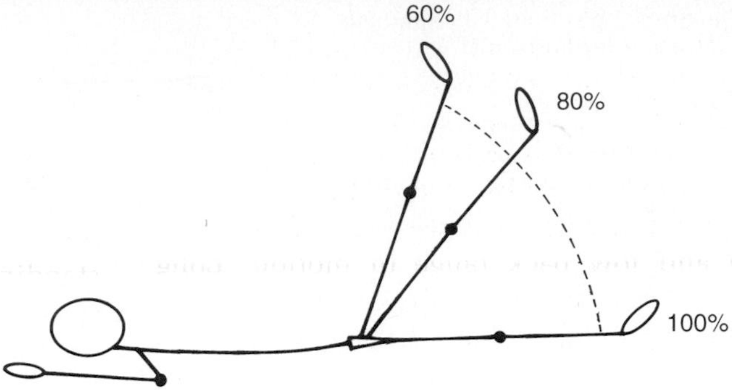
Sacroiliac provocation ASIS gapping (see Fig. 30–3*A*) and compression in supine position	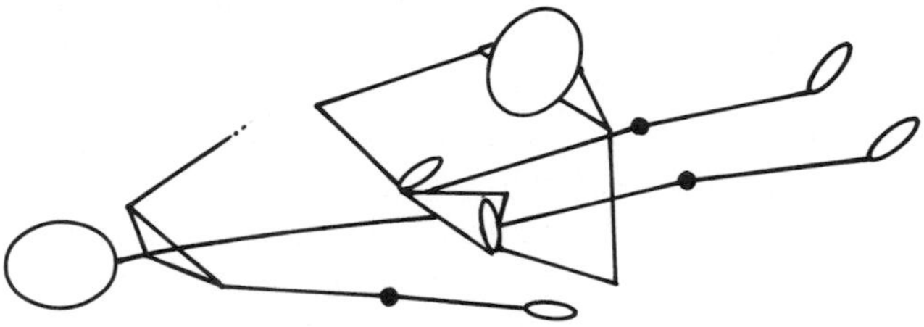

ASIS, anterior superior iliac spines; PSIS, posterior superior iliac spine.

standing, the patient is asked to drop her head forward, shoulders forward, and to lean forward from the waist as far as possible without discomfort. Three repetitions are ideal if tolerated. The practitioner should observe from posterior and lateral views for a reversal of the lumbar curve from the lordotic start position to a position of flexion at end range. A slight kyphotic curvature should result above the iliac crest; this should flatten out in the low lumbar area. Individuals with dysfunctional musculoskeletal adaptations to the TPP posture often present with severe limitation of lumbar forward bending because of shortening of the thoracolumbar fascia, iliopsoas, and lumbar extensors. A flat lumbar curve or maintenance of the lordotic curve noted on the forward bending active range of motion test indicates adaptive shortening of musculoskeletal structures. It is not necessary for a patient to be able to reach the floor with fingertips to have normal lumbar forward bending—the change in the curvature alone reflects lumbar motion. Hamstring length and other factors such as innate joint mobility contribute to the ability to reach the floor. Complaints of pain with movement should be followed by inquiry about the exact location and nature of the symptom.

Instability in the lumbar spine may be manifested on active movement as poorly coordinated halting or juddering movements.[33] Generalized articular hypermobility was reported in conjunction with pelvic floor dysfunction by Norton.[50] Patients with articular instability or hypermobility often present with limited active range of motion, thought to occur secondary to protective muscle activity in the lumbosacral region.[33]

Passive range of motion of hip rotation is recommended for screening the CPP population. The incidence of reduced hip rotation range in CPP and low back pain was mentioned earlier in this chapter, as well as the significance of decreased mobility in the etiology of DJD of the hip. Lack of motion in the hip may contribute to excessive movement in the sacroiliac and pubic symphysis articulations during gait and other functional activities. Screening of passive range of motion of the hip can be accomplished in a prone, supine, or sitting position. In the supine position, the hip and knee are brought to 90 degrees of flexion. While 90 degrees of hip flexion (in sitting or supine) is maintained, the tibia is passively moved medially and laterally in the frontal plane while 90 degrees of knee flexion is maintained. The tibia should move approximately 45 degrees in both directions (Fig. 24–7). Lateral movement of the tibia in this position is a test of internal rotation; medial movement tests external rotation. Pain elicited with this procedure indicates irritability of the hip articulation.

A straight-leg-raise examination may also be performed as an assessment of pain-free hip and low back range of motion. Long used to incriminate lumbar disk pathology, this test provides information about the general flexibility of the low back, pelvis, and lower extremity. Pain with straight-leg raising may have a diskogenic origin, but other musculoskeletal factors are likely as well.

The Thomas test is a well-known procedure for assessing the length of the hip flexors, commonly shortened in CPP. The patient is positioned supine with knees at the end of the examining table. Both knees are pulled to the chest and held in place by the patient. One leg is then lowered to the examining table. If the leg does not contact the table, contracture or shortening of the hip flexors is indicated (Fig. 24–8). The degree of hip flexion is noted and used to determine the results of stretching exercises at later visits.

Strength and Stability

Several procedures can be used to determine the relative stability and strength of the lumbar spine and pelvis. Muscle test results are usually recorded as either normal, good, fair, poor, or trace or on a corresponding 1 to 5 numeric scale. Trendelenburg's test is performed with the patient standing and the examiner's hands on the superior aspect of each iliac crest. The patient is then asked to lift one leg slowly and march in place. Lowering of the pelvis on the side of hip flexion indicates contralateral gluteus medius weakness. Shifting of the lumbar spine position and changes in lumbar muscle tone may also be noted, indicating strength or stability problems in that region. Individuals who cannot attain unilateral stance for brief periods should be referred to physical therapy for specific muscle strength and joint mobility testing.

The quadruped (all fours) position can used to further examine strength and stability in the trunk. In this position, the patient is asked to attain a neutral pelvic position (slight lordotic curve) and to maintain that position while raising each extremity individually to a position horizontal to the sup-

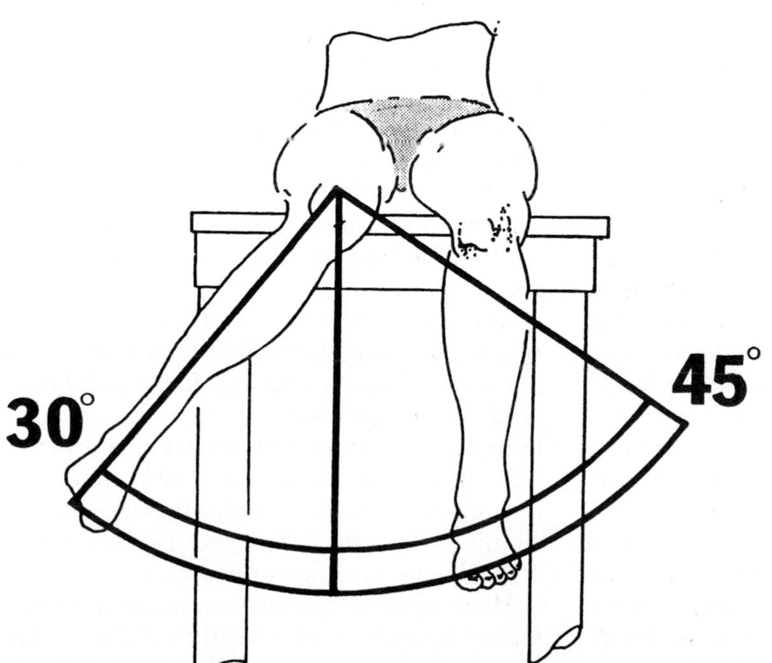

Figure 24–7. Hip: internal and external rotation range of motion testing. (From King PM, Myers CA, Ling FW, Rosenthal RH: Musculoskeletal factors in chronic pelvic pain. J Psychosom Obstet Gynaecol 1991;12:87.)

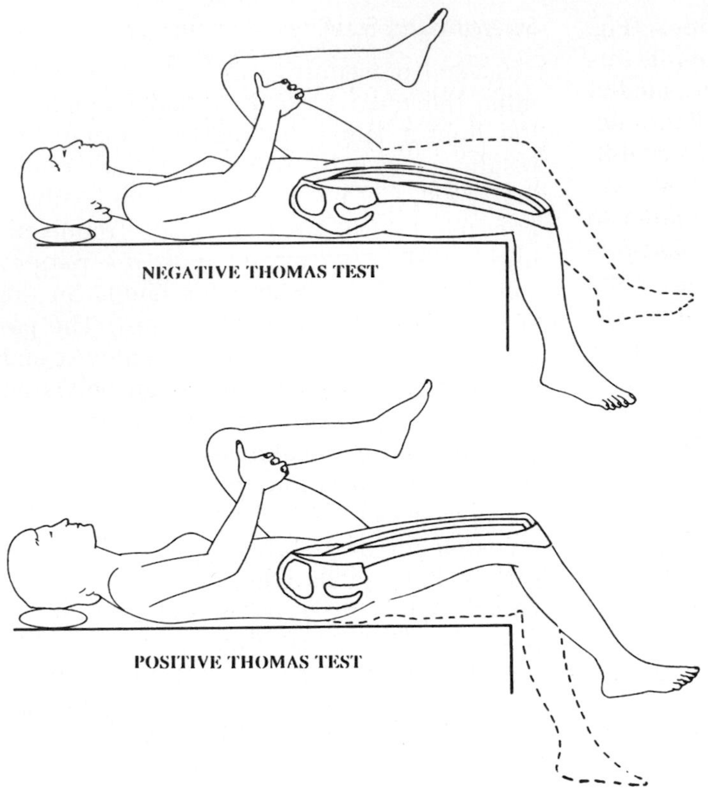

Figure 24–8. Thomas test for hip flexor contracture. (From King PM, Myers CA, Ling FW, Rosenthal RH: Musculoskeletal factors in chronic pelvic pain. J Psychosom Obstet Gynaecol 1991; 12:87.)

porting surface. Signs of instability include a unilateral drop in pelvic position or the inability to reach horizontal extremity positions without increasing the lumbar lordotic curve.

Strength of the pelvic floor is assessed through manual examination, biofeedback and electromyography, visual observation, and questioning the patient about continence and sexual function. Patients should be asked about their ability to start and stop the flow of urine while voiding and to contract the pelvic floor during intercourse. Manual examination for strength of the pelvic floor is described in Chapters 7 and 26. Manual strength of anterior, posterior, and lateral wall contractions is assessed by intravaginal palpation and resistance. A quick stretch applied by the clinician to either anterior, posterior, or right and left lateral walls of the vagina before contraction facilitates muscle activity. Visual observation is conducted for bulging of the pelvic floor and external genitalia during contraction. Rest position and movement of the perineal body, patency of the vagina and rectum at rest, and the presence of hemorrhoids should also be noted. The ability of the patient to contract the pelvic floor on cue and in isolation provides information about volitional control and proprioception. In response to a request for vaginal contraction, abdominals, hip, and low back extensors are frequently substituted owing to weakness and impaired proprioception. Electromyographic assessment is often conducted by physical therapists and provides information about muscle activity at rest and during contraction and about muscle strength and endurance.

Abdominal strength can be quickly assessed by asking the patient to perform a sit-up with hands behind the head and knees bent in supine position. Instruction to exhale gently with the attempted sit-up facilitates abdominal activity. The chin should be tucked to the chest and the patient asked to sit up just to the point that the shoulders clear the supporting surface.

More specific to the lower abdominals, which are often problematic in CPP, is the supine leg-lowering test. The patient raises both legs to 90 degrees hip flexion then slowly lowers the legs. Inability to lower the legs without lumbar lordosis indicates lower abdominal weakness. Care should be taken with this procedure because the raised legs provide a long lever arm of force that can exacerbate symptoms and possibly injure a patient who moves too quickly or with poor control.

Neurologic Assessment

Hyperalgesia may be associated with peripheral neuropathy; loss of sensation occurs with nerve compression. Flaccidity and atrophy in muscle and diminished deep tendon reflexes and strength occur with peripheral nerve compression. Peripheral entrapment sites likely to occur in patients with CPP are described elsewhere in this chapter. A screening of sharp/dull discrimination, deep tendon reflexes, and muscle strength for nerve roots T10–S4 is appropriate in this population. (Further discussion on neurologic assessment is provided in Chapter 25.)

Palpation

Palpation should be conducted to identify abdominal or pelvic floor trigger points. Palpation may also be used to identify tenderness and irritability in the low back musculature, lumbar intersegmental spaces, and sacroiliac articulations. (More detail on trigger point palpation is presented in Chapter 26.)

Special Tests

Sacroiliac Provocation. ASIS gapping and compression are special tests used to determine the irritability of the sacroiliac articulations. The clinician's hands are placed first lateral to then medial to the ASIS bilaterally. A slow stretch followed by a quick short stretch is applied to both sides simultaneously. Movement occurs at the sacroiliac joints and pubic symphysis. Positive signs include reproduction of the patient's symptoms, usually with specific local pain at either one sacroiliac or the pubic symphysis.

Diastasis Recti. Pelvic pain associated with pregnancy or the postpartum state may warrant a manual test for the presence of diastasis recti, described earlier.

Breathing Pattern. The clinician may also wish to observe a patient's breathing pattern, because I have found that diminished diaphragmatic breathing has been associated with musculoskeletal CPP.

Treatment

Physical Therapy

Exercise

Therapeutic exercise is the principal modality used in the management of musculoskeletal CPP. Stretching of the thoracolumbar fascia, piriformis, and iliopsoas is common, as well as strengthening of the abdominal, pelvic floor, and paraspinous muscles. Despite the presence of common themes, patterns and severity of dysfunction vary among individuals. Specific exercise prescriptions are developed on the basis of individualized assessments of function conducted by a physical therapist. In cases requiring pelvic floor strengthening, however, some type of biofeedback is always recommended, whether via patient's own intravaginal palpation or use of a technical device. The practitioner should spend ample time in individual instruction to ensure that patients understand the movement to perform well enough to contract and relax the pelvic floor volitionally. Instruction usually begins with requests to contract muscles as if stopping the flow of urine ("the faucet") and progressing to "elevators," in which the pelvic floor is lifted superiorly. The synergistic relationship between the abdominals and the pelvic floor should be capitalized on in training, with gentle exhalation to recruit abdominals added at the end of pelvic floor contractions. Endurance of contraction is still debated; however, frequency seems to be the key to success in restoring strength.

For most patients with CPP, excessive muscle tension in the pelvic floor is more likely an issue than pelvic relaxation. Manual myofascial release techniques applied externally are often used by physical therapists to reduce tension in the pelvic floor.

One such technique involves deep fingertip pressure applied medial to the ischial tuberosity to encourage muscle relaxation via deep pressure inhibition. Such techniques should be followed by relaxation education in which the patient volitionally relaxes the pelvic floor for 10 seconds, followed by brief 2-second contractions.

Joint Manipulation and Mobilization

Joint manipulation is defined here as "a skilled passive movement to a joint"[34] but is often used in reference to high-velocity short-amplitude thrust maneuvers used to snap articular adhesions. The term *mobilization* is used by many to describe more gentle passive movements. Manipulation is equated by many with chiropractic adjustments, which are essentially thrust maneuvers. I consider a thrust to be a type of manipulation and manipulation to apply to all passive joint movements including classic passive range of motion and various other means of articular stretching. Manipulation may be indicated to address restricted hip range of motion, displacements of the sacroiliac articulation, or restriction of lumbar mobility.

Massage, Myofascial Release, and Soft Tissue Manipulation

Massage, myofascial release, and soft tissue manipulation have subtle differences in definition, but all essentially refer to manual techniques of soft tissue lengthening, muscle relaxation, and stretching. Such techniques are commonly applied to the thoracolumbar fascia, multifidus, piriformis, and pelvic floor of patients with CPP. As with therapeutic exercise, technique should be individually selected to address specific problems of tone, extensibility, and state of inflammation of the involved myofascial structures. (See Chapter 26 for more information on myofascial treatment modalities.)

Biofeedback, Relaxation Training, and Muscle Reeducation

Muscle retraining or reeducation is often difficult to initiate owing to impaired proprioception due to trauma or disuse. Biofeedback instruments have been effectively used for many years in pelvic floor training. Simple pneumatic devices such as the perineometer, vaginal and rectal electric stimulation, and high-tech electromyography biofeedback units with computer-generated reports of muscle activity all are available and in routine use. Vaginal cones are an effective means of combined biofeedback and resisted exercise for the pelvic floor. The simplest biofeedback tool is a patient's own finger palpation of muscle activity via intravaginal contact. It has been clearly demonstrated that some means of biofeedback greatly enhances reeducation and strengthening of the pelvic floor.

Diaphragmatic breathing, progressive relaxation, or relaxation tapes may be important adjuncts to diminishing low back and pelvic floor hypertonicity associated with psychologic, gynecologic, and musculoskeletal problems.

Heat, Cold, Electrotherapeutic Modalities

Therapeutic heat is used to promote muscle relaxation and to facilitate stretching of connective tissue. Hot packs are the most common mode of therapeutic heat used for relaxation. Aerobic exercise is increasingly being used in physical therapy to raise tissue temperature before stretching in the less acute cases. Therapeutic cold is used to decrease joint and soft tissue inflammation. Electrotherapy modalities such as interferential current are used to enhance circulation, reduce pain, and stimulate muscle contraction. These modalities may be appropriate for managing pain and other signs and symptoms of inflammation common in the hips, pubic symphysis, and sacroiliac articulations of patients with pelvic pain.

External Supports

External supports such as lumbosacral corsets may be used to provide support early in the rehabilitation of patients with lumbar or pelvic instability. If therapeutic exercise programs are effective and posture and ergonomic suggestions followed, patients should graduate from the use of supports as their articular and myofascial strength and stability improve. The support may be useful during periods of exacerbation, however, and these are certain to occur because few patients never waver from their therapeutic program. Patients with significant irreversible degenerative disorders may benefit from long-term use of external supports. External supports designed specifically for pregnant clients are available.

Posture and Ergonomic Patient Education

Probably the most important part of the treatment regimen is the posture and ergonomic instruction provided by a clinician and then implemented by a patient. A detailed understanding of a patient's activities of daily living is required for an adequate program to be developed. Standing, sleeping, and sitting postures that encourage neutral lumbopelvic alignment and normal muscle length and strength are prescribed. Structural contributions to faulty posture such as leg length descrepancies have been noted in CPP populations[13] and may require external support such as a shoe lift in addition to posture instruction.

Pharmacology

Pharmacologic management of musculoskeletal dysfunction in CPP may be indicated to reduce inflammation or temporarily limit pain. NSAIDs are effective in reducing symptoms of most inflammatory musculoskeletal dysfunctions. Muscle relaxants may produce a generalized relaxation of tone. They may be counterproductive, however, when patients are actively involved in therapeutic exercise programs that focus on reeducation of muscle control as well as strengthening and stretching. In my experience, muscle relaxants have not appeared to reduce symptoms of CPP significantly.

Summary

Both local and referred CPP may frequently arise from musculoskeletal dysfunctions. Therapeutic interventions addressing musculoskeletal dysfunction can relieve symptoms of CPP. Physical therapy interventions such as exercise, massage, joint manipulation, biofeedback, posture education, and external supports all may be useful. Specific prescription for these interventions is based on a detailed assessment conducted by a musculoskeletal practitioner such as a physical therapist, including posture, range of motion and flexibility, strength and stability, neurologic status, and tissue irritability. A screening examination appropriate for use by gynecologic or family practice physicians was presented. The prevalence of musculoskeletal dysfunctions in CPP and the reported efficacy of the treatment of these conditions make a strong case for their inclusion in a physician's routine history and screening examination or at least for a routine physical therapy consultation. Collaboration among physicians, psychologists, and physical therapists in diagnostics, treatment, and research related to CPP should afford a clearer, more complete understanding of this often frustrating clinical problem.

References

1. Abbott J: Pelvic pain: Lessons from anatomy and physiology. J Emerg Med 1990;8:441.
2. Beard RW, Reginald PW, Pearce S: Pelvic pain in women. BMJ 1986;293:1160.
3. Guerriero WF, Guerriero CP III, Eward RD, Stuart JA: Pelvic pain, gynecic and nongynecic: Interpretation and management. South Med J 1971;64:1043.
4. Guzinski GM: Advances in the diagnosis and treatment of chronic pelvic pain. Adv Psychosom Med 1985;12:124.
5. Henker FO: Diagnosis and treatment of nonorganic pelvic pain. South Med J 1979;72:1132.
6. Hunter W, Zihlman AL: Abdominal pain from strain of intrapelvic muscles (letter). Clin Orthop Rel Res 1970;130:279.
7. Julian TM: Chronic pelvic pain part II: Management strategies. Female Patient 1989;14:19.
8. Weingold AB: Pelvic pain. In Kase NG, Weingold AB, Gershenson DM (eds): Principles and Practice of Clinical Gynecology, 2nd ed. New York, Churchill Livingstone, 1990, pp 479–508.
9. King Baker P: Musculoskeletal origins of chronic pelvic pain. Obstet Gynecol Clin North Am 1993;20:719.
10. King PM, Myers CA, Ling FW, Rosenthal RH: Musculoskeletal factors in chronic pelvic pain. J Psychom Obstet Gynaecol 1991;12:87.
11. Paradis H, Marganoff H: Rectal pain of extrarectal origin. Dis Colon Rectum 1969;12:306.
12. Reiter RC, Gambone JC: Nongynecologic somatic

pathology in women with chronic pelvic pain and negative laparoscopy. J Reprod Med 1991;36:253.
13. Sicuranza BJ, Richards J, Tisdal LH: The short leg syndrome in obstetrics and gynecology. Am J Obstet Gynecol 1970;10:217.
14. Sinaki M, Merritt JL, Stillwell GW: Tension myalgia of the pelvic floor. Mayo Clin Proc 1977;52:717.
15. Slocumb JC: Neurological factors in chronic pelvic pain: Trigger points in the abdominal pelvic pain syndrome. Am J Obstet Gynecol 1984;149:536.
16. Inman VT, Saunders JB: Referred pain from skeletal structures. J Nerv Ment Dis 1944;99:660.
17. Kellgren JH: On the distribution of pain arising from deep somatic structures with charts of segmental pain areas. Clin Sci 1939;4:35.
18. Kellgren JH: Observations of referred pain arising from muscles. Clin Sci 1939;4:35.
19. Gould SF: Anatomy. In Gabbe SG, Niebyl JR, Simpson JL (eds): Obstetrics: Normal and Problem Pregnancies, 2nd ed. New York, Churchill Livingstone, 1991, p 3.
20. Bowen V, Cassidy JD: Macroscopic and microscopic anatomy of the sacroiliac joint from embryonic life until the eighth decade. Spine 1981;6:620.
21. Walker J: The sacroiliac joint: A critical review. Phys Ther 1992;72:71.
22. Williams PL, Warick R (eds): Grays Anatomy, 36th ed. New York, Churchill Livingstone, 1980.
23. Weise H: The articular surface of the sacro-iliac joint and their relation to the movements of the sacrum. Acta Anat 1954;22:1.
24. Wilder DG, Pope MH, Frymozer JW: The functional topography of the sacro-iliac joint. Spine 1980; 5:575.
25. Basmajian JV, Nyberg R (eds): Rational Manual Therapies. Baltimore, Williams & Wilkins, 1993.
26. Egan N, Oisson TH, Schmid H, Selvik G: Movements of the sacroiliac joint demonstrated with roentgen stereophotogrammetry. Acta Radiol 1978; 19:833.
27. Weise H: The movements of the sacro-iliac joints. Acta Anat 1955;23:80.
28. Bookhout MM, Boissonnault JS: Musculoskeletal dysfunction in the female pelvis. Orthop Phys Ther Clin North Am 1996;5:1.
29. Kapandji IA: The Physiology of the Joints, vol III: The Trunk and Vertebral Column. New York, Churchill Livingstone, 1994.
30. Greenman PE: Principles of Manual Medicine. Baltimore, Williams & Wilkins, 1989.
31. Kessler RM, Hertling D: Management of Common Musculoskeletal Disorder: Physical Therapy Principles and Methods, 2nd ed. Philadelphia, JB, Lippincott, 1990.
32. Ellison JB, Rose SJ, Sahrmans SA: Patterns of hip rotation range of motion: A comparison between healthy subjects and patients with low back pain. Phys Ther 1990;70:7.
33. Paris SV: Physical signs of instability. Spine 1985;10:277.
34. Paris SV: Foundations of Clinical Orthopaedics. St. Augustine, FL, Institute Press, 1990.
35. Riczo DB: Spinal dysfunction in the female. Orthop Phys Ther Clin North Am 1996;1:47.
36. Benson JT (ed): Female Pelvic Floor Disorder. New York, North Medical Books, 1992.
37. DeLancey JOL: Anatomy and biomechanics of genital prolapse. Clin Obstet Gynecol 4:897.
38. Dunbar A: Physical therapy management of uterine prolapse. J Obstet Gynaecol Phys Ther 1993;17:3.
39. Santiesteban AJ: Electromyographic and dynamometric characteristics of female pelvic floor musculature. Phys Ther 68:344.
40. Gunn DR: Don't sit—squat! Clin Orthop Rel Res 1974;130:104.
41. Noble E: Essential Exercises for the Childbearing Years, 3rd ed. Boston, Houghton Mifflin, 1988.
42. Jull GA, Janda V: Muscles and motor control in low back pain: Assessment and management. In Twomey LT, Taylor JR (eds): Physical Therapy of the Low Back. New York, Churchill Livingstone, 1987, pp 253–278.
43. Aspinall W: Clinical implications of iliopsoas dysfunction. J Man Manip Ther 1993;1:41.
44. MacLennan AH, Green RC, Nicolson R, Bath M: Serum relaxin and pelvic pain of pregnancy. Lancet 1986;2:243.
45. Kendall FD, McCreary EK: Muscles—Testing and Function. Baltimore, Williams & Wilkins, 1983, p 160–165, 185–234, 269–315.
46. Kopell HP, Thompson AL: Peripheral Entrapment Neuropathies, 2nd ed. Huntington, NY, Kreigha, 1976.
47. Boissonnault JS, Blashack MJ: Incidence of diastasis recti abdominis during the childbearing years. Phys Ther 1988;68:1082.
48. Frahm J: Abdominal and pelvic floor muscle synergy in normal women. Research Presentation, Combined Sections Meeting, American Physical Therapy Association, New Orleans, LA, February 1994.
49. Dawson DM, Hallett M, Millender LH: Entrapment Neuropathies. Boston, Little, Brown & Co., 1983, pp 196–197, 221.
50. Travell JG, Simons DG: Myofascial Pain and Dysfunction: The Trigger Point Manual. Baltimore, Williams & Wilkins, 1983, pp 1–36.
51. Rosenthal RH, Ling FW, Rosenthal TL, McNeeley SG: Chronic pelvic pain: Psychological features and laparoscopic findings. Psychomatics 1984; 25:833.
52. Stout AL, Steege JF, Rupp SL: Comparison of personality profiles of premenstrual syndrome and chronic pelvic pain patients. J Psychosom Obstet Gynaecol 1989;10:121.
53. King PM, Ling FW, Myers CA: Screening for female urogenital system disease. In Boissonnault WG (ed): Examination in Physical Therapy Practice—Screening for Medical Disease, 2nd ed. New York, Churchill Livingstone, 1995.

25

Neuropathic Pain

J. Thomas Benson, MD

Neuropathic pain is pain mediated via a disturbed neuronal pathway. The definition itself is problematic because pain is not simply a sensation transmitted from the site of tissue damage to the brain. Pain perception is not the same as the transmission of pain impulses. Instead, the signal sent via nerves and neurotransmitters is entwined with signals from the limbic system, which contains the stored emotional experience of the individual. Hence, the pain experienced is affected by what an individual is thinking and feeling at the moment, the patient's personality, the presence or absence of a diagnosis, surrounding life circumstances, and secondary gain. Thus, pain is not objective but is always subjective and is always a conceptual state.

Throughout this chapter, it is necessary to keep in mind that although we are talking about abnormal pain mediation pathways and their treatments, pain is still a perception. There is no such thing as imaginary pain. However, pain can be felt in the absence of an observable abnormality in the neuronal pathway, and it is amenable to therapy. Pretended pain (malingering) is uncommon in medical situations.

Pain Pathways

Pain is generally perceived through naked nerve endings. The pain receptors (nociceptors) transmit impulses through two pathways: a lightly myelinated (Aδ fiber pathway) and an unmyelinated (C fiber) pathway. The small myelinated fibers supply the cold receptors and respond to mechanical stimuli, producing so-called sharp, stinging, "fast" pain. The unmyelinated C fibers supply polymodal or multisensitive nociceptors. They respond to mechanical and thermal stimuli, chiefly transmitting "warm" pain.

Other types of sensory stimuli are perceived through additional receptors: Meissner's corpuscles (texture recognition), Pacini's corpuscles (vibration, tickle, deep pressure), Merkel's disks (pressure, tactile), and Ruffini's organs (proprioception, warmth). These receptors transmit via neuronal structures that are more heavily myelinated and larger than the pathways transmitting pain.

The sensory pathways to the spinal cord are generally through the dorsal roots, although there are some ventral root afferents. The dorsal root ganglia contain the cell bodies for all the sensory nerves (somatic and visceral), each of which has a peripheral branch receiving afferent input and a central branch extending to the spinal cord (Fig. 25–1). Once reaching the spinal cord, secondary neurons convey the stimuli through the spinothalamic tracts (Fig. 25–2). These spinal sensory neurons are of two types: one specific to the nociceptive input and another of wide dynamic range, which responds to nociceptive and other inputs.

The fibers cross in the spinal cord and ascend to terminate in the ventroposterolateral nuclei of the thalamus. Afferents also end in the mediothalamic nuclei, where they have more involvement with motivational-affective components of pain. A few parallel pathways for transmission are found in the spinal-reticular and spinomesencephalic tracts. Visceral sensations are bilateral, because bilateral tractotomy (deep to spinothalamic tracts) has been found necessary to alleviate pain of visceral origin. In the cortex, pain is represented in the primary and secondary sensory cortex and the

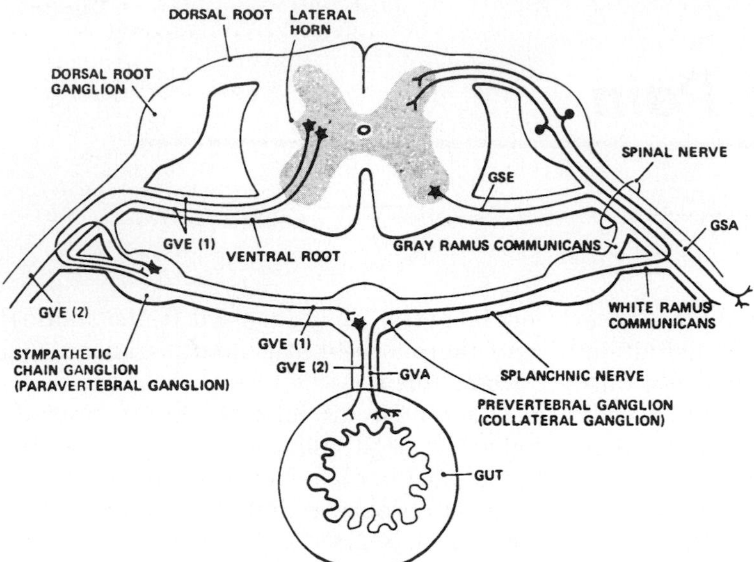

Figure 25–1. Functional components of a spinal nerve. General somatic afferent (GSA), general visceral afferent (GVA), and general somatic efferent (GSE) fibers and their cells of origin are illustrated on the right and are arbitrarily separated, for clarity, from the general visceral efferent fibers and cells GVE (1) and GVE (2) on the left. The autonomic (GVE) structures diagrammed here belong to the sympathetic division. (From Gilman S, Newman SW: Manter and Gatz's Essentials of Clinical Neuroanatomy and Neurophysiology, 8th ed. Philadelphia, FA Davis, 1992.)

cingulate gyrus, lesions of which sometimes ameliorate intractable pain.

In addition to the ascending pain system, a descending modulation system originates in the brainstem periaqueductal gray matter, projecting to the raphe nucleus and from there directly to the ventral and dorsal horns of the spinal cord, acting to inhibit nociception (see Chapter 2). These projections are joined by projections from the locus caeruleus.

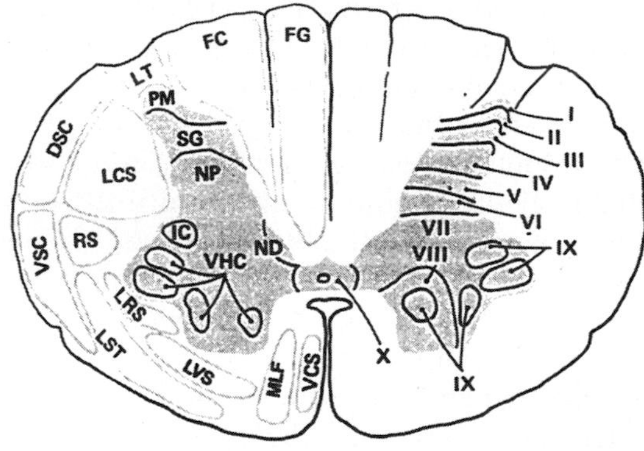

Figure 25–2. Cross section of the spinal cord at approximately the C8–T1 segmental level. Tracts and nuclei of the cord are illustrated on the left; Rexed's laminar organization of the gray matter is illustrated on the right. DSC, dorsal spinocerebellar tract; FC, fasciculus cuneatus; FG, fasciculus gracilis; IC, intermediolateral cell column; LCS, lateral corticospinal tract; LRS, lateral reticulospinal tract; LST, lateral spinothalamic tract; LT, Lissauer's tract; LVS, lateral vestibulospinal tract; MLF, medial longitudinal fasciculus; ND, nucleus dorsalis; NP, nucleus proprius; PM, posteromarginal nucleus; RS, rubrospinal tract; SG, substantia gelatinosa; VCS, ventral corticospinal tract; VHC, ventral horn cell columns; VSC, ventral spinocerebellar tract. (From Gilman S, Newman SW: Manter and Gatz's Essentials of Clinical Neuroanatomy and Neurophysiology, 8th ed. Philadelphia, FA Davis, 1992.)

Chronic Pain

Chronic neuropathic pain is associated with variable combinations of positive and negative sensory, motor, and vasomotor phenomena. The sensory phenomena may involve hyperalgesia (excessive sensitivity to pain), allodynia (pain sensation due to normally innocuous stimulation), paresthesia (spontaneous pricking or tingling), dysesthesia (impairment of sensitivity, especially touch), hyperesthesia (exaggerated tactile stimulation), hypoesthesia (diminished sensitivity), or anesthesia (absence of sensitivity). Sensory sensations may be spontaneous or induced.

Muscle pain is transmitted by the free nerve endings of fine myelinated and unmyelinated fibers found in fascia, tendon, and periosteum. Motor components of neuropathy may be characterized by muscle weakness or cramping. Muscle pain differs from cutaneous pain in that the muscle pain exceeds its nerve territory, often spreading to the areas supplied by nerve roots to other muscles (referred pain). In contrast, cutaneous pain tends to stay confined to the territory of the stimulated nerve. Most neuropathic muscle pain is progressively intense, increasing from pain with contraction, to soreness, to cramp. The most common neuropathic muscle pain is in calf muscles.

Vasomotor changes associated with chronic neuropathic conditions are characterized by localized areas that are either hot or cold. These skin changes typically occur as a result of chronic vascular abnormalities.

Models of Neuropathic Pain

Studies have succeeded in producing models of painful peripheral neuropathies in laboratory animals.[1] Although the initial neuronal trauma may be peripheral, the pain locus gradually becomes centralized owing to an excitotoxic effect on the spinal cord dorsal horn inhibitory interneurons. The role of the sympathetic nervous system varies, depending on the type of nerve injury and the temporal evolution of the syndrome. This chapter considers the pathophysiologic mechanisms, beginning with the periphery and progressing centrally. Discussion is focused on (1) peripheral effects, (2) effects at the dorsal root ganglion, (3) effects at the dorsal horn, (4) effects on central nervous system suppression, and (5) sympathetic effects.

Peripheral Neuropathy

Nerve injuries due to cuts, stretching, or compression yield neuromas-in-continuity—that is, sprouts trapped in intraneural scar tissue. The sprouts in the neuroma, as well as areas of demyelination, acquire abnormal and apparently spontaneous ectopic discharges that are probably due to an accumulation of newly developed ion channels (sodium, potassium, calcium, and others). The sprouts in the neuroma acquire an abnormal sensitivity to mechanical and cold stimuli and have been shown to acquire increased α-adrenoceptors on the primary afferent membrane, leading to abnormal response to norepinephrine. Both the lightly myelinated and unmyelinated pathways for nociception use L-glutamate as a neurotransmitter. The polymodal nociceptor units also use substance P and calcitonin gene–related peptide (CGRP) as neurotransmitters. Substance P and CGRP produce localized neurogenic inflammation. The polymodal nociceptors, in addition to responding to mechanical and thermal stimuli, also respond to chemical agents. Tissue injury releases potassium, bradykinin, and arachidonic acid metabolites including prostaglandins and leukotrienes. Prostaglandins sensitize tissues to the pain-producing effects of the other substances released by injury.

Treatment of the peripheral local site of neuroma formation can be directed toward the ion channels or the neurotransmitter/receptor. Increased sodium channel activity can be blocked with agents such as carbamazepine (Tegretol). Ion channel interruption can be accomplished with application of local anesthetics. Depletion of local transmission by substance P is theoretically possible using local applications of capsaicin applied three to four times daily for 2 to 4 weeks. Its use around mucous membranes, however, is too painful for effective therapy. Antiprostaglandins, such as aspirin and other nonsteroidal antiinflammatory drugs (NSAIDs), are effective systemically or locally as inhibitors of prostaglandin stimulation of polymodal nociceptors but are ineffective with leukotrienes.

Dorsal Root Ganglion Neuropathy

The neuronal sprout is not the only site of spontaneous ectopic discharges that may arise after peripheral nerve injury. The ectopic discharges may also arise in the afferent nerve cell bodies located in the dorsal root ganglion. This is an extremely important consideration because treatment aimed at the locus of the nerve injury (such as neuroma excision) does not correct the spontaneous discharge originating in the dorsal root ganglion. The neuropeptides that are released peripherally are also released centrally at the dorsal horn. The dorsal root ganglia are thought to be responsible for origin of tic or repetitive shock sensations, and carbamazepine is used for therapy of such shooting-type pain, presumably by acting primarily via its effect on sodium channel activity.

Dorsal Horn Neuropathy

Centralization of pain occurs because of spontaneous activity coming from the peripheral sensory neurons, leading to excessive excitation of secondary neurons at the dorsal horn. Glutaminergic synapses, acting on *N*-methyl-D-aspartate (NMDA) receptors, mediate the wind-up phenomenon responses. *Winding up* refers to the process in which noxious spontaneous stimulation leads to action potentials that increase in amount in apparently uncontrolled fashion. This process has a similarity to that which occurs in brain neurons in status epilepticus. Cells within the dorsal horn become damaged by this activity. Many of the damaged neurons are inhibitory neurons, and loss of this inhibition leads to exaggerated nociception in the spinal cord afferents.

Another function of dorsal horn neurons is to control nociceptive inputs that arrive from peripheral nerves in response to stimuli. Simultaneous stimulation of large, myelinated afferents blocks the stimulated nociceptor afferent activity through GABAergic interneurons (*gate control*). This blocking activity only occurs in response to stimuli and not in spontaneous C-nociceptor–induced pain. Distinguishing between the two types of neuropathy is important because only induced pain has a chance to respond to gate control therapy. Clinical testing involves administering large fiber sensory nerve stimulation, such as vibration, to determine if noxious stimulation appreciation is decreased.

These observations of dorsal horn function open opportunities for effective therapy. Therapeutic agents with anti-NMDA receptor activity are being developed. One possible though yet unproven agent, gabapentin (Neurontin), has been approved for use in adjunctive therapy of partial seizures and is currently in trials for dorsal horn effects in chronic neuropathic pain. Inhibiting the excessive excitation at the glutaminergic synapses may perhaps minimize the damage to inhibitory neurons and reverse or decrease the dorsal horn disinhibition of nociceptive input. Antiepileptic medications such as carbamazepine, phenytoin (Dilantin), and clonazepam (Klonopin) may be effective in dorsal horn activity, given its similarity to status epilepticus. Modulation of the dorsal root pain perception in hyperalgesia or allodynia may be obtained with electric stimulation through the GABAergic inhibition. GABA α-receptors may be activated by diazepam (Valium) and GABA β-receptors by baclofen. Muscle cramps are known to result from impaired GABA function and may be blocked by diazepam and baclofen. Baclofen has also been shown to improve spastic syndromes.

Central Neuropathy

The descending modulation system of the central nervous system acts on the dorsal horns of the spinal cord to inhibit nociception. This system principally acts via serotonin, norepinephrine, and opioids to inhibit pain transmission. Augmentation of the central modulation may be mediated by opiates (including methadone) and agents accentuating serotonin activities such as serotonin reuptake inhibitors (including paroxetine [Paxil] and amitriptyline [Elavil]). The latter must be used in fairly large doses and may also be helpful with depression and insomnia, the other common components of chronic pain syndromes.

Sympathetic Neuropathy (Reflex Sympathetic Dystrophy)

The role of the sympathetic nervous system in chronic pain is poorly understood, although animal models have facilitated a functional understanding of certain syndromes. In animal studies, chronic constriction of a nerve produces a reproducible evolution of skin temperature changes: The skin is abnormally warm for about 1 week, after which it evolves to a chronically cold status.

The late-stage cold skin is associated with an absence of norepinephrine staining of the nerve endings, implying that it is not due to excessive noradrenergic sympathetic vasoconstriction but more likely due to denervation supersensitivity to circulating catecholamines. It is well known that the sympathetic postganglionic cell body is dependent on a continuous supply of nerve growth factor from the tissue served by the nerve and transported retrogradely to the ganglion. Chronic constriction may well lead to symptomatic denervation by interfering with this transport. Sympathetically maintained pain and sympathetically independent pain may coexist and represent successive stages in the evolution of the disease process.

Patients may be divided symptomatically into those having warm and cold syndromes. The ABC syndrome[2] is the angry, backfiring, C-nociceptor syndrome. The skin is red and warm owing to antidromic vasodilatation with spontaneous burning pain and hyperalgesia to mechanical stimulation. Cooling the area abolishes the spontaneous pain and mechanical hyperalgesia. In this syndrome, the sympathetic system is intact and excessive sympathetic stimulation can lead to a slight cooling effect. Treatment that decreases sympathetic activity, such as medical or surgical sympathectomy, may actually accentuate the pain.

In contrast to the ABC syndrome, cold patients have burning pain and mechanical hyperalgesia with cold skin. The pain is provoked by cooling, whereas warming may decrease the pain. A subgroup of the cold patients may experience a loss of cold sensation. Both of these groups of patients have sympathetic denervation, with the skin chronically vasoconstricted owing to denervation supersensitivity. Local nerve block aids diagnosis of sympathetic denervation. If the cold skin is due to denervation hypersensitivity, the nerve block has no effect on the temperature of the part. If the cold skin is secondary to sympathetic stimulation, the nerve block stops the stimulation and the area vasodilates and warms.

Invasive therapeutic modalities for reflex sympathetic dystrophies have had almost universally disappointing results. For the most part, treatment is guided by the patient's response to sympathetic blockade. The placebo response, however, is of such significance that it is now strongly suggested that any such diagnostic block be placebo controlled. Treatment may be directed toward the central descending pain modulation system or the peripheral nervous system. Centrally acting agents include clonidine, which stimulates α-adrenoceptors in the brainstem, which inhibit the sympathetic outflow from the central nervous system. Clonidine has been found to be particularly effective in hyperhidrosis. Serotonin reuptake inhibitors, which include paroxetine, have an added benefit in the treatment of depression. Peripherally directed treatment either consists of blocking sympathetic activity, when the pain is sympathetically maintained, or is aimed at decreasing supersensitivity in sympathetic-independent pain. Sympathetic chemical blockade may be produced with parenteral administration of phentolamine (Regitine) or orally with phenoxybenzamine (Dibenzyline). Prazosin (Minipress) produces a blockade of postsynaptic α-adrenoceptors in sympathetically independent supersensitivity.

In an attempt to provide simplification for clinical guidance, Table 25–1 reflects pathophysiologically directed medical management of neuropathic pain. Current research activity is progressing in this area, and this information should soon be outdated. Expanded research efforts are definitely needed.

Pelvic Pathways

Neuropathic pain involving the pelvis and pelvic organs can be best understood in the context of its anatomic and functional organization. The chief nerve supply of the pelvis comes from sacral nerves, whose roots, because of the unequal growth of the vertebral column in comparison with the spinal cord, traverse a long distance from the termination of the spinal cord (at the level of the first lumbar vertebra) to the exit of the nerve root from the sacral foramina. The roots, forming the cauda equina (horse's tail), join to form nerves shortly before the

Table 25–1. **PATHOPHYSIOLOGICALLY DIRECTED MEDICAL MANAGEMENT OF NEUROPATHIC PAIN**

Site	Pathophysiology	Diagnoses	Management
Peripheral	Neuronal sprouting Spontaneous ectopic discharge	Sensory and vasomotor abnormalities detected by mechanical and thermal stimuli. Vasomotor abnormalities in nerve territory detected by temperature and color changes. Motor effects if motor nerve involved. Normal neurophysiologic test results proximal to periphery.	Ion channel blockade: Lidocaine Carbamazepine
Polymodal nociceptor units	Neurotransmitters: substance P, CGRP, prostaglandin sensitization		Anti–substance P Capsaicin Antiprostaglandins Nonsteroidal antiinflammatory drugs
Dorsal root ganglion	Spontaneous ectopic discharge	Tic or repetitive shock sensations; persistence of spontaneous sensory disturbances after local infiltration block at periphery; may have abnormal sensory nerve conduction studies.	Carbamazepine
Dorsal horn	Excess of glutaminergic synapses activating on NMDA receptors with spontaneous activity leads to damage of pain inhibiting neurons	Sensory, motor, and vasomotor abnormalities; allodynia; persistence of spontaneous pain after local infiltration; loss of gait control—check by detecting loss of reduction of hyperesthesia with noxious stimulation by simultaneous vibrating stimulation.	Anti-NMDA receptors (gabapentin); antiepileptic medications including clonazepam, phenytoin, carbamazepine
	Loss of GABAergic inhibition of induced pain; impaired GABA function in muscle pain and spasticity.		Electric stimulation (requires normal proximal nerve). Larger myelinated nerve activity to inhibit induced pain. Activate GABA receptors: baclofen, diazepam
Central antinociceptive network	Losses of catecholamine antinociception	Objective findings above, plus signs of pain, depression, insomnia cycle.	Augmenting central modulation: Opioids including methadone
	Serotonin receptor agonist		Tricyclic antidepressants: (amitriptyline), paroxetine
Sympathetic	Sympathetically intact—maintained pain	Vasomotor and temperature changes pronounced; sympathetically maintained pain; cold areas vasodilate and warm with nerve block; sympathetically independent pain, cold areas do not vasodilate and warm with block. Warm areas may have increased pain with sympathetic block; such areas demonstrate some pain relief with cooling. All blocks should be placebo controlled; neurophysiologic tests of sympathetic efferents are possible.	Medical "sympathectomy," phentolamine—parenterally, phenoxybenzamine, oral lidocaine
	Sympathetically denervated hypersensitivity		Postsynaptic α block (prazosin)
	Central brainstem α stimulation to reduce peripheral output		Clonidine

CGRP, calcitonin gene–related peptide; NMDA, *N*-methyl-D-aspartate; GABA, γ-aminobutyric acid.

nerve exits the vertebral column. The nerves are surrounded by a protective dense tissue called *perineurium*, which the nerve roots lack. The nerve roots are thus vulnerable to trauma, such as that which commonly occurs with disk herniation.

The terminal part of the spinal cord, giving rise to the pelvic nerves (conus medullaris), is subject to disk herniation, ankylosing spondylitis, ependymomas, lipomas, dermoid cysts, transverse myelitis, arteriovenous malformations, and congenital meningomyelocele, all of which may result in cord tethering. Pathology at the conus can also occur as a complication of abdominal aortic aneurysm surgery after prolonged aortic clamping and spinal cord ischemia. Cauda equina lesions are also very common. Central disk protrusion, congenital caudal aplasia (from diabetic mothers), congenital and acquired spinal stenosis (pseudoclaudication syndrome), ankylosing spondylitis, schwannomas, primary and metastatic malignancies, lymphomas, meningiomas, neural fibromas, chordomas, acquired immunodeficiency syndrome, and cytomegalic infection may be involved in the etiology of cauda equina lesions. Cauda equina lesions secondary to arachnoiditis occur in episodic fashion and may also develop after injections of oil contrast, alcohol, phenol, or very high doses of intrathecal penicillin. Diabetic lumbosacral radiculopathies most commonly involve the L3–L4 routes and are bilateral in half of the cases. This is so common that radiculopathy (nerve root disorder) should be considered before investigating visceral pathology in diabetic persons with chronic truncal pain.

As discussed in Chapter 5, the anterior rami of the nerves form the lumbosacral plexus after leaving the vertebral column. Plexus lesions are most commonly associated with malignancies (cervical, rectal, and lymphoma), radiation damage, or hematomas. Symptoms include patchy muscle weakness and sensory loss in the thighs and legs.

Isolated nerve injuries (mononeuropathies) occur commonly in the pelvis. The most common is the compressive and stretch injury that may affect the pudendal nerve during labor and delivery. Mechanical compressive nerve damage of a permanent nature may occur with 80 mm Hg pressure for 8 hours. The pressures generated during the second stage of labor normally reach a maximum of 240 mm Hg.[3] Stretch has also been shown to cause nerve demyelination if the nerve is stretched 15% of its length.[4] Because the pudendal nerve is fixed in the obturator fascia (Alcock's canal), descent of the pelvic floor readily causes stretch injury. The pudendal nerve is stretched 15% with only 1.35 cm descent of the pelvic floor during labor; thus, stretch injury is very common. Pudendal nerve injuries cause sensory deficits or paresthesias and sensory abnormalities (described earlier) over S2, S3, and S4 dermatomes and motor deficits in the external anal sphincter and periurethral and perineal musculature.

Ilioinguinal nerve injury is most frequently manifested as surgical damage, particularly with needle urethropexy.[5] Iliohypogastric and genitofemoral nerve injury is usually encountered after Pfannenstiel's incisions or use of self-retaining retractors or with formation of postoperative adhesions in the lower abdominal and inguinal area. Damage to these nerves typically causes sensory abnormalities in the inguinal area, upper anteromedial thigh, and a small portion of the genitalia.

Obturator nerve injury is commonly encountered now that more surgery is being performed in the space of Retzius. It is characterized by sensory abnormalities in the medial thigh with denervation in the thigh adductors, leading to weakness in thigh adduction (see Chaper 5).

Entrapment of the lateral femoral cutaneous nerve (meralgia paresthetica) occurs at the level of the anterior superior iliac spine, producing sensory changes over the lateral thigh. The site of entrapment is at the point where the nerve pierces the inguinal ligament or the fascia lata.

The femoral nerve is frequently damaged by overzealous use of retractors. The most common cause of femoral neuropathy, however, is diabetes. This produces weakness of the quadriceps with subsequent weakness of leg extension at the knee, as well as sensory impairment over the anterior medial aspect of the thigh and the medial aspect of the lower leg. If iliopsoas weakness is present, the damage is above the inguinal ligament area. This may occur after head compression of the lumbar roots as they enter the pelvic inlet during labor and delivery. Iliopsoas weakness is identified by weakness of thigh flexion at the hip.

Table 25–2 summarizes the findings in mononeuropathies involving the pelvic area.

Diagnosis

Treatment of neuropathic pain previously was universally disappointing. However, with the advent of increasing choices of therapeutic options, it is imperative that treatment be guided by specific clinical diagnoses. Subjecting patients to therapeutic interventions without determining the underlying pathophysiology can delay treatment and lead to treatment failure and disillusionment on the part of the patient and the health care team.

A carefully taken history is of utmost importance and should be directed toward obtaining temporal details of the associated sensory, motor, and vasomotor phenomena. Distinguishing between types of sensory disturbance and between spontaneous and induced pain is important.

The physical examination expands on the information obtained from the history and allows different diagnostic hypotheses to be tested and treatment to be determined. The peripheral manifestation of abnormal neuronal sprouting is suggested by finding areas with mechanical hyperalgesia or allodynia. The temperature of the area helps to distinguish the hot and cold syndromes. The effect of cooling and warming the area is helpful in directing therapy. For example, if the pain is increased by warming, then therapies directed toward reducing sympathetic input could be deleterious because the resulting vasocongestion would lead to warming and an increase in symptoms. The presence of localized inflammation would suggest activity of substance P and CGRP neurotransmitters.

As part of the diagnostic evaluation of patients with neuropathic pain, nerve blocks are helpful for diagnosis and treatment. Because of the significant placebo effect, it is imperative that the blocks be placebo controlled before using them to dictate therapy. If somatic nerve block improves

Table 25–2. **FINDINGS IN MONONEUROPATHIES INVOLVING THE PELVIC AREA**

Nerve	Motor	Sensory
Pudendal	Anal sphincter Perineal muscles Periurethral skeletal muscle	Dermatomes S2, S3, and S4 Perineum Paraanal
Ilioinguinal	Lower obliquus internus Transversus	Medial thigh and lateral labia majora Below inguinal ligament
Iliohypogastric	Obliquus internus Transversus	Iliac branch: posterior superior gluteal region; Hypogastric branch: anterior suprapubic area
Genitofemoral	Portion of lateral bulbocavernosus	Femoral branch (lumboinguinal nerve)—proximal anterior thigh Genital branch—with round ligament to labia majora
Lateral femoral cutaneous	None	Anterior branch: lateral and anterior thigh above knee Posterior branch: skin from greater trochanter to midthigh
Obturator	Adductores muscles of hip Articular branch to hip joint	Medial—proximal half of leg Medial thigh—distal to adductor longus
Femoral	Quadriceps Iliacus—supplied above inguinal ligament	Middle cutaneous: anterior thigh above knee Medial cutaneous: medial thigh, medial leg with saphenous nerve
Posterior femoral cutaneous	None	Skin over low, lateral gluteus maximum, groove between thigh and perineum to labia majora

spontaneous pain or mechanical hyperalgesia, then it is very likely that the nerve is intimately involved in the pathophysiology of the pain. Local blocks of peripheral nerves may also give an indication of the relative activity at the dorsal root ganglion and dorsal horn. If this activity is determined to be a significant component of a patient's pain (i.e., peripheral nerve blocks do *not* reduce pain), then treatment may be directed against spontaneous neuronal activity with anti-NMDA receptor medication (gabapentin) or antiepileptic medication (clonazopam, phenytoin, or carbamazepine). Conversely, treatment of induced neuronal activity can be accomplished with electric stimulation (TENS unit or skin magnets) or by enhancing GABA inhibition medically (diazepam, baclofen).

Proximal nerve blocks or sympathetic chain blocks may suggest the presence of sympathetically maintained pain if vasocongestion and warming occur after the block. Absence of this phenomenon may suggest sympathetic denervation, and tests for autonomic dysfunction and localized small fiber effects may be necessary. However, methadone, amitriptyline, and paroxetine are empirically used when treatment directed toward the periphery has not resulted in satisfactory response.

Conventional nerve conduction and electromyography (EMG) studies should be performed. These are very important in demonstrating neuropathic pain; however, it should be kept in mind that this testing checks for large fiber nerve function, and abnormality does not necessarily imply that it is the cause of the pain. Likewise, abnormal small fiber function can exist with normal large fiber function. Despite these nonspecific results, the screening is important because needle EMG has the ability to explicitly document a nonorganic origin for muscle weakness. Tests such as somatosensory quantitative thermal tests, which look at thresholds for cold and warm stimulation and for heat pain and cold pain, are helpful in difficult cases.[6] Current perception threshold quantitative sensory testing helps in evaluation of small fiber activity. Normal data have been collected for perianal and perineal cutaneous regions.[7] Several tests of autonomic function[8] may be useful in highly selected cases. These include quantitative sweat testing (Qsart), recording of potentials evoked in sweat glands (sympathetic skin responses), and fluctuations in pulse rate and blood pressure associated with Valsalva's maneuver, deep breathing, and positional changes.

Treatment Principles

Drug therapy, when used for pain, should be given on a time-contingent basis, not on an as-needed basis. Each drug should be given an adequate trial and taken to high doses or frequencies before changes are made.

Surgery for neuropathic pain has limited indications. In mononeuropathies aggravated by movement, translocation of nerves is sometimes possible. In compression neuropathies, decompression may be helpful. Surgical sympathectomy, as indicated, must be very carefully selected and in general has had less than satisfactory results. Dorsal rhizotomies and tractotomies may be considered in extreme cases. Neurolysis for pain relief generally is short lasting and of little use if centralization has occurred.

Selection of patients for neurolysis such as presacral neurectomy or uterosacral denervation (see Chapter 18) should be limited to those with definite neuropathic pain without established centralization. Thus, they must demonstrate objective sensory, motor, and vasomotor changes with dramatic relief with placebo-controlled nerve blocks and demonstration of a sympathetically maintained component to the pain either by sympathetic chain blocks or tests for localized small fiber effects. The pathways being interrupted in these procedures are visceral afferent and sympathetic efferent. If the sympathetic component is active, some vasodilatation and warming may be noted after nerve block. The warming can be objectively measured by skin surface thermometers. Thus, patients with midline pelvic sensory disturbance without pain centralization, with sympathetically maintained pain, would be the best candidates for presacral neurectomy. Such patients would demonstrate dramatic pain relief with warming and vasodilatation after the nerve block. In these patients, repeated nerve blocks may have beneficial therapeutic activity and could be used instead of surgery.

Most patients with chronic neuropathic pain can be treated by an interested primary care giver, specialist, or subspecialist. Careful examination of the sensory, motor, and vasomotor phenomenon does not require specialized equipment for baseline studies. Conservative management including pharmacologic adjuncts is within the scope of the primary caregiver. However, before suggesting invasive therapies for neuropathic pain such as organ removal or nerve surgery, referral to specialists who can conduct the associated neurophysiologic evaluations is appropriate.

Returning again to the premise indicated at the beginning of the chapter that pain is a subjective, conceptual state, treatment of neuropathic pain by necessity must consider a patient's surrounding life circumstances and frequently requires multidisciplinary approaches.

References

1. Bennett GJ: An animal model of neuropathic pain: A review. Muscle Nerve 1993;16:1040.
2. Fruhstorfer H, Lindblom U, Schmidt WG: Method for quantitative estimation of thermal thresholds in patients. J Neurol Neurosurg Psychiatry 1976;39:1071.
3. Rempen A, Kraus M: Measurement of head compression during labor: Preliminary results. J Perinat Med 1991;19:115.
4. Lundberg G: Nerve Injury and Repair. New York, Churchill Livingstone, 1988, p 54.
5. Miyazaki F, Shook G: Ilioinguinal nerve entrapment during needle suspension for stress incontinence. Obstet Gynecol 1992;80:246.
6. Ochoa J: The human sensory unit and pain: New concepts, syndromes and tests. Muscle Nerve 1993;16:1009.
7. Benson JT: Clinical neurophysiological techniques in urinary and fecal incontinence. In Ostergard D, Bent A (eds): Urogynecology and Urodynamics: Theory and Practice. Baltimore, Williams & Wilkins, 1996.
8. Low PA: Laboratory evaluation of autonomic failure. In Low PA (ed): Clinical Autonomic Disorders. Boston, Little, Brown & Co, 1993, p 171.

26

Myofascial Syndromes

Kristen Costello, PT, BCIAC

Reiter and Gambone[1] studied 183 women with chronic pelvic pain after nondiagnostic laparoscopy and found myofascial pain to be the most common somatic cause, followed by atypical cyclic pain; gastroenterologic, urologic, and infectious diseases; and pelvic vascular congestion. This chapter discusses myofascial pain syndromes (MPS) and their relationship to pelvic pain.

Pathophysiology of Myofascial Pain Syndrome

The formation of myofascial pain and its trigger points (TPs) has been explained as a progressive process with two specific stages: (1) the neuromuscular stage and (2) the organic musculodystrophic stage.[2]

Neuromuscular Stage

In the neuromuscular stage, muscle hyperactivity and irritability are sustained by many perpetuating factors that include nutritional inadequacies, mechanical and postural stressors, and prolonged constriction of muscle such as that caused by a tight belt around the waist or a tight bra strap that constricts the upper trapezius.[3, 4] Injury or microtrauma can cause a disruption of the muscle fiber, which then releases free calcium within the muscle and disturbs the sarcoplasmic reticulum.

In the presence of adenosine triphosphate (ATP), the free calcium ions stimulate the actin/myosin activity and increase metabolic activity. This sustained interaction then releases serotonin, histamine, kinins, and prostaglandins, which can fire the groups 3 and 4 muscle nociceptors, and sets up a neural circuit between the central nervous system, nociceptors, and motor units. The circuit is then perpetuated by the conscious awareness of pain, which provokes muscle guarding and splinting, which leads to the vicious cycle of decreased blood flow to the muscle and therefore decreased ATP and calcium pump action.[2, 4, 5] This cycle is also perpetuated by poor postural habits and by allowing the muscle to tighten further by avoiding stretching activities.[4] Lack of restorative sleep also leads to the vicious cycle owing to the inability of the already chronically fatigued muscle to relax fully during sleep.[2]

Musculodystrophic Stage

The second stage, organic musculodystrophic changes, occurs after this sustained contractile activity and further release of noxious byproducts. The muscle attempts to adapt to the increased metabolic activity and is unable to do so, resulting in localized fibrosis. The atrophied tissue is replaced by less metabolically active connective tissue, which accounts for the increased ground substance found in fibrotic tissue in biopsy samples.[2] Figure 26–1 summarizes the pathophysiologic stages in the formation of myofascial pain.

Differential Diagnosis of Fibromyalgia and Myofascial Pain Syndrome

Although fibromyalgia (FM) and MPS share certain features, they are distinct from each other. The literature is made confusing

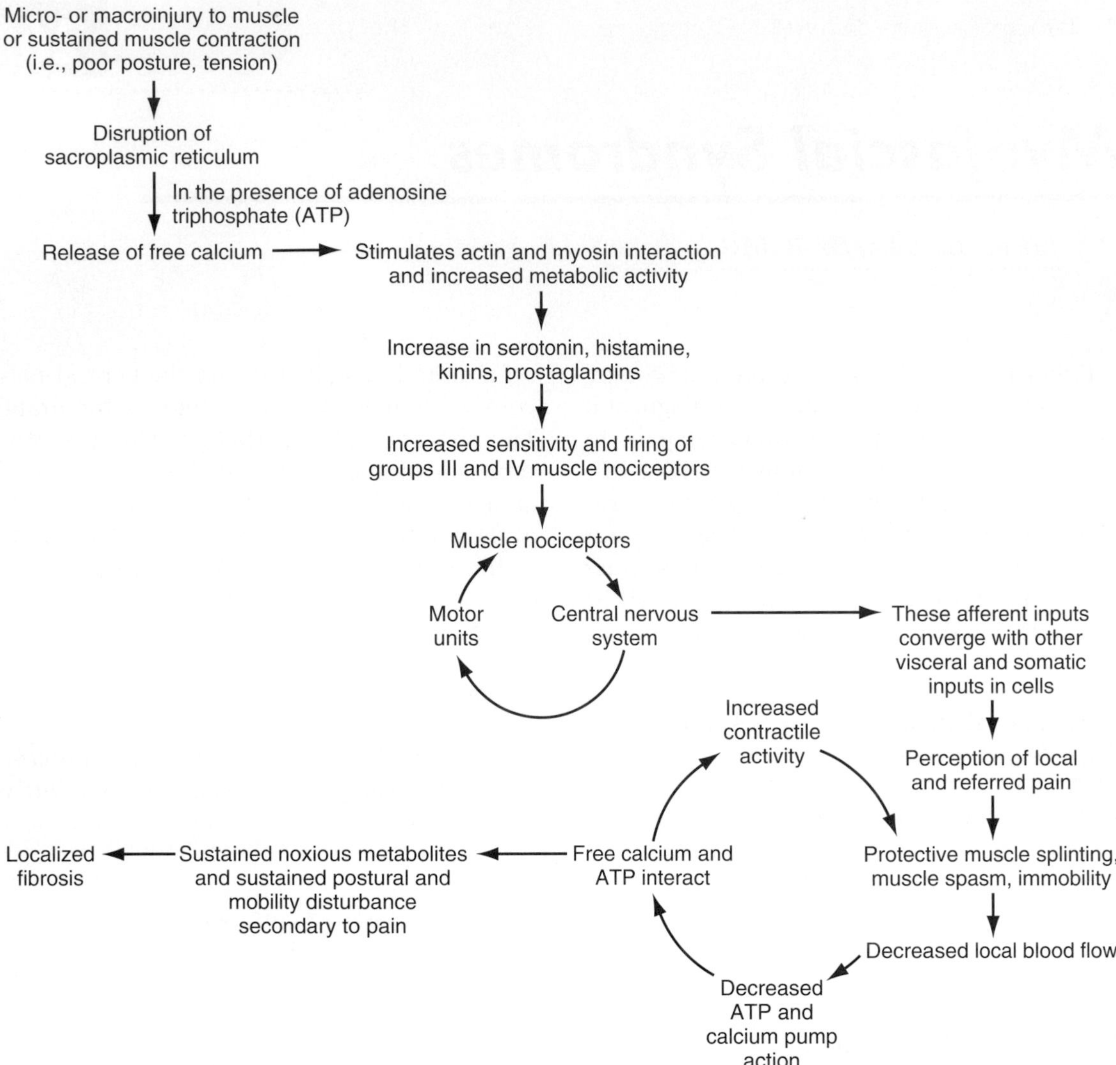

Figure 26–1. Pathophysiology of myofascial pain syndromes. (From Rachlin ES [ed]: Myofascial Pain and Fibromyalgia. St. Louis, CV Mosby, 1994, p 152.)

by the use of different terms to describe either FM or MPS, such as fibrositis, myofascitis, muscular rheumatism, myalgic spots, idiopathic myalgia, fibromyositis, and many others. This section discusses FM and MPS separately and then describes how to differentiate between them.

Fibromyalgia

When compared with a control group, patients with FM more often complain of coccygeal and pelvic pain, constipation, and diarrhea.[6] Hulme reported that 43% of patients with FM complain of pelvic pain, 70% complain of irritable bowel syndrome, 62% complain of global anxiety, and 12% complain of irritable bladder and female urethral syndrome.[7]

FM has been described as a form of nonarticular rheumatism characterized by widespread musculoskeletal aching and stiffness along with palpable tenderness of specific points.[8–10] The 1990 American Academy of Rheumatology criteria for FM included tenderness to palpation in at least 11 of 18 designated areas as one of the main signs.[11, 12] Wolfe and colleagues[13] listed the areas as follows:

1. Two centimeters distal to the lateral epicondyle of the elbow
2. Insertion of the nuchal muscles into the occiput
3. Intertransverse ligaments of C5–C7
4. Upper border of the trapezius (approximately midpoint)
5. Supraspinatus, medial aspect just above the scapular spine
6. Pectoralis, over the upper border of the second rib, about 2 cm from the sternum
7. Upper gluteal area, just below the iliac crest, in the outer quadrant
8. Insertion of the muscles into the greater trochanter of the femur, about 2 cm posterior
9. Medial condyle of the femur, about 2 cm above the joint line, on the anterolateral aspect of the bone

As any clinician understands, each individual is unique in his or her response to a pressure stimulus. "Psychological factors, factors related to secondary pain, individual pain perception, and pain behavioral patterns must all be considered in evaluating the subjective complaint of tenderness."[14]

Diagnosing FM on the basis of tender spots has been criticized because of its subjective nature and inability for pathophysiologic verification.[12, 15] Many studies have therefore attempted to objectify more precisely the tender spots by use of a dolorimeter or pressure algometer. The current criteria for abnormal pressure pain sensitivity diagnostic of FM tender spots is approximately 4 kg of pressure applied by the thumb.

Results of routine tests such as complete blood count, erythrocyte sedimentation rate, chemistry profile (including muscle enzymes), and rheumatoid factor are normal in FM.[9, 11] Antinuclear antibodies are not more prevalent than in a control group of similar age, race, and sex. Subjective dry mouth was more common in the fibromyalgic population.[11, 12, 16] Multiphase skeletal scintigraphy[11, 17] and electromyography (EMG)[11, 18, 19] also yield normal results in patients with FM.

Surface EMG measurements taken during specific work tasks did not differ between control groups and the fibromyalgic population, but the patients with FM perceived greater work effort and the quality of the task performed was inferior to that of the control group.[12, 19] Alert found that EMG muscle tension between active contractions was higher in fibromyalgic patients.[12, 20]

Goldenberg[12] stated that nuclear magnetic resonance spectrography studies have shown that the muscle is not the primary pathologic unit in FM. He reports that FM and chronic fatigue syndrome may follow well-treated Lyme disease or may mimic Lyme disease. Buchwald states that 70% of patients diagnosed with FM also met the criteria for chronic fatigue syndrome.[12, 21] (See Goldenberg[12] for a complete review of the literature on the subject of the relationship between FM, chronic fatigue, and MPS.)

Myofascial Pain Syndromes

Myofascial pain as characterized by Travell and Simons[3] defines an active myofascial TP as "a focus of hyperirritability in a muscle or its fascia that is symptomatic with respect to pain. It refers a pattern of pain at rest or on motion that is specific for the muscle. An active TP is always tender, prevents full lengthening of the muscle, weakens the muscle, usually refers pain on direct compression, mediates a local twitch response of muscle fibers when adequately stimulated, and often produces specific referred autonomic phenomena, generally in its pain reference zone."

Further differentiation can be made between an active and latent TP in that a latent TP may have all the characteristics of an active TP except that it is only painful on palpation and does not usually refer. A myofascial TP should also be distinguished from other TPs such as those arising from cutaneous, ligamentous, periosteal, and nonmuscular fascial tissue. Latent TPs are usually found coincidentally on palpation, and although they themselves do not cause pain except when palpated, they can inhibit complete muscle lengthening and cause weakness. This can lead to abnormal movement patterns and poor sedentary posture and can prevent comfortable exercise routines. For example, proximal adductor group latent TPs can interfere with comfortable intercourse.

When a TP is palpated, the patient may respond with either a positive jump sign or a local twitch response. A jump sign is present when pressure over a TP produces a patient's dramatic response such as the eyes widening, a quick inhalation, or the verbal response "right there." In contrast, a local twitch response is the transient contraction of muscle fibers containing a TP after stimulation by a snapping palpation or needling over that TP.[20] If the TP is the source of pain, palpating this point reproduces the pain complaint. Hubbard has found sustained spontaneous needle EMG activity at MPS TPs while adjacent nontender muscle fibers were electrically silent.[12, 22]

A TP can lead to abnormal movement patterns. For example, a patient may complain of high abdominal wall pain due to a TP located in the rectus sheath above the umbilicus. Such patients often show difficulty in taking a deep diaphragmatic breath because of pain on excursion of the diaphragm with stretching of the abdominal wall. They may not have been aware of this because pain had led to unrecognized limited diaphragm movement.

This deficit could then lead to a number of additional problems, which could include overuse tension of the accessory muscles of inspiration such as the scalenes and upper trapezius and decreased physical endurance due to poor oxygen exchange. Such patients may also have reproduction of pain with contraction of the affected muscles, often limiting their use of the abdominals for functional activities.

The clinical features associated with myofascial TPs include localized specific point tenderness over a taut band of muscle that on palpation causes a characteristically referred pain pattern. As stated by Travell and Simons, an individual muscle TP has a specific pattern of referred pain that is reproducible and predictable. These patterns can be a key to diagnosing an MPS and are used to locate the muscle most likely responsible for the pain pattern. Some muscles refer very locally, but others can have a much more extensive referral pattern.[3] Specific muscle groups that may contain TPs and refer pain in and around the abdominal wall or pelvic region include the abdominal obliques and rectus abdominis, hip flexors including the iliacus and psoas, adductor group, piriformis, quadratus lumborum, gluteals, and pelvic floor musculature. Figures 26–2 to 26–5 show some common pelvic TPs and their referred pain pattern. (For more detail, see Travell and Simons.[3])

The local twitch response can be elicited by placing the specific muscle group in a very slight passive stretch just past resting position, palpating the muscle perpendicular to the fibers, snapping or rolling over the fibers at the most tender spot containing the TP, watching the patient's response, and recognizing the characteristic referral pattern. Travell and Simons state that it is the change of pressure over the TP that causes the twitch response, and the closer to the TP, the more vigorous the response.[3]

Abdominal Wall Trigger Points

A more thorough discussion of abdominal wall TPs is important because of the various and frequent somatic symptoms. Early studies such as that by Melnick reported the presence of pressure and bloating along with heartburn, vomiting, and diarrhea in patients with abdominal TPs.[23] Travell and Simons[3] state that abdominal wall TPs can closely mimic visceral disorders. Diarrhea may be a concomitant of a TP in the rectus abdominis or obliques and may be a secondary autonomically controlled response of the smooth muscle and secretory activity.[3] Early studies showed that active myofascial abdominal wall TPs can simulate appendicitis symptoms.[3, 24, 25] Studies in the 1930s suggested that abdominal myofascial TPs can mimic pain associated with the urinary bladder,[3, 26] gallbladder disease,[3] diaphragmatic hernia and peptic ulcer,[3, 24, 27] gastric carcinoma, chronic cholecystitis, or gallstone colic.[3, 24]

In summary, Bennett[28] described FM and MPS as similar in that both have tender areas on palpation and both demonstrate naloxone sensitivity and αΔ sleep disturbances (discussed later). They differ from

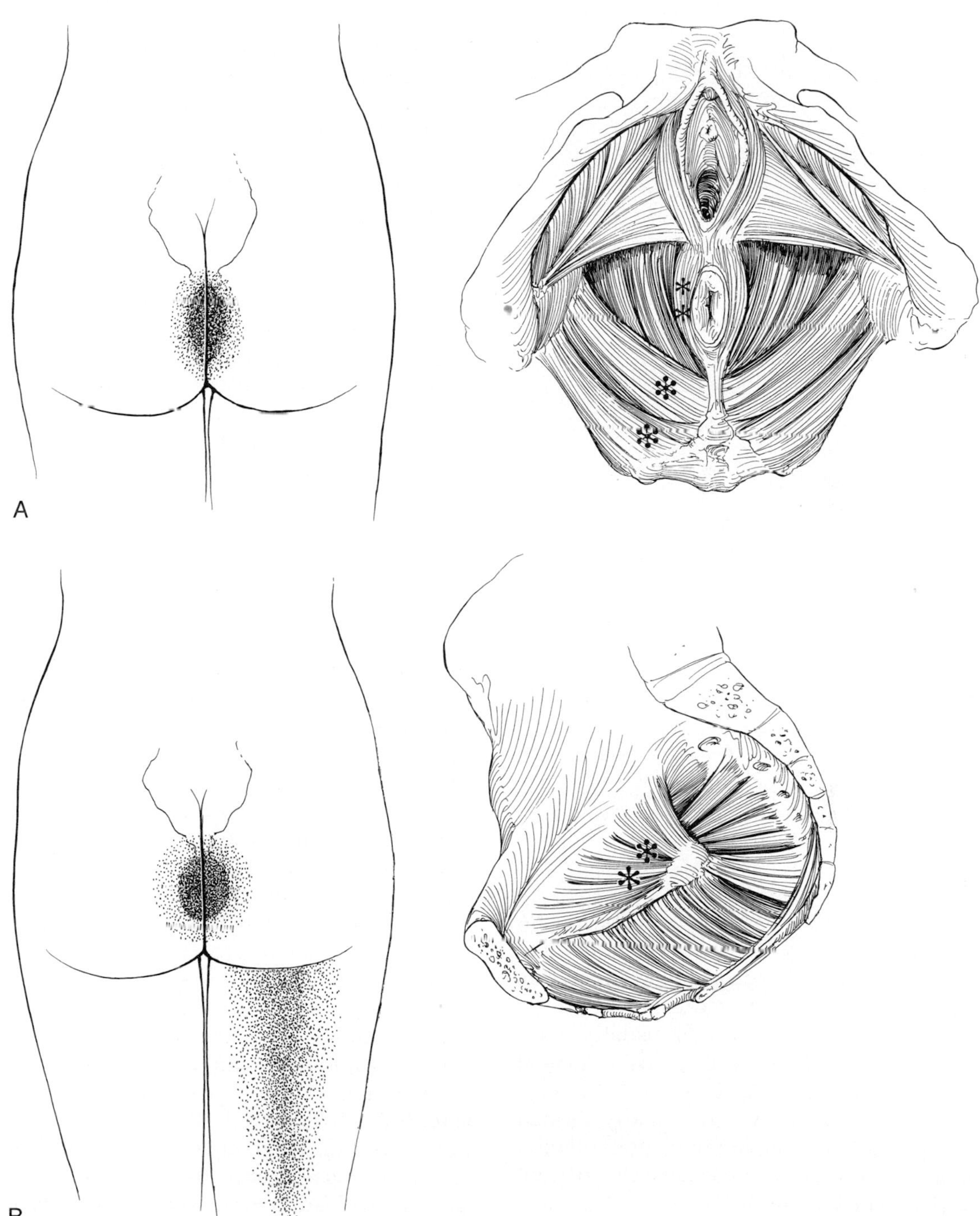

Figure 26–2. Referred pain patterns (solid and stippled) generated by trigger points (asterisks). *A*: In the right sphincter ani, levator ani, and coccygeus muscles. *B*: In the right obturator internus muscle. Pain referred from this muscle sometimes spills over to include the posterior proximal region of the thigh. (From Travell JG, Simons DG: Myofascial Pain and Dysfunction. The Trigger Point Manual, vol 2. Baltimore, Williams & Wilkins, 1983, p 112.)

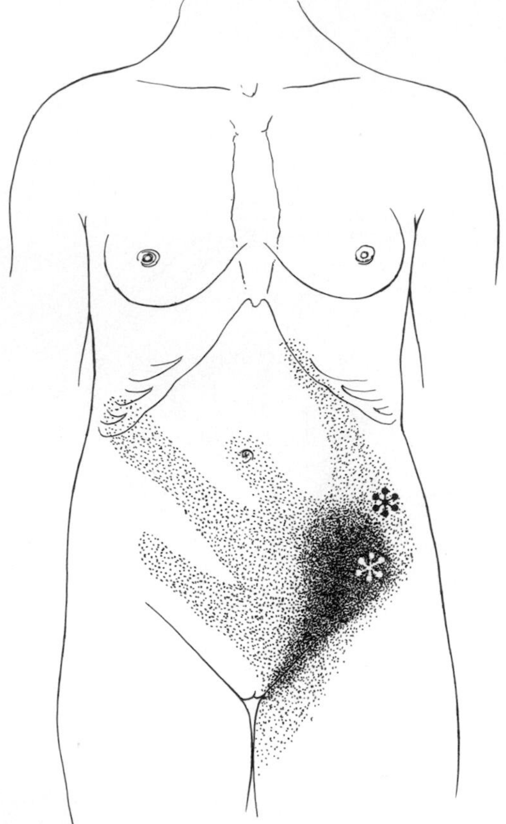

Figure 26–3. Referred pain pattern (solid) of trigger points (asterisks) in the oblique (and possibly transverse) abdominal muscles. Groin and lower quadrant pain, referred from trigger points in the lower lateral abdominal wall musculature of either side. (From Travell JG, Simons DG: Myofascial Pain and Dysfunction. The Trigger Point Manual, vol 1. Baltimore, Williams & Wilkins, 1983, p 662.)

each other in that total body pain and fatigue are present in FM whereas tenderness is more regional or localized in MPS; muscle biopsy specimens show reduced ATP in FM only. FM tender points do not usually cause referred pain and are symmetrically located at their specific multiple sites,[14] whereas MPS tender points are not usually located symmetrically and have few regional tender spots. Table 26–1 summarizes the different symptoms of FM and MPS.

Etiology of Myofascial Pain Syndrome

When a muscle is healthy and has active blood flow, normal flexibility, and normal strength and is not subjected to repetitive microtrauma or macrotrauma, it does not develop TPs. TPs are thought to occur in a muscle in response to acute or chronic stress caused by many factors, including chronic microtrauma, sleep disorders and fatigue, macrotrauma, systemic influences, and psychosocial stress and tension.

Psychosocial Correlates

It is important to consider the relationship between lifestyle and pain complaints in patients with chronic pelvic pain. Chronic pain syndrome (CPS) has been described as pain lasting more than 3 to 6 months; unresponsive to pharmacologic intervention, surgery, or medical treatment; and frequently associated with depression. Tait suggests that CPS should not be treated with narcotic analgesics.[29] Not all patients with persistent pain develop CPS, but those who do are more likely to have a history of developmental and psychosocial risk factors. Chronicity can lead to dysfunction in which virtually all areas of psychosocial function are compromised.[30]

With this in mind, careful consideration when questioning patients about their specific life circumstances not only can often aid the clinician in getting a clearer picture of the contributing causes of pain but also can increase a patient's awareness of causal factors and personal responsibility for management. Some predictors of chronic pain severity include depression, attention to pain, general health status, attributions or beliefs about pain, anxiety, social support, educational level, socioeconomic status (including employment and disability compensation), and familial models for chronic pain.[31, 32]

It is well understood that stress can lead to muscle tension and that chronic muscle tension can lead to pain. Many women have minimal outlet for this stress, which then leads to chronic patterns of muscle holding or bracing. In my experience, chronic bracing may follow a serious accident or surgery requiring prolonged immobilization, prolonged or repetitive positions at work, family and marriage conflicts, poor health and

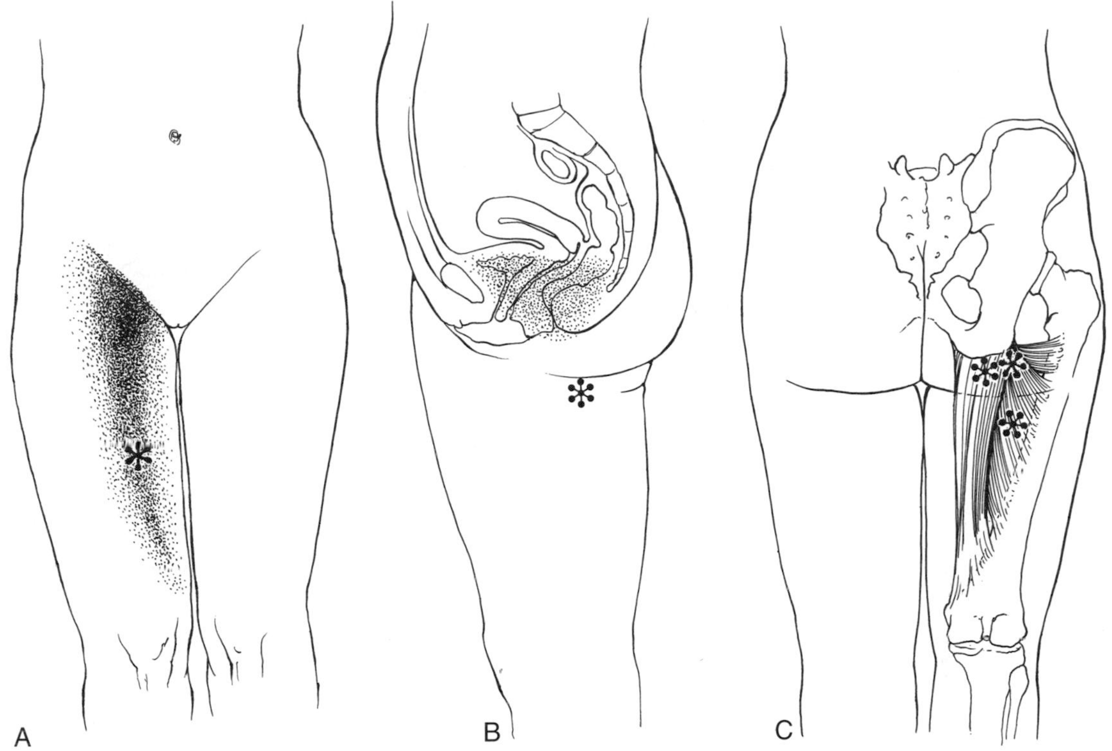

Figure 26–4. Pain pattern (solid) referred from trigger points (asterisks) in the right adductor magnus muscle (stippled). *A*: Anterior view of the referred pain pattern from the midthigh trigger point. *B*: Midsagittal view showing the intrapelvic pattern referred from the trigger point. These trigger points are found in the most proximal portion of the ischiocondylar part of the adductor magnus medial to or deep to the gluteus maximus muscle. *C*: Posterior view, anatomy of the muscle and location of its common trigger points. (From Travell JG, Simons DG: Myofascial Pain and Dysfunction. The Trigger Point Manual, vol 2. Baltimore, Williams & Wilkins, 1983, p 292.)

lifestyle habits, lack of adequate or appropriate exercise, poor posture, poor self-esteem and self-confidence, and a history of rape or childhood sexual abuse (see Chapter 3).

Much research in the literature supports the finding that pain and depression often coexist, and when the depression is treated, the pain often improves or disappears.[33] In many cases, when the pain is treated and resolved, depression diminishes.

Sleep Disturbances

Moldofsky and colleagues found that healthy subjects deprived of stage 4 sleep were more vulnerable to temporary musculoskeletal pain and mood disturbances. They postulated that a lack of brain serotonin might be responsible for the $\alpha\Delta$ sleep disturbances and might also be associated with increased sensitivity to pain.[3, 34] Sleep deprivation can lead to exhaustion. That patients may then become prone to accidents and less able to deal with stress is readily accepted by many clinicians. Sleep deprivation can also lead to increased levels of anger or depression, and early morning awakening is a common vegetative sign of depression.

Chronic Microtrauma

Chronic microtrauma can also be labeled a mechanical or postural stressor. This type of stress includes significant leg length discrepancies, walking or prolonged weight-bearing on high heels, tight pieces of clothing around the body, improper movement or breathing patterns, poor lifting habits, and poor dynamic or static body mechanics. Work positions held for prolonged periods and stress that accompanies many duties are major factors in perpetuating myofascial

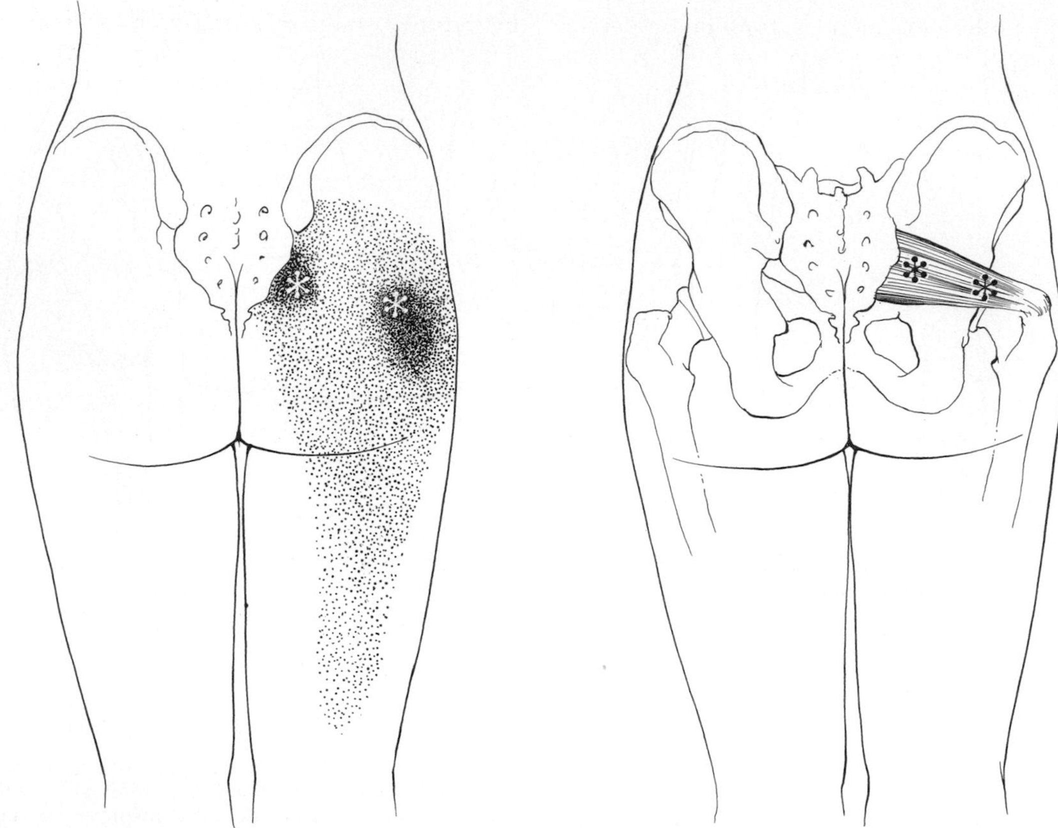

Figure 26–5. Composite pattern of pain (solid) referred from trigger points in the right piriformis muscle (asterisk). The lateral asterisk (trigger point 1) indicates the most common trigger point location. The stippling locates the spillover part of the pattern that may be felt as less intense pain than that of the essential pattern (solid). Spillover pain may be absent. (From Travell JG, Simons DG: Myofascial Pain and Dysfunction. The Trigger Point Manual, vol 2. Baltimore, Williams & Wilkins, 1983, p 188.)

pain and TPs. These can lead to a general deconditioning of the musculoskeletal system, resulting in muscle weakness, tightness, atrophy, or chronic bracing patterns.

Macrotrauma

Causative factors of myofascial pain and hypertonus dysfunction can include ortho-

Table 26–1. **COMPARISON OF VARIOUS FEATURES OF FIBROMYALGIA SYNDROME AND MYOFASCIAL PAIN SYNDROME (MPS)**

Features	Fibromyalgia Syndrome	Myofascial Pain Syndrome
Musculoskeletal pain	Widespread	Regional
Tender points	Multiple, widespread	Few, regional
Referred pain	+	+ +
Taut band	Similar to normal controls	Similar to normal controls
Twitch response	Probably similar to normal controls	Similar to normal controls
Fatigue	+ + + +	+ +
Poor sleep	+ + + +	+ +
Paresthesia	+ + +	+ +
Headaches	+ + +	+ +
Irritable bowel	+ +	+
Swollen feeling in tissues	+ +	+

+, 24% or less; + +, 25%–49%; + + +, 50%–74%; + + + +, 75%–100% of patients.
From Rachlin ES: Myofascial Pain and Fibromyalgia. St. Louis, CV Mosby, 1994, p 23.

pedic pathology such as trauma to pelvic structures or musculoskeletal dysfunctions such as those in the sacroiliac or iliosacral structures, thoracolumbar joints, joint capsules, ligaments, disks, and hip joints.[35] Neurologic factors that can lead to TPs include nerve root compression or peripheral nerve entrapments[5] (see Chapter 24).

Systemic Influences

Endocrine and metabolic imbalances include thyroid or estrogon deficiencies and anything that can create dysfunctions in energy metabolism.[3] Poor nutrition and faulty eating habits can cause a muscle to be vulnerable to TPs. Travell and Simons mention nutrients of special concern: the water-soluble vitamins B_1, B_6, B_{12}, C; folic acid; calcium; iron; and potassium.[3] Systemic infections such as viral diseases (e.g., influenza and herpes simplex) and especially chronic bacterial infections are likely to aggravate myofascial TPs.[3]

Psychosomatic causes such as fatigue, stress, tension, fear, or anxiety can bring on muscle involvement just as readily as can abnormal mechanical stress. These factors commonly coevolve as chronic pain develops. Understanding these interactions is an ongoing educational process for both clinicians and their patients.[36]

Specific Myofascial Causes of Pelvic Pain

Hypertonus

Hypertonus dysfunctions of the pelvic floor or abdominal wall can be caused or affected by any of the factors just mentioned. Hypertonus of the levator ani group (pelvic floor tension myalgia) produces pain poorly localized to the perivaginal area, perirectal area, lower abdominal quadrants, suprapubic regions, coccyx, and posterior thigh.[37] Other names for this syndrome include *proctalgia fugax, proctodynia, proctalgia*, and *diaphragma pelvis spastica*.[38] Piriformis syndrome is a similar problem in the adjacent piriformis muscle. Coccygodynia may result from spasm in surrounding muscles or from inflammation in the sacrococcygeal joint. All these disorders are similar in that they involve a high resting tone in specific musculature that attaches to the pelvic bony and fascial structures.

Interstitial Cystitis, Vulvodynia, and Urethral Syndrome

It has been shown that both intersititial cystitis[39–42] (see Chapter 22) and vulvodynia[43, 44] (see Chapter 21) can create pelvic floor tension myalgia, which may contribute to the pain associated with these conditions. Dyspareunia is also common in patients with interstitial cystitis.[40–42] When chronic pain is present, bracing or splinting around that painful region is common. The pelvic floor hypertonus common in patients with interstitial cystitis and vulvodynia can be and is often overlooked.

Spasm of urethral smooth muscle has been implicated as a possible cause of urethral syndrome.[41] Associated with this spasm are intermittent urinary flow patterns,[45] detrusor dyssynergia, postcoital voiding dysfunctions and incomplete voiding,[41] pubococcygeal tenderness,[41] and resting pelvic floor pain.[46]

Diastasis Recti

Diastasis recti, or separation of the rectus muscle bundles in the midline, may be caused by obesity or pregnancy and can cause suprapubic or lower abdominal pain in some instances. The six anterolateral abdominal muscles and the normally positioned rectus abdominis function to maintain posture and stabilize the abdominal wall during times of increased intraabdominal pressure.[47] The constant pulling apart of the rectus sheath could also cause pain at the pubis insertion.

Attempts to strengthen an already present diastasis can increase the dysfunction by pulling the rectus sheath apart instead of working to increase approximation of the rectus margins. Specifically, patients with diastasis should avoid trunk rotation, double leg lifts, and sitting straight from supine.[48] To prevent further separation, patients should splint the abdominal wall during abdominal strengthening exercise or Valsalva's maneuvers of any kind.[48, 49]

Pelvic Relaxation

Pelvic relaxation can also be a cause of myofascial pelvic discomfort. The symptoms can include a feeling of fullness or heaviness in the pelvic region, especially after prolonged standing or weight-bearing. Patients may also have associated stress incontinence. Norton[50] discusses two possible causes of pelvic relaxation: (1) after childbirth, the pelvic ligaments that support the genital organs fail to prevent genital prolapse, and (2) pelvic floor muscles fail to alleviate chronic straining of the pelvic ligaments and fascia, resulting in gradual lengthening and breakage. In cases of mild or moderate pelvic floor relaxation, increasing pelvic muscle strength can alleviate the symptoms.

Scar Tissue

Poor surgical scar mobility can also produce pelvic pain in the abdominal wall or the pelvic floor. Perineal surgical scars can affect sexual functioning if not sufficiently mobile. Incisional scars should have unrestricted mobility in all directions. Limitation in one or more directions produces pain when that limited direction is stressed. Reactive muscle contraction can produce secondary vaginismus.

Subjective and Objective Evaluation

Taking a complete subjective history of the pain, as it currently exists and as it developed chronologically, is the first step in clinical assessment. General physical examination techniques for musculoskeletal disorders and myofascial pain syndromes are discussed in Chapter 24.

Abdominal Wall

Abdominal wall evaluation should include checking for strength and flexibility as well as for TPs. It is often found that the presence of TPs over the abdominal wall causes pain with contraction of the affected muscle and prevents full lengthening of that muscle. Rectus abdominis TPs are found by palpating the muscle with a fingertip (see Chapter 7) from the lower rib cage to the pubic bone. Abdominal oblique TPs are most often found medial to the iliac crest. Psoas involvement can be found by slowly exerting pressure diagonally inward toward the muscle from outside the rectus margins. Diaphragmatic TPs are located by palpating along the lower rib margins and checking for diaphragmatic excursion with breathing.

Pelvic Floor Evaluation

The pelvic floor evaluation should include reflex testing along with internal and external assessment of the more superficial urogenital diaphragm musculature and the levator ani muscle group. For purposes of patient education, use models or pictures of the pelvis and have a patient view the external examination in a mirror that she holds for herself.

General skin integrity, mobility of episiotomy scars, and the condition of the introitus and location and excursion of the perineal body should be assessed. The excursion test is done by observing the resting position of the perineal body, asking the patient to squeeze and lift her perineum and then to release and bear down.

External palpation of the pelvic floor should include palpation of all quadrants to look for TPs and pain as well as asymmetries in sensation and tone. Herman and Wallace[52] describe an external examination called the pelvic clock examination, which represents the specific urogenital and pelvic diaphragm muscles as numbers on a clock face (Fig. 26–6).

Evaluation of strength and proprioceptive control of the pelvic floor muscles includes manual muscle testing during the internal examination by asking the patient to squeeze around your inserted finger while you watch for inappropriate substitution

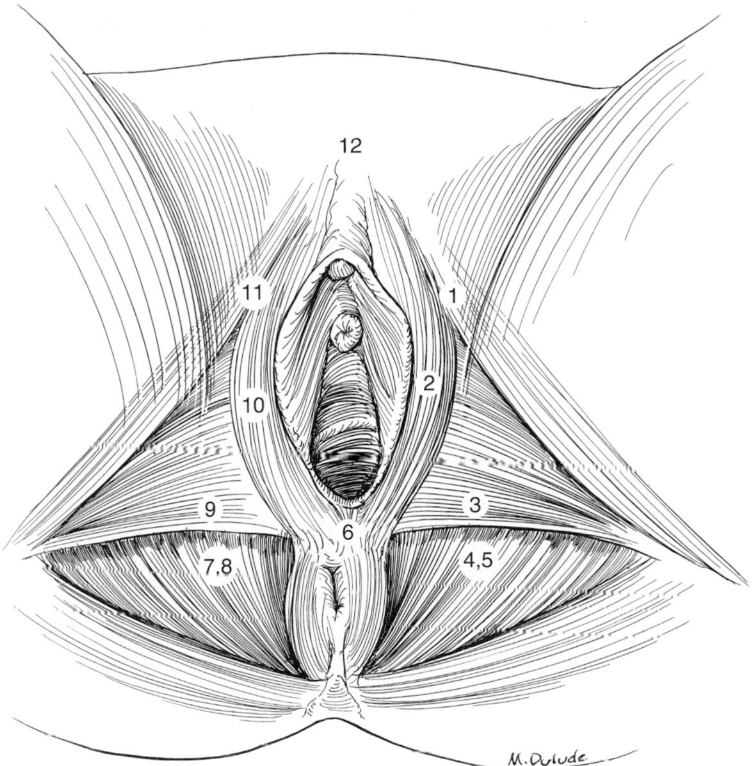

Figure 26–6. The symphysis pubis is at the 12 o'clock position, and the perineal body is at 6 o'clock. The 4, 5, 7, and 8 o'clock positions are below 6 o'clock and represent the right (7 to 8 o'clock) and left (4 to 5 o'clock) levator ani muscles; 3 and 9 o'clock represent the superficial transverse perineal muscles; 2 and 10 o'clock positions represent bulbocavernosus muscles; 1 and 11 o'clock represent ischiocavernosus muscles.

patterns such as abdominal overrecruitment or tightening of the adductors or gluteals. The use of biofeedback surface EMG to assess pelvic floor strength, hypertonus, and proprioceptive awareness, as well as patient education, is very useful and is discussed later. The manual muscle test should be performed in all four quadrants as you assess for asymmetries in strength, tenderness during contraction, appropriate relaxation after contraction, and endurance. Patients may be unable to follow your commands owing to poor awareness and proprioception of this body region.

It is easier to assess the deeper levator ani level musculature such as the piriformis and coccygeus by internal rectal examination. Ventral surface coccyx tenderness, coccyx position, and mobility can also be checked. About 30 degrees of pain-free coccyx flexion and extension is normal.[51]

Treatment

Patient Education

Patient education is vitally important and should begin with the first visit, using models and pictures to explain the role of the pelvic floor. It is important that a patient feel that she is participating in her own rehabilitation, which requires education and encouragement to learn all she can about her body.

Teaching pelvic floor relaxation techniques can be performed using various methods, depending on the individual patient and her learning style. General relaxation techniques such as breathing instruction, used frequently with patients with tension headaches, often facilitate relaxation of the pelvic floor musculature. Performing contract-relax exercises with the pelvic floor allows patients to learn what she must do to release a contraction, and emphasis on the relaxation phase gives her feedback on successful techniques.

Biofeedback

Biofeedback is used to obtain objective information about electric activity of the pelvic floor muscles, to detect increased resting tension levels of the pelvic floor, and even more importantly to give feedback to a patient about this physiologic process during both evaluation and treatment. Biofeedback is particularly useful when a patient has difficulty learning the relaxation exercises.

EMG biofeedback is done using surface EMG internally or externally. The external electrodes can be placed either over the skin of the urogenital diaphragm for the more superficial muscle layers, as in vaginismus due to bulbocavernosus spasm, or more posteriorly, closer to the anus for the deeper levator ani group. Single-user internal vaginal or rectal sensors can provide more specific information about the deeper levator layers and are the electrodes most often used in research on pelvic floor dysfunction. Contraindications to the use of internal vaginal sensors may include virginal status, youth (children), pain on insertion, and menstrual bleeding or pregnancy. A rectal sensor may be used for virginal patients or during menstrual bleeding. Figure 26–7 demonstrates placement of external surface electrodes for evaluation and treatment.

Teaching physiologic quieting and general relaxation techniques is helpful for patients with chronic pain. Biofeedback can make this learning process much easier for patients to grasp. This can be done with the use of surface EMG electrodes placed over general sites such as the upper trapezius and frontalis or the use of thermal feedback for temperature regulation. Using both muscle tension awareness training and relaxation techniques can aid patients' recognition of early signs of pain and tension.

Manual Soft Tissue Work

Hands-on treatment ranges from superficial massage to deep myofascial release techniques. Deep tissue work progresses slowly into the layers, not only for patients' tolerance but also for success in releasing the muscle and fascial layers. Myofascial releasing techniques used directly over the pelvic floor can be very effective in decreasing pelvic floor tension. Acupressure techniques or manual stretching during massage

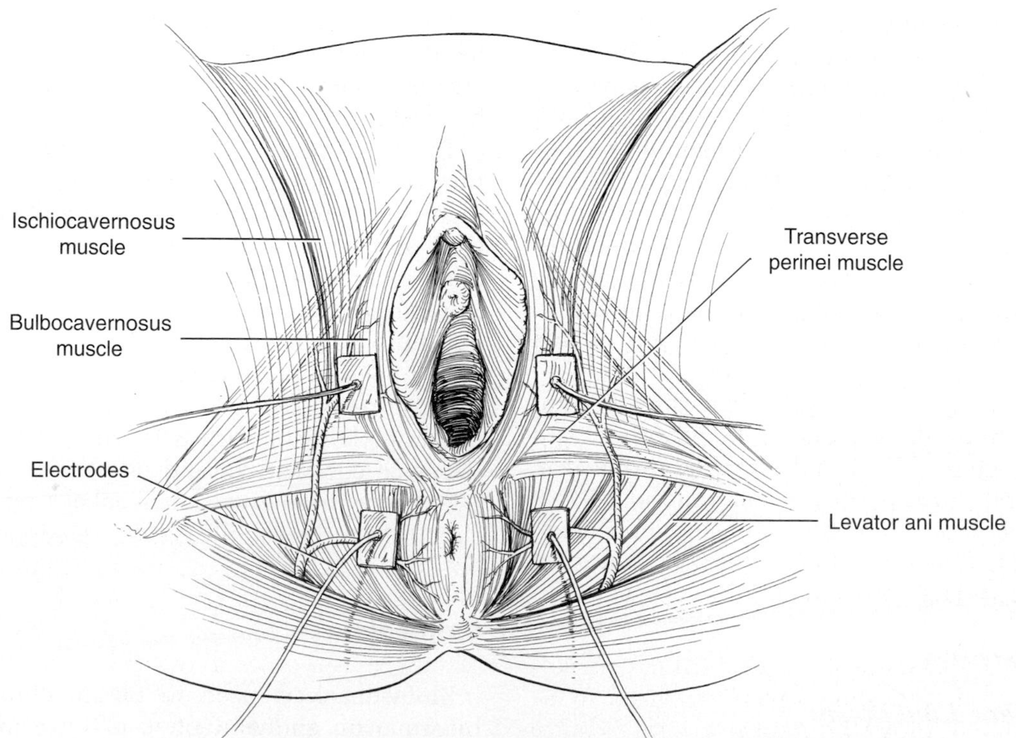

Figure 26–7. Electrode placement for external surface electrodes for levator biofeedback. Internal vaginal or rectal sensors can also be used.

over the affected muscles is effective for internal or external TP releases. Friction massage is used for decreasing scar tissue adhesions in episiotomy sites, which can occasionally cause pain with intercourse. Internal work such as acupressure for releasing internal TPs, Thiel's massage (transrectal levator massage), and coccyx mobilization techniques can be used when indicated.

Therapeutic Exercise

Musculoskeletal evaluation findings determine the individual therapeutic exercises prescribed. Correction of imbalances such as muscle weakness, tightness, spasm, and poor fine motor control especially related to the pelvis and trunk is necessary before any exercise program. It is also crucial to inactivate active TPs (discussed later) to restore the muscle to its normal resting length in preparation for strengthening. Developing appropriate fine motor control is necessary for eliminating chronic and habitual movement patterns that perpetuate myofascial dysfunctions. This sensorimotor control can be applied in movement therapy instruction such as through Feldenkrais, Alexander's technique, and Aston's patterning.[52a]

Assessing a patient's body mechanics as she gets in and out of the car, carries items such as heavy purses or portable baby car seats, and replicates her sitting postures and work positions can often give a clinician ample information for patient education.

An appropriate aerobic exercise program is strongly recommended for general conditioning, for reduction of daily stressors, and to prevent recurrence of myofascial pain symptoms. Some clinicians believe that aerobic exercise can decrease depression and aid pain relief owing to endorphin release. Rigorous exercise is not required.

Trigger Point Injections

TP dry needling or injection is not always indicated. This should be reserved for those cases that do not respond to an appropriate physical therapy program or after the development of fibrotic scar.[53] Rachlin describes the injection procedure used in management of TPs.[53] McCain believes that mechanical disruption of the TP, rather than the type of solution used with injection, is the critical factor and that precision in needling the exact point is necessary to accomplish inactivation.[54]

Spray and Stretch

Vapocoolant sprays such as ethyl chloride and Fluori-Methane have been widely used to inactivate TPs. The mechanism involves cooling the skin to create a sudden reduction in skin temperature by quick evaporation on contact. This causes stimulation of the skin sensory afferent fibers, which then act on the polysynaptic spinal cord reflexes, which close the gate, preventing sensation at the higher centers (see Chapter 2). This then allows for increased passive stretch during the temporary anesthesia period, which has a direct therapeutic effect on the TP.[5] Correct technique of spraying and stretching is important if pain relief and TP inactivation are to be achieved. Travell and Simons[3] detail this procedure, which involves stretching the muscle as the essential component and then spraying to facilitate that stretch. The investigators state that gentle, persistent stretching of the muscle without spray is more likely to inactivate a TP than spraying alone without stretch. It is important to remember that although correct spray and stretch technique can provide immediate inactivation of TPs and reduction of pain, a program designed to resolve the underlying causes(s) of those TPs is necessary for long-term benefit.

Electric Stimulation

A few studies have shown good results in using high-voltage galvanic stimulation (HVGS) in the treatment of levator ani syndrome. In one study, 45 patients with levator ani spasm were given HVGS at 80 Hz in an average of five sessions of 20-minute treatments; 91% showed excellent results.[54] Another study with 28 subjects using high-voltage pulsed electric stimulation at 120 Hz showed that 50% had symptom relief after an average of eight sessions of 60-minute treatments.[55] Both of these studies used rectal probes and intensities at patients' tolerance between 100 and 400 volts. External stimulation sites on the low back at S2–S4 are recommended for those patients who cannot tolerate use of internal probes.[56] Other forms of electric stimulation for pelvic pain include interferential current with conventional electrode placements over the lower abdomen, sacrum, low back, or adductors. A transcutaneous electric nerve stimulation (TENS) unit can also be used over TPs or over their referred pain zone.[57] Travell and Simons state that caution is needed when using high-amplitude TENS, which creates muscle contraction, because of the possibility of aggravating a myofascial TP.[3, 58] A TENS unit may also be used over specific acupuncture points.[58] The use of a TENS unit is contraindicated in the area of a demand-type cardiac pacemaker.[57, 58]

Ultrasound

Ultrasound's physiologic effects include an increase in skeletal muscle tissue temperature to depths up to 5 cm. The physiologic effects on tissue include an increase in collagen tissue extensibility, alterations in blood flow, changes in nerve conduction velocity, increases in pain threshold, increased enzymatic activity, and changes in contractile activity of skeletal muscle.[59] When pain threshold is increased after applying ultrasound to the pelvic floor musculature, patients have greater tolerance of manual soft tissue work such as manual stretching, myofascial release techniques, or friction massage.

Moist Heat and Ice

The use of external moist heat before any kind of soft tissue work is performed over pelvic and abdominal regions is helpful not only for tissue preparation but also for patients' comfort and tolerance. Using ice after deep tissue work such as myofascial release techniques and acupressure TP releases can be beneficial in decreasing any possible posttreatment discomfort. A vaginal ice pack to apply after internal TP work can be made by filling a condom about one third full of ultrasound gel and 1 tsp rubbing alcohol.[51]

Counseling

Psychologic counseling for some patients with chronic pelvic pain is necessary to achieve maximum results. Women with a history of sexual or physical abuse, marriage or relationship conflicts, psychiatric disorders such as clinical depression, or posttraumatic stress syndrome often benefit from psychotherapy focused on improving coping skills and decreasing psychosocial dysfunction.[31] No matter how appropriate the treatment or how professional the clinician, pain intervention techniques can fail if the underlying psychopathology is not addressed.[30]

Medications

Analgesics and psychotropic medications have been used in treating chronic pelvic pain. Tricyclic antidepressants (TCAs) administered in low doses may improve sleep disturbances. It has been postulated that low-dose TCAs may act by repletion of endorphins.[31] Other pharmacologic interventions include medications for dysmotility disorders, local anesthetics or steroids for TP injections, and ovarian cycle suppressants.[31] The use of narcotics is generally discouraged because of the increasing dose levels needed to attain pain relief, the potent side effects of smooth muscle relaxation, which may exacerbate concurrent dysmotility disorders, and the sedative effects, which may decrease cognitive functions.[31]

Integration of Myofascial Work into Total Clinical Care

Myofascial problems can start as a direct result of faulty body mechanics and the other factors discussed earlier and may be interpreted by patients as resulting from gynecologic problems, when no pelvic visceral pathology or dysfunction exists. Alternatively and perhaps more commonly, myofascial pain may develop gradually over time in response to transient or ongoing discomfort caused by gynecologic pathology or dysfunction. When first evaluated, the amount of pain attributable to each source may be impossible to assess. In most instances, a patient's needs are best served when a comprehensive treatment plan is devised through close collaboration between the gynecologist or other primary care physician and the physical therapist or other health care professional performing myofascial evaluation and treatment. Serial examination and review by the clinicians involved results in the clearest diagnoses and most effective treatments.

References

1. Reiter R, Gambone J: Non gynecologic somatic pathology in women with chronic pelvic pain and negative laparoscopy. J Reprod Med 1991;36:253.
2. Cantu R, Grodin A: Myofascial pain syndromes. In Lewis C (ed): Myofascial Manipulation—Theory and Clinical Application. Frederick, MD, Aspen Publishers, 1992.
3. Travell JG, Simons DG: Myofascial Pain and Dysfunction. The Trigger Point Manual, vol 1. Baltimore, Williams & Wilkins, 1983.
4. Friction JR: Myofascial pain syndrome. In Friction JR, Awad E (eds): Advances in Pain Research and Therapy, vol 17. New York, Raven Press, 1990, p 107.
5. Rachlin ES: Trigger points. In Rachlin ES (ed): Myofascial Pain and Fibromyalgia. St. Louis, CV Mosby, 1994, p 145.
6. Waylonis GW, Heck W: Fibromyalgia syndrome. New associations. Am J Phys Med Rehabil 1992;71:343.
7. Hulme JA: Fibromyalgia, A Handbook for Self Care and Treatment. Missoula, MT, Phoenix Publishing, 1995.
8. Wolfe F, Smythe HA, Yunus MB, et al: The American College of Rheumatology 1990 Criteria for Classification of Fibromyalgia: Report of the Multicenter Criteria Committee. Arthritis Rheum 1990;33:160.
9. Yunus MB, Masi AT, Calabro JJ, et al: Primary fibromyalgia (fibrositis): Clinical study of 50 patients with matched normal controls. Semin Arthritis Rheum 1981;11:151.
10. Smythe HA: Non articular rheumatism and psychogenic musculoskeletal syndromes. In McCarty DJ (ed): Arthritis and Allied Conditions: A Textbook of Rheumatology. Philadelphia, Lea & Febiger, 1979, pp 881–891.
11. Muhammad B: Fibromyalgia syndrome and myofascial pain syndrome: Clinical features, laboratory tests, diagnosis, and pathophysiologic mechanisms. In Rachlin E (ed): Myofascial Pain and Fibromyalgia. St. Louis, CV Mosby, 1994, pp 3–31.
12. Goldenberg DL: Fibromyalgia, chronic fatigue syndrome, and myofascial pain syndrome. Curr Opin Rheumatol 1995;7:127.
13. Wolfe F, Smythe HA, Yunus MB, Bennett RM: The American College of Rheumatology 1990 Criteria for the Classification of Fibromyalgia. Report of the Multicenter Criteria Committee. Arthritis Rheum 1989;33:160.
14. Rachlin ES: History and physical examination for regional myofascial pain syndrome. In Rachlin E (ed): Myofascial Pain and Fibromyalgia. St. Louis, CV Mosby, 1994, p 159.
15. Cohen ML, Quintner JL: Fibromyalgia syndrome, a problem of tautology. Lancet 1993;342:8876.
16. Bengtsson A, Ernerudh J, Vrethem M, et al: Absence of autoantibodies in primary fibromyalgia. J Rheumatol 1989;16:1466.
17. Yunus MB, Berg BC, Masi AT: Multiphase skeletal scintigraphy in primary fibromyalgia syndrome: A blinded study. J Rheumatol 1989;16:1466.
18. McBroom P, Walsh NE, Dumitro D: Electromyography in primary fibromyalgia syndrome. Clin J Pain 1988;4:117.
19. Svebak S, Anjia R, Karstad SI: Task induced electromyographic activation in fibromyalgic subjects and controls. Scand J Rheumatol 1993;22:124.
20. Elert J, Dahlqvist SR, Alamy B, Eisemann M: Muscle endurance, muscle tension and personality traits in patients with muscle or joint pain: A pilot study. J Rheumatol 1993;20:1550.
21. Buchwald D: Comparison of patients with chronic fatigue syndrome, fibromyalgia, and multiple chemical sensitivities. Arch Intern Med 1994;154:2049.
22. Hubbard DR, Borkoff GM: Myofascial trigger points show spontaneous needle EMG activity. Spine 1993;18:1803.
23. Melnick J: Treatment of trigger point mechanisms in gastrointestinal disease. N Y State J Med 1954;54:1324.
24. Gutstein RR: The role of abdominal fibrositis in functional indigestion. Miss Val Med J 1944;66:114.
25. Telling WH: The clinical importance of fibrositis in general practice. BMJ 1935;1:689.
26. Hoyt HS: Segmental nerve lesions as a cause of the trigonitis syndrome. Stanford Med Bull 1953,11:61.
27. Melnick J: Trigger areas and refractory pain in duodenal ulcer. N Y State J Med 1957;57:1073.
28. Bennett RM: Myofascial pain syndromes and the fibromyalgia syndrome: A comparative analysis. In Friction JR, Awad E (eds): Advances in Pain Research and Therapy, vol 17. New York, Raven Press, 1990, pp 43–67.
29. Tait RC: Psychological factors in chronic benign pain. Curr Concepts Pain 1983;1:10.
30. Grzesiak RC: Psychological considerations in myofascial pain, fibromyalgia, and related musculoskeletal pain. In Rachlin E (ed): Myofascial Pain and Fibromyalgia. St. Louis, CV Mosby, 1994, p 61.
31. Milburn A, Reiter R, Rhomberg AT: Multidisciplinary approach to chronic pelvic pain. Obstet Gynecol Clin North Am 1993;20:643.
32. Turk D, Meichenbaum D, Genest M: Pain and Behavioral Medicine: A Cognitive-Behavioral Perspective. San Diego, CA, Academic Press, 1983.
33. Rosenthal RH: Psychology of chronic pelvic pain. Obstet Gynecol Clin North Am 1993;20:627.

34. Muldofsky H, Scarisbrick P, England R, et al: Musculoskeletal symptoms and non-REM disturbances in patients with "fibrositis syndrome" and healthy subjects. Psychosom Med 1975;37:341.
35. Baker PK: Musculoskeletal origins of chronic pelvic pain. Obstet Gynecol Clin North Am 1993;20:719.
36. Mennell JM: Intricacies and interrelationships in the body systems. In Mennell JM (ed): The Musculoskeletal System Differential Diagnosis from Symptoms and Physical Signs. Frederick, MD, Aspen Publishers, 1992.
37. Wallace K: Female pelvic floor functions, dysfunctions, and behavioral approaches to treatment. Clin Sports Med 1994;13:459.
38. Sinaki M, Merritt JL, Stillwell GK: Tension myalgia of the pelvic floor. Mayo Clin Proc 1977;52:717.
39. Chaiken DC, Blaivas JG, Blaivas ST: Behavioral therapy for the treatment of refractory interstitial cystitis. J Urol 1993;149:1445.
40. Whitmore KE: Self care regimens for patients with interstitial cystitis. Urol Clin North Am 1994;21:121.
41. Summitt RL: Urogynecologic causes of chronic pelvic pain. Obstet Gynecol Clin North Am 1993;20:685.
42. Webster DC: Sex and interstitial cystitis: Explaining the pain and self care. Urol Nurs 1993;13:4.
43. Jones KD, Lehr ST: Vulvodynia: Diagnostic techniques and treatment modalities. Nurse Pract 1994;19:34.
44. Pomerantz E: Vulvodynia: Etiology and treatment strategies. J Obstet Gynecol Phys Ther 1994;18:10.
45. Kaplan WE, Firlit CF, Schoenberg HW: The female urethral syndrome: External sphincter spasm as etiology. J Urol 1980;124:48.
46. Barbalias GA, Meares EM: Female urethral syndrome: Clinical and urodynamic perspectives. Urology 1984;23:208.
47. Kotarinos RK: Diastasis recti and review of abdominal wall. J Obstet Gynecol Phys Ther 1990;14:8.
48. Rangelli D, Hayes SH: Vaginal birth after cesarean delivery: The role of the physical therapist. J Obstet Gynecol Phys Ther 1995;19:10.
49. Pauls JA: Therapeutic Approaches to Women's Health. A Program of Exercises and Education. Musculoskeletal Complaints During Pregnancy. Frederick, MD, Aspen Publishers, 1995, pp 2–1:18.
50. Norton PA: Pelvic floor disorders: The role of fascia and ligaments. Clin Obstet Gynecol 1993;36:926.
51. Barker S: Course notes from an integrated approach to pelvic pain syndromes. Sponsored by PhysioTherapy Associates, San Diego, CA, July 1995.
52. Wallace K: Hypertonus dysfunction. In Wilder E (ed): American Physical Therapy Association Section on Women's Health 1997 Gynecological Manual, Alexandria, VA, p 130.
52a. Miller B: Manual therapy treatment of myofascial pain and dysfunction. In Rachlin E (ed): Myofascial Pain and Fibromyalgia. St. Louis, CV Mosby, 1994, p 415.
53. Rachlin ES: Trigger point management. In Rachlin E (ed): Myofascial Pain and Fibromyalgia. St. Louis, CV Mosby, 1994, p 173.
54. McCain GA: Treatment of Fibromyalgia and Myofascial Pain Syndromes. In Rachlin E (ed): Myofascial Pain and Fibromyalgia. St. Louis, CV Mosby, 1994, p 31.
55. Morris L, Newton RA: Use of high volt galvanic stimulation for patients with levator ani syndrome. Phys Ther 1987;67:1522.
56. Dunbar A: An overview: Use of high volt galvanic stimulation for patients with levator ani syndrome. Physiotherapy Ob/Gyn Bulletin, Dec 1987.
57. Barr JO: Transcutaneous electrical nerve stimulation for pain management. In Nelson RM, Currier DP (eds): Clinical Electrotherapy, 2nd ed. Norwalk, CT, Appleton & Lange, 1991, p 261.
58. Kloth LC: Interference current. In Nelson RM, Currier DP (eds): Clinical Electrotherapy, 2nd ed. Norwalk, CT, Appleton & Lange, 1991, p 221.
59. Ziskin MC, McDiarmid T, Michlovitz SL: Therapeutic ultrasound. In Michlovitz SL (ed): Thermal Agents in Rehabilitation, 2nd ed. Philadelphia, FA Davis, 1990, p 134.

Selected Readings

Chirarelli P, O'Keefe D: Physiotherapy for the pelvic floor. Aust J Physiother 1981;27:4.

Fischer A: Pressure algometry (dolorimetry) in the differential diagnosis of muscle pain. In Rachlin E (ed): Myofascial Pain and Fibromyalgia. St. Louis, CV Mosby, 1994, pp 121–141.

Mersky H: Psychosocial factors and muscular pain. In Friction JR, Awad E (eds): Advances in Pain Research and Therapy, vol 17. New York, Raven Press, 1990, pp 213–225.

Millard R: The conservative management of urinary incontinence. Aust Physiother Obstet Gynecol Bull 1982;3:30.

Nicosia JF, Abcarian H: Levator syndrome: A treatment that works. Dis Colon Rectum 1985;28:406.

Ono K: Electromyographic studies of the abdominal wall muscles visceroptosis. Tohoku J Exp Med 1958;68:347.

Sandberg G, Quevillon R: Dyspareunia: An integrated approach to assessment and diagnosis. J Fam Pract 1987;24:66.

Smythe HA, Gladman A, Dagenais P, et al: Relation between fibrositic and control tenderness: Effects of dolorimeter scale length and footplate size. J Rheumatol 1992;19:284.

Whitman A, Bigler FC: Preoperative diagnosis. J Kans Med Soc 1977;78:411.

27

Psychiatric Illness

Robert A. Bashford, MD

In the diagnosis and management of chronic pelvic pain (CPP), it appears that approaching medical and psychologic aspects simultaneously is the most productive path. In most cases of chronic pain, psychologic determinants dictate how the pain is expressed and to a significant extent the impact of the pain on the person's life. This chapter reviews the psychiatric problems most often encountered in women with CPP and discusses diagnostic and treatment methods most appropriate in a primary care setting.

Responses to Pain

Pain responses are affective, cognitive, and behavioral.[1] The affective components include fear, depression, anxiety, irritability, and anger. The cognitive factors are the expectations and meaning of the pain to the patient, the patient's family, and society. Behavioral responses include changes in work, leisure activities, and sexual adjustment.

In addition, each patient brings individual constitutional factors into the pain event (i.e., the way of dealing with adversity such as loss or stress). Loss can be the loss of a limb or organ, loss of functioning, or loss of the sense of control over one's life. Stress is inherently part of chronic pain as it affects an individual's work, social, and sexual functioning.

Case 1: Mrs. X is a 24-year-old woman who has had CPP for 11 years and who has, as a result of it, missed 30 to 40 days of school or work per year. The pain is in the left lower quadrant. It is intermittent, increases with menses, and is not associated with gastrointestinal (GI) or urinary tract symptoms. Laparoscopy 5 years ago revealed "minimal endometriosis," which was cauterized. Work and sexual function improved for 2 years, but both have deteriorated since marriage 2 years ago.

Mrs. X married "the perfect husband." "He's good to me and understands my situation, but I'm afraid if I don't get better, he'll leave me. He wants a family, but I'm scared I won't be a good mother." Mrs. X grew up with her parents and a sister who was 5 years older than she. This sister was killed in an automobile accident 12 years ago, when Mrs. X was 12 years old. After that, her mother's emotional health fell apart. She had several bouts with depression and alcohol abuse and was emotionally unavailable to Mrs. X. They have been estranged for the past several years, although she maintains a good relationship with her father. She has never been in therapy and says "I cried at the funeral (sister's) and got all of that over, and it hasn't really bothered me since." Mrs. X guesses that she has had 75 physician and emergency room visits since the beginning of her pain 11 years ago (in the spring after her sister's death).

This case demonstrates fairly obvious psychologic events that seem temporally related to the pain. For her, pain appears a socially acceptable and recognized reason for physician visits. In other words, she can obtain medical help for pain symptoms much more easily than for complaints of overwhelming feelings of grief, anger, or abandonment. For her, endometriosis may have contributed to the somatic and visual nociceptive stimuli she felt, but her other needs influenced her illness behavior.

It is estimated that 30% to 40% of patients

presenting to a primary care physician's office have an agenda other than the stated complaint but because of shame, lack of understanding, or a history of not having been heard before, consciously or unconsciously, use a physical complaint to mask an emotional complaint. Mrs. X has recently begun to make strides again as her physician has acknowledged an emotional component to her pain, has told her that she is "not crazy," and has promised to stay with her even if he ends up doing a laparoscopy that shows little or no pathology. She is in psychotherapy and is receiving psychotropic medications concurrent with the medical evaluation of her pain.

Nature of Chronic Pain

In evaluating chronic pain, one must differentiate between nociception and pain. *Nociception* is a "sensory response that occurs specifically to tissue damage."[2] The taxonomy of the International Association of the Study of Pain describes "*pain* as the unpleasant sensory and emotional experience associated with actual or potential tissue damage or described in terms of such damage."[3] This definition dilutes the relationship between the pain experience and tissue damage and opens the door for a substantial emotional component in the expression of pain. Low back pain following a fall frequently frustrates the patient and physician because no pathology can be demonstrated. On the other hand, when we remove our finger from a hot stove, this reflex is nociception (response to tissue damages) without any emotional component. There is no advantage to dividing pain into nociceptive or psychogenic; rather, it is more useful to react as if all pain is a combination of factors.

As described in Chapter 2, an integrated approach assesses interplay between mind and body from the beginning of a patient's work-up. The patient and physician do not then have to retreat to a difficult referral to a mental health worker at the end of a nondiagnostic physical work-up. Referral in this belated manner deflates the patient and puts the mental health worker in an impossible position. Both the patient and physician should begin with the premise that pathologic pelvic findings may not be sufficient to explain chronic pain. Second, any pain that has existed for long enough generates significant emotional overlay.

Acute and chronic pain are very different disease entities (see Chapter 2). Chronic pain exceeds or outlasts the recognized stimulus, and patients appear more comfortable than one might expect from the description of their pain. Chronic pain may persist when evidence of physiologically or pathologically produced nociception has abated; when coupled with loss of function, this becomes a chronic pain syndrome. Chronic pain gradually evolves a life of its own. The pace and degree of this evolution are influenced by the patient's predisposition to react to stress emotionally and the ongoing behavioral and emotional patterns that develop because the "pain confers an advantage (emotional advantage beyond eliciting withdrawal from damaging stimuli) to the organism."[4] Behavior patterns are more likely to persist when operant learning occurs—that is, when a behavior is regularly followed by positive events (reinforcement), the behavior is more likely to occur again in similar circumstances.

In the family, the meaning of pain, the individual's personal experience and understanding of the pain, "why me" questions, and concerns about the future are important aspects of chronic pain. By the time patients with chronic pain see a primary care physician, they are already experiencing uncertainty that may be perceived as loss of control, helplessness, and social isolation.

This pain concept is demonstrated in a model suggested in Aronoff's text.[5] The scheme shows that nociception and pain are less important in chronic pain than are the suffering (the total experience and reaction to the pain) and pain behavior that follow. Pain behavior is related to the change that the pain initiates in social, family, and personal circumstances. Referral to a mental health worker is important when suffering and pain behavior become more time and energy consuming than the pain itself.

Engel's classic report in 1959 described "pain proneness."[6] From birth on, pain-prone patients, as he describes them, build a "library" of pain experiences that dictate later responses to pain. Engel states, "in a child's development, pain and relief of pain enter into the formation of interpersonal relations and of concepts of good and bad, reward and punishment, and success and failure." Even though there is not yet a sound epidemiologic measure of the prevalence of pain-prone patients, overrepresented in pain populations are patients with prior substance abuse, functional dyspareunia, inhibited sexual desire, and histories of sexual and physical abuse.[7]

Clinical Evaluation

The biopsychosocial approach to evaluation of pain recognizes mind and body as one functioning unit. First, a complete history and physical examination may disclose likely contributing physical and physiologic factors (see Chapters 6 and 7). Further inquiries are needed to investigate the premorbid functioning of a patient, such as a history of anxiety, depressive personality, or somatoform disorders. Self-report scales such as a Beck Depression Inventory[8] can help this process.

An important aspect of premorbid functioning is the way in which the patient expressed pain in childhood. Did she have words for emotions or was she alexithymic, using somatic symptoms instead of emotional language? This is typified by a child's being unconsciously afraid of failure and consistently refusing to go to school because of headaches or stomachaches.

An evaluation of marital distress is important in relation to CPP. One study showed that 56% of women evaluated for chronic pain scored in the maritally distressed range (< 100 on the Locke-Wallace Marital Adjustment Test).[9] It is important to understand the baseline level of sexual functioning, but it is sometimes difficult to determine whether the current sexual dysfunction is a result of the pain or was present before (and is unassociated with) the pain (see Chapter 9).

Finally, a patient's response to the pain is important. Is it exaggerated, appropriate, or minimized? How is the patient functioning at work, in the family, and in intimate relationships? Is the patient litigious?

The family's response to the patient's pain is most important. Melzack in 1985 described high-distress and low-distress spouses of patients who have chronic pain. Fifty percent of high-distress spouses ranked their own pain higher on the McGill Pain Questionnaire than did the identified patients themselves.[10] Payne and Norfleet described several possible styles of interaction among family members and the patient in pain: "(1) pain serving as a proxy for dysfunction in the family that is easier to tolerate than the dysfunctional relationships in the family, (2) the family acting as reinforcer for the pain by nurturing and caring for the patient, (3) the patient using pain to control the family (with this pattern unwittingly reinforced by the family), and (4) the stress of the family life producing psychological effects which predispose the patient to stress and pain."[11]

Case 2: A 14-year-old girl had an episode of acute cystitis 2 years previously. This was treated and cleared, but she had repeated episodes of lower abdominal and vaginal pain despite negative cultures and findings in the next $1^1/_2$ years. She had an extensive work-up including cystoscopy, laparoscopy, and computed tomography scans, with negative findings. She was unable to attend school and had become homebound because of her pain.

The family was a professional family and at first glance appeared to be functioning well, but it later became clear that the marriage was in jeopardy. The mother was suspicious that the father was having an affair. Although both the mother and child denied it, their relationship was rigid and enmeshed. As discussion focused on any family relationship issue instead of the urethritis, the child would become dysfunctional from pain. The family communication rotated around her pain.

This example meets all the criteria for a family interaction in which pain becomes the focus for the family's dysfunction. The pain was reinforced by the continued nurturing and caring for the patient. The patient gained control (unconsciously) over the family through this pain, and her pain hid the dysfunction in the family.

Finally, in evaluating a patient with CPP, a clinician needs to evaluate his or her own feelings (countertransference) about the patient and her disorder. Because the pain is sometimes intractable and unfixable and surrounded by difficult interpersonal relations, both clinicians and staff may find themselves acting in response to their own feelings about the patient. The actions of many patients, particularly those with personality disorders, are unconscious; the clinician's task is to be attuned (because the patient is not) to the impotence, anger, and frustration that he or she might feel when faced with a chronically ill, difficult patient. Because patients' actions are unconscious, it is rarely helpful for clinicians to be confrontative. Clinicians and their staff have to watch for *acting out* on patients, which is sometimes represented by a quick negative therapeutic intervention and sending patients on their way. What appears to be a perfectly reasonable procedure (e.g., a laparoscopy) may be interpreted by a patient as abandonment. The effectiveness of any intervention is increased if it is seen as part of an overall diagnostic approach, and the physician-patient relationship can continue regardless of the outcome.

Following is a brief description of the common psychiatric comorbidities of CPP and methods of treatment.

Depression

A clinician frequently wonders, Is CPP a manifestation of preexisting depression or does it result in (cause) depression or anxiety? Depressed individuals are overrepresented (about 60%) in any chronic pain population, and persons with chronic pain are overrepresented in surveyed populations of depressed patients. Forty-nine percent of individuals in one study of 63 patients with chronic pain met criteria for depression.[4] Part of the problem is in diagnosis. Depression by traditional criteria is represented by changes in cognitive, behavioral, and somatic areas. Depression, when associated with pain, is more likely to increase the sensitivity to pain (lower the pain threshold) and to be associated with irritability, blandness, and social withdrawal than with traditional symptoms of sadness, sleeplessness, and suicidal ideation.

A depressive disorder is twice as likely to occur in women as in men and has an 8% 6-month prevalence rate in women.[12] It is not just an adjustment reaction to a stressor. Adjustment reaction with depressed mood is a reaction to a recognizable stressor and has a limited life span without treatment. This is alluded to in Chapter 28, in distinguishing a depressive mood (changes associated with the stress of pain) from a freestanding (major) depression. Aspects of depression may be found in an adjustment disorder, but a major depression (*Diagnostic and Statistical Manual of Mental Disorders, Fourth Edition* [DSM-IV] definition)[13] lasts longer than 2 weeks and is marked by symptoms of sadness, anhedonia, guilt, irritability, decreased (or increased) mood and appetite, lack of concentration and energy, and suicidal thoughts. Table 27–1 is a mnemonic for diagnosing depression (Sig. E CAPS—Prescribe Energy Capsules). Five of the symptoms including *either* anhedonia (loss of interest or pleasure in activities) or sadness must be present.

In contrast, dysthymia is a long-duration, low-level depression that has been present

Table 27–1. **MNEMONIC FOR DIAGNOSTIC CRITERIA FOR DEPRESSION: SIG E CAPS (PRESCRIBE ENERGY CAPSULES)**

S	Sleep	Insomnia or hypersomnia
I	Interests	Loss of interest or pleasure in activities
G	Guilt	Feelings of excessive guilt, worthlessness, hopelessness, helplessness
E	Energy	Fatigue or loss of energy
C	Concentration	Diminished concentration ability, indecision
A	Appetite	Decreased or increased appetite, >5% weight loss or gain
P	Psychomotor	Psychomotor retardation or agitation
S	Suicidality	Suicidal ideation, plan, or attempt

most of the time for longer than 2 years. In other words, the symptoms are similar to those of major depression but are present at a lower, more chronic level. This problem often responds to antidepressant medication and psychotherapy.

It is important to recognize that a person can be depressed without being sad and can be sad without being depressed. Either sadness or anhedonia must be present to diagnose major depression, but both do not have to be present. Clinical evidence supports treating chronic pain with antidepressants whether a clear depression can be diagnosed or not. Neurotransmitters involved in pain transmission include substance P, enkephalins, endorphins, serotonin, and norepinephrine. The primary effect of most antidepressants on serotonin and norepinephrine is to inhibit their uptake and subsequent metabolism, thus increasing the availability.[2] Serotonin diminishes pain in an unknown way. Our evolving understanding is that common neurotransmitter pathways do appear to mediate pain and mood, and these may potentially explain why antidepressants are successful in treating pain. (See the detailed discussion of pain theories in Chapter 2, and see Chapter 28 for a discussion of tricyclic antidepressants in pain management.)

Case 3: This 34-year-old woman had an episode of regional ileitis 6 years ago, and 10 cm of her bowel was removed. Since that time, she had been plagued by abdominal pain. She had had three laparoscopies and two laparotomies, with findings of minimal endometriosis and adhesions. Most recently, she presented to the hospital with right lower quadrant pain *without* GI or genitourinary symptoms, fever, or positive laboratory or physical findings. She was taking large doses of methadone for the pain. She is a professional person who had been unable to work much in the past several months. She was having difficulty with sleep, poor concentration, and low energy and met some criteria for a major depression. She denied sadness but was taking no pleasure in any of her previously pleasurable work or relationships. She did not describe many somatic complaints before the onset of GI symptoms (i.e., she did not have somatization disorder). Her first husband had physically abused her.

By history, this is at least the third episode of major depression that she has had; none was previously treated. Her relationships (marriage and friends) were faring very poorly. Her previous depressions were not associated with somatization. This woman is likely to benefit from antidepressants even though she does not meet criteria for a full-blown free-standing major depression.

In treating depression associated with CPP, first look for an organic cause of the depression. Hyperthyroidism, multiple sclerosis, and lupus erythematosus (although they must be considered) are less likely causes of depression than are medications. These can be prescription medications, over-the-counter medications, or illicit drugs. Any medication or withdrawal from a medication is a possible culprit in the genesis of depression until proved otherwise.

The second important aspect of treating a depressed patient with pain is education. Such patients have often seen many doctors and have accrued many diagnoses. We should help put together the information in some comprehensible form as we try to understand patients' perception of what is wrong with them, what has been done, and what is to be done.

In the general pharmacologic treatment of depression (do not forget accompanying psychotherapy), tricyclic antidepressants have given way to the new selective serotonin reuptake inhibitors (SSRIs). It was initially thought that the SSRIs with their low side effect profile were still too expensive, but tricyclics with their anticholinergic and adrenergic side effect profile require physician visits, electrocardiograms, and laboratory data including blood level measurements that probably make them as expensive as SSRIs. The choice between SSRIs or tricyclics should be based on how their side effect profiles will influence a patient's symptoms. Tricyclics have annoying and sometimes dangerous anticholinergic side effects (constipation, dry mouth, urinary retention, hypotension, sedation, cardiac arrhythmia, and weight gain). For example, a woman with irritable bowel syndrome characterized predominantly by diarrhea may tolerate tricyclic antidepressants better than the SSRIs.

The SSRIs include fluoxetine (Prozac), paroxetine (Paxil), sertraline (Zoloft), and fluvoxamine (Luvox). Trazodone (Desyrel) and nefazodone (Serzone) are more pharmacologically similar and are often referred to as serotonin receptor modulators (SRMs). Venlafaxine (Effexor) has potent serotonergic and noradrenergic effects (i.e., like tricyclics) but lacks the anticholinergic, sedative, and hypotensive side effects. In high doses, it may cause a modest increase in blood pressure and GI disturbances.

Clinicians should be acquainted with the side effect profile (see Chapter 28), contraindications, and reasons for referral for psychiatric consultation before prescribing these drugs. Most, including GI and anxiety side effects, abate over time. We should be careful about treating anxious patients and older patients and use a small starting dose for both (e.g., 5 to 10 mg fluoxetine equivalent).

An underestimated side effect in women is sexual dysfunction, including both decreased libido and change in orgasm. Because decreased libido is often part of depression, it is frequently difficult to decide whether libido has changed because of the disorder (depression) or its treatment (antidepressant medications). Most of the antidepressants have been implicated in sexual dysfunction. Bupropion (Wellbutrin) and the newest SSRIs (nefazodone) are presented as being relatively devoid of sexual side effects.

Anorgasmia is most probably secondary to antidepressant therapy, not the depression itself. Treatment strategies include decreasing the dose of medication, omitting weekend doses or switching to another antidepressant. Giving a new additional agent such as bethanechol, cyproheptadine, yohimbine, or amantadine is the least desirable treatment of anorgasmy.[14]

Sexual side effects have been reported in as many of 40% of patients taking SSRIs. Physicians should describe them at the start of treatment so that patients can report them and physicians can change or decrease medications if they occur. Noncompliance because of sexual dysfunction can be minimized by anticipating the possibility at initiation of medications. Again, all antidepressants have the same approximate efficacy (70% to 80%) when used appropriately in correctly diagnosed cases, and thus the choice of drug should be made on the basis of the side effect profile.

Clinicians and patients should commit to 4 to 6 months of antidepressant use. Because of the long half-life of these medications (e.g., 9 days for fluoxetine and its metabolites), clinicians should wait 2 to 3 weeks at each dose level before making a change in type of medication. If a patient feels somewhat better, the clinician should wait 4 to 6 weeks, and if the patient has not had *significant* improvement of target symptoms (listed by the patient and the clinician before beginning medications), then the medication type should be changed. If the patient is achieving desired results, the clinician should treat for at least 4 to 6 months with 20 mg of fluoxetine or equivalent doses of other agents (Table 27–2).

No particular work-up other than taking a thorough medical history and performing a physical examination needs to be carried out before prescribing SSRIs. In overdose, their safety level, particularly compared with that of tricyclic medications, seems to be excellent.

Clinicians should probably ask for at least initial evaluation from a psychiatrist if a patient has a history of previously inadequately treated depression, personality disorder, significant anxiety, substance abuse, suicidal ideation, history of bipolar disorder in either the patient or family, or atypical

Table 27–2. **SEROTONIN-SELECTIVE REUPTAKE INHIBITOR DOSES**

Drug	Usual Adult Daily Dose (mg)	Range
Fluoxetine (Prozac)	5–20	10–100
Fluvoxamine (Luvox)	50–150	25–300
Paroxetine (Paxil)	20–30	10–50
Sertraline (Zoloft)	25–100	12.5–200
Venlafaxine (Effexor)	75–225	25–375

depressive symptoms such as hypersomnia and hyperphagia. Another indication for referral is the failure of single-drug treatment to lift the depression. Primary care physicians should be able to monitor patients after the consultation. Primary care physicians should acquaint themselves with a psychiatric colleague who is comfortable with and willing to care for their patients with CPP.

In large studies, antidepressants are most efficacious when part of an integrated approach.[15] An integrated approach (including psychotherapy, dietary, and environmental factors) addresses issues that antidepressants do not, such as long-term emotional conflicts, family chaos, or the primary and secondary gain of chronic pain.

Anxiety

Anxiety is a disorder frequently encountered in a primary care setting. The lifetime prevalence of anxiety disorders in the United States is estimated to be between 10% and 15%, with women affected more often than men. Anxious patients present to a physician with fearfulness, nervousness, worry, stress, conflict, and somatic complaints. Overactivity of the autonomic nervous system may result in diarrhea, dizziness, sweating, palpitations, syncope, tachycardia, tingling in the extremities, upset stomach, and urinary frequency. Equally important to patients and physicians is the awareness of being nervous or frightened—patients fear that people will see their anxiety.

Pathologic anxiety (as opposed to adaptive alerting anxiety) is probably underdiagnosed in primary care physicians' offices because of lack of clear definitions in practitioners' minds and a reluctance for anxious patients to be forthcoming about obsessive rituals, fears of leaving the house, fears of social encounters, or terrifying flashbacks about trauma. In women dealing with CPP, an anxiety disorder can complicate treatment, although it seldom is the primary cause of the pain syndrome.

As in all psychiatric disorders, an organic cause should be ruled out, especially when symptoms first appear after the age of 35 years. This can be part of the medical history and includes systemic conditions such as cardiovascular disease, pulmonary insufficiency, and anemia that result in hypoxia; neurologic disorders such as cerebrovascular accidents, epilepsy, multiple sclerosis; endocrinopathies; and probably most important, illicit and prescription drug intoxications, withdrawals, abuse, and dependence. Commonly implicated are benzodiazepines, alcohol, amphetamines, nicotine, cocaine, theophylline, marijuana, and vasopressor agents.

Psychiatrists divide anxiety disorders into panic disorder, social and simple phobias, obsessive-compulsive disorder (OCD), posttraumatic stress disorder (PTSD), and generalized anxiety disorders.

A panic episode often begins as a completely spontaneous event with a crescendo of symptoms including tachycardia, palpitations, nausea, numbness, chest pain, fear of dying, and fear of going crazy or doing something uncontrolled. The attack often begins with a sense of terror or impending doom. A stressful event sometimes is a precipitant, but more often the attack is unexpected. After an attack, the anticipation of a recurrence, with the resultant anxiety, becomes as important as the attack itself. Complications of panic attacks include depression (with a significant suicide risk, particularly in untreated, frightened, uninformed patients), substance abuse, and agoraphobia.

Agoraphobia (literally "fear of the marketplace") is a common problem in persons with panic attacks. Patients become fearful of being anywhere outside of the home where it would be difficult to get help, such as on streets, in stores, on bridges, and in tunnels. Patients insist on accompaniment by a close friend or family member for all of their activities. Patients and their families quickly lose their ability to cope.

If a firm diagnosis of panic disorder is made and the practitioner elects to treat the patient, medical treatment would involve antidepressants for patients with a history of substance abuse. If a patient has no history of substance abuse, benzodiazepines are a reasonable treatment (Table 27–3). The

Table 27–3. **TREATMENT FOR PANIC DISORDER**

Drug	Dose
Tricyclic Antidepressants	
Imipramine, desipramine	Start 10–25 mg qhs Target 100 mg (Increase 10–25 mg every 2–3 days)
Benzodiazepines	
Alprazolam (Xanax)	Start 0.25 mg tid Target 2–6 mg qd (Increase 0.25 mg every 1–3 days)
Clonazepam	Start 0.25 mg bid Target 2–3 mg qd (Increase 0.25 mg every 1–2 days)
Selective Serotonin Reuptake Inhibitors (SSRIs)	
Fluoxetine (Prozac)	Start 5 mg qd Target 10–20 mg qd (Increase after 2–3 weeks—rapid increase or high dose of SSRIs may provoke panic symptoms.)
Sertraline (Zoloft)	Start 25 mg qd Target 50–100 mg qd (If no response in 2–3 weeks, increase to 25 mg bid or 50 mg qd)
Paroxetine (Paxil)	Start 10–20 mg Target 20–30 mg qd (If no response in 2–3 weeks, increase to 20–30 mg)

Note: It may be advisable to begin with a benzodiazepine for several days for immediate response while waiting for a SSRI to become effective.

target should be a major reduction in symptoms, and if improvement continues, it is reasonable to continue these medications for 6 to 12 months, tapering over 2 to 4 months. Pharmacologic treatment frequently reduces panic attacks, but a concurrent behavioral desensitization program (probably conducted by a psychologist or by trained office personnel) allows a more permanent approach after the medications are discontinued. Physicians should be acquainted with side effects of the foregoing medications, but in the doses used, they are relatively mild and uncommon (see Chapter 28). Large doses of any of these medications can precipitate more panic attacks. If the three approaches outlined do not result in a major reduction in symptoms, it would seem appropriate to reassess the diagnosis of panic disorder or refer the patient to a psychiatrist.

Social phobias affect 3% to 5% of the population. Social phobias are persistent fears in which a person is afraid of acting in a humiliating or embarrassing way. Examples include a fear of speaking in public, fear of choking on food in public, hand trembling in public, inability to urinate in a public lavatory, or fear of saying foolish things or not being able to answer questions in social situations. A simple phobia is a persistent fear of a specific or circumscribed object or situation. These frequently begin in childhood with fears of animals, needles, storms, or injuries. Neither phobia requires treatment if a patient has no work or social impairment.

If treatment is indicated, the simplest approach is use of β-adrenergic blockers such as propranolol as needed or three times daily (30 to 180 mg per day). In addition to allowing single dosing, atenolol is said to have fewer central nervous system effects. Another option is clonidine (Catapres), 0.1 to 0.6 mg per day.

When these medications are used, patients frequently improve on their own as their physiologic response to anxiety decreases. Adding behavior therapy, in which patients are exposed in a hierarchic fashion to provoking stimuli and taught to relax simultaneously, improves long-term results, especially with simple phobias. Primary care physicians might well treat occasional social phobias if results are good, but the more pervasive, complicated, and crippling phobias should be referred to a psychiatrist.

Generalized anxiety disorder is what nonpsychiatrists usually think of as anxiety. It is a nonspecific, chronic, often lifelong disorder in which people seem to be pathologically worried about everything. It is defined as a chronic syndrome encompassing motor symptoms of trembling, twitching, restlessness, easy fatigability; autonomic hyperactivity such as sweating, dizziness, shortness of breath, frequent urination; and hypervigilence resulting in trouble falling asleep, exaggerated startle response, and irritability. It is more frequent in women than men and, unlike panic, is not limited to discrete time periods and, unlike phobic disorder, is not focused on discrete stimuli. The treatment is psychotherapy with psychopharmacologic support. The danger in general practitioners' treating generalized anxiety is its lifelong chronicity and the potential for lifelong antianxiety drug use, abuse, and dependence. If the disorder is resulting in significant work or social impairment, psychiatric evaluation is indicated.

OCD is either increasing in prevalence or more likely is better recognized. Patients were previously secretive about their crippling ritualistic behavior, but as magazines, newspapers, and talk shows have publicized the disorder, patients are much more forthcoming about their symptoms. OCD and depression frequently coexist. The diagnosis of OCD requires either obsessions with persistent thoughts and ideas that one cannot ignore (the need to wash or order one's room or unrealistic unremitting fear of catastrophe or illness) or a compulsive or motor component (rituals such as checking doors, hand-washing, counting steps, or ordering or arranging objects) to ward off the anxiety-provoking obsession.[16] Anorexia nervosa and bulimia have obsessive-compulsive ritualistic components.

The age of onset of OCD is often before 20 years and frequently follows stressful events such as a death or pregnancy. SSRIs such as fluoxetine are much more effective than psychotherapy. If the diagnosis is made in a primary care physician's office, a psychiatric opinion is useful to rule out comorbid symptoms of panic, generalized anxiety disorder, depression, and even delusions (fixed false beliefs), which would each require a different pharmacologic approach. Successful treatment of OCD frequently requires larger doses of SSRIs (40 to 80 mg fluoxetine equivalents) than does the treatment of depression.

When dealing with PTSD, the place of primary care physicians is probably in diagnosis and referral.[17] PTSD occurs in persons who have experienced an event outside the range of usual human experience. This can be a threat to one's own life or one's children's lives, an actual disaster, serious injury, or physical or sexual abuse. The trauma is frequently ongoing when the patient is seen. The patient frequently (1) reexperiences the trauma through dreams and flashbacks, (2) tends to be emotionally numbed to past experiences, and (3) has increased arousal (or autonomic instability) such as frequent angry outbursts, hypervigilance, an exaggerated startle response, and difficulty falling asleep.

A primary care physician is one of the first to encounter the disorder in a patient, particularly in sexually and physically abused patients. Treatment usually includes psychotherapy with supportive pharmacotherapy. The goal of pharmacology is to treat comorbid symptoms such as depression, persistent flashbacks, persistent anger and hypervigilence, and even psychotic episodes. The outcome of PTSD is related to the severity of the stressor, the degree of psychologic soundness before the stressor, and the extent of ongoing stress.

Finally, benzodiazepines deserve special comment. Benzodiazepines do cause sedation, decrease visual and motor coordination, impair memory, and potentiate the effects of alcohol and other drugs. Most importantly, tolerance, dependence, and thus addiction may occur with benzodiazepines without a patient's showing behavioral pathology. Self-medication and alarmingly high doses may result in an addicted patient who is at risk for seizures unless careful detoxification occurs. Abuse can be prevented if they are used in a carefully symptom-targeted manner and their use is frequently (as often as weekly) monitored and reassessed. Physical dependence can develop in low-dose use (10 to 40 mg per day) for several years or high-dose use over weeks, and individuals can develop tolerance to diazepam doses up to 1000 to 1500 mg per day.[18] Benzodiazepines with a long half-life such as diazepam (60 hours) may not present withdrawal symptoms until 7 to 10 days after cessation. Withdrawal may first present with seizures, which can be lethal if untreated.

The prevalence of anxiety disorders in women with OCD is unknown, but clinical experience suggests that they are relatively common. Of the various anxiety disorders, PTSD and generalized anxiety are perhaps the most common.

Personality Disorders

Table 27–4 lists personality disorders as described in DSM-IV.[19] Personality disorders are disorders that are not listed on Axis I but frequently coexist with and contribute to Axis I disorders. The five categories (or Axes) in DSM-IV separate and describe diagnoses, stressors, and functioning. Axis I is used to describe thought disorders such as schizophrenia or mood disorders such as depression or substance abuse. Axis II describes personality disorders (personality traits that have become rigid and result in work and relationship dysfunction). Axis III describes medical disorders. Axis IV describes the severity of psychosocial stressors, and Axis V describes the level of functioning of a patient.[20] In part, the spirit of Axis II was to define disorders marked by interpersonal difficulties. Affected individuals would probably fare well on a deserted island, as opposed to Axis I patients, who suffer when alone or when with people.

Personality disorders are marked by chronicity, inflexibility, and maladaptation. People with personality disorders adjust poorly to stress, regress in behavior when stressed, and tend to externalize their problems as the fault of someone else (particularly cluster B disorders). Some personality disorders probably have a biogenetic component, but the etiology is equally psychodynamic and developmental.[21]

Table 27–4. **THREE CLUSTERS OF PERSONALITY DISORDERS**

Cluster A (Odd)	Cluster B (Dramatic)	Cluster C (Anxious)
Schizotypal	Histrionic	Avoidant
Schizoid	Narcissistic	Dependent
Paranoid	Antisocial	Obsessive-compulsive
	Borderline	

Personality disorders develop at an early age because of a genetic predisposition or dysfunction in relationships with caregivers, resulting in a child (later adult) with maladaptive patterns of functioning. The most dramatic of these disorders is a borderline personality disorder (discussed later).

One of the benefits of understanding these disorders is the ability to recognize the feelings they evoke in a clinician (countertransference). These are the patients who are irritating to deal with, who become annoyingly clingy. The more you try to do, the less you are able to achieve. They seem insatiable, and most that goes wrong feels as if it were your fault. Ideally, experienced clinicians acknowledge their own personality traits (e.g., tendency to self-blame, use of denial, need for positive regard), particularly under the stress of caring for difficult patients, and come to understand how certain patients can arouse strong feelings in them. In doing this, it is easier to manage their patients, the staff, and their own feelings.

The diagnosis of personality disorder is made by self-report, observation, or semistructured interview.[21] If clinicians are paying attention to their own feelings, the diagnosis frequently becomes obvious when they are acting or feeling in an exaggerated way toward a patient. If, in fact, clinicians are acquainted with their own emotional baseline, this exaggerated response is a red flag that a patient has a personality disorder or has *regressed to* a personality disorder in the presence of stress (chronic pain). Again, this may be a patient who functions without any sign of personality dysfunction when pain free.

In the beginning, clinicians need to acknowledge that these ways of dealing with individuals are unconscious and therefore not available to immediate verbal correction, that they are to be managed, not cured, and that this is the way some patients deal with the world, particularly under stress.

Clinicians can then plan treatment specifically addressing a patient's personality needs.

Case 4: A 28-year-old woman is referred for evaluation of chronic right lower quadrant pain with diffuse, vague accompanying symptoms. She begins the office visit by telling you that you are her "hope for a cure." She has seen many other physicians who have been unable to help her. By the time she sees you, she's already angered some of your office staff. She relates their incompetence at drawing blood.

Further history reveals several jobs as a midlevel executive in the publishing business, which she left for vague reasons. She describes few successful relationships with either sex. While in college, she had symptoms of an eating disorder. She also describes long-term symptoms consistent with dysthymia, or a low-level depression. At the end of the visit, she requests an alprazolam (Xanax) refill, and when you defer that, she becomes agitated. By the end of the visit, she is angrily talking about suicidal ideation as you try to understand her pain.

Confrontation does not work with this patient, but understanding her interpersonal dysfunction (and its effect on you) allows better care and possibly clues to her pain. If you understand her probable cluster B diagnosis, you set limits rather than confront; expect extreme anger at any hint of abandonment, and describe *realistic* expectations from the beginning. The issue of safety is frequently relevant to these patients when they are stressed. They may be suicidal or at least have suicidal ideation. Either should be taken very seriously, probably with a psychiatric evaluation.

In considering personality disorders, cluster A as described in Table 27–4 is usually more obvious.[22] These are odd, eccentric, paranoid, withdrawn personalities that genetically may have a relationship to Axis I disorders such as schizophrenia. While evaluating the pain in these patients, it is useful to obtain an initial psychiatric consultation to rule out frank psychosis. Some patients with a cluster A diagnosis are delusional about the origin of their pain. That is, they have a fixed false belief that demonstrates psychotic thinking about processes that lead to their pain. An example is a patient who believes that a difficult boss has done something to cause her pain (idea of reference).

Cluster B patients are more likely to visit our office with pain complaints. A definite relationship is noted between cluster B patients and mood disorder. All patients in each cluster have overlapping characteristics, and it is uncommon for a single diagnosis to be made. Patients with a histrionic personality are especially threatened when illness causes the loss of function or attractiveness. Their very self-worth depends on superficial attractiveness. Awareness of this helps clinicians in managing a patient's pain in a nonconfrontive yet firm way that avoids the histrionic emotions that patients express if they sense impending loss.

Patients with antisocial personality disorder (sociopaths) show patterns of behavior that disregard other people. These are the individuals who come to the attention of clinicians as manipulative, malingering patients who may have factitious symptoms and are trying to avoid an obligation through their chronic pain. Direct confrontation and limit setting are the only approach in this situation.

Narcissistic and borderline personality disorders are on a spectrum of personality disorders, with borderline the more chaotic and dysfunctional. Narcissism is represented by a lack of empathy and manipulativeness in a person with a fragile ego. Patients with a borderline personality (see Case 4) are probably the most difficult to handle in a clinical setting. Again, these patients may not have a borderline personality disorder when not stressed, but the vicious cycle of pain and regression to primitive character behavior is present when they are seen in the office.

By definition, patients with a borderline personality disorder are anxious, angry, suicidal, and impulsive and have the potential for substance abuse. They have intense chaotic relationships and are easily overwhelmed by stress. Their most confusing and difficult mechanisms of adaptation (maladaptation) are splitting and projection. Splitting is a defense that defines people (e.g., staff and physicians) as all good or all bad, with no in-between. They also project, or see everyone else as the source of the problem. The staff needs to be educated about these defenses, because patients with borderline characteristics make others furious.

It is important to recognize that individuals with borderline personality structures perceive any distancing as abandonment. This includes not being on call for them at all times. Therefore, clinicians need to approach such patients by setting limits in a frank manner: "I will stay with you through your disorder. There will be times when I will not be available to you, but that doesn't mean I've left you. I will return to be able to take care of you." The chaotic, intense encounters that these patients create can result in litigiousness when a physician does not understand the power and depth of these patients' personality dysfunction.

The final cluster (C) of personality disorders includes dependent, avoidant, obsessive-compulsive, and passive-aggressive personalities. In the setting of a physician's office, dependent patients approach illness with few good relationships and low self-esteem. A hint of this was seen in a previous case in which a patient presented to a physician who, she hoped, could "cure it all." This could be interpreted as a splitting, but it could also be looked at as dependence in which the entire treatment is placed in the physician's hands. These patients have unreasonable expectations of physicians (which is, of course, a trap for both) and express anger and hurt when the expectations are not met.

Patients with an obsessive-compulsive personality might require more detail in a description of their illness and treatment plans. This common trait in the population is often exaggerated during illness. Wise clinicians approach rigid obsessive-compulsive patients with just enough detail, allowing patients to be a part of their own care plan. This approach takes into account patients' need to have a sense of control over themselves and their care. This situation is the opposite of that with patients with dependent personality, and one in which physicians and patients can easily engage in power struggles if physicians do not take these needs into account. As in all personality disorders, it is the duty of clinicians, not patients, who are relatively unaware of their problems, to choreograph the relationship.

Finally, patients with a passive-aggressive personality are distinguished by overt cooperation and covert sabotage. These patients undermine their own treatment and need more direct confrontation to facilitate appropriate care.

Psychiatric treatment of patients with personality disorder consists of both psychopharmacologic treatment of symptoms and insight-oriented psychotherapy. This level of treatment is often beyond the scope of primary care clinicians. In fact, emotional "uncovering" in such patients may cause a great deal of harm. If patients are capable of some insight and psychologic perspective, referral to a mental health professional can be helpful. It is a clinician's job in caring for these patients with CPP to get along with them, minimizing regression and maximizing compliance. These are patients who are accustomed to dysfunction and describe strain in interpersonal relationships as someone else's fault. Clinicians who understand this are better able to treat these patients' pain. CPP by definition is frequently vague, diffuse, and difficult to diagnose. In patients with personality disorder, uncertainty and delay may promote regression and maladaptive physician-patient relationships.

Somatization

"Somatoform disorders are characterized by physical complaints lacking known medical basis or demonstrable physical findings in the presence of psychological factors judged to be etiologic or important in the initiation, exacerbation, or maintenance of the disturbance."[23] In any physical illness, including pain disorders, the diagnosis of somatization implies a process by which a person substitutes (consciously or unconsciously) physical symptoms for psychologic purposes. This should be differentiated from disorders traditionally thought to have psychophysiologic components, such as asthma, Crohn's disease, ulcer disease, hypertension, arthritis, and neurodermatitis.

Somatization is encountered more often by primary care physicians than by specialists. The most obvious and dramatic form is a conversion disorder in which psychologic distress is converted to a physical presentation that has important unconscious symbolic meaning to the patient. It is encountered in most fields—neurology with paresthesias, dyskinesias, hysterical seizures; otorhinolaryngology with swallowing difficulties or aphonia; ophthalmology with tunnel vision; and GI disorders such as pain, gas, and vomiting. The difficulty with diagnosing conversion disorder is that as many as 30% to 40% of patients with diagnosed conversion disorders are found to have a diagnosable physical or psychiatric disorder when observed for several years.[24]

It is important to identify the primary and secondary gain in conversion disorders. The primary gain represents the conflict and a partial solution to the conflict. An example is pelvic pain that is due to sexual abuse and that results in inability to have sexual relations (which are dreaded). The secondary gain avoids responsibility, gets support, manipulates others, and is important to understand in addressing the disorder.

The best understanding of somatization is often gained from a developmental standpoint. Children generally have emotional reactions (bad, sad, glad, mad), and communication of emotion begins and is facilitated by the acquisition of language. Children are then able to identify and verbalize emotions. A family that does not label and communicate emotions begins to resolve conflict (mad, sad, bad) with somatic language; the family and child become stuck at the somatic level of experiencing. Such children rely on a headache or upset stomach instead of their real fear of failure to keep them from school. They have learned to substitute somatic symptoms for all emotions. In somatization, the major conscious or unconscious motivation is achievement of the sick role.

Somatization was long thought to occur in low socioeconomic, rural, poorly educated, fundamentally religious groups, but it is becoming clear that the sophisticated somatization disorders of the 1990s more closely duplicate organic disease. They are not the obvious diagnoses of tunnel vision or hand-in-glove numbness.

Somatization (Briquet's syndrome or hysteria) has been studied more than any other somatoform disorder. To diagnose somatization disorder, a clinician must establish that a patient with CPP has a history of many symptoms in several organ systems. The diagnosis of somatization disorder requires diagnostic criteria including pain and GI, sexual, and pseudoneurologic symptoms (Table 27–5). The diagnosis has a high degree of stability, and this is usually a lifelong disorder. Comorbidities of depression, anxiety, drug and alcohol use, and OCD are significant. This is an expensive disorder that requires much medical care. If physicians recognize the disorder and monitor their countertransference, they can develop controlled dependence of patients to take better care of them and keep them out of the hospital and operating room.

The new DSM-IV deleted somatoform pain disorder and added "pain disorder associated with psychological factors," which requires that (1) the pain should be present in one or more anatomic sites; (2) the pain causes a significant *impairment* in the patient's social or occupational functioning; (3) psychologic factors appear to be operative in the onset, severity, exacerbation, or maintenance of the pain; and (4) the patient's pain is not primarily due to a

Table 27–5. **SUMMARY OF DIAGNOSTIC CRITERIA FOR SOMATIZATION DISORDER**

Many physical complaints with onset before age 30 years and long-standing occurrence for several years. Results in medical intervention and significant impairment in social or occupational functioning.

Symptoms have occurred within each of the following categories and are not entirely due to a known medical condition or are not fully explained by clinicial findings:

1. Sexual symptoms
2. Gastrointestinal symptoms
3. Pseudoneurologic symptoms
4. Pain symptoms

mood, anxiety, or psychotic disorder. If a medical disorder, such as pelvic adhesions, has a significant role in the patient's pain complaints (with exaggerated symptoms), then it may be "pain disorder associated with both psychological factors and a general medical condition." The more difficult pain syndrome is the one in which psychologic factors are predominant and medical factors are minimal. Such patients are unlikely to gain complete relief. It is important in the physician-patient relationship that both have reasonable expectations and that physicians manage their countertransference toward patients. Clear therapeutic contracts that minimize positive reinforcers of the pain help control symptoms and minimize continued searching for a physician.

Hypochondriasis

All pain syndromes need to be differentiated from hypochondriasis, which usually begins in later decades than does somatization disorder (which usually begins in late adolescence). Hypochondriasis is an overconcern with health or disease with misinterpretation of bodily symptoms. Medical evaluation and reassurance are frequently not therapeutic. The preoccupation is not delusional—that is, patients when confronted do not believe that they have disease, but their concern about disease and their fear consume enormous energy. Of course, the most important first step in treating hypochondriasis is to rule out a subtle presentation of disease such as multiple sclerosis, myasthenia gravis, or systemic lupus erythematosus. Patients with hypochondriasis "amplify somatic style."[25] Comorbidities of anxiety and depression are often present, but the most treatable and important comorbidity is that of OCD. Hypochondriac patients often have obsessive, intrusive thoughts about illness. SSRIs are very helpful but sometimes must be used in large doses equivalent to 40 to 80 mg of fluoxetine.

Factitious disorders must be ruled out or at least considered in anyone presenting with pain. Factitious disorder is the voluntary production of signs or symptoms of disease for no reason other than to achieve the sick role. There are no external incentives such as avoiding responsibility, as in malingering. The majority of patients are women and are employed in the health professions. Diagnosis requires a high index of suspicion and is frequently made by retrieving a history from the chart or family and identifying repeated illness episodes without pathology. Surprisingly, these individuals respond reasonably well to direct confrontation.

The treatment of all these somatoform disorders requires managing the transference of patients, because they have positive and negative feelings toward physicians, nurses, and hospitals. They are often unconsciously repeating unresolved childhood conflicts. Again, we may understand that perspective long before a patient does. It is important in dealing with families to identify and address the secondary gain of patients. Establish one physician as the one in charge, schedule regular visits, and identify stresses and conflict that exacerbate the situation. For some patients, providing a language (i.e., psychotherapy) in which they can say in words what they were attempting to say in body language is helpful. A physician, of course, must be alert for signs of real disease, which can occur concurrently with somatoform disorders. Comorbidities of anxiety, depression, or psychosocial stress should be addressed. When physicians understand and appreciate the psychologic significance of symptoms and establish an empathic therapeutic alliance with patients, patients can be more easily maintained and kept out of the sick role. It is the awareness of these disorders that allows us to address them.

Summary

Neither primary care physicians nor their patients with CPP are likely to be overwhelmed by pain symptoms if at the outset they consider the importance of the emotional component in precipitating and maintaining symptoms.

If the pain is the core, years of pain result in surrounding layers of suffering and pain behavior that often become more important than the pain.

Addressing suffering and pain behavior and looking for comorbidities of depression, anxiety, somatoform symptoms, and personality disorder greatly increase physicians' and patients' chances of achieving successful pain management.

References

1. Tyrer SP (ed): Psychology, Psychiatry, and Chronic Pain. Oxford, Butterworth-Heinemann, 1991, pp 25–43.
2. Tyrer SP (ed): Psychology, Psychiatry, and Chronic Pain. Oxford, Butterworth-Heinemann, 1991, p 9.
3. Tyrer SP (ed): Psychology, Psychiatry, and Chronic Pain. Oxford, Butterworth-Heinemann, 1991, p 4.
4. Aronoff GM: Evaluation and Treatment of Chronic Pain, 2nd ed. Baltimore, Williams & Wilkins, 1992, p 57.
5. Aronoff GM: Evaluation and Treatment of Chronic Pain, 2nd ed. Baltimore, Williams & Wilkins, 1992, p 400.
6. Engel GL: Psychogenic pain and the pain-prone patient. Am J Med 1959;42:899.
7. Harrop-Griffiths J, Katon W, Walker E, et al: The association between chronic pelvic pain, psychiatric diagnoses, and childhood sexual abuse. Obstet Gynecol 1988;71:589.
8. Beck AT: Depression Inventory. Philadelphia, Center for Cognitive Therapy, 1978.
9. Locke MJ, Wallace KM: Short marital adjustment and prediction tests: Their reliability and validity. Marriage Fam Living 1959;21:251.
10. Melzack R: The McGill Pain Questionnaire. In Melzack R (ed): Pain Management and Assessment. New York, Raven Press, 1983.
11. Payne B, Norfleet M: Chronic pain and the family: A review. Pain 1986;26:1.
12. Talbott JA, Hales RE, Yudofsky SC: Textbook of Psychiatry. Washington, DC, American Psychiatric Press, 1988, p 409.
13. American Psychiatric Association: Diagnostic Criteria from DSM-IV Quick Reference. Washington, DC, author, 1994, p 161.
14. Seagraves RT: Treatment of emergent sexual dysfunction in affective disorders: A review and management strategies. J Clin Psychiatry Update Monogr 1994;1:8.
15. Kames LD, Rapkin AJ, Naliboff BD, et al: Effectiveness of an interdisciplinary pain management program for the treatment of chronic pelvic pain. Pain 1990;41:41.
16. American Psychiatric Association: Diagnostic Criteria from DSM-IV Quick Reference. Washington, DC, author, 1994, p 207.
17. American Psychiatric Association: Diagnostic Criteria from DSM-IV Quick Reference. Washington, DC, author, 1994, p 209.
18. Talbott JA, Hales RE, Yudofsky SC: Textbook of Psychiatry. Washington, DC, American Psychiatric Press, 1988, p 328.
19. American Psychiatric Association: Diagnostic Criteria from DSM-IV Quick Reference. Washington, DC, author, 1994, p 275.
20. American Psychiatric Association: Diagnostic Criteria from DSM-IV Quick Reference. Washington, DC, author, 1994, p 37.
21. Stoudemire A (ed): Clinical Psychiatry for Medical Students, 2nd ed. Philadelphia, JB Lippincott, 1994, pp 175–176.
22. American Psychiatric Association: Diagnostic Criteria from DSM-IV Quick Reference. Washington, DC, author, 1994, p 276.
23. Stoudemire A (ed): Clinical Psychiatry for Medical Students, 2nd ed. Philadelphia, JB Lippincott, 1994, p 277.
24. Talbott JA, Hales RE, Yudofsky SC: Textbook of Psychiatry. Washington, DC, American Psychiatric Press, 1988, p 539.
25. Stoudemire A (ed): Clinical Psychiatry for Medical Students, 2nd ed. JB Lippincott, Philadelphia, 1994, p 290.

28

General Principles of Pain Management

John F. Steege, MD

The management of chronic pelvic pain (CPP) has much in common with the management of pain involving other organ systems. Regardless of the organ focus of the pain, substantial efforts are required to educate a patient and her family about the nature of chronic pain, the potential role of many classes of medications, the need to treat components of the pain arising from several organ systems, the role of psychologic and behavioral approaches, and specific treatments for any organic pathology found.

Gynecologic surgeons have a particular challenge: to present any potential surgery to patients in a balanced fashion. Patients with pelvic pain commonly hope a straightforward surgical approach will fix the problem, and surgically trained gynecologists are prone to offer the approach they understand and use best.

Only sparse data describe the ability of gynecologic surgery alone to relieve pain. Although the data on hysterectomy suggest that pain is relieved and patients are satisfied with the surgery in the majority of cases,[1, 2] between 10% and 30% have either incomplete or no relief after surgery. These figures leave room for improvement. Follow-up data on the surgical treatment of endometriosis (see Chapter 14) and adhesive disease (see Chapter 13) are equally few.

Women with CPP often live in hope of a simple (or, at least, certain) cure. Especially in patients who demonstrate some of the hallmarks of the chronic pain syndrome (see Chapter 2), the education of a patient and her family should have the goal of helping them accept a rehabilitation approach instead. Realistic goals for a patient as an individual should be established early in the process. Although complete pain relief is often hoped for, the more reasonable goal may be pain management with improved function.

This chapter addresses the process of patient education, medication management, the role of psychologic and behavioral approaches, and additional approaches such as biofeedback and physical therapy and refers briefly to specific management approaches for individual pain syndromes. It concludes with a discussion of primary care management versus treatment at interdisciplinary pain clinics.[3]

Patient Education

After a complete chronologic pain history has been taken (see Chapter 6) and a thorough pain-oriented physical examination performed (see Chapter 7), a treatment plan can be outlined for a patient. In order for your suggestions to make more sense to a patient and to be better accepted, it is useful to address directly some ideas about pain and some common fears about what physicians say to patients with pain.

When someone with chronic pain seeks medical help, along with the details of the particular pain problem, several concerns are usually uppermost in the patient's mind: "I hope the doctor finds enough wrong to explain the pain" and "I know this pain is not in my head." These two ideas operate as a filter through which must pass all communications in the office.

Exceptions to this generalization certainly exist. Most physicians have seen cases in which persons attributed their symptoms to emotional distress and thus pursued psychologic help when they were really having problems from worsening organic disease. How individuals interpret their symptoms no doubt influences their choice of helping professional.

The basis for a more effective discussion of chronic pain rests on a consideration of theories of pain perception (see Chapter 2). Although the gate theory is certainly not the last answer in our understanding of pain, it does provide a useful metaphor for explaining the integrated function of body and mind in the development of pain. Discussing gate theory and explaining it with a diagram of the brain and spinal cord and its connections to the tissues of interest can help patients understand your approach. It directly confronts their concerns that you may indeed have a private agenda for determining whether or not the pain is physically or psychologically based. When a patient understands that you will not make this judgment at the end of your evaluation, she and her family will be far more open about sharing personal and emotional concerns and, it is hoped, will be more open to accepting the suggestion of psychologic support or psychotropic medication when that is appropriate.

As detailed in Chapter 2, the gate theory can be described very simply using a diagram of the brain and spinal cord. The notion that central processes contribute significantly to, in a physiologic sense, the transmission of nociceptive signals up to the brain is usually new information and makes logical sense to a patient and her family. The diagrammatic model can be extended to include contributions of nociceptive signals from several organ systems, such as the intestines, and from musculoskeletal activity and organic gynecologic pathology.

As described later, this naturally leads to a "shopping list" approach to treatment of many factors (Table 28–1). On this list is often a compendium of physical and emotional concerns. Once the approach is discussed in this manner, however, a patient and her family are firmly reassured that even the best clinician cannot assign a percentage value for each contributing factor; at best, the list simply describes items that are of significant importance. It is then the task of the physician and patient to decide together which treatments seem most important and are likely to be most cost-effective.

Table 28–1. **PATIENT EDUCATION: LISTING CONTRIBUTING CAUSES OF PAIN AND THEIR TREATMENT**

- Adhesions
  - Pulling on the bowels?
  - Attaching bowels to the ovaries?
  - Treatments
    - Bowel regulation: fiber, water, and so on
    - Pain medication
    - Laparoscopy: 70% chance of improving pain due to adhesions
- Irritable bowel syndrome
  - Diet (fiber and water)
  - Exercise
  - Stress reduction: relaxation training, therapy?
  - Medications: antispasmodics (see Chapter 23), amitriptyline
- Muscles
  - Levators: reverse Kegel's exercises, "let it fall out," physical therapy
  - Vaginal opening: tightening, relaxing exercises, crosswise position for sex, lubrication
- Chronic pain syndrome
  - Antidepressants to help pain-inhibiting systems ("gate")
  - Counseling

This said, it becomes more apparent to a patient and her family that the process of working through the treatment of the different components of the pain takes time. A series of regularly scheduled appointments facilitates this process, as opposed to asking a patient to call back if the pain continues. The latter approach often involves delays that serve only to dilute the gains that may have been made.

Make your list of contributing factors (see Table 28–1) with the patient and give her a copy. The list describes further diagnostic measures that might be useful as well as potential treatments and the prognosis for each particular component of the pain.

Although the example cited deals with adhesive disease, the list would look very similar for a person with endometriosis, adenomyosis, or other difficulties. I usually discuss the more obvious physical components first, because these are more often easily accepted by patients. I leave discussions of mood, marital conflict, and sexual dysfunction until later in the discussion, when I hope to have established credibility and rapport.

It is most useful for this discussion to take place with a family member present, particularly the spouse. The entire notion of integrating body and mind factors may be somewhat novel to a patient and her extended family when your patient goes home and tries to report to the family what the doctor said. The written list and the corroborating opinions of a family member who has heard your discussion are very helpful. Friends and relatives sometimes have more credibility in terms of the medical advice they offer than does the physician. If the message and the plan you are outlining contradict these assembled opinions, your effect is likely to be diluted.

The role of the more organically based components of pain is specifically discussed in other chapters (adhesions, see Chapter 13; functional bowel disease, see Chapter 23; musculoskeletal problems, see Chapter 24). This chapter focuses on discussion of more sensitive issues, such as mood disturbance, marital conflict, and sexual adjustments.

Depression is certainly more common in persons dealing with chronic pain (see Chapter 27). In many instances, it appears that physical illness must also occur to prompt the beginning of a chronic pain syndrome in someone who is depressed. Functional disease is certainly more common in depressed individuals, but there is less evidence that depression can be the entire source of a pain syndrome all by itself.

For the purposes of discussion with a patient and her family, it is useful to legitimize depression as an appropriate and expected reaction to the process of being in chronic pain. Referring to the gate theory model, it is then relatively easy to connect the affective changes a person acknowledges with their possible and even probable physiologic effects on pain perception itself. I often use the example that a broken arm might be far more uncomfortable to someone who has been in chronic pain for other reasons than it would be to an otherwise healthy individual. Some of this worsening response to pain can be a function of simply being in chronic pain, and some might be due to the accompanying depression.

When the impact of chronicity on pain threshold is described, some persons disagree, replying that they feel they have developed a great resistance to their pain over time, have learned ways to cope with it and ignore it when possible, and therefore fear the expansion of organic pathology as the reason for their recent increases in pain. This is a difficult part of the discussion, because their reasoning sometimes is certainly accurate. In such cases, a full exploration of the extent of organic pathology should certainly be carried out to clarify this discussion. When appropriate, pain mapping by microlaparoscopy can calibrate a person's pain threshold to a standard stimulus—for example, applying a tenaculum to the cervix or probing internal nongynecologic structures.

When discussing mood changes (i.e., depression and anxiety), it is important to distinguish depressive mood changes from a free-standing diagnosis of depression. Many people think of a depressed person as one who entirely withdraws from normal activities, continuously demonstrates a sad affect, has frequent crying spells, and so on. It is important to point out that mood disorders occur in all degrees of severity and that you are not labeling a patient as chronically depressed in a classic sense unless the history indeed documents that such is the case. This is a sensitive discussion, because it is very often the interaction that leads to a concerned or even angry reply that you are really telling her that the pain is all in her mind. This concern is usual and if not expressed should be brought up and dealt with directly.

Next, it is useful to discuss the ways in which pain typically intrudes on a family. It indeed acts like an unwelcome guest that has moved into the house and become a third member in the couple relationship or perhaps an undesirable member added to the entire family. The partner's reactions to the woman's pain are often complicated. The response to the beginnings of the pain problem are typically those that are most appropriate for acute pain. The partner offers support, reassurance, tactical help with assuming some of the tasks that the woman might ordinarily do, and in general postpones discussion of emotionally difficult topics in order to relieve the stress in the environment. The expectation is that once the pain resolves, attention can then be redirected to these recognized issues.

The discussion with a patient and her partner should focus on the idea that when pain continues chronically, this kind of support may work to their disadvantage. The longer the pain continues, the more this well-intentioned help may serve to reduce the pain victim's sense of functionality and erode her roles within the relationship and within the family. It may help to suggest gently that in this setting, a partner can help the pain victim to pace her activities and to slowly and gradually resume more of her functions within the relationship and the family. In many conditions, this allows a gradual return of function, hence an improvement in self-esteem, without adversely affecting the intensity of the pain itself. Put briefly, the partner's role becomes one of helping the pain victim to do things, rather than doing things for her.

In pelvic pain, the area of disability that perhaps most commonly prompts a search for medical care is a deterioration of sexual function. At least in terms of those who seek help at a gynecologist's office, this is the area of dysfunction that a patient often most wants to remedy. It is usually possible to tailor to the couple's needs your comments about supplemental lubrication, sexual stimulation, and changes in sexual position (see Chapter 9).

Medications

Physicians have traditionally been taught to minimize the number of medications as much as possible. In many situations dealing with chronic pain, this usually laudable principle may be a disadvantage. If indeed the etiology is multifactorial, then treatment of single components with medication or other approaches may be less than completely successful. When this happens, a patient's response to the results is often to discredit the appropriateness and the effectiveness of the medication prescribed. Later, it may be more difficult to incorporate this medication into an overall list of suggestions.

In many circumstances, it is indeed appropriate to prescribe a list of medications all at the same time, always keeping in mind the potential for medication interactions. At the same time, it is, of course, appropriate to review a patient's list of medications periodically to look for redundancies that might be eliminated or substitutions that might be made to allow an equally effective but perhaps less risky and less expensive medication regimen.

A review of specific categories of medications useful for chronic pain follows.

Analgesic Medications

The use of pain medications in chronic pain is very different from that which is most appropriate for acute pain. For patients with acute pain, it is most appropriate to start off with the strongest medication necessary to relieve the pain. Postoperative medication with narcotics is perhaps the clearest example. In that setting, a patient and her family appropriately try to taper off the medication as quickly as possible. The patient tries to postpone using the medication until the pain is more severe, and then she takes it. In this setting, she usually either voices some complaint or demonstrates some pain behavior (diminished activity, lying down, grimacing, and so on) that communicates to herself and to others the need for taking the medication.

When pain becomes chronic, it is often more useful to approach analgesic medication in a very different fashion. First, it is seldom possible to find a medication that relieves the pain completely, short of continuous narcotics at high doses. Even these medications, with time, tend to lose their effectiveness (tachyphylaxis). This may explain why pain medication demands can escalate over time even though the organic disease or even the functional components may indeed be stable. The escalation occurs because the patient's expectation is one of complete relief. She and her family should be encouraged to think of analgesics as attenuating the pain rather than relieving it completely.

The second difference related to use of analgesic medications when dealing with chronic pain is that they should be prescribed to be taken on as regular a basis as possible, taking into consideration the pharmacodynamics of the individual agent prescribed. This provides the greatest degree of pain relief over time and counteracts the tendency for pain to become intractable before the medication is taken. The out-of-control feeling comes from increased intensity of the primary pain source itself and often from the recruitment of surrounding organ systems, such as the intestines or the musculoskeletal systems, which contributes to the overall pain problem.

Prescription of analgesics on a schedule is called *noncontingent* scheduling. This means that taking the medication is not contingent on either voicing a pain complaint or demonstrating a pain behavior. These behaviors tend only to reinforce further the disability a patient might be experiencing and to reinforce her role as the sick person within the family (see Chapter 2). Noncontingent scheduling takes a patient's partner and family out of the role of having to acknowledge her pain before she takes medication and hence inadvertently reinforcing her pain. Breaking this pattern is often a relief to the family and to the patient and may be a very positive step.

It is always most appropriate to use nonnarcotic analgesics as a first choice. This is often difficult for a patient and her family to accept, because they have usually tried them on their own and found that they provide incomplete relief. Nevertheless, many are willing to try them again when it is explained that partial relief is the goal and that gradual improvement over time is the expectation, as other components of the overall treatment strategy begin to demonstrate their benefits.

Table 28–2 lists the most reasonable nonnarcotic choices. All have their side effects and toxicities. It may be useful to rotate among drug classes at intervals to avoid some of the more long-term toxicities listed.

Narcotic use in chronic pain is often avoided like the plague by physicians and patients alike. Judicious use is reasonable, and careful regular use of narcotics can greatly indeed improve functional capacity. Pharmacologically, narcotics can sometimes worsen depression. When this occurs, the patient may mistakenly interpret the change as a worsening of her pain and how she feels in general as signaling the need for even more or stronger medications. Similarly, an anxious patient may find that narcotic medication calms her tension and may develop a pattern of using narcotic medication inappropriately for this problem.

Table 28–3 lists the customary doses and toxicities of the more commonly used narcotic agents. Particular note should be made of methadone. Although its use as a substitute for street narcotics in addiction control programs is well known, its role as an effective analgesic is less commonly understood. With proper monitoring, methadone can be quite safely used for long periods without substantial dose escalation and without tachyphylaxis in terms of its analgesic effect. Perhaps the greatest barrier to its effective use is the attendant social stigma.

The problem of abuse of narcotic medications and overt drug-seeking behavior is of occasional concern to practicing primary care physicians and gynecologists dealing with CPP. Dependence on narcotic medication can grow slowly and insidiously. When more classic drug-seeking behaviors start to develop, they become a bit more obvious: Calling for prescription refills late in the day or on weekends, claiming that prescriptions for bottles of pills have been lost or stolen, and so on. To discover if drug-seeking behavior is taking place, it is prudent to check with a patient's pharmacist whenever calling in a prescription by asking the pharmacist to check the patient's profile for the prescription of other controlled substances. In most states, sharing this information is protected by law. In these circumstances, it is not legally considered a breach of patient confidentiality to learn of your patient's other prescriptions for controlled drugs written by other physicians. In some states, legal penalties exist for a patient who seeks out a new physician specifically for the pur-

Table 28–2. **NONSTEROIDAL ANTIINFLAMMATORY DRUGS COMMONLY USED IN CHRONIC PAIN MANAGEMENT**

Drug Name	Usual Dose Range	Side Effects
Ibuprofen 200 mg OTC: Advil, Nuprin, Motrin IB, Bayer Select Pain Relief Formula Motrin 400 mg, 600 mg, or 800 mg	400 mg q4–6h 600 mg q6–8h 800 mg q8–12h	Long-term use can result in serious GI toxicity such as bleeding, ulceration, and perforation. Minor upper GI symptoms such as dyspepsia are common early in therapy. Patients who smoke or drink >3 alcoholic beverages per day are at increased risk of GI bleeding. Does increase bleeding time, but less than ASA. Though rare, ibuprofen has been found to cause acute renal failure, renal papillary necrosis, and other signs of renal toxicity.
Naproxen Naprosyn 250 mg, 375 mg, or 500 mg	250–500 mg bid	Side effect profile very similar to ibuprofen.
Naproxen sodium Aleve (OTC), 220 mg per tablet Anaprox, 275 mg per tablet Anaprox DS, 550 mg per tablet	220 mg q12h for mild pain For moderate to severe pain, dosage can range between 220 mg q8h to 550 mg q12h	
Nabumetone Relafen, 500- or 750-mg tablets	1000 mg/d, either qd or 500 mg bid 2000 mg/d, highest dose	Although nabumetone has the usual side effects listed for all NSAIDs, the incidence of GI ulceration is significantly lower. It has much less effect on collagen-induced platelet aggregation and no effect on bleeding time. Most common side effects are diarrhoea, dyspepsia, and abdominal pain.
Ketorolac Toradol, 10-mg tablets	10 mg q4–6h prn pain for limited duration Not to be given for chronic use. 5–14 days is maximum duration.	Side effect profile similar to ibuprofen but incidence of serious GI tract adverse effects increases to rate higher than ASA 650 mg qid if given for longer than 2 weeks.

GI, gastrointestinal; ASA, acetylsalicylic acid (aspirin); NSAIDs, nonsteroidal antiinflammatory drugs.

pose of obtaining controlled drugs. When a patient reports her drugs as stolen, my colleagues and I replace the medication only after receiving a copy of the police report.

To attempt to put some bounds around the use of narcotic medication, we often find a narcotics contract useful (Table 28–4). By reading and signing this agreement, a patient acknowledges your concern about the use of narcotic medications and is also made aware of your vigilance about her behaviors. This contract, although it has no legal power, can serve to curtail excessive controlled substance use if it is initiated in the earliest stages of narcotic prescription.

Antidepressants

The tricyclic antidepressant medications have been a mainstay of chronic pain management for decades. An extensive meta-analysis concluded that substantial clinical series suggest the efficacy of amitriptyline, although true controlled trials either are lacking or are not sufficiently rigorous in

Table 28–3. **NARCOTICS COMMONLY USED IN CHRONIC PAIN MANAGEMENT**

Drug Name	Usual Dose Range	Side Effects
Hydrocodone bitartrate with acetaminophen Lortab 2.5/500, 5/500, or 7.5/500 Vicodin 5/750 Lorcet 10/650 Lorcet Plus 7.5/650 (all are scored tablets)	5–10 mg hydrocodone either q6h or q8h. Can use additional acetaminophen between doses to potentiate effect.	Lightheadedness, dizziness, sedation, nausea and vomiting, and constipation. (These are common side effects of all narcotics.)
Oxycodone hydrochloride Percocet 5 mg with 325 mg acetaminophen Percodan 4.5 mg with 325 mg aspirin (also contains 0.38 mg oxycodone terephthalate)	1 tablet q6h or q8h Additional acetaminophen between doses may serve to potentiate effect.	Common effects.
OxyCodone controlled release OxyContin	10–40 mg q12h	Common effects.
Methadone hydrochloride Dolophine 5- or 10-mg scored tablets	2.5 mg q8h to 10 mg q6h Commonly 15–20 mg qd	Common effects. Lower extremity edema or joint swelling may occur and require discontinuation. Concurrent use of desipramine may increase methadone blood level. Cautious use in patients on monoamine oxidase inhibitors.
Acetaminophen with codeine Tylenol No. 3, 300 mg acetaminophen with 30 mg codeine	1–2 tablets q6–8h	Common effects. Constipation very likely. Nausea and vomiting more common than with other narcotics. More common allergy—rash.
Morphine sulfate MS Contin or Oramorph	15–60 mg q12h; controlled-release tablets	Common effects. Higher doses increase risk of respiratory depression.
Fentanyl transdermal system Duragesic	25-μg patch, 1 q72h Also available in 50 or 75 μg. Always start with lowest dose.	Common effects. Patch must be kept from heat sources or dose may be increased. Extreme caution in patients on other central nervous system medications. Respiratory depression can occur.

design to prove a definite therapeutic effect of this class of drugs.[4] Nevertheless, treatment with antidepressants is clinically reasonable in many situations, especially when a biologic marker of depression such as early morning awakening has begun to appear. The effectiveness of antidepressants may be influenced to some degree by a person's genetic vulnerability to depression itself. In pain victims with a family history of depression, antidepressants may be more effective, even in the absence of overt clinical depression in the pain sufferers themselves.

In many series describing amitriptyline use, doses between 50 and 75 mg qhs are used. These are one half to one third of the usual therapeutic dose prescribed for a true clinical depression. The mechanism of action of these medications is uncertain, but it is hypothesized that they may operate by a central mechanism to alter the pain threshold of a person with chronic pain. In the past 15 years of work in our pelvic pain clinic, we have witnessed many examples of dramatic responses to this medication. The greatest drawbacks to the use of the tricyclic antidepressants are the side effects of constipation and morning drowsiness. In practice, then, we usually prescribe amitriptyline only for people who do not have significant constipation already. For patients

Table 28–4. **SAMPLE NARCOTICS CONTRACT**

What You Should Know About Narcotic Medications

Narcotic medications such as methadone or Tylenol No. 3 are potent pain killers that can sometimes be helpful in managing the discomfort due to various chronic painful disorders. The use of narcotic pain killers for chronic pain not due to cancer is controversial because of the possibility of addiction to these types of medications. Based on recent evidence and our own clinical experience, we believe that some narcotic medicines have a legitimate role in chronic pain management.

Your doctor may recommend a narcotic medication for you. It is important to understand that these medications should be used only if they provide an overall benefit to you, usually by increasing your activity tolerance. Side effects may include drowsiness, nausea, or constipation. If any of these occur, it is important to notify your physician. Caution must also be exercised in driving or operating heavy machinery because of the possibility of drowsiness. The likelihood that you will become addicted or "hooked" on a narcotic prescribed to control pain is *extremely low,* provided you do not have a prior tendency toward addiction. You should not drink alcohol while you are taking narcotic medications.

Because of the special considerations relating to narcotic use, the Pelvic Pain Clinic has developed the following policies, which you should carefully note:

1. No narcotic prescriptions will be refilled on weekends or during the evening hours. Patients should anticipate the need for renewal of their narcotic medications in advance and call for renewal during office hours, Monday through Friday, from 8:30 AM to 12 noon and 1:00 PM to 4:30 PM. Patients should allow enough time for prescriptions to be mailed.
2. Prescriptions that are lost or stolen will not be refilled. It is up to the patient to be sure that such incidents do not occur. In the event that drugs are stolen, we will consider refilling the prescription when a copy of the police report is faxed to our office.
3. You should obtain narcotics and other pain medications from the Pelvic Pain Clinic staff only. Patients who obtain narcotics from other physicians without our knowledge or who knowingly misrepresent their previously prescribed doses may be discharged from our clinic.
4. Any patient who uses narcotic medications for a long period may develop some degree of tolerance to them. When this occurs, higher doses of narcotics may be needed to achieve the same degree of pain relief. If tolerance should occur to a significant degree, rather than continue to increase the dose prescribed, we may discontinue or switch the narcotic for a period of 1 to 2 months.
5. Under no circumstances may patients increase their dose or frequency of narcotic use without a physician's approval. Patients may certainly decrease or gradually discontinue use in the presence of undesired side effects or improved pain control, but any unauthorized increase in dosing will lead to the possibility of discharge from our clinic. Narcotic medicines should never be abruptly discontinued.
6. As with any other medication, questions or concerns should be directed to the prescribing physician. We will be happy to receive your questions at (000) 000-0000.

with substantial irritable bowel syndrome or significant bladder irritability, the anticholinergic side effects of the tricyclic antidepressants may produce clinically useful results (Table 28–5).

The selective serotonin uptake inhibitors (SSRIs) are a newer class of antidepressants that in general are much better tolerated than the tricyclics. Although this application has not been systematically explored, it is tempting to think that subtherapeutic doses of these agents might also be effective for treating chronic pain, in a manner analogous to the results noted with the tricyclic antidepressants. In general, they are activating medications that do not aggravate constipation. In fact, side effects such as diarrhea and intestinal cramping may be limiting, as can the sense of hyperexcitability that sometimes occurs with their use. As a matter of practicality, once we have decided to prescribe an antidepressant, we choose the agent on the basis of a patient's bowel habit: amitriptyline for those with diarrhea and an SSRI for those tending to be more constipated.

The commonly available SSRIs are listed in Table 28–5, along with their dose ranges and toxicities. Although combinations of the SSRIs with the other antidepressants are widely used, their prescription in combination is more hazardous and needs to take into account drug interactions, as well as the age and general mental health of the patient. Formal psychiatric consultation may be more appropriate, especially when combinations of medications are contemplated.

Regardless of the agent prescribed, careful inquiry should be made about the patient's reaction to the idea of taking an antidepressant drug. Countless patients who have been prescribed such medications with all good intent have never filled the prescription because they felt insecure about taking such medications or resented their prescription.

Table 28–5A. **PHARMACOLOGY OF ANTIDEPRESSANT DRUGS**

Drug	Therapeutic Dosage Range (mg/d)	Average (Range) Elimination Half-Lives (h)*	Potentially Fatal Drug Interactions
Tricyclics			
Amitriptyline (Elavil, Endep)	75–300	24 (16–46)	Antiarrhythmics, MAO inhibitors
Clomipramine (Anafranil)	75–300	24 (20–40)	Antiarrhythmics, MAO inhibitors
Desipramine (Norpramin, Pertofrane)	75–300	18 (12–50)	Antiarrhythmics, MAO inhibitors
Doxepin (Adapin, Sinequan)	75–300	17 (10–47)	Antiarrhythmics, MAO inhibitors
Imipramine (Janimine, Tofranil)	75–300	22 (12–34)	Antiarrhythmics, MAO inhibitors
Nortriptyline (Aventyl, Pamelor)	40–200	26 (18–88)	Antiarrhythmics, MAO inhibitors
Protriptyline (Vivactil)	20–60	76 (54–124)	Antiarrhythmics, MAO inhibitors
Trimipramine (Surmontil)	75–300	12 (8–30)	Antiarrhythmics, MAO inhibitors
Heterocyclics			
Amoxapine (Asendin)	100–600	10 (8–14)	MAO inhibitors
Bupropion (Wellbutrin)	225–450	14 (8–24)	MAO inhibitors (possibly)
Maprotiline (Ludiomil)	100–225	43 (27–58)	MAO inhibitors
Trazodone (Desyrel)	150–600	8 (4–14)	
Selective serotin reuptake inhibitors			
Fluoxetine (Prozac)	10–40	168 (72–360)†	MAO inhibitors
Paroxetine (Paxil)	20–50	24 (3–65)	MAO inhibitors‡
Sertraline (Zoloft)	50–150	24 (10–30)	MAO inhibitors‡
MAO inhibitors§			
Isocarboxazid (Marplan)	30–50	Unknown	For all three MAO inhibitors: vasoconstrictors,‖ decongestants,‖ meperidine, possibly other narcotics
Phenelzine (Nardil)	45–90	2 (1.5–4.0)	
Tranylcypromine (Parnate)	20–60	2 (1.5–3.0)	

MAO, monoamine oxidase.
*Half-lives are affected by age, sex, race, concurrent drugs, and length of drug exposure.
†Includes both fluoxetine and norfluoxetine.
‡By extrapolation from fluoxetine data.
§MAO inhibition lasts longer (7 days) than drug half-life.
‖Including pseudoephedrine, phenylephrine, phenylpropanolamine, epinephrine, norepinephrine, and others.
From Depression Guideline Panel: Depression in Primary Care: Detection, Diagnosis, and Treatment. Rockville, MD: U.S. Department of Health and Human Services, Public Health Services, Agency for Health Care Policy and Research, 1993.

Careful discussion about the prescription must be undertaken, reinforcing the notion that these medications are used because they may work at a brain level to alter pain perception and facilitate the body's natural ability to block out pain signals. It should be strongly emphasized that the prescription of antidepressants does not necessarily imply that the pain is largely a psychologic issue. Here again, it is most useful to have at least one family member present during your discussion when dealing with such difficult issues.

Organ-Specific Medications

Practitioners dealing with CPP problems must become skilled at the effective use of gastrointestinal agents. (The details of thorough assessment and treatment of irritable bowel syndrome are discussed in Chapter 23.)

Medications and treatments for bladder irritability are commonly useful for treating CPP (see Chapter 22). A person with bladder spasms typically reports a history of intermittent muscle cramping pain sometimes triggered by the emptying of an overfilled bladder but many times appearing purely at random. In those who have developed a habit of frequent voidings, bladder capacity may diminish to the point that overfilling and resultant spasm occur easily. As is true with functional bowel disease, functional bladder disease of this type seldom interrupts sleep, unless the frequent voiding pattern has become established. Antispasmodic medications are useful to a degree but are difficult to use owing to their anticholinergic side effects. In general, sedation seems to be the most limiting of these.

Table 28–5B. **SIDE EFFECT PROFILES OF ANTIDEPRESSANT DRUGS**

Drug	Side Effect*						
	Central Nervous System*			Cardiovascular		Gastrointestinal	
	Anticholinergic†	*Drowsiness*	*Insomnia, Agitation*	*Orthostatic Hypotension*	*Cardiac Arrhythmia*	*Gastrointestinal Distress*	*Weight Gain >6 kg*
Amitriptyline	4+	4+	0	4+	3+	0	4+
Desipramine	1+	1+	1+	2+	2+	0	1+
Doxepin	3+	4+	0	2+	2+	0	3+
Imipramine	3+	3+	1+	4+	3+	1+	3+
Nortriptyline	1+	1+	0	2+	2+	0	1+
Protriptyline	2+	1+	1+	2+	2+	0	0
Trimipramine	1+	4+	0	2+	2+	0	3+
Amoxapine	2+	2+	2+	2+	3+	0	1+
Maprotiline	2+	4+	0	0	1+	0	2+
Trazodone	0	4+	0	1+	1+	1+	1+
Bupropion	0	0	2+	0	1+	1+	0
Fluoxetine	0	0	2+	0	0	3+	0
Paroxetine	0	0	2+	0	0	3+	0
Sertraline	0	0	2+	0	0	3+	0
Monoamine oxidase inhibitors	1+	1+	2+	2+	0	1+	2+

*Numbers indicate the likelihood of side effect occurring, ranging from 0, absent or rare, to 5+, relatively common.
†Dry mouth, blurred vision, urinary hesitance, constipation.
From Depression Guideline Panel: Depression in Primary Care: Detection, Diagnosis, and Treatment. Rockville, MD: U.S. Department of Health and Human Services, Public Health Service Agency for Health Care Policy and Research, 1993.

As described elsewhere (see Chapter 24), muscular problems such as levator spasm, piriformis spasm, and vaginismus are common in women with pelvic pain. It is tempting to believe that muscle relaxants may be of value in these circumstances. Unfortunately, the sedative side effects are again a limiting aspect of these medications (Table 28–6). Perhaps more importantly, the long-term therapeutic benefits are derived from helping patients to establish a better sense of personal control over the involved muscles rather than relinquish control to a pharmacologic agent. This is perhaps most true when dealing with muscular elements of dyspareunia; specifically, vaginismus is a problem that needs to be solved by teaching voluntary control rather than by taking medication (see Chapter 9).

Many conditions that cause pelvic pain have substantial negative impact on sexual function (see Chapter 9). In reaction to deep dyspareunia with either a functional or organic basis, sexual response may diminish, causing new discomforts due to insufficient vaginal lubrication. With time, these responses progress to the point that involuntary spasm of the levators and the introital musculature takes place, bringing on the additional problem of vaginismus. In approximately 25% of cases of vaginismus, the diagnosis is made on historical grounds alone, because the patient may be able to relax sufficiently to allow comfortable pelvic examination despite clear evidence that vaginismus occurs at home during sexual encounters.

To make matters worse, women with diminished sexual response find that the vaginal expansion that is a normal part of sexual arousal (see Fig. 9–1) is not taking place. When organic causes of deep dyspareunia are present, these anatomically tender areas remain closer to the vaginal introitus, thus making them more vulnerable to pain stimulation during coitus. With this combination of changes, a patient and her partner get into a vicious cycle. Less arousal leads to more pain, and more pain leads to still less arousal.

Therapeutic measures useful for managing this part of the problem include supplemental vaginal lubrication with any of a growing list of commercially available lubricants (e.g., Comfort, Replens, Astroglide, and K-Y jelly). For a less expensive though possibly

Table 28–6. **MUSCLE RELAXANTS COMMONLY USED IN CHRONIC PAIN MANAGEMENT**

Drug Name	Usual Dose Range	Effects and Side Effects
Cyclobenzaprine HCl Flexeril 10 mg	10 mg qhs up to 10 mg q8h	Most common side effects are drowsiness, dry mouth, and dizziness. Drug is closely related to tricyclic antidepressants—may interact with MAO inhibitors. Likely to enhance effects of alcohol and other CNS depressants. Recommended for short-term use only (i.e., 2–3 wk). Beware of atropine-like action—potential for urinary retention, etc. Action occurs at the brainstem, not at the muscle.
Methocarbamol Robaxin 500 mg Robaxin-750, 750-mg tablets Robaxisal: 400 mg methocarbamol with 325 mg aspirin	Robaxin: initial dose, 3 tablets qid (48–72 h) maintenance, 2 tablets qid Robaxin-750: initial dose, 2 tablets qid maintenance, 1 tablet q4h or 2 tablets tid Robaxisal: 2 tablets qid	Most common side effects are lightheadedness, dizziness, drowsiness, and nausea. Enhances effect of alcohol and other CNS depressants. Not indicated for long-term use. Mechanism of action is unknown—no direct effect on the contractile mechanism of striated muscle, the motor end plate, or the nerve fiber. Usual precautions apply regarding salicylates if prescribing Robaxisal.
Chlorzoxazone Paraflex 250-mg caplet	250–750 mg tid to qid. Usual dose is 500 mg tid to qid. Parafon Forte is scored.	No direct effect on skeletal muscle. Action may be related to sedative properties. Drug is usually well tolerated. Not indicated for long-term use. Drowsiness, dizziness, etc. are less frequent than with Robaxin and Flexeril.
Baclofen Lioresal 10-mg or 20-mg scored tablets	Must be tapered up. Begin at 5 mg tid × 3 d. Then 10 mg tid × 3 d, etc, until optimal dose is achieved. Usually effective between 40 and 60 mg qd. Maximum dose is 80 mg/d. Hallucinations and seizures may occur with abrupt withdrawal. Drug must be tapered off as well.	Baclofen is a muscle relaxant and antispastic drug, useful for relief of flexor spasms and concomitant pain, clonus, and muscle rigidity. Action occurs at the spinal level. Most common side effect is transient drowsiness. Patients may also experience dizziness, weakness, fatigue, confusion, and nausea, although these are all fairly rare. Can be used safely for a long period.

CNS, central nervous system; MAO, monoamine oxidase

slightly more messy alternative, ordinary vegetable oil serves well.

In many circumstances, couples find the need to alter their usual position for sexual intercourse. The crosswise position (see Fig. 9–2) is particularly useful in a number of obstetric and gynecologic situations. Because it does not require either partner to support his or her weight for any length of time, couples can learn to take their time in their efforts to find comfortable and pleasurable ways of experiencing sexual arousal. Because this position places no pressure on a woman's abdomen, she may feel more comfortable during pregnancy, postpartum, postoperatively, or whenever she has abdominal discomforts. The direction and depth of penile insertion can be easily controlled by either partner, allowing partners to adjust to any focal discomforts due to bladder irritability, vaginal apex pain, or any other focally tender area. For couples dealing with vaginismus, gentle and gradual approximation of vaginal entry can be attempted, and these attempts can be readily coupled with vaginal relaxation exercises (see Chapter 9) to accomplish comfortable intromission.

Effective use of this information of course relies on a couple's ability to communicate comfortably about sexual matters. In the course of suggesting such things as lubrication and position changes, one must tactfully ask if this is information that can be incorporated into their sexual interactions. It often helps to set up regularly scheduled appointments at fairly close intervals with a patient for whom sexual counseling suggestions have been offered. This legitimizes the importance of the issue and circumvents the embarrassment a patient might feel when calling back for another appointment, having to explain to the administrative personnel the nature of the need.

Psychotherapeutic Approaches to Chronic Pain

To many health care providers not directly involved with mental health fields and perhaps especially to surgically oriented specialists, the recommendation of mental health assistance often comes as a last resort. One often hears the phrase, "Give the patient the benefit of the doubt," which roughly translates to the effect that all possible and even many remotely possible physiologic causes of pain should be explored before one approaches psychologic issues with any level of detail or intensity. One senses that the feelings of the health care providers behind this notion are that mental health evaluation and treatment is a murky area at best, with suspect efficacy, and that suggesting it will anger a patient.

Although there certainly is truth to all of these concerns in many clinical situations, some general guidelines may help. As implied by the discussions in Chapter 2, it makes sense to include discussion of emotional issues from the very beginning of the discussion of a pain problem. This conveys a very important message to a patient and her family: that emotional and psychologic concerns are an integral part of your evaluation and treatment. Discussing the mechanisms of pain perception as we currently understand them may facilitate this communication.

Second, if a clinician has the sense that suggesting mental health evaluation would be useful, I think it is more easily accepted if it is included as one item on a list of suggestions (see Table 28–1) rather than a suggestion left to the end of an extensive and expensive organically oriented evaluation. In this context, mental health evaluation can be described as an exploratory or diagnostic inquiry, similar to the magnetic resonance imaging or the laparoscopy that looks for organic components. You do not have the answers to the questions at the beginning but simply suggest that a mental health consultant can help better define the emotional needs of the individual and the family and help them to cope with some needs that have perhaps been left unmet during the course of the patient's pain problem.

A successful mental health consultation also depends on having a receptive mental health consultant. Some mental health professionals are reluctant to start to work with a patient until all organic components have been evaluated and treated to the maximum degree possible. Given current theories of pain perception, this approach is far less useful and in fact limits the impact of the consultant. It also requires that patients be much more ready to accept psychologic approaches than is usually possible in the real world. Beginning mental health consultation before a patient is "medically cleared" does require more frequent communication between the mental health consultant and the primary care physicians. This consultation is often logistically difficult and requires repeated telephone calls, but it can be most clinically productive.

Selection of the appropriate mental health consultant is often difficult for a primary care physician. Therapists have highly individualized styles, and many primary care physicians are not fully acquainted with the training background and experience requirements of certification for the various types of mental health professionals.

The training and licensing requirements for psychologists, counselors, and so on also vary from state to state within the United States and certainly among countries. Within the United States, some national organizations (e.g., American Psychological Association, American Psychiatric Association, American Association of Marriage and Family Therapists) may be able to help locate the sources of information within each state that can provide a listing of licensing and training requirements.

As financial pressures become ever greater in medical care, a growing tendency of managed care providers is to try to provide therapy at increasingly lower cost. This usually means lowering the fees charged by doctoral level mental health professionals and encouraging or requiring therapy to be given by personnel with less training. Although the skill and personality of the individual therapist are a substantial ingredient in the construction of the successful therapeutic alliance, thorough training is certainly paramount. Primary care physicians have a responsibility to be attentive to the outcome of treatment given by less qualified personnel.

The types of therapies available also span a broad range. Individual psychotherapy that is psychodynamically oriented was the gold standard for decades. In more recent times, both clinical practice and outcome data suggest that behavioral measures may be applicable to many situations in which a patient is not predisposed to insight-oriented therapy. Time-limited behavioral paradigms may also be more cost-effective, although direct comparisons with insight-oriented therapy are relatively limited and well beyond the scope of this discussion. As these various therapeutic schools of thought have matured, many therapists have borrowed from each of them and provided an eclectic approach. Here again, the more highly trained and skilled the therapist is, the more he or she will be comfortably able to incorporate the strong points of various styles of therapy.

Marital and family therapy may have pivotal roles in the treatment of CPP in women. As defined in Chapter 2, one of the criteria for the chronic pain syndrome is that the identified patient's pelvic pain be one of the most important problems her family faces. The impact of the patient's pain may indeed ripple throughout the family dynamic structure and significantly alter all of the interpersonal relationships with the family. Family dysfunction of various degrees may ensue and may require the assistance of a marital or family therapist. In the experience of many clinicians, restoration of the family's integrity is one of the most difficult parts of recovery from a chronic pain syndrome of any type affecting any family member (see Chapter 4). This may be especially true in the problem of pelvic pain, which so often affects the marital and sexual relationship of a couple.

One of the most difficult psychologic and emotional problems to deal with in clinical practice is the problem of sexual and physical abuse (see Chapter 3). A substantial volume of literature suggests that sexual abuse during childhood may be associated with negative sequelae in adult life. Problems positively associated with histories of childhood sexual abuse include increased prevalence of every psychiatric disorder, with the exception of schizophrenia; sexual dysfunction; irritable bowel syndrome; chronic headache; premenstrual syndrome; and the inability to maintain stable interpersonal relationships.

When a history of sexual abuse is obtained, it is often extremely difficult to decide whether or not the feelings about this abuse remain an active ingredient in the present everyday life or whether they remain an impediment to, in Freud's terms, the ability "to love and to work." For a clinician struggling to assess a CPP problem, eliciting a history of sexual abuse is certainly important, but the decision about what then to do about it is even more problematic.

The literature dealing with treatment of the sequelae of sexual abuse is not encouraging. It appears that the best outcome one can hope for is for the abuse victim to have successfully pushed the events and the feelings far enough into the background that they remain a painful memory but somewhat removed from everyday life and relationships. The intense pain of these experiences can never be totally removed, it appears. As a matter of clinical practicality, then, perhaps it is useful to recommend therapeutic intervention when the impact of the abuse is still very much felt in the present and appears to be an obstacle to functioning, regardless of the degree to which one suspects it may be involved in the development of the pain syndrome. If the memories and the feelings about the abuse are in fact more distant, then bringing them back into the foreground may cause more pain than is clinically productive and may contribute little to resolution of the pain problem. Clinical judgments of this type are always very difficult; it can only be hoped that further investigation in clinical work in the next decades will provide more reliable information to guide clinicians.

General Measures for Pain Treatment

Clinicians are confronted with a baffling array of possible pain treatments. Each of these stems from its own particular philosophy and is offered by a wide variety of practitioners. Most of these treatments are supported by very few data to back up their application, specifically in the area of CPP. Although it is beyond the scope of this discussion to provide a detailed assessment of each of these approaches, a listing and brief description might be useful.

Physical therapy is the approach that I have personally found most useful in my practice (see Chapter 24). A growing subgroup of physical therapists is becoming still more knowledgeable about pelvic floor musculoskeletal function and is skilled in evaluating and treating the problems originating from these structures. In a manner analogous to the suggestions made earlier about the interaction with mental health professionals, the most productive role for a physical therapist is in collaborating with the primary care provider to establish a communicative relationship centered on the care of individual patients. This can perhaps best begin with a primary care physician's visit to the physical therapist's office to witness the type of evaluation and treatments offered for patients with pelvic pain. One can then have a better sense of what is practical and cost-effective in terms of the type, frequency, and duration of physical therapy treatments. When a patient is being comanaged by a physician and physical therapist, communication should occur regularly (perhaps monthly) to ensure that all the components of her pain problem (see Table 28–1) are continually addressed. This is an area in which much learning is taking place, and it is hoped that better information will be available within the next decade.

Of the tools used by physical therapists and others, the transcutaneous electric nerve stimulator (TENS) unit and biofeedback are perhaps the ones most familiar to the general medical community. In general, TENS units are most useful for treating somatic (as opposed to visceral) pain and are most effective when the somatic pain is over a fairly well-defined anatomic area. Some use has been made of a transvaginal TENS unit device, which provides electric stimulation to both the pelvic floor musculature and the surrounding visceral structures. The mechanism of action in this setting is uncertain, but the initial results are sufficiently encouraging to suggest the need for more complete evaluation and continued experimentation with their use.

Biofeedback has been shown to be quite effective for treating headaches and perhaps somewhat less effective for low back pain. Its use in treating pelvic pain is relatively undocumented. The trend in the past decade has been to recognize that generalized relaxation training may be as effective as biofeedback itself. However, for a patient who is skeptical of general psychologic or behavior approaches and is more receptive to treatments that using electronic gadgetry, biofeedback can provide a useful beginning for treatment of pain problems. In this setting, the best outcome is often obtained when the biofeedback is administered by someone with clinical therapeutic training as well, as opposed to a biofeedback technician. In the course of the biofeedback sessions, a therapeutic relationship may be developed, and this may lead to greater clinical utility and clinical improvement than the biofeedback itself.

Massage therapy has many advocates. For patients with more diffuse musculoskeletal problems, massage therapy can be extremely effective. It may have less direct clinical utility for pelvic pain problems, because the levator plate can be massaged externally only in thin patients. Transvaginal massage is practiced by relatively few therapists but may be an effective avenue for those appropriately trained.

Many physical therapists and massage therapists note that the process of massage can be associated with the awakening of past memories and the emergence of intense emotions. As a patient reaches a sense of comfort and trust at a physical level with the massaging therapist, trust also develops in terms of sharing emotional concerns. This can be extremely therapeutic in itself and in the hands of an appropriately skilled therapist can lead to emotional growth and healing or to referral to other forms of therapists and mental health clinicians. Little is reported about the negative potential for such interactions, but one must suppose that this may be a concern as well, especially in more emotionally fragile individuals.

Acupuncture is an approach with thousands of years of history and a philosophy of pain perception different from much of traditional Western medicine. Its effectiveness is variable, but its therapeutic impact in many clinical situations cannot be denied. As with other forms of treatment that are nontraditional, the certification process for acupuncturists is often unknown to clinicians. In the United States, each state has its own certification process, often including a written examination. A national certifying organization publishes a yearly listing of certified practitioners (National Commission for Certification of Acupuncturists, P.O. Box 97075, Washington, DC 20090). Because not all states recognize the National Commission's certification process, clinicians should contact the appropriate agency within their own state for information pertinent to that state.

In addition to these treatment modalities, numerous other approaches are available to patients, including herbal remedies, osteopathy, chiropractic, meditation, yoga, and so on.

The ways in which all of the treatment methods described in this chapter are specifically applied to individual clinical problems are discussed throughout this book in the chapters devoted to those specific clinical entities.

Survival Skills for Health Care Providers

Most gynecologic problems have solutions; hence, their treatment is professionally rewarding and satisfying. When treating chronic pain problems, if you feel you have helped more than half of the chronic pain victims you see, you are probably doing reasonably well. These discrepant outcomes often make the treatment of chronic pain difficult for health care providers to tolerate. How can a provider tolerate the frustrations of limited success? Consider the following suggestions:

1. For very difficult patients, set up regular visits, with a time limit for each visit. Focus each visit, as much as practical, on one complaint on the list. Preventive visits defuse much anger and frustration and convey your ongoing concern.
2. As appropriate, comanage the problems with one or more consultants. Offer support to the others involved in your patient's care.

3. Change your definition of success. (This often also means helping a patient to change *her* definition of success.) Instead of defining success as complete pain relief, use the following criteria:
   a. Stable medication needs
   b. Stable or gradually improving pain reports
   c. Containment within the originally involved organ systems or reduction in the number of organ systems involved
   d. Improved mood and mental outlook despite continued pain
   e. Improved function at work and home despite continued pain
   f. Improved marital and sexual adjustment despite continued pain
   g. A continuing positive physician-patient relationship
   h. Keeping her out of the operating room
   i. Keeping her away from unnecessary medical tests

With appropriate goals set, the care of a woman with CPP can be extremely rewarding. The complete successes are just that much better.

References

1. Stovall TC, Ling FL, Crawford DA: Hysterectomy for chronic pelvic pain of presumed uterine etiology. Obstet Gynecol 1990;75:676.
2. Carlson KJ, Miller BA, Fowler FJ: The Maine Women's Health Study: II. Outcomes of nonsurgical management of leiomyomas, abnormal bleeding, and chronic pelvic pain. Obstet Gynecol 1994;83:566.
3. Kames LD, Rapkin AJ, Naliboff BD, et al: Effectiveness of an interdisciplinary pain management program for the treatment of chronic pelvic pain. Pain 1990;41:41.
4. Goodkin K, Gullion CM: Antidepressants for the relief of chronic pain: Do they work? Ann Behav Med 1989;11:83.
5. Depression Guideline Panel: Depression in Primary Care: Detection, Diagnosis, and Treatment. Rockville, MD: US Department of Health and Human Services, Agency for Health Care Policy and Research, 1993.

29

Taking Care of Patients: The Caregiver's Perspective

Barbara S. Levy, MD

The treatment of a disease may be entirely impersonal; the care of a patient must be completely personal . . . the secret of the care of the patient is in caring for the patient.

Dr. Francis Peabody

We in medicine need to restore our patients' confidence in the most powerful healer in the world: the human body.

Dr. Paul Brand

Approaching a patient with chronic pain appears overwhelming to many practitioners initially; however, with a systematic approach and specific endpoints in mind, it may prove extraordinarily rewarding despite the challenge. Many patients with chronic pain have traveled from office to office and frequently from specialist to specialist without finding relief. They view their bodies with detachment and resentment, feeling hostile, hopeless, and angry. To them pain is a signal that something is "broken," and they seek a mechanic to fix the broken part. Our first challenge is to overcome this viewpoint and create a therapeutic partnership with patients. This may seem an insurmountable task; however, with active listening, validation, and education, rapport may be established and patients may become empowered to participate with the physician in the healing process.

Establishing a Therapeutic Relationship

Set the tone for the relationship at the beginning. Questionnaires completed by a patient before the initial physician interaction send a message that the caregiver is interested in the patient's own description of her symptoms. This document may then form the outline for the first encounter. Several visits may be required to establish a trusting relationship. Early in the process, focus on a patient's physical symptoms. A thorough history includes not only a description of the pain but also a patient's interpretation of these symptoms. What does the patient think is wrong? What are her fears about these symptoms? What are her expectations of the physician? This is the time to shift the focus from curing to caring. A patient must begin to believe that (1) the physician believes her symptoms are real and (2) the physician cares enough about her to work with her to improve the quality of her life. Management of chronic pain is a long-term process. Quick fixes are ultimately doomed to failure. Only through a therapeutic partnership, with a patient's beginning to participate in her care and to become knowledgeable about the process of healing, can long-lasting relief be achieved.

It is important at this juncture to establish what both the patient and the physician will define as success in this endeavor. The primary goal of therapy for patients with chronic pain is not elimination of all pain. That would render a person vulnerable to injury, as in those who lack sensation secondary to diabetic neuropathy or Hansen's disease. The primary therapeutic endpoint is the elimination of suffering—the adverse emotional response to pain experienced by a patient. Maximization of the quality of life is what we are striving for. A patient must understand that removal of the pain generators, the source of pain, does not necessarily cure the condition. The response, both physical and emotional, of the body to that long-standing pain requires modification and conditioning as well.

Educating a patient about the consequences of chronic pain is essential to establishing the appropriate therapeutic relationship. For a patient to become a partner in healing, she should be introduced to the physiology of pain—the neurologic pathways involved in the perception of pain and the physical and chemical mechanisms that interact to cause chronic pain and the chronic pain syndromes. We, on the other hand, must learn about the patient as a person. It is critical for us to understand her roles as daughter, mother, wife, worker, and friend. *Harrison's Principles of Internal Medicine* tells us that a "physician needs to consider the terrain in which an illness occurs—in terms not only of the patients themselves but also of their families and social backgrounds. . . . Without this knowledge it is difficult to develop insight into the patient's illness. Such a relationship must be based on thorough knowledge of the patient and on mutual trust and the ability to communicate with one another."[1]

The key to working with patients with chronic pain is to approach them as unique individuals whose problems reach far beyond their presenting complaints. Their anxiety and fear about their physical symptoms must be transcended for true healing to occur. Such a patient frequently sees herself as a victim and as an experimental subject for the experts to work on, not as a partner in her own recovery and health. Altering this outlook is the goal in establishing the therapeutic relationship. If this does not occur, long-term success in managing chronic pain is unlikely. This may be quite difficult, because these patients are understandably frustrated with and distrustful of medical providers. Their long-standing efforts to achieve a cure have often been met with a multitude of interventions, surgery, and expensive drugs and little if any success.

It is useful to share some insights with a patient at the first visit:

1. There are *no* magic bullets, pills, or operations.
2. Healing is a process, not a single event in time.
3. The patient herself is in control of that process, not the provider.

It is also critical to ask a patient what her goals are in seeking treatment at this time. A patient's purpose may sometimes surprise us. Despite her complaint of chronic pain, she may simply seek reassurance that she has no serious illness rather than treatment or cure of the pain. If we are unaware of her issues, we are unlikely to be successful in ultimately satisfying her needs.

Practical Guidelines for Care—Back to Basics

Treatment of chronic pain cannot begin until a therapeutic relationship is established (Table 29–1). The first visit with a patient must validate her symptoms and create an atmosphere in which she feels comfortable, safe, and accepted. Obtain as much clinical information as possible. Have your office request previous medical records in advance from these patients so that the interview time may be spent learning about patients' perceptions of their diagnoses and treatments rather than establishing a time line of events. Review the data objectively. Videotapes of prior laparoscopic procedures are especially helpful. These should be viewed with the patient and your comments shared with her as you look at the tapes together.

Form your own conclusions. In an effort to explain the extent of prior surgery, physicians may have created a mental picture for a patient of extensive and damaging disease. Showing her the anatomy and discussing the extent of disease with her may be beneficial in shifting a patient's mindset from

Table 29–1. **GOALS OF THE PHYSICIAN-PATIENT ENCOUNTER**

Validation	Empowerment
Education	Maximize the quality of life
Reassurance	

illness and disability to wellness. Objective evaluation of the extent of underlying disease is critical; however, the approach to a patient varies little despite the severity of underlying pathology.

Focus initially on a patient's physical symptoms and her emotional responses to those symptoms. Find out what is currently making her daily life miserable and choose to address one specific problem that will make a significant impact on her quality of life. Success in this first endeavor will make further intervention and interruption of the cycle of chronic pain easier. Remind yourself and the patient that the goal of treatment is improvement in the quality of life and not necessarily cure of the underlying condition.

Educate a patient about the physiology of pain. When she begins to understand the biologic purpose of pain and how this system has gone awry in her condition, she will become less fearful. The perception of pain consists of three phases: a noxious stimulus—the signal; transmission of the message; and a physical and emotional response to the message. When a pain pathway becomes chronic, any physical sensation in the region of pain—even nonnoxious stimulation—will likely be transmitted along the same neural pathways and be interpreted by the brain as painful. For patients who have difficulty understanding this concept, I frequently use the example of phantom pain to help illustrate the function of the central nervous system in this process. Phantom pain is excruciating pain that is interpreted by the brain as coming from a limb that has been removed. Disease in that limb clearly is not responsible for this sensation. Understanding this concept frequently permits a patient to accept treatment for the aberrant signal processing without feeling that her pain is being interpreted as in her mind. Tricyclic antidepressants in low doses work well in blocking the pathways responsible for these hard-wired pain messages. A patient must be informed about the nature of these drugs and their purpose in this particular clinical situation. Otherwise, when she discovers the nature of the drug prescribed, she may feel betrayed and deceived that a psychotropic medication was recommended.

Narcotics are generally not appropriate drugs for management of chronic pain syndromes. Most patients who resort to narcotic medication for relief are delighted when you recommend alternate methods for management of their pain. Drug seekers reveal themselves quickly when the integrated approach to chronic pain is outlined at the initial visit.

Recommend regular physical exercise to stimulate endorphin release and improve stress management. The regimen varies depending on the physical capabilities of the patient, but this is as important as any medication we may prescribe. Therefore, write out your recommendations for the type, duration, and frequency of exercise on a prescription blank. This reminds a patient that this is a serious suggestion and one that is as likely to benefit her as any medication. Similarly, discuss diet and lifestyle habits that may influence her general physical health. Busy people in our culture frequently ignore the needs of their bodies in their hectic daily schedules. Beginning to love and care for oneself is an essential step in the process of recovery from chronic pain. This may begin with attention to proper nutrition, exercise, and rest.

Learn about a patient's fears, concerns, and expectations. I like to end the first visit with a patient by asking her what she had hoped to gain from her appointment and whether her goals have been achieved. This serves to focus her attention on her expectations and allows her to communicate with me if they have not been adequately addressed. Patients are often unsure about the purpose of their consultation. Their real concerns sometimes are not obvious to them any more than they are to us. A careful social, family, and medical history may elucidate an area of concern that can be easily addressed. If a patient leaves without a satisfactory explanation of her concerns, however, she will be unhappy with the encounter and is less likely to have a favorable response to your treatment regimen whatever it may be.

Reassurance is key in managing these patients. They need constant reassurance that their pain does not represent a life-threatening condition and that their pain can be managed successfully whether or not the underlying factors that may have initiated the chronic pain syndrome are cured. This concept is foreign to many who approach medicine as a hard science with a classic Cartesian split between mind and body, but acceptance of the holistic approach is crucial to success in management of chronic pain. We must constantly remind ourselves and our patients, as well as referring physicians, that our goal is to maximize the quality of life and eliminate suffering, not necessarily to cure disease. We may be objectively successful in treating endometriosis or pelvic adhesions only to discover that our patients continue to suffer from the consequences of long-term pain—a chronic pain syndrome.

Pain Intensifiers

In approaching patients with pain, a clinician must be alert for those elements in a patient's environment that serve to intensify her pain (Table 29–2). Fear and helplessness are commonly identified in careful interviews of pain sufferers. Fear may be related to concern about the underlying cause of the pain or fear that the pain will never be adequately controlled. Helplessness occurs when patients perceive themselves as victims unable to control their own bodies. Loneliness and isolation also serve to intensify the perception of pain. When a patient has nothing to distract her from her discomfort, she tends to focus on it. Clearly a rich and full life helps to ameliorate the emotional overlay attendant with chronic pain. Excess stress, on the other hand, serves to increase muscle tension and the body's physical reaction to pain. Attention to stress management skills and stress reduction is important in the overall approach to patients with chronic pain.

Table 29–2. **PAIN INTENSIFIERS**

Fear	Loneliness/isolation
Anger/dismissal	Helplessness
Guilt	Stress

Guilt and anger also serve to intensify the perception and interpretation of pain. These emotions may be well hidden by a patient both from herself and from the care provider. They must be uncovered and appropriately addressed before long-term management of the pain can be successful.

The Integrated Approach

Once a therapeutic relationship has been established with a patient, in which both her needs and expectations and the clinician's outlook and approach have been accepted, the care of a chronic pain sufferer becomes an easy partnership. When a patient has been validated and believes that her physician truly cares for her welfare, it is not difficult to work with her to accomplish your mutual goals. It is important for us as care providers to assemble a team of like-minded practitioners to provide coordinated care for a patient. This team is likely to include a physical therapist and psychologist in addition to medical specialists with an interest in chronic pain. Pain clinics have been established specifically to address the needs of chronic pain victims and are excellent resources for the communities they serve. Unfortunately, not all pain services are geared to provide coordinated care. At my hospital, the pain service is administrated by our anesthesiologists and is noticeably unidimensional in its approach to chronic pain. Basically, if it cannot be blocked with local anesthetic agents, they cannot address it. Referral to a service such as this does not substitute for the integrated approach necessary to manage chronic pelvic pain fully. It is important that the team you assemble to care for your patient be coordinated in its approach. A patient cannot receive different messages from each care provider and remain confident about her treatment. One person must accept primary responsibility for coordinating a patient's care and modifying the regimen on the basis of the results of the care program.

Conclusion

With this basic approach to patients presenting with chronic pain complaints, a clinician can treat these patients with confidence and success. Addicts seeking only prescription refills and patients who are not motivated to get well will drop out and do not return. These are individuals who are not truly interested in care, and continued efforts to treat them serve as only a source of frustration both for them and for us. In order for us to feel successful, we must learn to allow these patients to seek care elsewhere. Ultimately, nothing we do can improve their quality of life until they are prepared to accept responsibility for themselves and their care. We cannot force that change, but we can facilitate it if a patient is open to the shift from curing to caring. Treatment of a patient requires dispassionate application of the science of medicine while exercising compassion, warmth, and understanding. We must not become so absorbed in the disease that we forget the victim. It is not only the treatment itself but the physician's words and behavior that are capable of healing or causing harm. Our goal is treatment of the patient and improvement in the quality of her life; this does not always mean cure of disease.

Reference

1. Braunwald E, Isselbacher KJ, Martin JB, et al: Harrison's Principles of Internal Medicine, 11th ed. New York, McGraw-Hill, 1987, p 1.

Selected Readings

Brand P, Yancey P: The Gift Nobody Wants. New York, HarperCollins, 1993.

Siegel BS: Love, Medicine, and Miracles. New York, Harper & Row, 1986.

30

Pain Medicine and the Role of Neurologic Blockade in Evaluation

William S. Blau, MD, PhD, and William E. von Kaenel, MD

Pain Medicine Approach to Chronic Pelvic Pain

Characteristics of Chronic Pelvic Pain

For many physicians, chronic pelvic pain (CPP) is "one of the most frustrating and controversial areas of [clinical] practice."[1] As detailed in other chapters of this book, the potential organic causes of CPP are numerous and include many organ systems. In some cases, diagnosis by standard techniques is difficult. To many practitioners, the term implies a syndrome in which the organic source of pain is obscure and psychologic/behavioral features predominate. Patients are often somatically focused and may have other unexplained physical complaints, such as digestive symptoms, headache, or back pain. These complaints may be intermixed with objective pathology, but often, no definitive physical, radiologic, laboratory, or pathological abnormalities can be found to explain the complaints fully. If no specific source of pain is identified or specific treatment offered after conventional diagnostic evaluation, referral to a specialist in pelvic pain or an interdisciplinary pain management center may be indicated.

Pain Medicine and the Interdisciplinary Approach

In the past 20 years, pain medicine has emerged as a relatively distinct medical specialty, although the background and therapeutic approach of specialists can vary considerably. The specialty continues to define itself, with ongoing development of processes for credentialing, accreditation, and standards of practice.[2–5] The need for a separate specialty is driven by the complexity of chronic pain disorders and the need for interdisciplinary therapeutic approaches that include attention to organic pathology, psychologic dysfunction, and rehabilitation needs. An interdisciplinary approach has been shown to be superior to a single specialty approach in chronic pain in general[6] and in CPP in particular.[7–10]

Various chronic pain practice models currently exist, with variable emphasis on patient screening, comprehensive versus modality-oriented care, and inpatient versus outpatient management (Table 30–1).[11] Primary therapy may be directed toward the underlying organic disorder, behavior modification/psychologic management, or rehabilitation. An existing accreditation process emphasizes comprehensive outcome-oriented approaches with inpatient capability.[12] Pain medicine facilities may provide a variable level of expertise and interest in CPP, and the resources of any local facility for managing CPP should be explored before a referral is made.

Role of the Anesthesiologist in Pain Medicine

Surveys reveal that the majority of pain management practices in the United States

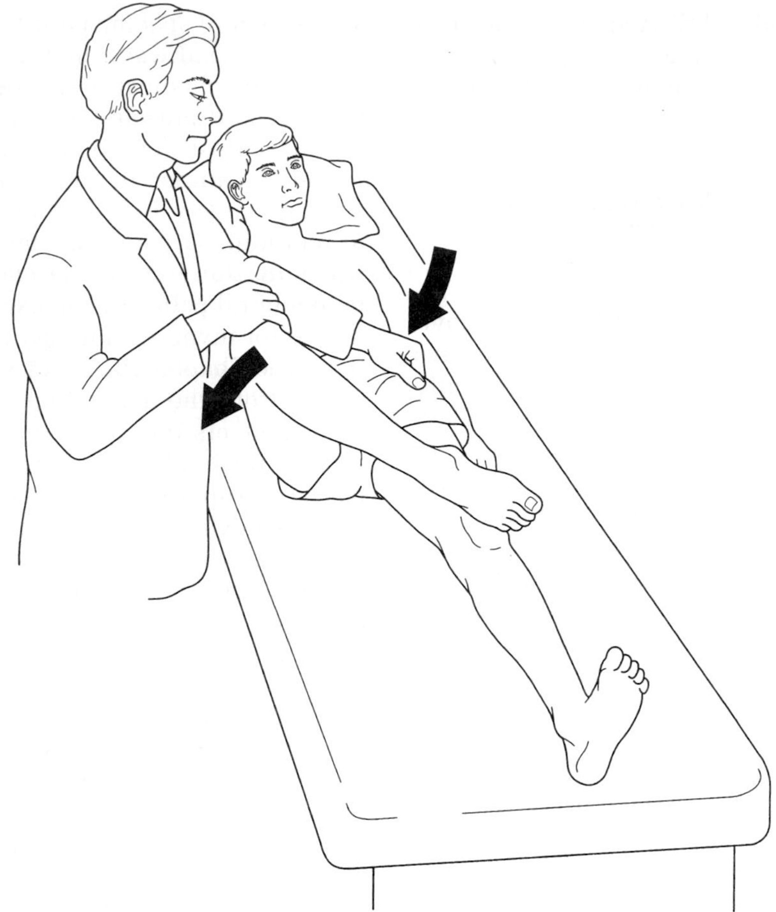

Figure 30–1. Patrick's maneuver. The leg is externally rotated and abducted, with the knee flexed and the heel on the contralateral knee. Referral of pain anteriorly to the groin in the absence of back pain may reflect pathology of the hip joint; primary referral posteriorly to the low back or buttock is more consistent with a sacroiliac source of pain. (In Magee DJ: Orthopedic Physical Assessment, 3rd ed. Philadelphia, WB Saunders, 1992, Figure 11–8. Redrawn from Beetham WP, et al: Physical Examination of the Joints. Philadelphia, WB Saunders, 1965.)

to identify patients with primary or contributing anxiety, depression, or somatization; maladaptive coping styles; or a history of physical or sexual abuse that would predispose to the development of CPP (see Chapters 3 and 8). A pain diary is often helpful for identifying temporal trends, correlates, and behavioral responses to severe pain. Selected patients may undergo further evaluation during a personal interview with a psychiatrist or clinical psychologist to determine whether they might benefit from relaxation training, biofeedback, cognitive-behavioral therapy, pharmacologic therapy, or psychotherapy.

Diagnostic Studies

Various diagnostic studies and procedures are obtained during the primary evaluation of CPP to rule out urologic, gynecologic, and gastrointestinal disorders (see Chapter 11). On referral to a pain management center, all prior films and reports are obtained and reviewed. Other studies may be obtained to rule out less common sources of pelvic pain, as indicated by the clinical assessment. Various radiologic studies are available for evaluation of mechanical causes of low back or pelvic pain. These include plain radiographs (flexion and extension), bone scans,

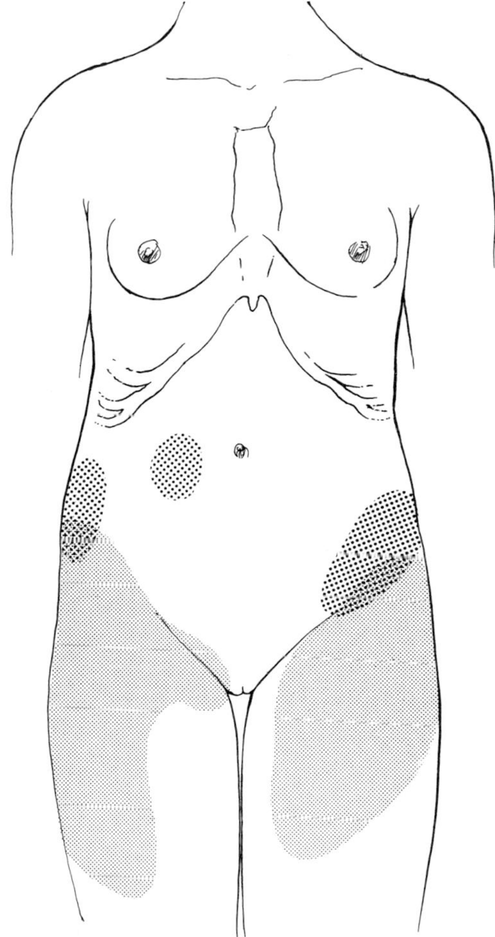

Figure 30–2. Anterior referral of pain from the zygapophyseal joints at L1–L2 (diagonal lines) and L4–L5 (cross-hatching). (From McCall IW, Park WM, O'Brien JP: Induced pain referral from posterior lumbar elements in normal subjects. Spine 1979;4:441.)

computed tomography (CT), magnetic resonance imaging (MRI), and myelography. Suspected neurologic dysfunction at the spinal or peripheral level may be evaluated by electromyography/peripheral nerve conduction velocities.

Differential Diagnosis

The diagnosis of CPP can be approached in various ways. Medical and surgical specialists such as gynecologists often seek a diagnosis based on tissue pathology. Diagnostic tests are used to discover visible anatomic pathology to which the pain condition can be ascribed. This approach is effective if explanatory pathology exists and is causative of the pain state. However, for many of the causes of CPP (e.g., myofascial pain, neuralgias), the pain generator can be neither visualized nor identified on biopsy. Persistent diagnostic evaluation in a search for tissue pathology can be futile, as well as costly and potentially hazardous.

The pain medicine approach centers around the pain state and is often used after an exhaustive medical and gynecologic evaluation has failed to demonstrate tissue pathology. The clinical characteristics of the pain are elucidated, and diagnosis is based on these. Pain states or conditions are classified in many different ways—for example, acute versus chronic, nociceptive versus neuropathic, malignant versus nonmalignant, and so on. The outline shown in Table 30–2 describes a useful classification scheme for CPP.

The first distinction must be made between central and peripheral pain sources. Central refers to the neuraxis (the brain and spinal cord) and includes psychologic diagnoses as well as neural pathology. Peripheral pain refers to nociception in the tissues or neuropathic pain in peripheral nerves. Peripheral pain sources may be somatic (pain in the tissues supplied by the spinal nerves, such as the abdominal wall) or visceral (tissues supplied by visceral afferent fibers, such as the uterus or ovaries). Somatic and visceral pain can be either nociceptive or neuropathic. Neuropathic pain is pain that arises from damaged or dysfunctional nerves (e.g., pudendal neuralgia). Visceral neuropathic pain is less well characterized but certainly exists,[21] one possible example being endometrial implants that invade visceral neural tissue.

Table 30–2. **CLASSIFICATION OF CHRONIC PELVIC PAIN**

I. Central
    1. Neurogenic
    2. Psychogenic
II. Peripheral
    A. Somatic
        1. Neuropathic
        2. Nociceptive
            a. Myofascial
            b. Skeletal
            c. Cutaneous
    B. Visceral
        1. Neuropathic
        2. Nociceptive
            a. Gynecologic
            b. Urologic
            c. Gastrointestinal

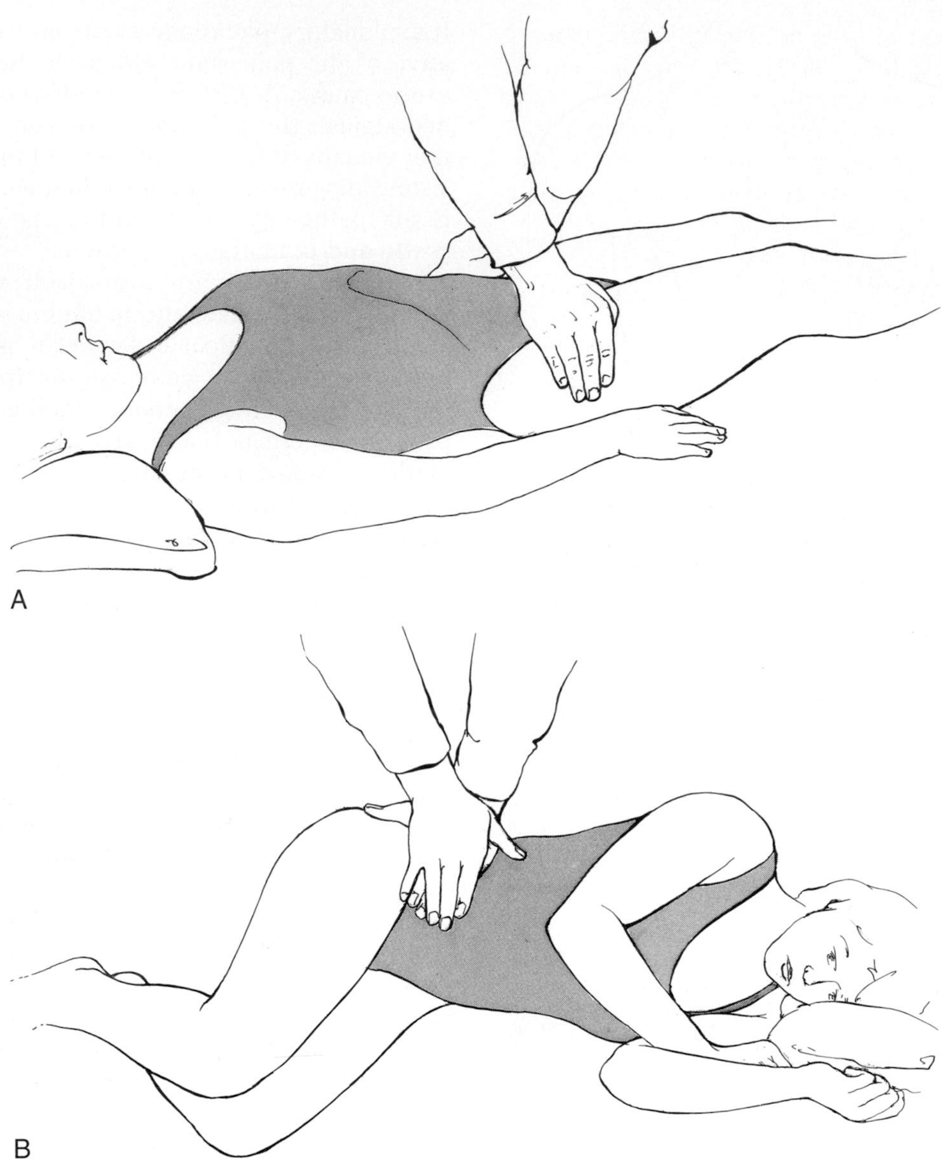

Figure 30–3. Maneuvers to elicit sacroiliac joint pain. *A*: The distraction or gapping test: Bilateral pressure is applied posterolaterally over the anterior superior iliac spines ("prying") with the patient in a supine position. *B*: The compression test: Downward pressure is applied over the lateral iliac crest with the patient in a lateral position. Unilateral pain in the low back or buttock is suggestive of sacroiliac joint origin.

It is often not possible to arrive at a specific diagnosis on the basis of an initial evaluation. It may be possible, however, to determine if the primary pain problem is likely to be somatic, visceral, or central. More specific diagnoses can be then entertained. A somatic pain source is suspected when the pain is localized, sharp, or near a surgical scar. The pain is more or less constant but may be increased with activity. Painful trigger points or structures of the lumbosacral spine can refer pain to the pelvis when stimulated. Visceral pain is characteristically vague, poorly localized, diffuse, dull, and aching. Pain can be referred to a distant site and may be associated with autonomic symptoms such as nausea, vomiting, sweating, and bradycardia. Visceral pain tends to be episodic and related to internal bodily processes rather than activity or position. Reflex muscle spasm in the spinal cord segments affected by the visceral pain can produce a somatic pain source that complicates pain symptoms.[22] A peripheral pain source can almost always be identified in patients with CPP; thus, purely psychogenic pain is an uncommon occurrence. However, it is not at all uncommon for a patient's psychologic makeup to be a major or even dominant factor in the clinical picture. In some patients, the ratio of positive psychologic findings to negative physical findings suggests a primarily central explanation for a patient's pain state.

Based on a thorough review of results of a patient's history, physical examination, psychologic screens, and studies, a diagnostician is often able to make a preliminary judgment about the relative importance of visceral, somatic, or central sources of pain. However, many of the anatomic and neurologic causes of chronic pain have no diagnostic gold standards. Conventional diagnostic maneuvers vary widely in their sensitivity and specificity.[23] Pain arising from muscles, joints, intervertebral disks, or peripheral nerves cannot be visualized on radiographs or scans and may not be detected with electromyography or peripheral nerve conduction velocity tests. Conversely, radiographic abnormalities or alterations in nerve function do not reliably identify sources of pain.[24]

In this setting, anesthetic blockade of suspected pain-generating nerve pathways or structures can provide specific diagnostic information that can lead to more focused or appropriate therapy. In the simplest sense, a structure may be considered to be a pain generator if interruption of afferent nociceptive pathways from that structure, by the injection of local anesthetic, produces pain relief.

Neurologic Blockade

Basic Considerations

Definitions

Physicians are sometimes unclear about what blocks achieve. An important distinction is between local anesthetic blocks and neurolytic blocks. A local anesthetic block is temporary, with direct effects lasting only as long as the duration of the local anesthetic (e.g., lidocaine). Such a block can have a therapeutic effect, with pain relief outlasting the local anesthetic pharmacologic effect. Other therapeutic agents are sometimes added to the local anesthetic for additional effect, such as steroids in lumbar epidural injections for low back pain. Neurolytic (or neuroablative) blocks involve the destruction of nerve tissue using phenol, alcohol, electrothermy, or cryoablation. These are less commonly performed, more often in malignant pain when life expectancy is limited. Neurolytic blocks have been advocated for many different nonmalignant pain conditions but are controversial owing to the risk of permanent complications such as motor block and neuropathic pain. For the purposes of this chapter, *block* refers to the use of regional anesthesia with local anesthetics.

Uses of Neurologic Blockade

Conduction blockade has a long history in the diagnosis and management of chronic pain.[25] As a diagnostic aid, it has been used for identifying anatomic sources of nociception or nociceptive pathways; to differentiate pains of visceral, somatic, central, and peripheral origins; and to determine the relative role of nociception in patients who have complex chronic pain syndromes. It can also provide a prognostic value in allowing patients to experience sensory changes and other possible effects of neuroablative procedures, as well as to predict the outcome that procedures such as presacral neurectomy may have on pain. Finally, blockade can have a number of potential therapeutic benefits by providing for more effective application of physical therapy and functional restoration, through a direct therapeutic effect for certain types of neurogenic disorders, and by improvement in blood flow by sympathetic blockade. It cannot be overemphasized that anesthetic approaches to pain diagnosis and management must be effectively incorporated into a comprehensive interdisciplinary approach that is tailored to the needs of an individual patient.

Interpretation of Diagnostic Blocks: Pitfalls

Although the concept of using neurologic blockade to clarify a diagnosis is appealing, the conduct of diagnostic anesthetic blocks is fraught with potential for errors in interpretation, and very few of these procedures have been validated by studies of sensitivity and specificity.[26, 27] Placebo effects or the failure of specificity of the block may lead to false-positive results. Technical failure of the block or failure of the patient to reliably report changes in their pain intensity can lead to false-negative interpretations. It is essential that those performing and interpreting such procedures be technically proficient and aware of the possibilities for misinterpretation, in order to avoid drawing inappropriate and possibly harmful conclusions.

Placebo Effect

Thirty percent or more of normal subjects can be expected to manifest a placebo effect in response to sham pain therapy.[28] The effect most likely represents a complex and involuntary alteration in central processing of nociceptive afferent signals in response to the expectation of pain relief. It cannot be overemphasized that such a response does not necessarily imply malingering, somatization, or any other aberrant psychologic state. The relevance of the placebo effect to this discussion is that it can provide one mechanism by which one may arrive at a false-positive conclusion—that is, that a structure is a pain generator when, in fact, it is not.

Failure of Specificity

One way to compensate for the possibility of inaccurate needle placement during a block is to use larger volumes of local anesthetic to facilitate spread of anesthetic throughout tissue planes or anatomic spaces and increase the likelihood of reaching the target nerve or structure. Increased spread may compromise specificity of the block, however. For example, evidence shows that local anesthetic injected during standard techniques of stellate ganglion block fails to reach the stellate ganglion and is likely to block other neural structures.[29] Similarly, use of more than 2 to 3 ml of anesthetic in the blockade of a lumbar nerve root may result in spread of anesthetic solution into the epidural space or to adjacent nerve roots.[30] Larger volumes or doses of local anesthetic may also raise the potential for significant symptomatic relief of certain types of neurogenic pains by systemic absorption. Significant systemic levels of lidocaine may occur after stellate ganglion block, for example.[31] Finally, poorly understood characteristics of central nervous system processing of nociceptive afferent impulses may lead to reduction in pain report even if a block is performed distal to a known site of pathology.[32]

Technical Failure

Proper interpretation of a diagnostic block presumes technical success—that is, that the targeted neural pathways were in fact subjected to an anesthetic conduction block. Technical failure of a block occurs most commonly because of failure to place the needle in close enough proximity to the target neural structure or to insert the needle tip in the wrong anatomical space (e.g., intravascular). Many blocks are performed on the basis of knowledge of surface anatomy and its relationship to neural structures. However, there is ample opportunity for inaccurate needle placement[30] or interindividual variability in the relationships between neural and other anatomic structures. For blocks of most somatic nerves, failure can be readily detected by the lack of onset of cutaneous anesthesia, but for some autonomic blocks, failure may go undetected unless special attention is paid to measurement of temperature, skin resistance, or capillary blood flow.[33] For some autonomic blocks, there may be no readily measurable index of success (e.g., superior hypogastric plexus). Failure rates of commonly used blocks may vary from nearly 0% (e.g., saphenous nerve at the ankle) to 40% or more.[30, 33]

Failure of the Patient to Reliably Report Alterations in Pain

Some patients may be unwilling to admit to pain relief from a successful neural blockade for psychologic reasons or secondary gain. Others may have such a high level of anxiety or may be so distracted by the pain of the procedure that they are unable to assess the result of the block accurately; in these cases, the true severity of the underlying pain may be subject to question.

Techniques to Enhance the Reliability of Diagnostic Blocks

Maximize Accuracy

Despite the limitations described earlier, diagnostic blocks remain useful for guiding therapy, provided techniques are used by an experienced diagnostician to minimize errors in interpretation. Physicians who perform diagnostic blockades must undergo specialized training to ensure the most accurate and safest needle placement, so that only small amounts of local anesthetic are required. For blockade of nerves that contain efferent motor fibers, the proper use of a nerve stimulator to produce muscle contraction in the distribution of the target nerve can help to confirm accurate needle positioning. Inadvertent intravascular injection is detected by including epinephrine 1:200,000 with the anesthetic and monitoring for an abrupt increase in heart rate. Accuracy can be enhanced further by the use of ultrasonography, image-intensified fluoroscopy, or CT scan to guide and confirm needle placement. Injection of radiopaque contrast after needle placement can confirm both proper location (e.g., radiculogram or arthrogram) and spread of the anesthetic. Whenever possible, the success of the block must be confirmed by objective testing of sensory or autonomic function (e.g., loss of pinprick sensation or increase in temperature, respectively). More sophisticated methods are also available.[34]

Rule Out Placebo Effect

Ruling out the possibility of a placebo effect can be technically and ethically problematic. The most conventional test would require performance of a sham procedure, in which a needle would be placed under circumstances identical to those of an active injection, up to and including the use of radiologic guidance, if indicated. The time, effort, cost, and discomfort involved in order to conduct a rigorous test for placebo response makes this an unattractive option. For procedures that present the opportunity for placement of indwelling catheters (e.g., epidural or plexus blocks) sequential injections with crossover between active and inactive agents may be an acceptable means of ruling out placebo effect. A technique we have used for more minor procedures is simply to raise a skin wheal with a 25-gauge needle using about 0.25 ml of 0.5% lidocaine, after setting the patient's expectation for the active block. Once a placebo response is ruled out, after several minutes, we proceed to place the larger block needle through the skin wheal for the active procedure. Alternatively, a saline injection may be used.

An additional approach has been suggested to preclude placebo response and enhance specificity during performance of medial branch nerve blocks for the diagnosis of zygapophyseal joint pain.[27] The test is performed in two stages. During one stage, an injection is performed with an anesthetic of either short or long duration (e.g., lidocaine or bupivacaine, respectively), and if pain relief is obtained, the patient is instructed to make careful note of the quality and duration of relief. On a different day, the procedure is repeated with an anesthetic of different duration. A positive diagnosis of zygapophyseal pain is made if the patient again obtains relief and is able to distinguish the difference in duration of relief without knowing that a different anesthetic was used. Positive predictive values greater than 95% were obtained using this technique. In general, return of pain after only a brief period of relief relative to the duration of the local anesthetic used (e.g., after 1 hour with bupivacaine) is suggestive of a placebo response.

Meticulous Evaluation of Patient Response

For diagnostic procedures, it is important to avoid or minimize systemic administration of anxiolytics or analgesics to avoid confounding the interpretation of the results (e.g., patients with primary myofascial pain associated with muscle spasm could obtain relief from the muscle-relaxing effects of a benzodiazepine). With a minimally sedated subject, the entire process of neural blockade can be diagnostic. One frequently derives a sense of a patient's pain tolerance, level of anxiety, and pain behaviors. Valuable information is also gained in some cases from reproduction of a patient's pain during needle placement or injection. This is especially true of diagnostic injections of myofascial trigger points, intervertebral disks, or zygapophyseal joints. Reproduction of a typical pattern of referred pain that correlates with a patient's symptoms by stimulation of a structure is highly suggestive of that structure's being the source of pain.

Obviously, relief of pain after a diagnostic block is essential for confirming a diagnosis. Diagnostic blocks can be performed only if a patient has pain. The often episodic nature of some pain (e.g., visceral) mandates that scheduling of such blocks be flexible. One may question the severity of pain in a patient who focuses more on the residual soreness from a diagnostic injection than on the relief obtained. The specificity of a block is enhanced if complete pain relief is obtained. Partial pain relief after a block is more problematic and is suggestive that more than one structure or pathway may be contributing to the symptoms. A 50% reduction in pain may be required as a minimum for making therapeutic decisions that rely on a positive block outcome. Even more significant than the reported pain relief may be an objectively documented increase in functional ability after a diagnostic block. It is essential to document changes in both spontaneous and elicited pain, when the patient is brought through full range of motion or asked to assume positions that were previously intolerable because of pain.[26]

Ultimately, we await more rigorously conducted investigations in order to better understand the true predictive value of nerve blocks as diagnostic tools in various situations. Pending such studies, carefully conducted and interpreted blocks may provide useful diagnostic information when used judiciously as part of a comprehensive interdisciplinary program.

Types of Diagnostic Procedures

Trigger Point Injection

A trigger point may be defined as a hyperirritable spot, usually within a taut band of skeletal muscle or in the muscle's fascia, that is painful on compression and that can give rise to characteristic referred pain, tenderness, and autonomic phenomena.[16] Trigger points in the muscles of the low back, abdominal wall, and pelvis can be a significant and often overlooked source of pain in the pelvic region (see Chapter 26). Injection of anesthetic into a trigger point is generally considered to be a therapeutic rather than a diagnostic procedure, but if the source of pelvic pain is uncertain and a trigger point is considered as one possibility, relief of pain after a trigger point injection can provide confirming evidence.[10, 35]

Peripheral Nerve Block

Some types of diagnostic blocks may serve to identify the anatomic region of a source of pain, even if a specific diagnosis is not obtained. For example, relief of pain after diagnostic blockade of peripheral nerves such as the intercostals or ilioinguinal may help to preclude a visceral source of pelvic pain. In the case of a peripheral neuralgia, appropriate neural blockade may be truly diagnostic, as well as therapeutic.

Segmental Nerve Block

Some pains may derive from nerve pathology at the level of the spine, with pain referral to the pelvic region. Any inflammatory or neuropathic process affecting the T11–L1 nerve roots, as may occur in herpetic neuralgia or diabetic radiculopathy, can refer pain in a dermatomal pattern to overlie the pelvic region. In such cases, the involved spinal level may be identified by selectively blocking individual nerve roots and observing the effect on pain report. Far lateral nerve root compression at L5–S1 has been linked to the signs and symptoms of interstitial cystitis,[36] and pain relief after prognostic anesthetic block at this level may lend support for surgical decompression of the L5 nerve root. T10 nerve root block may have utility for identifying ovarian pain when a visceral source of pain is suspected and only minimal or partial pain relief is obtained from blockade of the superior hypogastric plexus.[37]

Superior Hypogastric Plexus Block

The superior hypogastric plexus block was originally described as a neurolytic treatment for malignant pelvic pain.[38] The technique has been refined subsequently, and its efficacy for cancer related pain documented.[39–41] The superior hypogastric plexus is located anterior to the sacral promontory and provides visceral innervation to the uterine fundus; the medial third of the fallopian tubes, the connective tissue of the mesosalpinx, and the broad ligaments; the bladder fundus; and the distal colon[37] (see Chapters 5 and 18). Needles are directed bilaterally from near the iliac crest under fluoroscopic guidance to the area of the sacral promontory. Radiocontrast is injected to confirm placement in the appropriate tissue plane. For diagnostic blocks, 8 to 10 ml of 0.25% to 0.5% bupivacaine is injected bilaterally to provide coverage of the entire superior hypogastric plexus.

Differential Subarachnoid/Epidural Block

The primary value of differential subarachnoid or epidural blocks is for distinguishing peripheral versus central nervous system origins of CPP, especially for patients in whom the central cause is suspected on the basis of psychologic assessment[7] or in whom peripheral findings are lacking. The technique is presented to a patient as a trial of therapy that will lead to a better understanding of the origins of the pain, without raising any specific expectations about when or how much pain relief should be obtained. For the spinal (subarachnoid) approach, a needle is placed in the subarachnoid space via a lumbar approach, followed by injection of saline or aspirated cerebrospinal fluid as a placebo. After a placebo response is ruled out (lack of pain relief), a dose of local anesthetic adequate to create a total sensorimotor blockade of the pelvic region is given. Cutaneous sensation and temperature, as well as spontaneous and elicited pain on a visual analogue scale, are assessed before and 5 minutes after each injection. If the patient fails to report relief of pain during complete sensorimotor blockade of the affected body region, the cause of the pain may be concluded to be proximal to the block (i.e., of central origin). In the broadest sense, this could include patients with pathology of the central nervous system above the level of the blockade (e.g., postthalamic stroke syndrome) or with altered central processing of nocicoptive information (e.g., activation of phantom limb pain under subarachnoid block).[42] It is more often associated with malingering or psychosomatic disorders. In any case, continuing to attempt to diagnose or treat the syndrome at the peripheral level is fruitless, and further invasive treatments such as nerve blocks or surgery are contraindicated. Subarachnoid blocks can be incomplete (e.g., unilateral or patchy), and objective means must be used to demonstrate that sensation in the area of interest is completely absent in order to avoid drawing false conclusions.

Epidural blockade can be used in a manner similar to differential spinal blockade. Advantages include avoidance of dural puncture and the ability to thread a catheter for subsequent injections. However, the slower onset of the block leads to a more prolonged procedure and a greater possibility of errors in interpretation due to unilateral blockade or hot spots. Adequate blockade of all pelvic spinal levels may require large volumes of anesthetic. Assessments may occur at 15-minute intervals owing to the slower onset of blockade. Differential epidural block may also be used to aid in clarifying the segmental level of origin of a pain, when sequential doses are administered through an indwelling catheter to produce blockade at sequentially higher segmental levels.

An alternative approach to ruling out a

central cause of pain uses the intravenous pentothal test (discussed later).

Skeletal Structures

Skeletal structures of the spine and pelvis—zygapophyseal joints, intervertebral disks, sacroiliac joint—can produce patterns of referred pain that may mimic visceral pelvic pain. A carefully taken history and thorough physical examination can usually distinguish these sources of pain, but definitive diagnosis can be made only after diagnostic blockade of these structures.[43, 44]

Intravenous Injection/Infusion

Intravenous injection of general anesthetics such as sodium thiopental can be used to help identify malingering or other central types of pain.[45] In the so-called pentothal test, enough drug is administered to create a transient depth of anesthesia adequate to inhibit conscious manifestations of pain behavior (unresponsive to verbal command) but allow the patient to remain responsive to truly painful stimuli. Under these circumstances, a patient's response to nonpainful stimulus, painful stimulus unrelated to the patient's chronic pain, and maneuvers that elicit the patient's usual pain under normal conditions are compared. Absence of response during attempts to elicit the usual pain are suggestive of malingering or psychogenic pain. This test depends on a means of eliciting the usual pain (e.g., by palpation) and can be safely conducted only with cardiorespiratory monitoring by a practitioner proficient in airway management and resuscitation.

Chronic neuropathic pains may be sympathetically maintained or sympathetically independent.[46] Intravenous infusion of phentolamine, a nonselective α-blocker, has been shown to correlate with pain relief after selective sympathetic block and may be used as an alternative diagnostic technique to sympathetic blockade.[47] This would be of particular value for investigation of visceral nociceptive pains, because blockade of sympathetic efferent pathways (e.g., lumbar sympathetic chain, superior hypogastric plexus) would also interrupt visceral afferent fibers, which also course through these structures; therefore, relief of pain after blockade would not be specifically diagnostic for sympathetically maintained pain. To perform a phentolamine infusion, intravenous access is obtained and normal saline is infused for 10 to 15 minutes until the pain score at rest and with provocation has stabilized, to rule out placebo effect. As much as 1.5 mg/kg of phentolamine is then infused (with the patient unaware of when the true infusion begins) over 20 to 30 minutes, with repeated pain assessments at regular intervals during and after the infusion is completed. Greater than 50% pain reduction is suggestive of a significant component of sympathetically maintained pain.

Numerous studies and case reports have confirmed the observation that systemic levels of lidocaine far below those required to interfere with normal afferent neural transmission (such as would occur during a nerve block) are effective in reducing pain in some neuropathic syndromes, and pain relief may be relatively long lived.[48] The mechanism seems to involve suppression of spontaneous ectopic nerve impulses, which may be noted in some neuropathic disorders.[49] The physiologic effect and interpretation of systemic lidocaine infusion are therefore different from that of a peripheral nerve block, when local concentrations of anesthetic are sufficient to inhibit normal transmission of nerve impulses. For example, pain relief obtained during conduction blockade of the pudendal nerve would be consistent with either a pudendal neuralgia or a nociceptive source of pain within the distribution of the pudendal nerve (e.g., a trigger point). Relief with intravenous lidocaine, however, would be highly suggestive of a neuralgia, because abnormal spontaneous neural activity is primarily affected. The technique may be used for the purposes of clarifying a diagnosis,[50] as a prognostic test for the efficacy of an oral sodium channel blocker such as mexiletine, or as primary therapy. Placebo effect is ruled out as described earlier for phentolamine infusion. Then, 5 mg/kg of lidocaine is infused over about 30 minutes while the patient is closely monitored for any signs of toxicity. Evidence suggests that higher systemic levels associated with more rapid infusion may produce a better therapeutic result.[51]

Role of Blockade in the Evaluation and Treatment of Chronic Pelvic Pain

Overview

Figure 30–4 illustrates a simplified schema for the use of blocks in the evaluation and treatment of CPP. This schema clearly oversimplifies the clinical reality of CPP, which is often complicated and enigmatic. For example, psychologic factors are involved in all CPP states, and visceral and somatic pain can appear together. We find it useful, however, to have a framework so that the physician can attempt to proceed from the known to the unknown. Although the psychologic makeup of a patient with CPP may be such that it makes pain mountains out of nociceptive molehills, it is nonetheless useful for a physician to identify the molehill. It is much easier to approach psychologic issues after having gained the credibility of identifying—and temporarily alleviating—a tissue pain source. At the same time, we would not suggest that neurologic blockade is indicated for the assessment of every patient with CPP. Its value as a diagnostic aid is most clear for patients for whom a diagnosis is not established after conventional evaluation by a gynecologist or other specialists.

The approach depicted in Figure 30–4 follows the preliminary judgment of the clini-

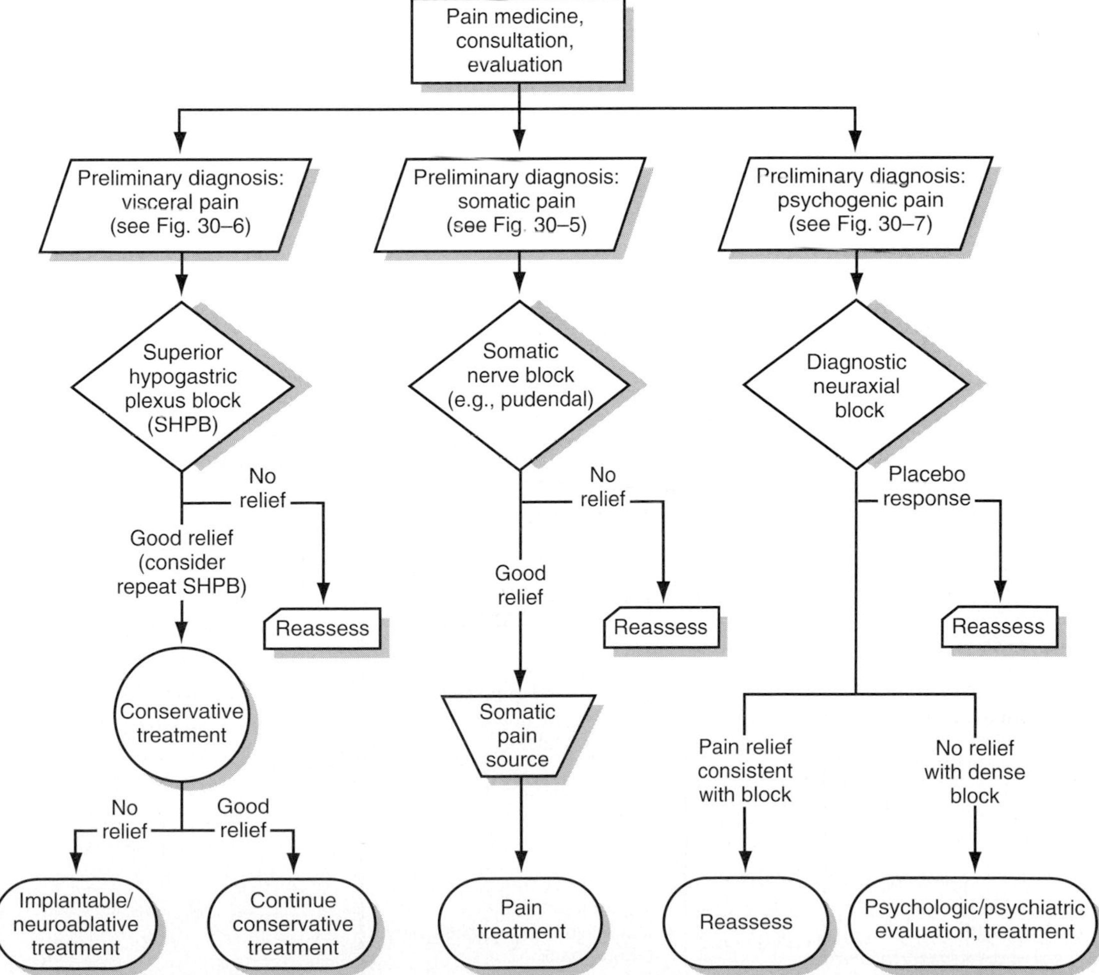

Figure 30–4. Overview of the approach to a patient with chronic pelvic pain of uncertain cause.

cian in terms of whether a visceral, somatic, or central pain source is most likely. The first step in clarification of the diagnosis is to provide temporary analgesia for the suspected condition. For those patients thought to have a visceral pain source, a diagnostic block of visceral afferent pathways (e.g., superior hypogastric plexus) is performed. If the pain source appears to be somatic (e.g., pudendal neuralgia) a somatic block (pudendal nerve block) is performed. With a lack of physical findings or a surfeit of psychologic findings, a diagnostic spinal or epidural block is performed to determine the extent of a peripheral nociceptive pain source. These steps are represented in greater detail in Figures 30–5 to 30–7.

Suspected Somatic Pain Source
(Fig. 30–5)

Patients with somatic pain may undergo one of several possible diagnostic blocks with the goal of achieving temporary complete relief. If evidence suggests a myofascial pain syndrome, for example, specific trigger points are injected with local anesthetic. Alternatively, a somatic nerve block (e.g., pudendal block) or block of one of the structures about the spine (e.g., zygapophyseal joint) may be performed, depending on the degree of clinical suspicion about the source of pain. The amount of pain relief is assessed, and any remaining pain is evaluated for quality and location. It is important to assess for any residual spontaneous pain, elicited pain, or tenderness, because somatic pain may be referred from an underlying visceral source—that is, a successful somatic block can unmask underlying visceral pain or uncover another somatic source. The patient's reaction to pain relief is noted, with special attention paid to pain migration or exaggerated symptoms.

Complete temporary relief from a somatic block supports a diagnosis of a somatic pain

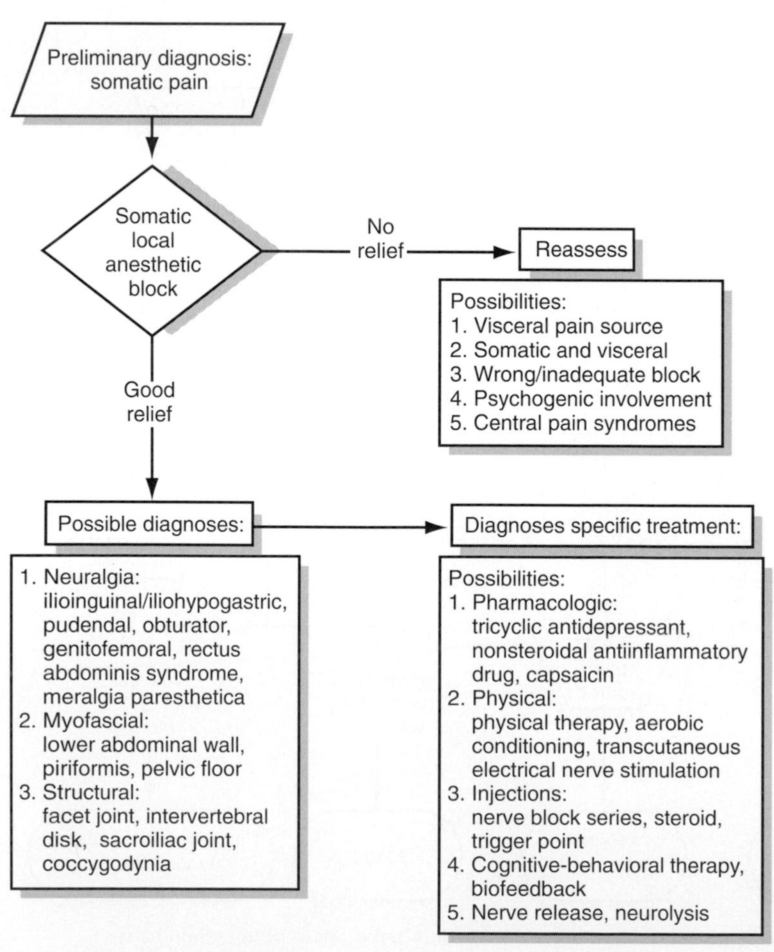

Figure 30–5. Evaluation and treatment of suspected somatic pain.

source. Most common is myofascial pain syndrome, localized to muscles such as the rectus abdominis or levator ani. In such patients, history and physical examination may also reveal regional pains in the shoulder and neck or the more generalized condition of fibromyalgia.[52] Other common possibilities include entrapments or neuralgias of peripheral somatic nerves. Treatment for somatic pain includes repeated somatic nerve blocks, trigger point injections, physical therapy, aerobic conditioning, transcutaneous electric nerve stimulation (TENS), tricyclic antidepressants, and analgesics.

Suspected Visceral Pain Source
(Fig. 30–6)

It is helpful to provide confirmation of a visceral pain source through neural blockade. This is because (1) no pathology has often been found, and pain relief through regional anesthesia confirms a nociceptive source; (2) the nociceptive source can be serious and treatable; (3) treatment of visceral pain differs markedly from that of somatic pain; (4) pain relief with a superior hypogastric plexus block raises the possibil-

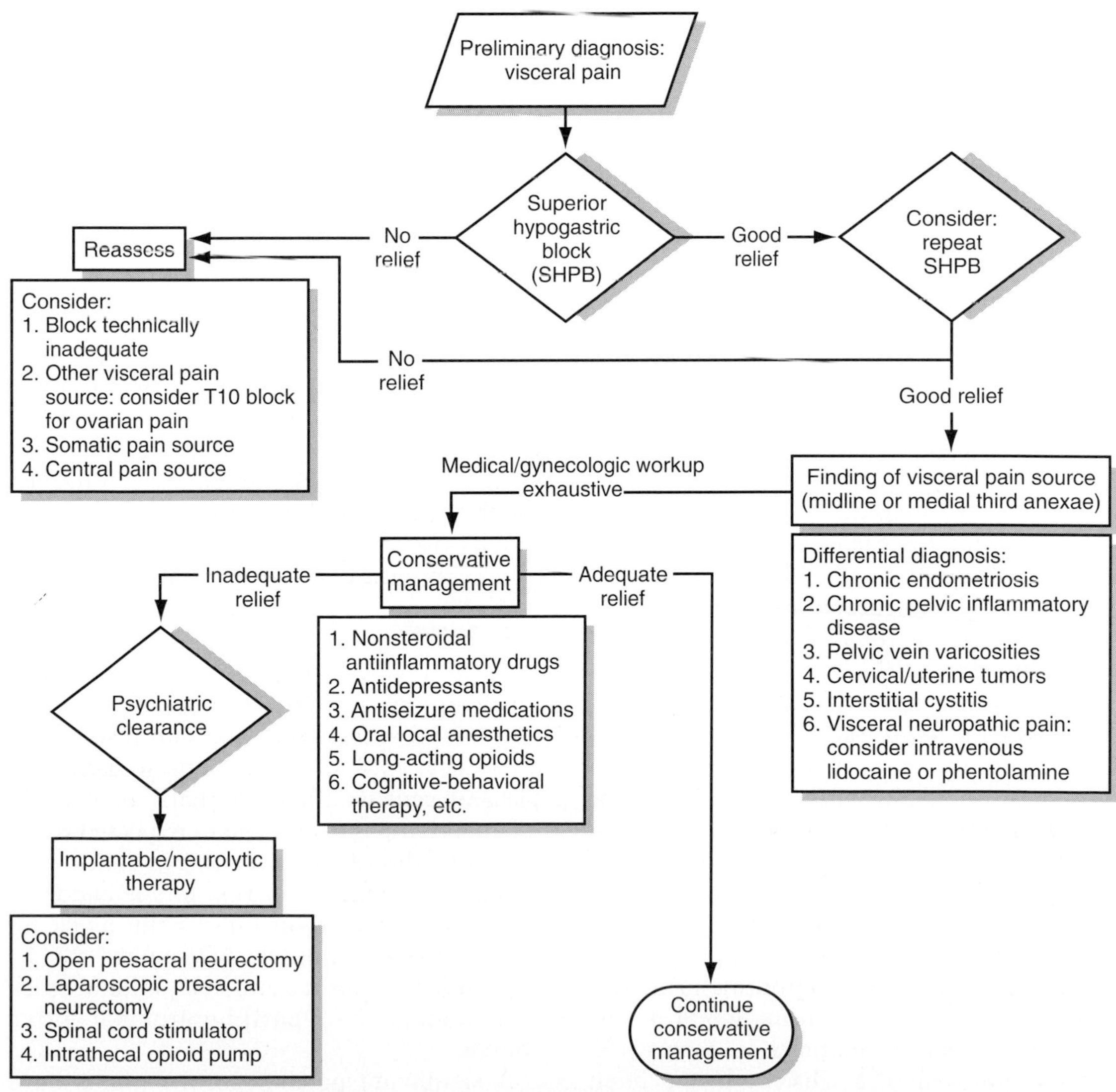

Figure 30–6. Evaluation and treatment of suspected visceral pain.

ity that long-lasting relief may be obtained through a presacral neurectomy.

Pain relief after superior hypogastric plexus block is consistent with a visceral nociceptive source in the midline or the medial adnexa. Pain originating from the ovaries may not be completely blocked, because afferent fibers also travel with the ovarian plexus, ultimately traversing the aortic plexus to enter the spinal cord at the T10 level. Therefore, blockade of the spinal nerve root at T10 may be considered in addition to the superior hypogastric plexus block if an ovarian source of pain is to be ruled out. If pain relief is obtained, a more specific visceral diagnosis may be considered on clinical grounds, and the gynecologist may wish to investigate further (e.g., by diagnostic laparoscopy under local anesthesia) or to treat a suspected gynecologic source of pain. If a thorough evaluation of a patient with a visceral pain source reveals no explanatory pathologic abnormality, the patient is treated as if she had a visceral neuropathic pain, using treatment protocols adopted from other neuropathic pain conditions (e.g., postherpetic neuralgia). The pharmacologic approach may include tricyclic antidepressants, smooth muscle relaxants (e.g., nifedipine), anticonvulsants (e.g., carbamazepine), oral local anesthetics (e.g., mexiletine), and long-acting opioids such as sustained-release morphine. Psychologic consultation is often quite helpful.

If conservative measures are ineffective or lead to intolerable side effects, consideration is given to neuroablation of the superior hypogastric plexus. The conventional approach is to perform an open presacral neurectomy (*superior hypogastric plexus* and *presacral nerves* are synonymous). Although performance of a chemical neurolytic superior hypogastric plexus block for nonmalignant CPP has been advocated,[53] no published series to date attests to its efficacy or safety. The efficacy of presacral neurectomy for CPP is in itself controversial. All would agree, however, on the importance of patient selection; pain originating primarily from the ovaries, for example, might not be entirely eliminated. Patients in many previously published series had not been screened by multidisciplinary evaluation, and no series has screened for response to a prognostic superior hypogastric plexus block.[54–56] It is our impression that the efficacy of presacral neurectomy is much greater among carefully selected patients who have responded positively to prognostic superior hypogastric plexus block. Certainly, the likelihood of success would be low in patients who failed to respond to anesthetic block.

Patients suspected of having visceral pain and who do not respond to a superior hypogastric plexus block or T10 nerve root block should be reassessed. It may be worthwhile to repeat the block. Patients with evidence of somatic pain should have the appropriate somatic nerve block. If the pain source is completely unclear or if psychologic factors appear to play a major part, performing a differential spinal or epidural may help to confirm the presence of a peripheral nociceptive source.

Psychogenic Pain (Fig. 30–7)

In the opinion of some experts, the complaint of patients with CPP is largely attributable to psychopathology or psychologic factors.[57] In our experience, a visceral or somatic pain source is usually demonstrable but with psychologic factors also having a significant role. For some patients, however, relief is provided by neither somatic nerve blocks nor a superior hypogastric plexus block, or they have predominant psychologic findings. For such patients, the most relevant question is whether a source of peripheral nociception is a factor. A diagnostic spinal or epidural block seeks to determine whether pain relief can result from a simultaneous block of both somatic and visceral sensory fibers. Somatic or visceral nociceptive pain sources are expected to respond to the block, with the patient's pain level diminishing as the block becomes more dense and returning as the block resolves over 60 minutes. A response consistent with the sensory and sympathetic block is evidence of a peripheral nociceptive source.

A significant percentage of patients have a placebo response—that is, their pain di-

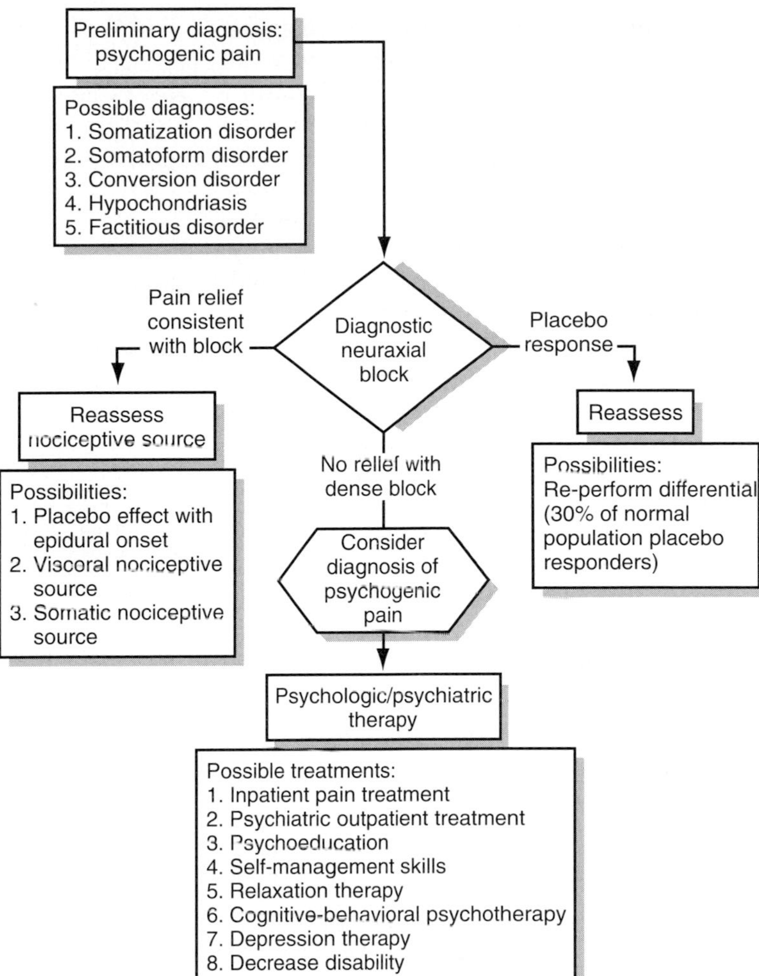

Figure 30–7. Evaluation and treatment of suspected psychogenic pain.

minishes with injection of saline. In such patients, pain often returns over a short time and the study can be continued. If the placebo response persists, the procedure is halted and the patient reassessed. It is difficult to draw conclusions in this setting, because the placebo response is common among patients with demonstrated pathology. A response of increased pain or no relief with a dense high block is consistent with a central pain source, a category that includes both psychologic diagnoses and neurologic pathology. In patients with positive psychologic findings, a diagnostic spinal or epidural can assess the relative importance of peripheral nociception contributing to the pain complaints. In patients without psychologic findings, a finding of a central pain source may prompt suspicion of neurologic pathology such as spinal cord tumors. In either case, failure to obtain relief would contraindicate further nerve blocks or operations targeted at possible peripheral sources of pain.

Summary

Patients with CPP without a clear-cut diagnosis can present a vexing problem for a gynecologist, urologist, or gastroenterologist. Because of frequent psychologic overlay and a physician's inability to confirm a peripheral diagnosis, these pains often become categorized as psychogenic or factitious. Evidence suggests, however, that many if not most of these patients do have true peripheral pathology. If initial conventional evaluation fails to produce a diagnosis, we recommend early consultation with a gynecologic pain specialist or an interdisciplinary pain management center. Comprehensive assessment with attention paid to organic, psychologic, and functional issues can provide important diagnostic information for the primary physician and may serve to prevent unnecessary or misguided attempts at surgical intervention. Anesthesiologists as specialists in pain medicine can use a rational progression of diagnostic procedures, taking care to avoid errors in interpretation, in order to arrive at a more specific diagnosis that serves to reassure patients and leads to more rational therapy.

References

1. Stout AL, Steege JF, Dodson WC, et al: Relationship of laparoscopic findings to self-report of pelvic pain. Am J Obstet Gynecol 1991;164:73.
2. Abram SE, McCreary C, Rosomoff RS, et al: Certification in pain management. Am Pain Soc Bull 1992;2:5.
3. Parris WCV: Credentialing in pain medicine. Am Pain Soc Bull 1992;2:6.
4. Chapman S: Outpatient chronic pain management programs. In Tollison CD, Satterthwaite JR, Tollison JW (eds): Handbook of Pain Management, 2nd ed. Baltimore, Williams & Wilkins, 1994, pp 676–685.
5. Sanders SH: An image problem for pain centers: Relevant factors and possible solutions. Am Pain Soc Bull 1994;4:17.
6. Flor H, Fydrich T, Turk DC: Efficacy of multidisciplinary pain treatment centers: A meta-analytic review. Pain 1992;49:221.
7. Kames LD, Rapkin AJ, Naliboff BD, et al: Effectiveness of an interdisciplinary pain management program for the treatment of chronic pelvic pain. Pain 1990;41:41.
8. Gambone JC, Reiter RC: Non-surgical management of chronic pelvic pain: A multidisciplinary approach. Clin Obstet Gynecol 1990;33:205.
9. Reiter RC, Gambone JC: Nongynecologic somatic pathology in women with chronic pelvic pain and negative laparoscopy. J Reprod Med 1991;36:253.
10. Peters AAW, van Dorst E, Jellis B, et al: A randomized clinical trial to compare two different approaches in women with chronic pelvic pain. Obstet Gynecol 1991;77:740.
11. American Pain Society: 1996 Pain Facilities Directory. Glenview, IL, American Pain Society, 1996.
12. Chapman SL: CARF accreditation for chronic pain programs. Am Pain Soc Bull 1991;1:8.
13. Reiter RC: Occult somatic pathology in women with chronic pelvic pain. Clin Obstet Gynecol 1990;33:154.
14. Steege JF, Stout AL, Somkuti SG: Chronic pelvic pain in women: Toward an integrative model. Obstet Gynecol Surv 1993;48:95.
15. Kellner R, Slocumb JC, Rosenfeld RC, et al: Fears and beliefs in patients with the pelvic pain syndrome. J Psychosom Res 1988;32:303.
16. Travell JG, Simons DG: Myofascial Pain and Dysfunction: The Trigger Point Manual, vol II. Baltimore, Williams & Wilkins, 1992.
17. Thomson H, Francis DMA: Abdominal-wall tenderness: A useful sign in the acute abdomen. Lancet 1977;2:1053.
18. Beatty RA: The piriformis muscle syndrome: A simple diagnostic maneuver. Neurosurgery 1994; 34:512.
19. Sinaki M, Merritt JL, Stillwell GK: Tension myalgia of the pelvic floor. Mayo Clin Proc 1977;52:717.
20. Laslett M, Williams M: The reliability of selected pain provocation tests for sacroiliac joint pathology. Spine 1994;11:1243.
21. Gebhart GF: Visceral nociception: Consequences, modulation and the future. Eur J Anaesthesiol Suppl 1995;10:24.
22. Zimmerman M: Peripheral and central nervous mechanisms of nociception, pain and pain therapy: Facts and hypotheses. In Bonica JJ (ed): Advances in Pain Research and Therapy, vol III. New York, Raven Press, 1979, pp 3–32.
23. Deyo RA, Rainville J, Kent DL: What can the history and physical examination tell us about low back pain? JAMA 1992;268:760.
24. Jensen MC, Brant-Zawadzki MN, Obuchowski N, et al: Magnetic resonance imaging of the lumbar spine in people without back pain. N Engl J Med 1994;331:69.
25. Bonica JJ: The Management of Pain, 2nd ed. Philadelphia, Lea & Febiger, 1990.
26. Boas RA: Nerve blocks in the diagnosis of low back pain. Neurosurg Clin North Am 1991;2:807.
27. Barnsley L, Lord S, Wallis B, et al: False-positive rates of cervical zygapophyseal joint blocks. Clin J Pain 1993;9:124.
28. Turner JA, Deyo RA, Loeser JD, et al: The importance of placebo effects in pain treatment and research. JAMA 1994;271:1609.
29. Hogan QH, Erickson SJ, Haddox JD, et al: The spread of solutions during stellate ganglion block. Reg Anesth 1992;17:78.
30. Ferrer-Brechner T, Brechner VL: Accuracy of needle placement during diagnostic and therapeutic nerve blocks. In Bonica JJ, Albe-Fessard D (eds): Advances in Pain Research and Therapy, vol I. New York, Raven Press, 1976, pp 679–683.
31. Backonja M, Gombar K: Serum lidocaine levels following stellate ganglion sympathetic blocks and intravenous lidocaine injection. J Pain Symptom Manage 1992;7:2.
32. Xavier AV, McDanal J, Kissin I: Relief of sciatic radicular pain by sciatic nerve block. Anesth Analg 1988;67:1177.
33. Malmqvist EL-Å, Bengtsson M, Sörensen J: Efficacy of stellate ganglion block: A clinical study with bupivacaine. Reg Anesth 1992;17:340.
34. Chado HN: The current perception threshold evaluation of sensory nerve function in pain management. Pain Digest 1995;5:127.
35. Slocumb JC: Neurological factors in chronic pelvic pain: Trigger points and the abdominal pelvic pain syndrome. Am J Obstet Gynecol 1984;149:536.
36. Gillespie L, Bray R, Levin N, et al: Lumbar nerve root compression and interstitial cystitis—response to decompressive surgery. Br J Urol 1991;68:361.
37. Guerriero WF, Guerriero CP, Eward RD, et al: Pelvic pain, gynecic and nongynecic: Interpretation and management. South Med J 1971;64:1043.
38. Plancarte R, Amescua C, Patt RB, et al: Superior

hypogastric plexus block for pelvic cancer pain. Anesthesiology 1990;73:236.
39. de Leon-Casasola OA, Kent E, Lema MJ: Neurolytic superior hypogastric plexus block for chronic pelvic pain associated with cancer. Pain 1993;54:145.
40. Plancarte R, Velazquez R, Patt RB: Neurolytic blocks of the sympathetic axis. In Patt RB (ed): Cancer Pain. Philadelphia, JB Lippincott, 1993.
41. Waldman SD, Wilson WL, Kreps RD: Superior hypogastric plexus block using a single needle and computed tomography guidance: Description of a modified technique. Reg Anesth 1991;16:286.
42. Tessler MJ, Kleiman SJ: Spinal anaesthesia for patients with previous lower limb amputations. Anaesthesia 1994;49:439.
43. Derby R, Bogduk N, Schwarzer A: Precision percutaneous blocking procedures for localizing spinal pain. Part 1: The posterior lumbar compartment. Pain Digest 1993;3:89.
44. Schwarzer AC, Aprill CN, Bogduk N: The sacroiliac joint in chronic low back pain. Spine 1995;20:31.
45. Krempen JF, Silver RA, Hadley J: An analysis of differential epidural spinal anesthesia and pentothal pain study in the differential diagnosis of back pain. Spine 1979;4:452.
46. Stanton-Hicks M, Jänig W, Hassenbusch S, et al: Reflex sympathetic dystrophy: Changing concepts and taxonomy. Pain 1995;63:127.
47. Raja SN, Treede R-D, Davis KD, et al: Systemic alpha-adrenergic blockade with phentolamine: A diagnostic test for sympathetically maintained pain. Anesthesiology 1991;74:691.
48. Paggioli JJ, Racz GB: Intravenous and oral anesthetics in pain management: Reflections on intravenous lidocaine and mexiletine. Pain Digest 1995;5:69.
49. Devor M, Wall PD, Catalan N: Systemic lidocaine silences ectopic neuroma and DRG discharge without blocking nerve conduction. Pain 1992;48:261.
50. Marchettini P, Lacerenza M, Marangoni C, et al: Lidocaine test in neuralgia. Pain 1992;48:377.
51. Chaplan SR, Bach FW, Shafer SL, et al: Prolonged alleviation of tactile allodynia by intravenous lidocaine in neuropathic rats. Anesthesiology 1995;83:775.
52. Wolfe F, Smythe HA, Yunus MB, et al: The American College of Rheumatology 1990 criteria for classification of fibromyalgia: Report of the Multicenter Criteria Committee. Arthritis Rheum 1990;33:160.
53. Patt RB: Celiac and superior hypogastric plexus block. In Nineteenth Annual Meeting Refresher Course Syllabus. Richmond, VA, American Society of Regional Anesthesia, 1994, pp 56–68.
54. Candiani GB, Fedele L, Vercellini P, et al: Presacral neurectomy for the treatment of pelvic pain associated with endometriosis: A controlled study. Am J Obstet Gynecol 1992;167:100.
55. Vercellini P, Fedele L, Bianchi S, et al: Pelvic denervation for chronic pain associated with endometriosis: Fact or fancy? Am J Obstet Gynecol 1991;165:745.
56. Nezhat C, Nezhat F: A simplified method of laparoscopic presacral neurectomy for the treatment of central pelvic pain due to endometriosis. Gynaecology 1992;99:650.
57. Guzinski GM: Gynecologic pain. In Bonica JJ (ed): The Management of Pain, 2nd ed, vol II. Philadelphia, Lea & Febiger, 1990, p 1364.

31

Research Directions

Deborah A. Metzger, PhD, MD

The subject of chronic pelvic pain (CPP) represents a rich and open realm for further exploration through research. Few systematic studies have adequately captured the essence of CPP and all of its complexities. In fact, this book just scratches the surface of single-discipline observations of CPP. The future is ripe for interdisciplinary research and treatment approaches that may prove to have a common base with chronic pain of nongynecologic origin.

In the repertoire of clinical exploration, the scientific method (i.e., experimental validation of a phenomenon) is the gold standard means of developing clinical theory and practice. Information that is gathered by other methods is deemed less reliable. However, the use of the scientific method has limitations when dealing with issues as complex as CPP. These limitations are rarely considered in designing research studies and include the nature of the questions we ask, the type of methods we use to answer those questions, and the ways these questions and our belief systems influence outcomes, inferences, and generalizations. In developing clinically valid research, striving to approximate the elegance of the randomized placebo-controlled experimental research model is ideal. However, in aiming for an integrated understanding of CPP, it may be that we need to sacrifice some of this elegance in the spirit of capturing the essence of the interrelationship of factors in women with CPP. Field research, clinical observations, exploratory research, and phenomenologic study conducted retrospectively on women with CPP may yield greater understanding of this condition than that afforded by strictly controlled laboratory paradigms. Furthermore, the social, cultural, and familial influences that are interwoven into the lives of women with CPP impose significant independent variables that may defy measurement. Because pain cannot be studied in a vacuum, we need to modify our experimental approaches to obtain valid and applicable data.

Difficulties in Designing Research on Chronic Pelvic Pain

To achieve the goals of obtaining meaningful data, we need to examine critically the research that has been published so that we may better design future studies. Most current approaches are imperfect. Experimental studies suffer limits in generalizability, whereas descriptive studies are limited by the difficulty in corroboration and clarity of interpretation of results. Moreover, various social and political factors have interfered with honest scientific and clinical observations, usually without scientists' and clinicians' having any awareness of what their prejudices were. These same forces continue to exist. Future research needs to take into account not only our ignorance (what we know that we do not know) but also our biases (what we do not know that we do not know).

Investigator Bias

Widespread, deep-seated assumptions have been made about cause-and-effect relationships in CPP, the most pervasive being that pelvic pain is a psychosomatic disorder. Even the most open and progressive of clinicians may sometimes find it emotionally difficult to deal with the realities of CPP. It is certainly understandable that we may at times need to distance ourselves emotionally by putting blame on a patient. To a greater or lesser extent, these assumptions guide investigators in forming hypotheses that they want to test experimentally.

Other biases may be cultural. For example, observations have been made in simian animal models that endometriosis can be prevented by frequent pregnancies and brought on by periods of nonfertile menstrual cycling. This observation can be extended to women in that the apparent increased prevalence of endometriosis may be a consequence of changes in childbearing and the availability of effective contraceptives that generally do not alter the occurrence of regular menstrual bleeding. Unlike our predecessors, who had a few menstrual periods interrupted frequently by long periods of amenorrhea related to pregnancy and lactation, our culture now assumes that menstrual bleeding every 28 days is the norm, with only rare interruptions for pregnancy. This assumption is so ingrained in our culture that birth control pills are given so that withdrawal bleeding occurs every 28 days even though this is unnecessary for contraceptive efficacy. Why not have withdrawal bleeding every 2 months, 6 months, or never? Are we putting women unnecessarily at risk for the development of endometriosis by continuing this cultural assumption? Can we prevent or delay the development of endometriosis?

Selection of an Appropriate Control Group

Observational studies generally include a control group that defines the population norm. However, an important issue is, What is an appropriate control group for women with CPP? Some studies have used infertile patients, gynecologic patients without pain, or patients with pain other than pelvic pain. When selecting an appropriate control group, it is important to assess the likelihood that the control groups will be as likely to divulge sensitive issues such as sexual abuse, drug use, and family issues as women with CPP. Women with infertility issues may consider questions about sexual abuse as irrelevant to their treatment and may withhold information. The control groups chosen may differ substantially from the CPP group in socioeconomic status, education, and self-esteem. These independent variables are not routinely considered in selecting a control group.

An example of difficulties in control group selection is illustrated by the experiences of a clinic specializing in the treatment of individuals with chronic pain. The goal of the study was to assess the presence of an abuse history in patients using staff members as a control group. The researchers hypothesized that the staff members who participated in the survey would have a low prevalence of sexual abuse, representative of the general population. However, staff members actually reported higher rates of sexual, physical, and emotional abuse than did those seeking treatment for pain.[1] This study demonstrates the need to investigate assumptions about the prevalence of abuse (or any other characteristic) not only in the general population but also in the specific control groups selected to help answer a research question.

Methods of Data Collection

Methods of data collection have included in-person interviews, telephone interviews, and written questionnaires—all of which have unique strengths and weaknesses. In-person interviews may allow a better overall understanding of a patient and may also allow a climate that would encourage divulging sensitive information. However, they are labor intensive and expensive.

The person who conducts the interview may also influence the validity of the data collected. For example, a woman who is interviewed by a social worker may make the assumption that her caregivers believe that her pain is due to social problems or somatization. Thus, she endures the interview in a defensive posture. Because many of the studies dealing with CPP are multidisciplinary, this interviewer bias may be magnified if each group is interviewed by a person from a different discipline.

Data from women with CPP are generally

collected at a single point in time. Unfortunately, the lack of cross-sectional studies that evaluate women over time has limited our understanding of how fluctuations in social issues affect the level of functioning of women with CPP.

The scores from standard questionnaires are often used to compare women with CPP with controls. However, the chosen instrument may not be valid for women with CPP and significant psychosocial issues. In other words, differences in independent variables may be affecting a woman's ability to provide meaningful data.

Controlling for Psychosocial Issues

CPP has complex relationships with poverty, substance abuse, levels of intelligence, family structure, abuse history, education, sexuality, and marriage—all of which influence adaptability and development of coping skills. How do you define the positive and negative effects of family structure? Childhood sexual abuse appears both to have sustained impacts on psychologic functioning in many survivors and to have the potential for motivating the development of behaviors that, although immediately adaptive, often have long-term self-injurious consequences such as selection of an abusive marriage partner, drug use, and promiscuous sexual behavior.

In contemporary culture, the link between stress and illness has almost become a cliché, yet we are only beginning to acknowledge the ramifications of this association in the diagnosis and management of CPP. The introduction of the diagnosis of posttraumatic stress disorder is an important stepping stone in helping to define how extreme environmental stress affects soma and psyche. New data on the effects of emotional and physical trauma on the immune system are beginning to emerge, and these may help provide some new avenues for understanding and treating somatic disorders.

Defining a Diagnosis

The difficulty in defining a diagnosis is illustrated by a patient who was evaluated and treated by an overwhelming number of pain experts. This 35-year-old multiparous woman had a 2-year history of incapacitating left lower quadrant pain with associated pain in her left lower back. She had a history of many surgical procedures: four cesarean sections and two laparotomies for ectopic pregnancies. She and her husband had literally traveled the world in search of an expert who could diagnose and treat her pain, and in the process they accumulated a 6-inch-thick notebook of reports from orthopedists, gastroenterologists, physical therapists, gynecologists, general surgeons, and so on. Four gynecologists experienced in the evaluation and management of CPP came to four different conclusions about the cause of her pain: (1) ovarian vein varicosities, (2) neuropathy, (3) adhesions, and (4) inguinal hernia with associated piriformis muscle spasm. Some of these diagnoses were subsequently eliminated on the basis of her response to treatment. Neither ovarian vein embolization, ovarian vein ligation, nor lysis of adhesions had any impact on the pain. She underwent laparoscopic pain mapping with conscious sedation, which seemed to suggest a nonpalpable hernia. However, at the time of publication of this book, she had not yet gathered the courage to undergo yet another surgical procedure and is attempting a trial of gabapentin (Neurontin) for presumed neuropathy.

This patient illustrates many important points. One of the difficulties in comparing results of research is that the definitions of CPP differ among different groups. Moreover, great variability in referral bias, treatment approaches, and treatment styles is noted among different groups, making direct comparisons or generalizations difficult. Although it is unlikely that uniform agreement on what constitutes CPP will be obtained, it is crucial that researchers specifically address the issue of defining the characteristics (nature, severity, and context) of the pain under study so that comparison of etiologies and treatments is possible.

Women with CPP are a heterogeneous group, even when they share the same diagnosis. It is unusual indeed to identify "pure" diagnostic groups (i.e., women who only have a single definable cause of their pain). Because of their ease of diagnosis, they are often treated by a nonspecialist. Thus, most patients who are referred for management of CPP have more than one physical reason for pain, are disabled because of the length of time that they have been in pain, or have emotional/social/developmental issues that interfere with coping ability.

Placebo Effect

The placebo effect is one of the most acknowledged confounding variables in research design and interpretation and is the single most important reason for including a control group in a randomized clinical trial of a treatment. Placebo effects are found with drugs, medical treatments, surgery, biofeedback, psychotherapy, and even diagnostic tests. It is essential for investigators to understand the extent to which placebo effects account for improvements observed in clinical studies to avoid erroneous claims of efficacy. Factors that influence the placebo effect include a patient's expectations of treatment and a provider's attitude toward the patient and the treatment. Only independently evaluated, randomized controlled trials can establish an effect of a treatment above and beyond the natural history of the condition being studied. Placebo effects are likely to be strongest when the patient is anxious, the physician is perceived as having great expertise, the patient and physician believe the treatment is powerful, and the treatment is impressive and expensive.[2] These effects are likely to be substantial, may be sustained for long periods, and may explain some or all of the benefits attributed to treatment.

In their review of the placebo effect, Turner and colleagues[2] conclude, "There are important implications for research and clinical training in all areas of medicine. The quality of the interaction between the physician and patient can be extremely influential in patient outcomes and in some (perhaps many) cases, patient and provider expectations and interactions may be more important than specific treatments. . . . The body's capacity to modulate symptoms and suffering involves more than simply 'psychological factors,' where those are seen as traits or personality characteristics. Symptoms, illness, and their changes over time reflect complex interactions between anatomical and neurophysiological processes, on the one hand, and cognitive-behavioral and environmental factors on the other. These findings support the thesis that these factors are inextricably intertwined."

As pervasive as the placebo effect is, we have little information about how we can use this phenomenon. If the belief in a procedure, treatment, or physician is so strong that pain is diminished for a time, how can this be used clinically? Which women are particularly susceptible to placebo effects? Over what period of time is the placebo effect expressed? What causes the beneficial effect to disappear?

Scope of the Research

Research in CPP has generally been interpreted through a single discipline (i.e., gynecology). However, many of the syndromes described in this book could not exist in isolation from other specialties, and perhaps even the designation into chapters is arbitrary. For example, one way of viewing and organizing information on CPP is according to neuropathic syndromes, but so is a chapter devoted to left lower quadrant pain that encompasses not only neurologic disease but urologic, gynecologic, orthopedic, and general surgical disease. As emphasized in this book, just as CPP cannot be treated in isolation, it also requires input from a multidisciplinary team to study it.

Attention is currently focused on the possibility that endometriosis is a systemic disease and that the endometriotic implants seen at surgery are but one manifestation. Alterations in humoral and cellular immunity have been described, but are these responsible for the growth of ectopic endometrium or a consequence of it? Women with endometriosis commonly report fatigue, bowel problems, muscle aches, low-grade fever, and low resistance to infections. Other health problems are more prevalent among those with endometriosis, including lupus, atopic diseases, autoimmune thyroid disease, fungal disease, chronic fatigue syndrome, and fibromyalgia. Does this indicate that systemic changes have occurred? Clearly, fresh ideas will arise from the different perspectives of other fields of research.

Defining Successful Treatment

In the past, we have defined successful treatment by a specific endpoint (i.e., change in pain scores, need for pain medications, and so on). However, this often reflects a researcher's criteria of success, not necessarily a patient's. Medical research has traditionally focused on clinical and physiologic indicators such as skin temperature, blood pressure, and hematocrit. These outcomes were chosen because they are easy and inexpensive to measure, are reproducible, and do not require large numbers of subjects to show a statistically significant change. Unfortunately, they avoid much more difficult but relevant outcomes such as patient satisfaction, quality of life, and functional status.

Quality of life, although seemingly one of the most crucial aspects of any treatment, has seldom been measured as a study outcome. This lack of attention stems not from lack of importance but from tremendous methodologic difficulties. In particular, it is often difficult to define what constitutes quality of life, and even when agreement is reached about the components of quality of life, a problem is how to convincingly and reproducibly measure these components so that different treatments can be compared.

Another area of concern is to define which procedures used to treat women with CPP are effective. Randomized clinical trials have traditionally been used, but they are becoming less practical for a number of reasons. First, they are prohibitively expensive. Second, procedures developed in an academic environment with a small subset of patients may not be directly applicable in general clinical practice. Third, more than one treatment modality is commonly used, making it difficult to determine the independent contributions of any one therapy. Finally, randomized trials frequently do not address the patient-specific issues that are an important endpoint in outcomes research.

The Future of Research in Chronic Pelvic Pain

It is clear from the discussion in the first part of this chapter that our current research approaches are inadequate for an area as complex and poorly understood as CPP. Novel methods are necessary to approach this area from a number of different perspectives and disciplines. Outcomes research offers expanded capabilities for studying CPP that are not possible with the more traditional research approaches. To date, outcomes research studies have been composed of multidisciplinary teams of researchers and clinicians who study complex chronic medical problems such as back pain, prevention of low birth weight, ischemic heart disease, and management of diabetes. Outcomes research includes the measurement of traditional clinical endpoints such as pain scores, blood loss, and length of stay but also encompasses a wider range of possibilities. It attempts to measure the quality of care by examining such aspects as cost, patients' satisfaction, quality of life, complications, and other outcomes that are truly relevant to patients.

Defining Outcomes Research

Outcomes research attempts to study medical interventions on a large scale as they are happening. Procedures and results are assessed as they are actually performed, a process that has been described as "the epidemiologic surveillance of medical care." Because patients are not randomized, they receive the integrated treatment that is believed to be appropriate for their particular situation. Assessment of outcome, which may be periodically tested over time, is based on quality of life measures, cost, patient satisfaction, and complications.

The technology to store and analyze such a complex database requires sophisticated computerized databases to organize information on patient demographics, disease mix, clinical interventions, clinical outcomes, and quality of life. Furthermore, data need to be stored in a standard fashion so that patients at different sites can be compared. At present, no such integrated data entry and retrieval systems exist, except for small-scale databases designed for use by health maintenance organizations.

Examples of Outcomes Research

One of the goals of outcomes research is to define which of the procedures in practice are effective by studying procedures as they are actually performed. This is described as "the epidemiologic surveillance of medical care."[3] An example of how these data can be used is a study comparing open and laparoscopic cholecystectomies using discharge data from Maryland hospitals.[4] Although laparoscopic cholecystectomy was initially believed to be cheaper and to have lower mortality because of its minimally invasive nature, the results showed that the costs were similar and the same number of patients died after both types of surgery. Because of the way in which the data were collected, it was possible to analyze the altered practice patterns that resulted in these unexpected findings. These results occurred because in the community, patients who were not as sick and would have been treated medically were instead candidates for surgery and the 33% decrease in operative mortality per case was countered by the 28% increase in number of procedures performed per year. Thus, the new procedure was applied to a different group of patients than the traditional procedure was, an important piece of information noted by outcomes research that would not have been detected by traditional clinical trials.

Another study from Maine assessed a prospective cohort of women undergoing hysterectomy for benign disease.[5] These researchers found that patients had marked improvements in a number of symptoms, including pelvic pain, urinary symptoms, fatigue, and sexual dysfunction. In addition, improvements were noted in indices of mental health, general health, and activity at 6 months and 1 year. In a companion study, similar improvements were noted in patients treated medically, although a large fraction of patients eventually needed surgical therapy.[6] The value of this study was to dispel the assumption that medical therapy is an equivalent but preferable alternative to surgery. Surgical management of these common benign gynecologic problems truly enhances quality of life.

Research Questions

In anticipation of the development of a multicenter outcome research center for CPP, we need to develop a standard patient questionnaire to assess pain severity, location, degree of disability, living situation, past treatments, and so on. This questionnaire would be appropriate for a wide range of specialties that currently manage the different components of CPP. The addition or expansion of questions would allow specialty-specific data tracking. This multidisciplinary project would be quite an undertaking but would also expand the dialogues that have been taking place on a very limited scale.

Regardless of the research techniques, many questions are begging for attention:

1. Does surgical lysis of adhesions add anything to the overall integrated management of CPP? How do you determine who is an appropriate candidate for surgery?
2. What criteria should be used for prescribing antidepressants in CPP? Does one use pain syndrome criteria, personality criteria, psychometrically defined depression, or empirical treatment of all patients?
3. What is the role of pain specialists in the management of CPP, especially in this era of managed care? Would *one* consultation visit early in the course of the problem ultimately lead to less resource use and better outcomes, compared with the current practice of referring only in the most desperate and refractory cases? If we attended to the *source* of the pain early, would we have a condition called CPP?
4. How do we integrate CPP management in residency programs? Pain is perhaps the

most common presenting problem, yet a disproportionately small proportion of time and attention is paid to pain management.

The study of CPP is in its infancy. With new and better research tools, we will have the ability to make significant advances in diagnosis and treatment.

References

1. Karol RL, Micka RG, Kuskowski M: Physical, emotional and sexual abuse among pain patients and health care providers: Implications for psychologists in multidisciplinary pain treatment centers. Prof Psych Res Pract 1992;23:480.
2. Turner JA, Deyo RA, Loeser JD, et al: The importance of placebo effects in pain treatment and research. JAMA 1994;271:1609.
3. Caper P: The epidemiologic surveillance of medical care. Am J Public Health 1987;77:669.
4. Steiner CA, Bass EB, Talamini MA, et al: Surgical rates and operative mortality for open and laparoscopic cholecystectomy in Maryland. N Engl J Med 1994;330:403.
5. Carlson KJ, Miller BA, Fowler FJ Jr: The Maine women's health study: I. Outcomes of hysterectomy. Obstet Gynecol 1994;83:556.
6. Carlson KJ, Miller BA, Fowler FJ Jr: The Maine women's health study: II. Outcomes of nonsurgical management of leiomyomas, abnormal bleeding and chronic pelvic pain. Obstet Gynecol 1994;83:566.

Selected Readings

DeNardis MC: The relationship between chronic pelvic pain and childhood sexual abuse. Clinical research project submitted in partial fulfilment of the requirements for the degree of doctor of psychology at the Alhonor School of Professional Psychology, 1994.

Ellwood PM: Outcomes management: A technology of patient experience. N Engl J Med 1988;318:154.

Tarlov AR, Ware JE, Greenfield S, et al: The medical outcomes study: An application of methods for monitoring the results of medical care. JAMA 1989;262:925.

32

General Surgical Aspects

Ibrahim Daoud, MD

Pain of enterocolic origin is one of the most common complaints encountered by physicians in their medical practice. A skillfully taken history and meticulous physical examination of the abdomen result in a diagnosis in about 75% of cases.[1, 2] The remaining 25% of patients may require more extensive diagnostic efforts.

The cause of chronic pelvic pain (CPP) is often enigmatic. Of women seeking gynecologic help for CPP, from 7% to 60% may have a gastroenterologic diagnosis, depending on the practice setting.[3] Because the cervix, uterus, and adnexa share innervation from the hypogastric plexus with the distal ileum, colon, rectosigmoid, and bladder, determining whether pelvic pain is of gynecologic or enterocolic origin is often difficult.[2] Pain sensation from the gastrointestinal (GI) tract is often diffuse and poorly localized, and the referred component of visceral pain from the GI tract is often to the same dermatome as referred pain originating from the reproductive organs.[4]

Enterocolic disorders causing CPP include irritable bowel syndrome, infectious diarrhea, chronic or recurrent appendicitis, inflammatory bowel disease, intestinal ischemia, abdominal wall hernias, and diverticular disease. In this chapter, the discussion is limited to those causes of CPP requiring surgical intervention: abdominal wall hernias, chronic or recurrent appendicitis, diverticular disease, and adhesions interfering with bowel function.

General Diagnostic Approach

A thorough medical history should include the pattern of pain (constant, intermittent, or cyclic); its intensity, location, radiation, and duration; and the relationship of the pain to eating and bowel movements. The physician should ask about blood or mucus in the stool, bowel habit changes, and if the pain is associated with nausea, vomiting, and abdominal distention.

Physical examination should note scars, masses, and distention. Examine for groin (inguinal, femoral), incisional, epigastric, umbilical, and spigelian hernias. Inspect the perineum and the rectum digitally and the rectum with the anoscope to rule out perineal hernias, rectal masses, hemorrhoids, fissures, and fistulas. Pelvic examination should be included.

Useful diagnostic studies include flat and upright abdominal radiographs to detect calcifications or distended bowel. Ultrasound examination of the abdomen can rule out gallstones, abdominal masses, or pancreatic enlargement. The stool should be checked for occult blood in patients with a history of rectal bleeding and in patients older than 40 years. In patients with lower GI signs, flexible sigmoidoscopy with barium enema or colonoscopy should be performed to rule out colorectal disease. Similarly, an upper GI series with small bowel follow-through can detect inflammatory bowel disease.

Sometimes, despite a complete history and physical examination and reasonable radiologic evaluation, no definitive diagnosis emerges. If the symptoms persist despite medical therapy and if examination findings are reproducible, a diagnostic laparoscopy might be indicated. The patient should consent to an appendectomy, repair of any hernias found, lysis of adhesions, and possible laparotomy. A thorough laxative bowel preparation and preoperative intravenous antibiotics diminish complications in the event of bowel injury or indicated segmental resection. Preoperative review by a gastroenterologist, urologist, or psychiatrist may be necessary in some cases. At laparoscopy, the entire abdomen should be examined, with special attention to the areas of pain and tenderness.

Abdominal Wall Hernias

The differential diagnosis of lower abdominal pain in women includes hernias. These are less often suspected, however, because of the relatively low incidence of hernias in women.

The most common hernias in women are inguinal (indirect or direct) and femoral, in that order, just as in men. However, femoral hernias are relatively more common in women than men, accounting for 20% of all groin hernias found in women. Indirect inguinal hernias are congenital, and direct inguinal and femoral hernias are considered acquired. External and internal views of the locations of these hernias are shown in Figure 32–1.

If a patient has a typical history of a hernia (i.e., a mass in the groin and pain or discomfort with straining, lifting, or when changing from sitting to standing) and the examination fails to reveal a hernia, the diagnosis should not be ruled out. Repeated examination may disclose a hernia, but diagnostic laparoscopy should be considered to evaluate persistent symptoms even if the examination is unrevealing.

Inguinal and Femoral Hernias

Laparoscopically, an indirect inguinal hernia is evident as an opening adjacent to the round ligament (Fig. 32–2). However, a direct or femoral hernia may not be clearly seen until the peritoneum is opened; the hernia is usually found after dissecting the preperitoneal fat. A direct inguinal hernia can sometimes be clearly seen as a defect or indentation in the peritoneum in the area of Hesselbach's triangle (rectus abdominis, medial umbilical ligament medially, epigastric vessels or lateral umbilical ligament laterally, iliopubic tract or inguinal ligament inferiorly) (Fig. 32–3). If it is not clear, the peritoneum in Hesselbach's triangle can be grasped and pulled cephalad, and a redundant peritoneum or sac is identified.

A femoral hernia is usually seen below the iliopubic tract and above Cooper's ligament just medial to the iliac vein (Fig. 32–4). If it is not readily visible, a gentle push with a blunt instrument reveals weakness in the peritoneum. Once the diagnosis is established intraoperatively, the peritoneum is incised transversely at the level of the apex of Hesselbach's triangle from the medial umbilical ligament to about 3 to 5 cm lateral to the internal ring or round ligament. The peritoneum is then dissected bluntly downward, and fat is removed from the preperitoneal space to expose the hernia.

All the hernias described so far can be diagnosed more easily by laparoscopy than by exploration via external incision. They can be repaired either laparoscopically or through a skin incision. If the diagnosis can be established without laparoscopy, then an external incision under local anesthesia usually allows adequate repair and prompt return to function. Laparoscopic repairs of several types have been devised and appear to have acceptably low rates of recurrence at this time. Longer follow-up is needed, because 50% of recurrences appear after 5 years. Laparoscopic surgery may have advantages in the repair of recurrent or bilateral hernias.

Spigelian Hernia

Spigelian hernia is a protrusion through the transversalis fascia lateral to the edge of the rectus muscle but medial to the spigelian line and at the level of the semicircular line of Douglas midway between the umbilicus and the pubis (Fig. 32–5*A*). The hernia sac can protrude through one, two, or three layers of the spigelian aponeurosis (Fig. 32–5*B*). These hernias occur primarily in adults between 40 and 70 years of age but can be found at any age. The hernia is usually small but can present with incarceration and strangulation of bowel in about one fourth of cases.

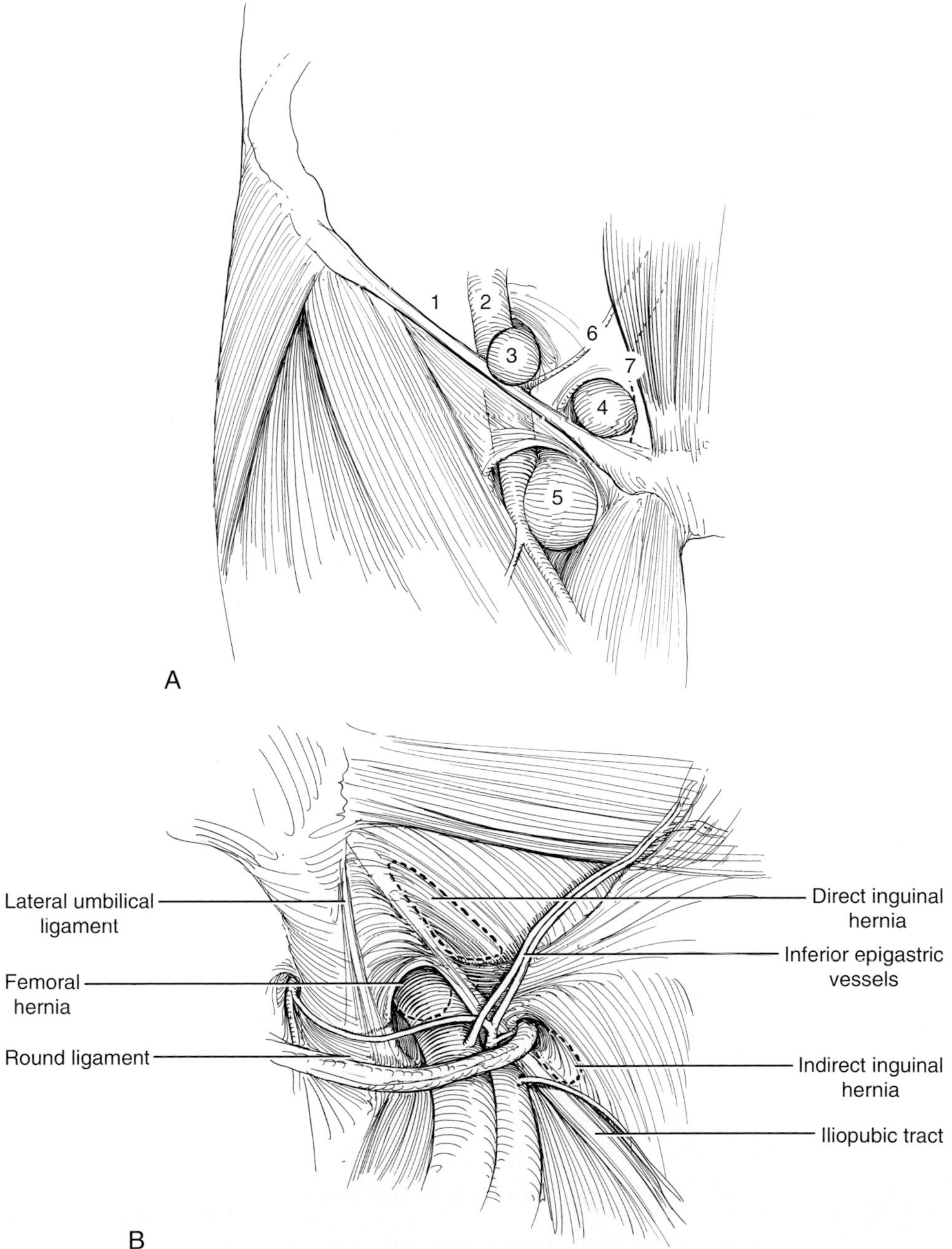

Figure 32–1. *A*: Three types of groin hernia and some important landmarks: 1, inguinal ligament; 2, femoral artery; 3, indirect hernial sac; 4, direct hernial sac; 5, femoral sac; 6, inferior epigastric artery; 7, lateral umbilical ligament. (Modified from Rowe JS Jr, Skandalakis JE, Gray SW: Multiple bilateral inguinal hernias. Am Surg 1973;39:269.) *B*: Internal view of the groin demonstrating anatomic landmarks for the identification of direct and indirect inguinal hernia and femoral hernia.

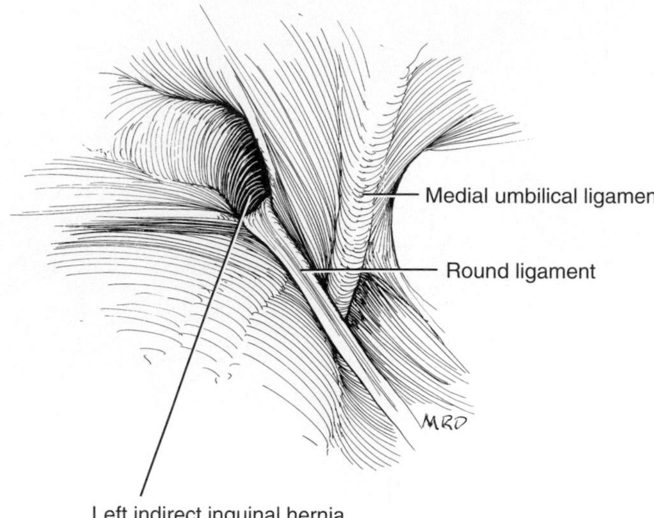

Figure 32–2. Laparoscopic view of left indirect inguinal hernia.

Incisional Hernia

Incisional hernias are especially common in vertical incisions of the abdomen and are more common in patients with a history of wound seroma, hematoma, or postoperative wound infection.

Obturator Hernia

Obturator hernias are very rare hernias that are about five times more common in women than in men and present between ages 50 and 90 years. A peritoneal pouch, usually with accompanying small bowel, follows the course of the obturator vessels through the obturator fossa. The loop of intestine can become incarcerated, prompting presentation with symptoms of bowel strangulation. Emergency surgery is usually necessary.

Epigastric Hernia

Epigastric hernias present as small defects in the linea alba between the xyphoid and

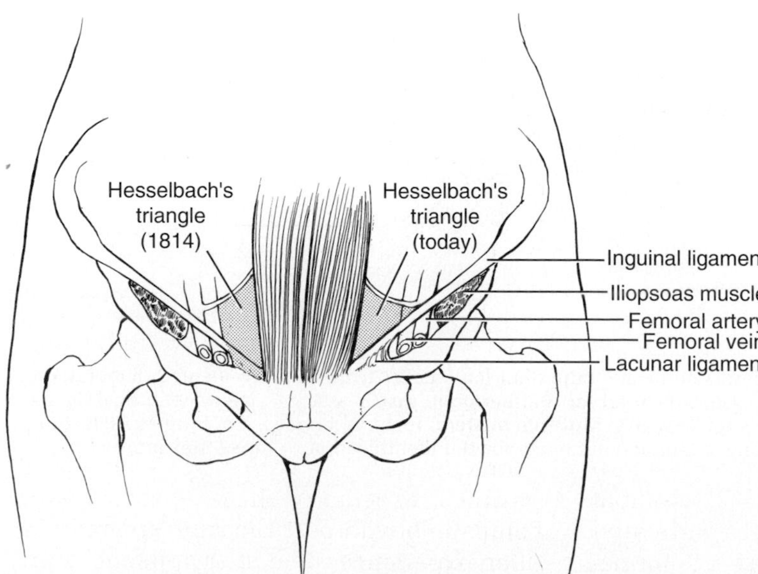

Figure 32–3. Hesselbach's triangle.

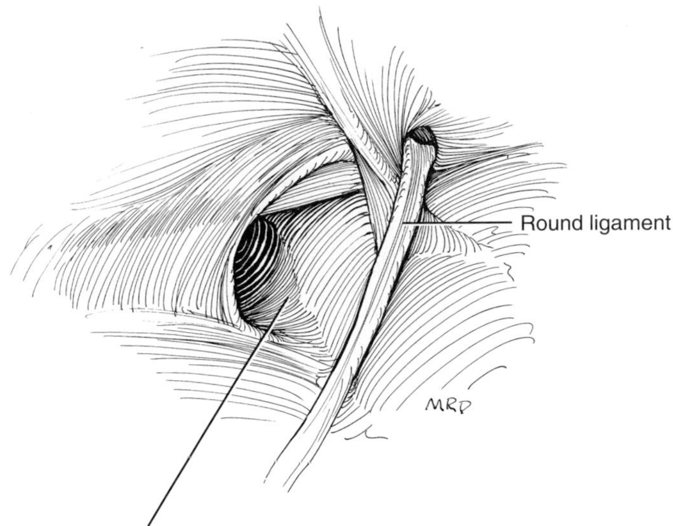

Figure 32–4. Right femoral hernia.

the umbilicus and represent about 5% of all abdominal wall hernias.[5] Patients usually complain of pain after exercise, local tenderness, and occasionally nausea or vomiting. Bowel rarely becomes incarcerated in this type of hernia, because it usually contains omentum or fat.

Umbilical Hernia

Representing 3% of all hernias,[5] the umbilical hernia is typically congenital but often enlarges during and after pregnancy. It presents as protrusion at the umbilicus and local pain or vague generalized abdominal pain. Any patient who has an umbilical hernia, who is older than 3 years, and who is symptomatic should have the hernia repaired.

Chronic or Recurrent Appendicitis

Until the mid-1970s, elective appendectomy for CPP or chronic right lower quadrant abdominal pain was commonly performed via laparotomy.[1] Between the mid-1970s and early 1990s, it was believed that elective appendectomy was not indicated because of the high percentage of normal appendices noted and because of possible increased morbidity, such as infertility due to postsurgical adhesions. Laparoscopic appendectomy for chronic right lower quadrant pain now is increasingly performed.

Chronic appendicitis may be caused by incomplete luminal obstruction secondary to inspissated fecal material and may be responsible for severe recurrent cramping abdominal pain in the right lower quadrant.[4] Lee and colleagues believe that chronic appendicitis occurs in 0.6% of patients. The findings are those of fecalith in 36% of patients, torsion in 27%, fibrotic lumen in 27%, and inspissated material in 9%.[6]

Recurrent appendicitis refers to the patterns of symptoms and not to abdominal findings, although a correlation may exist. Patients being evaluated for acute appendicitis report a 4% to 25% incidence of previous abdominal pain in the right lower quadrant.[7] Chronic appendicitis is more rare and presents with chronic localized abdominal pain that is usually relieved by appendectomy.

During laparoscopy, if the appendix is indurated, enlarged, hyperemic, or kinked, it should be removed, especially if the patient has right lower quadrant pain or tenderness at McBurney's point, or at the location of the appendix. Patients with these examination findings, especially those with a history compatible with past subacute appendicitis, often experience relief after appendectomy.[6]

My experience with this disease includes

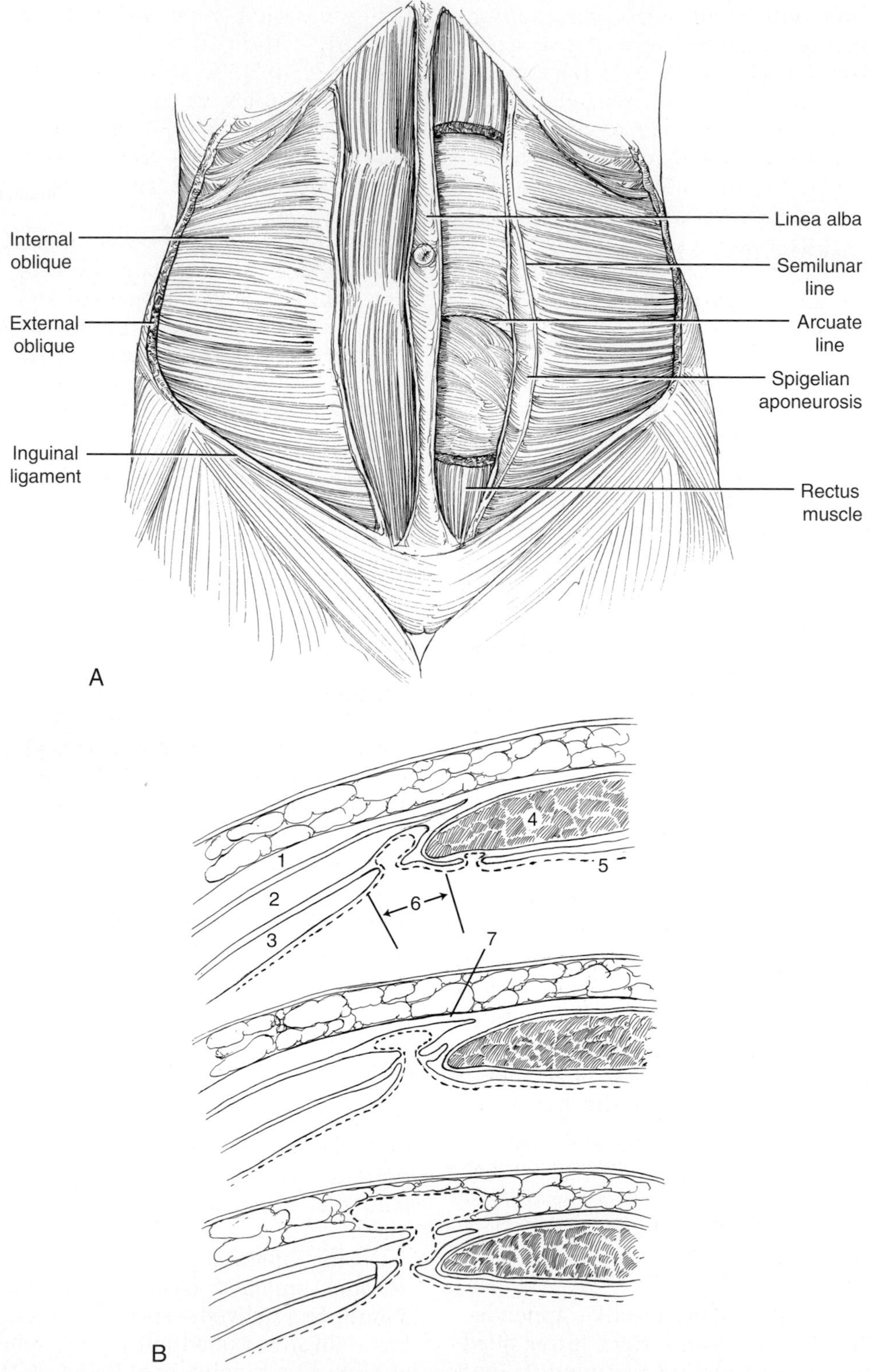

Figure 32–5. *A*: Ventral view of the abdominal wall, showing the relationships among the semicircular line of Douglas, the semilunar line, and the spigelian aponeurosis, through which a spigelian hernia protrudes. *B*: Schematic cross section of the ventral abdominal wall cephalad to the semicircular line of Douglas, indicating possible locations of spigelian hernias: 1, external oblique muscle; 2, internal oblique muscle; 3, transversus abdominis muscle; 4, rectus abdominis muscle; 5, peritoneum; 6, spigelian aponeurosis; 7, external oblique aponeurosis.

10 patients with recurrent or chronic right lower quadrant pain treated by laparoscopic appendectomy. Of the 10, 2 were male and 8 were female. Their ages ranged from 13 to 49 years. The pathology report revealed subacute appendicitis in one, early appendicitis in two, chronic inflammation in two, lymphoid follicular hyperplasia in two, and luminal obstruction and fecal material in three. Only 1 patient of 10 continues to have symptoms after surgery. Review of the literature reveals an incidence of inflammation of about 0.5% to 0.6% of all elective appendectomy specimens.[6] Hattei and colleagues concluded that acute appendicitis can resolve spontaneously and recur repeatedly in the same person.[7] Others reported an incidence of recurrent appendicitis of 16% in the general population and chronic appendicitis in 1%.[8]

Recurrent and chronic appendicitis are clearly controversial entities. They are comparatively infrequently reported, and they are so unusual that there are no well-defined and well-accepted clinical or pathologic criteria for the diagnosis.[9] Most patients are dismissed as having psychosomatic pain or are diagnosed as having irritable bowel syndrome.[4] We believe that chronic or recurrent appendicitis should be included in the differential diagnosis of CPP.

Diverticular Disease

Diverticulosis is an acquired condition that appears as early as the age of 35 years even though it most commonly affects those in the fifth through the seventh decades of life. In 70% of cases, the sigmoid colon is the major focus of the process, and the rectum is always spared. It is a disease occurring above the peritoneal reflection, because the rectum has no serosa. Diverticula are produced by increased intraluminal pressure, which causes the mucosa to protrude or herniate through the circular muscle of the bowel wall. It is essentially a false or pulsion diverticulum, in contrast to Meckel's diverticulum, which is a full-thickness diverticulum of congenital origin involving the terminal ileum.

Most patients with diverticulosis are asymptomatic (about 85%). Treatment is generally conservative and includes a high-fiber diet. In 15% of patients, attacks are recurrent and are usually treated with antibiotics and elective segmental resection. About 5% of patients present with complications such as abscesses, fistulas, or perforations.[1]

Any patient who is older than 35 years and who has left lower quadrant pain associated with changes in bowel habit including alternation of constipation with diarrhea, straining, or decreased caliber of stool should be considered possibly to have diverticulitis. Evaluation includes sigmoidoscopy plus barium enema, or colonoscopy. At laparoscopy, the sigmoid colon may have obvious diverticulosis with induration or may be inflamed, with formation of a mass or abscess. All patients with a history of diverticulitis should have bowel preparation before any diagnostic laparoscopy.

Adhesions

Patients with intestinal adhesions and chronic abdominal pain that is intermittent and crampy in character and associated with nausea or vomiting should be considered candidates for laparoscopic lysis of adhesions (see Chapter 13). The impact of laparoscopic adhesiolysis of pelvic disease has been studied; the chances for relief of pain after intestinal adhesiolysis are less well understood. Anecdotal experience suggests that patients with adhesions severe enough to cause bowel obstruction are more likely to develop recurrent adhesions after surgery. Patients undergoing extensive laparoscopic adhesiolysis should be told that although the procedure reduces that adhesion burden by about 50%, some adhesions are likely to recur and their symptoms may recur.

References

1. Jones NC, Sturdy DE: Surgical and orthopedic causes of pelvic pain. In Rocker I (ed): Pelvic Pain in Women. New York, Springer-Verlag, 1990, pp 136–150.
2. Hightower NC, Roberts JW: Acute and chronic lower abdominal pain of enterocolic origin. In Renaer M (ed): Chronic Pelvic Pain in Women. New York; Springer-Verlag, 1981, pp 110–137.

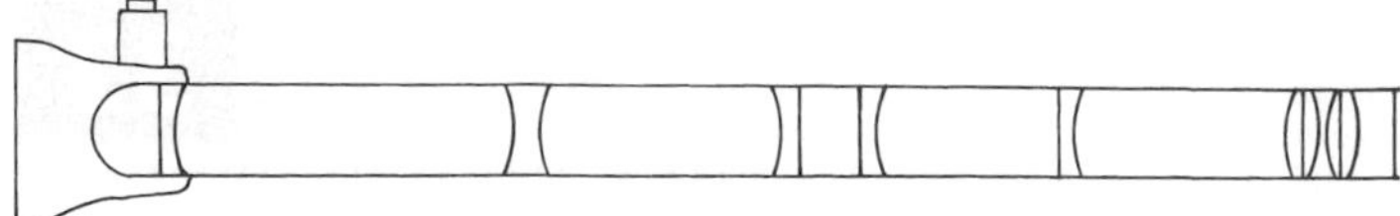

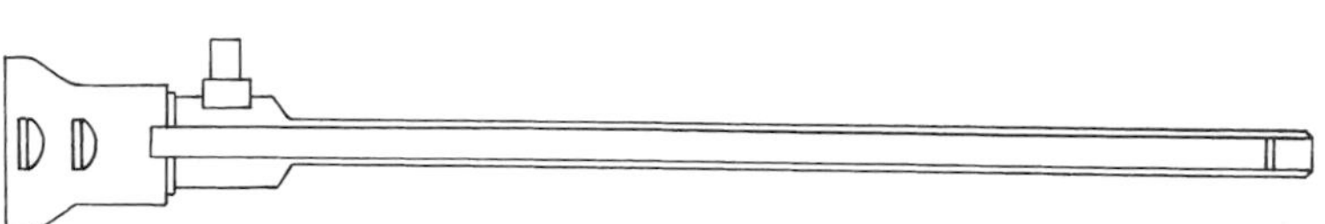

Figure 33–1. Design of the flexible microlaparoscope. Lens systems at either end of the instrument are connected by a fused fiber bundle.

similarly sized operative instruments. Here we must recall the history of the 1970s, when a large array of 3-mm instruments was made available but was gradually discarded in favor of 5-mm instruments. The 3-mm versions simply did not have the mechanical advantage sufficient to successfully clamp, cut, or perform biopsy. Because the 3-mm and 5-mm instruments are all designed for use under general anesthesia, the change in diameter was of little importance.

The present 2-mm instruments have limitations that are reminiscent of their 3-mm predecessors. Gentle grasping is possible, although firm retraction is far more difficult. The narrow-diameter instruments also have the disadvantage of concentrating all of the force applied into a small area, thus increasing their propensity for traumatizing serosal surfaces.

Similarly, the smaller the laparoscope diameter, the more it can act like a needle, potentially causing inadvertant visceral or vessel injury. Again, 2 mm would seem to be a size that when used with appropriate caution is less likely to inflict injury.

In addition to these concerns, perhaps the greatest limitation at present is the lack of a practical energy source for coagulation and hemostasis. Bipolar coagulation instruments tested at this diameter are too small to deliver cautery over a sufficient area and are fragile and unreliable. A monopolar needle can be used but has the disadvantage of sometimes provoking as much trouble as it solves. Prototypes are being developed for a 2-mm diameter argon beam coagulator, which may avoid some of these limitations.

With time and ingenuity, some of these shortcomings will no doubt be overcome and microlaparoscopy will find its niche. Along with these developments, we must devise the office laparoscopy environment that will combine safety with optimum cost-effectiveness.

Cost-Effectiveness

The experience of the past several years has clearly demonstrated that during and after outpatient laparoscopy under local anesthesia, a patient's recovery and comfort are excellent. Properly selected patients virtually without exception prefer this to a procedure performed under general anesthesia in an operating room. Assuming that office microlaparoscopy can adequately replace the need for an operating room procedure in a patient's care, the cost of the laparoscopy can be reduced by as much as 80%.

Logistically, once the details are worked out in each individual office setting, the ability to perform this procedure in the office diminishes the need for duplication of information and record keeping and simply diminishes the number of people involved in accomplishing the same end result. When kept under the control of the office staff, the procedures can be scheduled in a way that suits the purposes of that office, rather than suiting the schedule of another facility. In some states, regulations governing billing for the overhead connected with office procedures may be problematic, making it administratively simpler to perform such procedures in an ambulatory surgery setting. Even if such a facility if used, the speed of the procedure may result in lower cost than standard laparoscopy.

In certain chronic and troubling situations, such as endometriosis and adhesive disease, the increased cost-effectiveness of the individual procedure may very well allow more aggressive treatment approaches to these difficult problems without unduly escalating the cost of medical care.

Equipment

A microlaparoscopy tower can be constructed to closely imitate the standard operating room endoscopy tower. This contains the camera unit and light source as well as a high-resolution monitor and a gas insufflator as the minimum equipment necessary. A videocassette recorder for video recording and a freeze-frame recorder for making still photographs are desirable. A small side table or Mayo's stand is needed to hold the sterilized microlaparoscopy instruments and trochars or inserters (Fig. 33–2). (The size of table needed will expand as the technology advances.) Sterilization bins for soaking instruments in Cidex and a small autoclave are necessary. Monitoring equipment needed for conscious sedation is listed in Table 33–1.

Patient Selection

Patients of American Society of Anesthesiologists class I and some of a class II rating

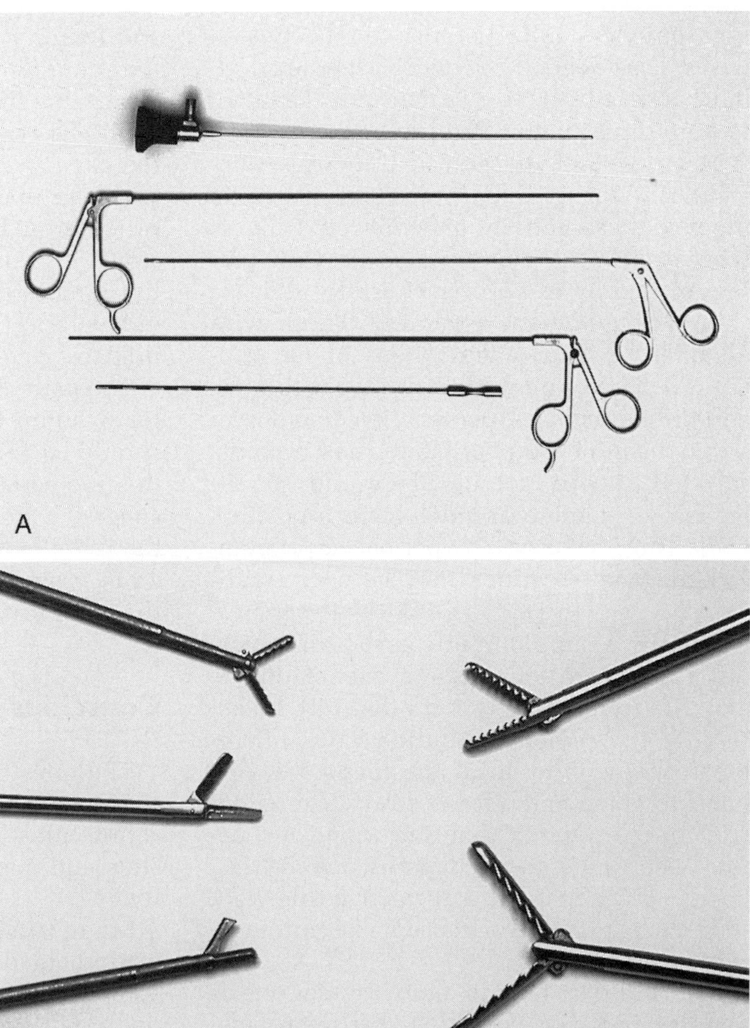

Figure 33–2. *A*: Two-millimeter microlaparoscope with assorted instruments. *B*: Two-millimeter microlaparoscopy instruments (left) compared with 3-mm laparoscopic grasping instruments.

Table 33–1. **MONITORING AND EMERGENCY EQUIPMENT FOR LAPAROSCOPY UNDER LOCAL ANESTHESIA**

Electrocardiogram
Blood pressure (automated preferable)
Pulse oximeter
Nasal and oral airways
Suction
Ambu bag
Oxygen supply
Reversing agents for narcotics and sedative-hypnotics (drawn up in syringes)
Full emergency cart nearby

(mild medical conditions) are appropriate. Contraindications to the conscious sedation technique in the office include pulmonary conditions such as chronic obstructive pulmonary disease, pulmonary hypertension, acute bronchitis, and apnea. Patients with asymptomatic mild asthma can be treated with an as-needed bronchodilator (e.g., albuterol nebulizer) two to four puffs about 15 to 30 minutes before the procedure.

Mean arterial pressure can increase substantially during these procedures owing to the anxiety sometimes experienced. Patients with significant hypertension or with previously known coronary artery disease should therefore be excluded. Those with allergies to many medications or environmental agents or with severe psychiatric conditions such as personality disorder or panic disorder are poor candidates. Patients selected should not be obese and should be able to tolerate Trendelenburg's position well. Those who have experienced prior anesthetic complications may be poor candidates.

Finally, a simple "belly grab" diagnostic test performed on a supine patient on the examination table is very helpful in assessing the patient's candidacy for microlaparoscopy under local anesthesia: Use one hand to grasp and lift the lower abdominal wall in the manner that one would use before inserting a 2-mm laparoscopic Verres' needle. If the patient can tolerate this well, then she is probably an acceptable candidate for the procedure.

If a candidate fails to qualify under one or more of these criteria, then her microlaparoscopy can be attempted under conscious sedation technique in an operating room setting. General anesthesia can be induced if it should be unsuccessful.

Patient Preparation

Certainly equal in importance to all of the foregoing medical considerations is the value of preparing a patient. She should have a reliable support person and transportation mode available to her and should be fully informed about the limitations of the surgery itself and the anesthesia techniques used. Detailed orientation to the events of the procedure itself does much to allay anxiety. This means communicating to her either verbally, pictorially, or by walking her through the procedure room, entire equipment setup, position of the table, number and identity of the people expected to be in the room, and so on. It is useful to provide a step-by-step written outline of exactly what she will experience. She should have the expectation of continued verbal contact with the operating surgeon throughout the procedure. During any instructional sessions, it is useful to have a family member listening to the conversation as well to provide support to the patient as she mentally prepares herself.

The patient should take nothing by mouth for 6 hours before the procedure, and she should be advised to avoid smoking because this increases gastric volume. Some centers suggest a mild laxative bowel preparation the night before. If this is done, an intravenous preload of fluids may be desirable if the patient has become dehydrated.

Conscious Sedation

The anesthetic method is a combination of intravenous anxiolytic and opioid medication, plus a local anesthetic at the trochar sites and sometimes in the peritoneal cavity.[6]

Monitoring for the procedure includes the equipment described earlier (see Table 33–1). Most importantly, one person should be dedicated to the administration of medications and observation of the patient, with no other responsibilities during the procedure.

Table 33–2. **ANXIOLYTICS**

Drug (Concentration)	Dosing	Suggested Maximum Dose/kg	Suggested Maximum Dose/Patient
Diazepam (5 mg/ml)	2.5 mg every 5–10 minutes (0.5 ml)	0.05–0.15 mg/kg	3.5–10.5 mg
Midazolam (1 mg/ml)	1.0 mg every 5 minutes (0.5–1.0 ml)	0.02–0.07 mg/kg	1.0–5.0 mg

A second person is necessary to hand the surgeon the requisite endoscopic equipment.

Intravenous medications given for conscious sedation should be given one at a time by slow intravenous push. It is generally not advisable to combine oral anxiolytics with intravenous medications of this type, because their summation may yield somewhat unpredictable levels of drug. Anxiolytics such as those listed in Table 33–2 may be used.[7] The opioid medications listed in Table 33–3 should be administered several minutes after the anxiolytic medication has had a chance to equilibrate.[8, 9] It is perhaps most useful to select one or two drugs of each class and to use those exclusively to establish comfort with their use.

The person providing medication is responsible for observing cardiopulmonary function, as well as the mental status of the patient. Signs of overmedication may include respiratory rate less than 10 per minute; signs of airway obstruction, such as snoring, rocking, and use of accessory expiratory muscles; the appearance of central apnea; and oxygen saturation less than 95%. Significant alterations of electrocardiographic rate and rhythm are also warnings.

The reversing agents for the anxiolytics and narcotics should be drawn up in syringes and ready for administration. It is not sufficient to make them included in an emergency cart, because they must be administered quickly when needed. The agent most often used is naloxone (Narcan), which is provided in the strength of 400 μg/ml. This should be diluted 1:10 and given as repeated 40-μg IV boluses as needed. This medication should not be given to known narcotic addicts, because it may precipitate severe withdrawal symptoms that may be hazardous in the course of a laparoscopy.

The reversing agent for the benzodiazepine class of compounds is flumazenil (Reversed), mixed in a dilution of 0.1 mg/ml and titrated to reversal of sedation, usually a total dose of 0.2 to 1.0 mg IV. The drug is provided in ampules containing 5 mg/ml. The duration of action of flumazenil is shorter (30 to 40 minutes) than that of midazolam (Versed) or diazepam (Valium). Resedation is possible after the flumazenil has worn off. Therefore, when this drug is used, the patient should be observed for a longer period in the recovery area before being discharged.

Various local anesthetics are applicable for this procedure (Table 33–4). My personal choice is bupivacaine because of its longer duration of action. The discomfort from the injection of a local anesthetic can be re-

Table 33–3. **NARCOTICS**

Drug (Concentration)	Dosing	Suggested Maximum Dose/kg	Suggested Maximum Dose/Patient
Fentanyl (50 μg/ml)	25–50 μg every 5 minutes (0.5–1.0 ml)	1–3 μg/kg	70–210 μg IV
Alfentanil (500 μg/ml)	250–500 μg every 5 minutes (0.5–1.0 ml)	5–20 μg/kg	350–1750 μg IV
Demerol	10–20 mg every 5 minutes	1.0–1.5 mg/kg	50–100 mg IV
Morphine	1–2 mg every 5 minutes	0.1–0.15 mg/kg	5–10 mg IV

Table 33–4. **LOCAL ANESTHETICS**

Agent	Concentration (%)	Plain Solution (Maximum Dose—mg)	Plain Solution (Maximum Dose—mg/kg)	With Epinephrine (Maximum Dose—mg)	With Epinephrine (Maximum Dose—mg/kg)
Short Duration					
Procaine	1–2	800	11	1000	14
Chloroprocaine	0.5–1				
Moderate Duration					
Lidocaine	0.5–1	300	4	500	7
Mepivacaine	0.5–1	300	4	500	7
Prilocaine	0.5–1	500	7	600	8
Long Duration					
Bupivacaine	0.25–0.5	175	2.5	225	3

duced by adding 0.3 ml of a 1 mEq/ml solution of sodium bicarbonate to each 10 ml of local anesthetic.[10] Local anesthetics with short or moderate duration of action can also be used for dripping on pelvic viscera. This is discussed later in terms of its diagnostic value, but it can also be used during biopsies or lyses of adhesions during laparoscopy under local anesthesia.

Procedure

The patient is asked to empty her bladder and change from street clothes into an appropriate washable or disposable hospital gown. The surgeon or the nursing assistant walks the patient into the procedure room and orients her again to the equipment and the people involved. She assumes a comfortable reclining position on the operating room table, and an intravenous line is started, preferably in her nondominant hand. A blood pressure cuff is placed on the opposite arm, and Po_2 and electrocardiogram leads placed conveniently. When all of the laparoscopic equipment is sterilized and ready, the patient is positioned in stirrups that support her knees with her thighs horizontal and her legs abducted. Her abdomen and vagina are prepared and draped, and a speculum is used to expose her cervix. A paracervical block is placed with 8 to 10 ml 1% lidocaine or 0.5% bupivacaine, using a total volume of about 8 to 10 ml divided among injection sites at 2, 4, 8, and 10 o'clock on the cervix. A cervical tenaculum is then attached to the anterior lip of the cervix, and a Cohn's cannula or similar manipulating device is attached to the cervix itself.

The surgeon then stands next to the patient and, while continually talking her through the procedure, anesthetizes the umbilicus with 2 to 4 ml of the local anesthetic of choice. With upward traction on the anterior abdominal wall, a 2-mm incision is then made with a scalpel and the umbilical port placed. Most available systems use a combination of a Verres' needle with a surrounding external sheath. When this sheath is placed and insufflation is complete, the laparoscopy can begin. A controlled study[11] has not shown a substantial difference in discomfort when using nitrous oxide versus carbon dioxide. Most patients can tolerate from 1.5 to 2.0 L before feeling discomfort from intraabdominal pressure. The patient is placed in 15 to 20 degrees of Trendelenburg's position, allowing the intestines to fall cephalad. The anesthetic is then placed at the lower midline port, assuming the abdominal wall is not obscured by any pathology. The second 2-mm port is then placed suprapubically, being careful to aim the port in the direction that the operator anticipates being most used in this procedure. This minimizes the amount of torsion placed on the parietal peritoneum during manipulation of the probe, thus diminishing discomfort (Fig. 33–3). The thicker the abdominal wall, the more discomfort is felt with manipulation of the lower probe; this is an intrinsic limitation of the technique.

In the presence of a previous midline incision or in any case in which open laparoscopy is considered, safe trocar placement can often be accomplished in the left upper

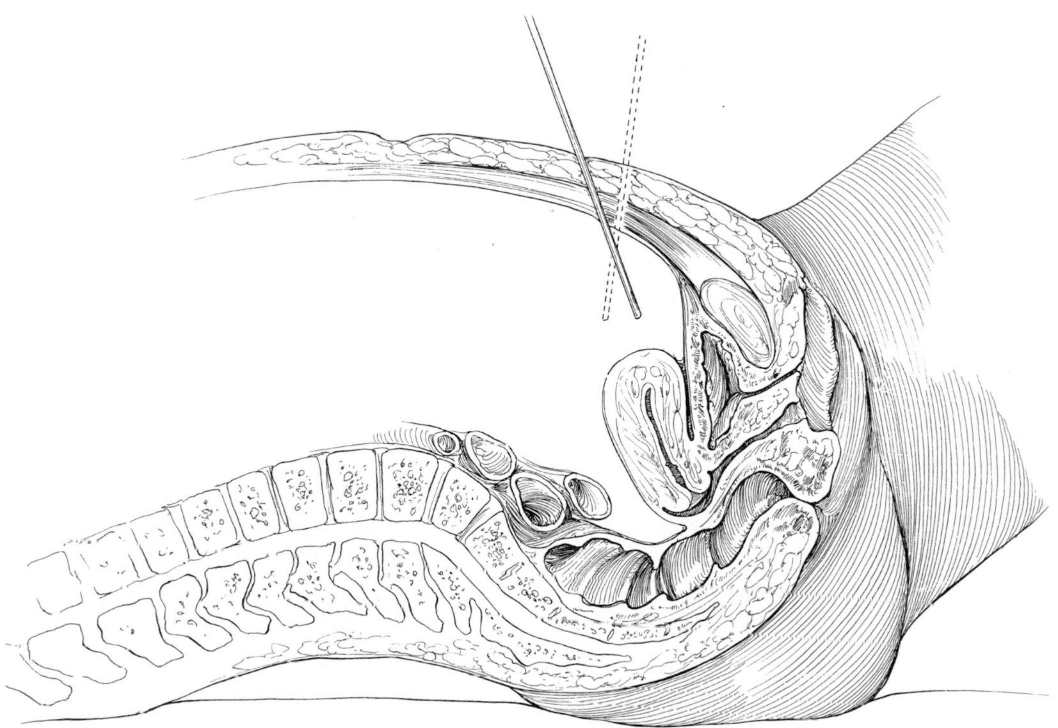

Figure 33–3. direction of insertion of the lower abdominal probe in microlaparoscopy.

quadrant. Simply place the introducer/Verres' needle just below the costal margin in the anterior axillary line. Propping the patient up to elevate her left side (partial right lateral decubitus position) allows slightly easier introduction of the pneumoperitoneum.

The smooth-tipped suprapubic probe can be used to complete any bowel manipulation necessary to provide a clear view of the pelvis. During the course of this manipulation, the patient should be queried about any discomfort that may mimic her clinical complaints.

When the procedure is complete, the operative instruments are removed, with as much insufflating gas expelled from the abdomen as possible. When the ports are removed, the incisions do not need suturing.

When the patient is sufficiently comfortable and alert after this procedure, she can walk to a recovery area with assistance or may be transported by a wheelchair. Monitoring in the recovery room usually requires about a half an hour to an hour. Before discharge, the patient should be capable of moving all her extremities, should be able to breathe deeply and cough, and should have normal consciousness and peripheral circulation. Her PaO_2 should be greater than 95%, and she should be able to void and take oral nourishment.

In an office setting, a simple one-page record can be constructed to record the essentials of the procedure, including the times and doses of medications and summary statements about vital sign recording. Many automatic blood pressure monitoring devices have a built-in printer that provides a written record of pulse and blood pressure readings. Still photographs can be taken during the procedure for later review with the patient and her family. Of course, when appropriate, it may be useful to place the video monitor in such a position that the patient can view the monitor herself. This may be less advisable when performing a pain-mapping procedure as described later.

Indications

All of the suggested indications discussed here are relative: No single procedure is uniquely suitable to microlaparoscopy, and in no category of procedure is microlaparoscopy appropriate in every clinical situation. Perhaps the most obvious applications for this procedure are conscious pain mapping, evaluation and treatment of endometriosis, and treatment of adhesions.

Conscious pain mapping is an extremely useful technique for evaluating patients with CPP. A patient should be carefully instructed that she will need to respond during the laparoscopy using a 1 to 10 rating scale to score the discomfort she feels as various portions of the pelvic floor and reproductive anatomy are touched. In dealing with such a patient, I usually palpate areas that are often nontender in order to assess the patient's general level of comfort with this procedure. If the first areas palpated are those that are likely to be tender, the patient may become so sensitized that subsequent examination does not yield useful information.

I find it generally useful to map the entire pelvis three complete times, looking for consistency of response. Most individuals rate the discomfort of palpation of the normal ovary at between 3 and 5 on a scale of 10 and offer similar ratings for other areas on the pelvic sidewalls, the psoas muscles, and so on. Readings of palpations of the intestines are usually less than that, although there certainly are exceptions. A systematic study of such readings is the ongoing subject of a multicenter investigation.

In addition to asking a patient to rate each probed area, she should also be asked whether or not such probing reproduces the pain she experiences clinically. Particular techniques that may be useful for difficult chronic pain cases include using the uterine manipulator to place the cervix in anterior traction and then using the probe to touch the uterosacral ligaments. Focal areas of tenderness that may be due to endometriosis can be discovered in this way. In particular, a determination can be made about whether areas of endometriosis are incidental findings or are indeed part of a woman's clinical pain syndrome (see Chapter 14).

Similarly, adhesions that are present can be placed on traction and the patient asked if such traction replicates her clinical pain. This is especially useful when dealing with bowel adhesions to the adnexal areas or adnexal adhesions to the pelvic sidewalls.

With the palpation complete, biopsy samples of either adhesions or endometriosis may then be taken as needed. If adhesions are clearly avascular, they can be anesthetized by dripping 1% xylocaine or chloroprocaine (Nesacaine) on them and then severed with the operative scissors.

Any fibroids suspected of contributing to clinical pain should be probe palpated, as should the appendix and the large bowel. It has been speculated that adhesions of the cecum area and the sigmoid may be more common in individuals with pelvic pain.[12] Further studies using the conscious pain-mapping technique may provide information about the true role of these alterations in the pain syndrome. They may indeed be variations of normal anatomy that have developed sensitivity because of a patient's chronic pain syndrome.

A significant number of patients who have had severe CPP with a chronic pain syndrome (see Chapter 2) may develop the problem of generalized visceral hyperalgesia. Such patients rate pain at an 8 or higher everywhere that the pelvic floor or surrounding viscera are touched. Such information is extremely useful because it suggests that the role of any organic pathology visualized should be carefully evaluated before attributing a patient's entire complaint to that pathology. It remains to be seen whether generalized hyperalgesia detected during the pelvic examination accurately predicts this type of laparoscopic observation. Even if this should be the case, it might be that laparoscopic documentation of this response pattern might help convince the patient and her family of the value of nonsurgical alternatives.

The second area of the greatest application of microlaparoscopy under local anesthesia is for the treatment of endometriosis. Patients currently are often changed from one expensive and uncomfortable medication to another on the presumption that continued endometriosis is at the root of their pain (see Chapter 14). Studies are needed to investigate the role of microlaparoscopy in assessing the response of endometriosis as it relates to the relief of pain associated with the disease. These data may allow more informed decisions about pregnancy planning and medication management.

Further studies are needed to compare surgical versus medical therapy for the early stages of endometriosis. If indeed medical therapy can be shown to be equivalent in results and if it can be further demonstrated that the stage of identified endometriosis influences the decision, then office laparoscopy to confirm the diagnosis and establish stage would be a cost-effective way to guide a patient toward medical therapy as a less expensive treatment modality.

The third area of most obvious application for this technology is in the treatment of adhesive disease. As discussed in Chapter 13, the role of adhesions in causing pelvic pain is controversial. Nevertheless, the vast body of clinical experience and a much smaller volume of true clinical studies have shown that lysis of adhesions may be effective in many cases. At best, current laparoscopic techniques reduce the adhesion burden by about 50%, which certainly leaves room for improvement.

The development of the adhesion prevention agents has been typified by one general observation: Many of the agents that appear to be very effective in animal models fail to meet expectations when used in women. Before any agent can be widely accepted, it must therefore undergo rigorous trials in patients. The expense, discomfort, and risk of repeated operating room laparoscopy have slowed and limited the evaluation of adhesion preventive agents. The development of microlaparoscopy should substantially accelerate the pace of this research. I would hypothesize that the ultimate adhesion prevention protocol involves careful operating room laparoscopy with adhesion barrier placement, followed at short intervals (about 1 week) by repeated mechanical interruption of newly reforming adhesions, together with repeated application of one or more adhesive preventive agents. Microlaparoscopy will have a key role in this progress.

In similar fashion, the microlaparoscopy approach will be joined with other pelvic surgery approaches, such as laparotomy for myomectomy. Second-look procedures have already been demonstrated to be useful in reducing the adhesion burden at the time of myomectomy,[13] and the microlaparoscopic approach should make this more practical.

Finally, one of the great difficulties in treating pelvic adhesions is determining prospectively the severity of the adhesions before laparoscopy is performed. In patients having undergone many previous operations, the microlaproscopic approach would allow office evaluation of the severity of disease, thus prompting appropriate referral if the surgeon encounters a degree of adhesive disease beyond his or her experience.

Other potential applications for microlaparoscopy have been suggested. Each of these may be applicable to a limited degree and is less likely to be useful than in the clinical situations described earlier. For example, it has been suggested that the bleeding from an ectopic pregnancy can be confirmed in order to decide between use of methotrexate versus operative laparoscopy. In practical terms, this is a relatively uncommon dilemma, given our present ability to detect ectopic pregnancy at very early stages using a combination of quantitative β-human chorionic gonadotropin levels and transvaginal ultrasound examination.

The role of microlaparoscopy in evaluating second-look procedures for patients with ovarian cancer has been widely debated.[14] Advocates suggest that in approximately 50% of cases, diffuse carcinomatosis can be demonstrated and thus an unnecessary laparotomy avoided. Opponents suggest that even in such cases, laparotomy with debulking of residual disease may be beneficial to a patient, although this approach remains unproven.

Documentation of a ruptured corpus luteum cyst may certainly be accomplished by microlaparoscopy. The combination of pregnancy tests with clinical examination, history, and transvaginal ultrasound examination almost always establishes a high probability of this diagnosis. The decision about whether or not to operate is based on the patient's clinical course and hemodynamic condition, rather than simply documenting that the cyst is bleeding. Microlaparoscopy might therefore have occasional utility but is not generally applicable for this problem.

A common emergency room dilemma is trying to distinguish between appendicitis and pelvic inflammatory disease. Microlaparoscopy in such cases might make earlier confirmation of diagnosis possible and thus might diminish patient morbidity by allowing earlier treatment. Patient selection may prove difficult in this setting, because a patient's anxiety level and acute discomfort are usually already high. Monitoring pelvic inflammatory disease by microlaparoscopy may occasionally be useful, but again, other clinical indicators most often provide the necessary information. In cases in which significant doubt remains, surgical intervention rather than simple observation is likely to be needed; hence, the microlaparoscopy procedure has relatively little value.

In the area of infertility, gamete intrafallopian transfer and zygote intrafallopian transfer will very likely be able to be accomplished using the microlaparoscope. This will be of substantial benefit to the degree that it reduces the long-term cost of these procedures.

In summary, microlaparoscopy under local anesthesia holds promise for wide application to various clinical situations. As a beginning, wider use of local anesthesia for laparoscopic sterilization procedures would provide opportunities for physicians to become more comfortable with the technique. Careful selective use of the procedure, as an emerging technology, is appropriate. Extensive further clinical research is needed to define more clearly the role of this new technology in women's health care. The challenge to the medical world is to use this procedure in place of operating room laparoscopy rather than in addition to it. Cost analyses must be carried out to develop the appropriate role for this procedure in the management of endometriosis. As with any new technology, the potential for overuse certainly exists.

References

1. Fishburne JI: Office laparoscopic sterilization with local anesthesia. J Reprod Med 1977;18:233.
2. Peterson HB, Hulka JF, Spielman FJ, et al: Local versus general anesthesia for laparoscopic sterilization: A randomized study. Obstet Gynecol 1987;70:903.
3. Love BR, McCorvey R, McCorvey M: Low-cost office laparoscopic sterilization. J Am Assoc Gynecol Laparosc 1994;1:379.
4. Palter SF, Olive DL: Office micro-laparoscopy under local anesthesia for chronic pelvic pain: Utility, acceptance, and cost-benefit analysis. J Am Assoc Gynecol Laparosc (in press).
5. Steege JF: Repeated clinic laparoscopy for the treatment of pelvic adhesions: A pilot study. Obstet Gynecol 1994;83:276.
6. Wetchler BV: Outpatient anesthesia. In Barash PG, Callen BF, Stoelting RK (eds): Clinical Anesthesia, 2nd ed. Philadelphia, JB Lippincott, 1992, pp 1389–1416.
7. Magni VC, Frost RA, Leung JWC, Cotton PB: A randomized comparison of midazolam and diazepam for sedation in upper gastrointestinal endoscopy. Br J Anaesth 1983;55:1095.
8. Stoeckl H, Schuttler J, Magnussen H, Hengstmann JH: Plasma fentanyl concentrations and the occurence of respiratory depression in volunteers. Br J Anaesth 1982;54:1087.
9. White PF, Coe V, Shafer A, Sung ML: Comparison of alfentanil with fentanyl for outpatient anesthesia. Anesthesiology 1982;57:435.
10. McKay W, Morris R, Mushlin P: Sodium bicarbonate attenuates pain on skin infiltration with lidocaine, with or without epinephrine. Anesth Analg 1987;66:572.
11. Lipscomb GH, Summitt RL, McCord ML, Ling FW: The effect of nitrous oxide and carbon dioxide pneumoperitoneum on operative and postoperative pain during laparoscopic sterilization under local anesthesia. J Am Assoc Gynecol Laparosc 1994;2:57.
12. Olive DL: Personal communication, 1996.
13. Myomectomy Adhesion Multicenter Study Group: An expanded polytetrafluoroethylene barrier (Gore-Tex Surgical Membrane) reduces post-myomectomy adhesion formation. Fertil Steril 1995;63:491.
14. Childers JM, Hatch KD, Surwit EA: Office laparoscopy and biopsy for evaluation of patients with intraperitoneal carcinomatosis using a new optical catheter. Gynecol Oncol 1992;47:337.

Appendix: Resources for Help with Pain

Lay Groups

American Chronic Pain Association
P.O. Box 850
Rocklin, CA 95677–0850
916-632-0922
Support organization, information pamphlets

Endometriosis Association
8585 N. 76th Place
Milwaukee, WI 53223
Support organization, information, newsletter

Fibromyalgia Network
5700 Stockdale Hwy, Suite 100
Bakersfield, CA 93309
Newsletter, contacts

HeadWay Migraine Newsletter
800-377-0282

Interstitial Cystitis Association
P.O. Box 1553
Madison Square Station
New York, NY 10159
212-979-6057

National Chronic Pain Outreach Association, Inc. (NCPOA)
7979 Old Georgetown Rd., #100
Bethesda, MD 20814–2429
301-652-4948
Bimonthly newsletter, index of available resources

National Headache Foundation
428 W. St. James Place, 2nd floor
Chicago, IL 60614–2750
800-843-2256; FAX 414-355-6065
Membership, newsletter

National Vulvodynia Association
P.O. Box 4491
Silver Springs, MD 20914–4491
703-319-0054

Peripheral Neuropathy National Network
19579 Temescal Canyon Rd., #1002
Corona, CA 91719
909-687-8026

Vulvar Pain Foundation
P.O. Drawer 177
Graham, NC 27253
910-226-0704

Professional Organizations

American Pain Society
4700 W. Lake Ave.
Glenview, IL 60025–1485
847-375-4715
http://cedar.cic.net:80/-apa/.
Membership, newsletter, copy of "Principles of Analgesic Use" and "Pain Facilities Directory," conferences

American Society of Pain Management Nurses
2755 Bristol St., Suite 110
Costa Mesa, CA 92628
714-545-1305
Networking, publications, directory, conferences

International Association for the Study of Pain (IASP)
909 NE 43rd St., Rm. 306
Seattle, WA 98105–6021
206-547-6409
Membership, journal Pain, *conferences*

International Pelvic Pain Society
Suite 402 Women's Medical Plaza
2006 Brookwood Medical Center Dr.
Birmingham, AL 35209
205-877-2950; FAX 205-877-2973
Conferences

National Commission for Certification
of Acupuncturists
P.O. Box 97075
Washington, D.C. 20090

Index

Note: Page numbers in *italics* indicate figures; those with a t indicate tables.